Brain Imaging in Substance Abuse

FORENSIC SCIENCE AND MEDICINE

Steven B. Karch, MD, SERIES EDITOR

BRAIN IMAGING IN SUBSTANCE ABUSE: *RESEARCH, CLINICAL, AND FORENSIC APPLICATIONS*
edited by ***Marc J. Kaufman,*** *2001*

TOXICOLOGY OF HERBAL PRODUCTS,
edited by ***Melanie Johns Cupp,*** *2000*

A PHYSICIAN'S GUIDE TO CLINICAL FORENSIC MEDICINE,
edited by ***Margaret M. Stark,*** *2000*

CRIMINAL POISONING: *INVESTIGATIONAL GUIDE FOR LAW ENFORCEMENT, TOXICOLOGISTS, FORENSIC SCIENTISTS, AND ATTORNEYS,*
by ***John H. Trestrail, III,*** *2000*

Brain Imaging in Substance Abuse

Research, Clinical, and Forensic Applications

Edited by

Marc J. Kaufman PhD

Harvard Medical School and McLean Hospital, Belmont, MA

Foreword by

Joseph Frascella PhD

National Institute on Drug Abuse, Rockville, MD

Humana Press **Totowa, New Jersey**

999 Riverview Drive, Suite 208
Totowa, New Jersey 07512

This publication is printed on acid-free paper. ∞
ANSI Z39.48-1984 (American Standards Institute) Permanence of Paper for Printed Library Materials.

Cover design by Patricia F. Cleary.

For additional copies, pricing for bulk purchases, and/or information about other Humana titles, contact Humana at the above address or at any of the following numbers: Tel: 973-256-1699; Fax: 973-256-8341; E-mail: humana@humanapr.com, or visit our Website at www.humanapress.com

Printed in the United States of America. 10 9 8 7 6 5 4 3 2 1

Library of Congress Cataloging in Publication Data

Brain imaging in substance abuse: research, clinical, and forensic applications/edited by Marc J. Kaufman.
p.; cm—(Forensic science)
Includes bibliographical references and index.
ISBN 0-89603-770-3 (alk. paper)
1. Substance abuse—Diagnosis. 2. Brain—Imaging. 3. Brain—Effect of drugs on. 4. Diagnostic imaging. I. Kaufman, Marc J. II. Series.
[DNLM: 1. Substance-Related Disorders—diagnosis. 2. Brain—drug effects. 3. Brain—physiology. 4. Diagnostic Imaging. 5. Forensic Medicine. WM 270 B814 2000]
RC386.6.D52 B74 2000
616.86'0754—dc21

99-054063

Foreword

The last two decades have seen prodigious growth in the application of brain imaging methods to questions of substance abuse and addiction. Despite considerable advances in our understanding of the central effects of drugs provided by preclinical data, relatively little direct evidence was known of how substances of abuse affect the brain and other CNS processes in humans. Brain imaging techniques have allowed access to the human brain and enabled the asking of questions never before imagined.

The positron emission tomography (PET) data of Volkow and her colleagues in the late 1980s, showing the uptake and time course of cocaine's binding in the human brain, revealed for the first time the distinct sites of action of this drug. This work was extremely important because it showed clearly, through imaging a drug in the brain of a living human, that the time course of its action paralleled the behavioral state of "high." This study marked a turning point in our understanding of drug-brain-behavior interactions in humans. Many more investigations of drug effects on the structure and function of the human brain were soon to follow, leading to much better insights into brain systems. Brain imaging allowed for the direct assessment of structural and functional anatomy, biology, and chemistry in substance abusers. The effects of both acute and chronic exposure could be assessed through imaging in the awake, behaving human, and these drug-induced changes in brain processes could be correlated effectively with increasingly more complex behavioral states. We now know much more about the subtle as well as distinct ways in which drugs influence brain-behavior interactions.

Despite the tremendous advances revealed over the last several years, most of which are described in detail within this book, early applications of brain imaging techniques were met with some skepticism. Questions were raised regarding the large expense of such clinical studies. For example, early PET work was sometimes criticized as being a very expensive autoradiographic method that could be done more effectively in preclinical models. Experimenter control was seen as being somewhat compromised because human drug abusers typically are not single-substance abusers; thus, brain imaging findings might not be directly attributable to abuse of one drug. Further, brain changes noted in imaging studies might have represented abnormalities associated with a preexisting condition, rather than resulting from the effects of drug use. Fortunately, clinical imaging researchers addressed these and other issues and persisted through these early times. The field has blossomed to include other imaging methods, and now includes studies that integrate findings across multiple modalites. The research findings detailed in this book are the product of this perseverance.

Brain Imaging in Substance Abuse: Research, Clinical, and Forensic Applications is an outstanding and in-depth compilation of the state-of-the-science in the clinical neurobiology of substance abuse. This book will be an extremely useful resource to the field and will provide an excellent overview to the more casual reader. The review chapters are comprehensive and include most abused substances for which findings have been obtained. All major brain imaging techniques are covered in this book, and importantly, the methods chapters are written in clear language so that even those with nontechnical backgrounds will understand these highly complex technologies. These methods chapters include discussions of strengths, weaknesses, and future directions of each modality. The review chapters are critical examinations of the methods and findings, and include discussions of experimental design factors that complicate clinical substance abuse research. Overall, what makes this book special and sets it apart from the usual text is its organization. A remarkably complete and structured bibliography with over 1350 citations is included. Detailed Tables of Contents and the extensive index facilitate access to topics and findings of interest. Thus, in addition to being a complete collection of critical reviews of the field, this book will serve as a particularly useful reference.

Rapid developments in brain imaging technology, as well as the integration of findings from individual brain imaging methods and combinations thereof, will lead us to a much better understanding of the neurobiology of substance abuse and addiction. The science presented in this book will form a firm foundation for future successes in this research endeavor.

Joseph Frascella, PhD
Chief, Clinical Neurobiology Branch
Division of Treatment Research and Development
National Institute on Drug Abuse

Preface

Brain imaging techniques are increasingly being used by clinical researchers, physicians, forensics experts, and lawyers to evaluate mechanisms and consequences of brain changes associated with acute and chronic substance abuse. Because of the technical nature and high costs historically associated with most brain imaging modalities, access to these technologies, and their practical applications in substance abuse research have been limited. However, the number of clinical research sites implementing brain imaging modalities is multiplying, and the techniques themselves are becoming less invasive and less expensive. This evolution will ensure expanded use of brain imaging in substance abuse-related research, diagnosis, and litigation.

The goal of *Brain Imaging in Substance Abuse: Research, Clinical, and Forensic Applications* is to describe the methods and to review the research findings generated by clinical brain imaging modalities most commonly used in the study of substance abuse and dependence. These include electroencephalography, emission tomography, and magnetic resonance. By themselves, each of these powerful techniques has the ability to measure a number of parameters that indicate brain function, including electrical activity, metabolism, hemodynamics, receptor and neurotransmitter levels, neurochemistry, and structure. It is the consensus of the contributors to this volume that the most comprehensive view of the mechanisms and consequences of drug abuse and dependence will be achieved by those who can understand and synthesize the research findings from all of these brain imaging modalities.

Pursuit of an integrated understanding of the literature from all of these fields is by no means a trivial goal, since each modality has numerous technical complexities. This book has been organized to assist in this effort. The first three chapters of the book describe the technical foundations for electroencephalography, emission tomography, and magnetic resonance. These chapters also discuss the strengths and weaknesses of each method. Chapters 1–3 are written so that readers with nontechnical backgrounds will be able to appreciate how these technologies work.

Chapters 4–6 present comprehensive reviews of the electroencephalographic, emission tomographic, and magnetic resonance research findings in substance abuse, and also discuss the methodological factors that complicate the interpretation of results from studies of chronic substance abusers. These factors include the confounds of polydrug abuse, medical and/or psychiatric comorbidity, premorbid disease, and genetic or sociologic predisposition to substance abuse. A concise, comprehensive list of the many confounds that confront all clinical brain imaging studies of chronic substance abusers is presented as a part of Chapter 4.

Chapter 7 focuses on the neuropsychology of substance abuse. While neuropsychological assessment is not strictly a form of brain imaging, it offers standardized and reliable methods for relating neuroimaging findings to higher levels of brain function. Accordingly, it is increasingly being required by peer-review committees, journal referees, and courts, to provide functional context for neuroimaging findings. This chapter reviews the extensive neuropsychology literature in substance abuse, lists and describes the most commonly used neuropsychological tests, and also discusses the strengths and weaknesses of this discipline.

There is a nexus between substance abuse and crime, and as a result, it is expected that brain imaging findings will see expanded use (and misuse) in legal contexts. Chapter 8 discusses these issues and proposes guidelines for appropriate use of brain imaging findings in the courtroom. This chapter also contains a discussion of the scientific and legal definitions of "evidence," and of how differences in these definitions between the professions contribute to problems when science (and scientists) enter the courtroom. This chapter is particularly relevant to judges who must render legal decisions based on legal *and* scientific precedents, because, according to Supreme Court rulings regarding the presentation of scientific evidence, they must serve as "gatekeepers," scrutinizing the relevance of expert scientific testimony.

The last part of the book is a comprehensive bibliography of clinical brain imaging and neuropsychological research in substance abuse. The bibliography is structured by technique and by substance abuse topic, and has a detailed table of contents to facilitate rapid access to topics of interest.

It is my hope that *Brain Imaging in Substance Abuse: Research, Clinical, and Forensic Applications* will help to foster a more complete understanding of the effects of substance abuse on the human brain, by providing better access to the methods and findings in this field.

Acknowledgments

I am grateful to my distinguished colleagues who contributed chapters to this volume, and to the following individuals for their contributions:

J. T. Arnold, PhD
Linda Chang, MD
Bruce M. Cohen, MD, PhD
Eileen Connolly, RTR
Lyn Dietrich, MSLS, AHIP
Kerstin Dostal, BA
Richard R. Ernst, PhD
Thomas Ernst, PhD
Joseph Frascella, PhD
Håkan Hall, PhD
Arnold R. Kriegstein, MD, PhD
Paul C. Lauterbur, PhD

Edythe D. London, PHD
Peter R. Martin, MD
Nancy K. Mello, PHD
Jack H. Mendelson, MD
Rabbi Donald J. Pollock, DAPA
Perry F. Renshaw, PHD
John J. Resnik, JD
Anne M. Smith, RTR
Edith B. Stern
Lawrence L. Wald, PHD

I would also like to thank the National Institute on Drug Abuse for generous grant support.

Additionally, I would like to acknowledge Bertha K. Madras, PHD, for a decade of wonderful mentorship, friendship, and insight.

Finally, I am indebted to my wife Rebekah, who spent many hours assisting in the preparation of this volume. My life and work have always benefited from her touch.

Marc J. Kaufman, PHD

Contents

List of Figures

Chapter 1

Chapter 2

Chapter 3

Chapter 4

Chapter 5

Chapter 6

List of Tables

Contributors

LANCE O. BAUER, PhD • *Professor of Psychiatry, Director, Neural Dynamics Laboratory, University of Connecticut School of Medicine, Farmington, CT*

BLAISE DEB. FREDERICK, PhD • *Instructor in Psychiatry, Harvard Medical School, Assistant Biophysicist, McLean Hospital, Brain Imaging Center, McLean Hospital, Belmont, MA*

STACI A. GRUBER, EdM • *Clinical Investigator, Cognitive Neuroimaging and Neuropsychology Laboratories, Brain Imaging Center, McLean Hospital, Harvard Medical School, Belmont, MA, and Department of Psychology, Tufts University, Medford, MA.*

DOUGLAS W. JONES, PhD • *National Institute of Mental Health, NIMH SPECT Lab, Clinical Brain Disorders Branch, DIRP, Bethesda, MD*

MARC J. KAUFMAN, PhD • *Assistant Professor of Psychiatry, Harvard Medical School, and Associate Research Pharmacologist, Brain Imaging Center, McLean Hospital, Belmont, MA*

ELENA M. KOURI, PhD • *Assistant Professor of Psychiatry, Harvard Medical School, and Associate Director, Behavioral Psychopharmacology Research Laboratory, McLean Hospital, Belmont, MA*

JENNIFER J. KULYNYCH, JD, PhD • *Health Practice Group, Hogan and Hartson, LLP, Washington, DC*

JONATHAN M. LEVIN, MD, MPH • *Assistant Professor of Psychiatry, Harvard Medical School, and Director, Laboratory of Cerebral Blood Flow, Brain Imaging Center, McLean Hospital, Belmont, MA*

SCOTT E. LUKAS, PhD • *Associate Professor of Psychiatry, Harvard Medical School, and Director, Behavioral Psychopharmacology Research Laboratory, McLean Hospital, Belmont, MA*

LUIS C. MAAS III., MD, PhD • *Research Associate in Neuroimaging, Brain Imaging Center, McLean Hospital, Belmont, MA*

ROBERT T. MALISON, MD • *Associate Professor of Psychiatry, Yale University School of Medicine, New Haven, CT*

PERRY F. RENSHAW, MD, PhD • *Associate Professor of Psychiatry, Harvard Medical School, and Director, Brain Imaging Center, McLean Hospital, Belmont, MA*

DEBORAH A. YURGELUN-TODD, PhD • *Associate Professor of Psychiatry, Harvard Medical School, and Director, Cognitive Neuroimaging and Neuropsychology Laboratories, Brain Imaging Center, McLean Hospital, Belmont, MA*

Chapter 1

Electroencephalography, Topographic Mapping, and Event-Related Potentials in Substance Abuse Research

Elena M. Kouri, PhD and Scott E. Lukas, PhD

History of the Electroencephalogram

Scientific interest in the ability of organisms to generate electrical activity dates back to the late eighteenth century when an Italian physiologist, Luigi Galvani, discovered that frogs' leg muscles were excitable tissues. It was not until the mid-nineteenth century, however, that scientists realized that the electrical activity of living tissue could be used as a sign of its function, when the German physiologist Du Bois-Reymond demonstrated that an electrical signal occurred concurrently with nerve impulses. This observation motivated a British physiologist, Richard Caton, to demonstrate in 1875 that brains from animals also generated electrical impulses.

More than 50 years later, in 1929, the German neuropsychiatrist Hans Berger was the first to record the electrical activity of the human brain. Berger discovered that the human brain produced regular electrical current oscillations that were rhythmic in nature and could be recorded from the scalp of individuals with intact skulls (Berger, 1929). He named the entire record of the brain's electrical activity the "Electrenkephalogramm" and abbreviated it EEG.

Berger's findings were not readily accepted by the scientific community at the time, mainly because neurophysiologists could not accept the notion that regular oscillations of quasi-sinusoidal form could represent the electrical activity of an organ as complex as the brain and, even less, that it could be recorded over the scalp. After years of skepticism, in 1934, the British scientists Edgar Adrian and B. Matthews replicated Berger's findings on the human electroencephalogram (EEG) (Adrian and

From: *Brain Imaging in Substance Abuse: Research, Clinical, and Forensic Applications*
M. J. Kaufman, ed. © Humana Press Inc., Totowa, New Jersey

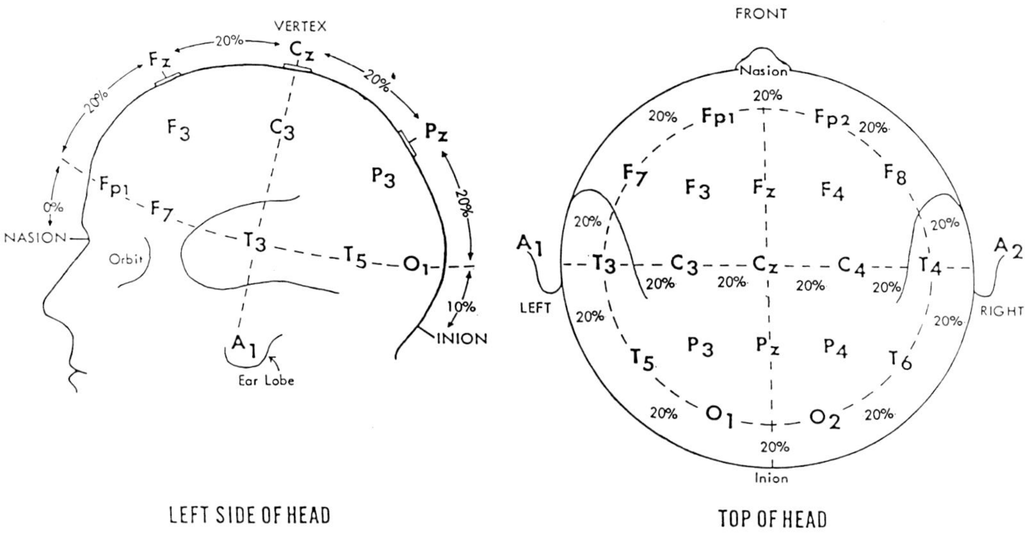

Fig. 1. Schematic diagram of the 10-20 International System for Electrode Placement.

Matthews, 1934), and Berger's work was finally accepted by the scientific community. Shortly thereafter, interest in brain electrical activity became widespread among scientists, and, since then, the EEG has become a conventional clinical procedure with significant diagnostic value and an important research tool in neuroscience.

Recording the Electroencephalogram

The technique of recording EEG involves obtaining a sample of brain electrical activity from a number of electrodes placed on the subject's head. Generally, a set of 21 electrodes is used, and the electrodes are placed over the scalp according to the 10-20 International System of electrode placement (Jasper, 1958). The 10-20 International System specifies the actual position in which the electrodes should be placed over the cerebral cortex by measuring standard landmarks on the skull. The placement of the 21 electrodes covers virtually the entire skull, and the position of each electrode is specified by a letter and a number according to the area of the brain to which it corresponds. The identifying letter of each electrode represents the brain area that it underlies: F denoting frontal, C denoting central, P denoting parietal, and O denoting occipital. The identifying number further refers to the location of the electrode with even numbers representing the right hemisphere and odd numbers representing the left hemisphere (Fig. 1).

The International System for electrode placement is called the 10-20 system owing to the placement of electrodes at a distance of either 10% or 20% from specific landmarks on the skull. The use of percentages to determine electrode placement allows for differences in skull sizes and shapes, and it ensures that the placement of electrodes is accurate with respect to the specific individual's skull. The initial step in determining the placement of electrodes is to determine, with a measuring tape, the distance between the nasion (the indentation where the nose joins the forehead) and inion (a prominent protrusion at the back of the head located at the nape of the neck)

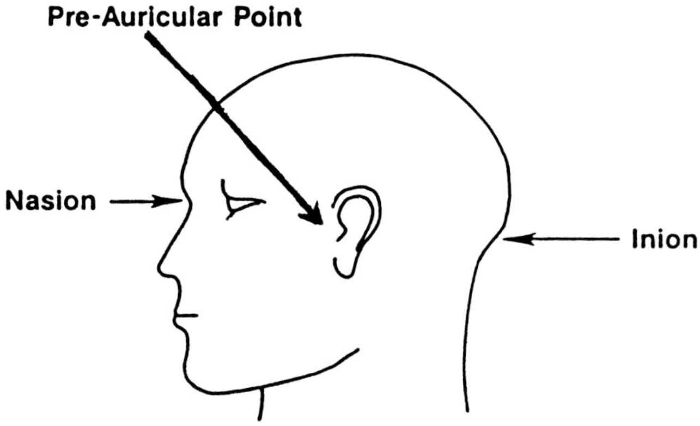

Fig. 2. Diagram of the landmarks of the 10-20 International System for Electrode Placement.

over the midline (Fig. 2). Then, 10% of the nasion-to-inion distance above the nasion is marked for placement of the frontal pole electrode F_{pz}, and locations at 20% of the nasion-to-inion distance along the midline are marked for placement of the midline electrodes F_z, C_z, P_z, and O_z (Fig. 1).

Once the midline electrode locations are established, the lateral measurements are made in the central coronal plane using the distance between the left and right preaurical points as the landmarks. The preaurical points are located in the front of the ears just above the triangular piece of cartilage that covers the opening of the external ear canal. Five points are located at different percent distances between the preaurical points. T_3 and T_4 are located above the preaurical landmarks at 10% of the total distance between the two preaurical points. C_3 and C_4 are at 20% above T_3 and T_4, respectively. The central electrode, C_z, should mark the midline or 50% distance between the two preaurical points. This electrode is also located at the 50% mark of the distance between the nasion and inion.

After the placement of the electrodes in the midline and coronal line is established, the electrodes around the circumference of the head are attached. In order to do this, the circumference of the head is determined by placing the measuring tape around the head and over the frontal, temporal, and occipital marks already established. Electrodes F_{p1} and F_{p2} are located at a distance of 5% of the total head circumference to the left and right of F_{pz}, respectively. All other circumference electrodes (F_7, F_8, T_3, T_4, T_5, T_6, O_1, O_2) are placed at a distance of 10% of the head circumference measurement between each one.

To determine the location of the electrodes in the parasagittal rows, the distance between F_{p1} and O_1 is measured with the measuring tape placed over the C_3 electrode. The placement of electrode F_3 is 25% of the distance between F_{p1} and O_1 backward from F_{p1}. Similarly, the location of electrode P_3 is 25% of the distance between F_{p1} and O_1 in front of O_1. The same measurements are taken for the right hemisphere to place F_4 and P_4.

The final step in following the 10-20 International System of electrode placement is to attach reference electrodes. Reference electrodes are critical because the voltage recorded at each electrode site is a measure of the difference in electrical potential between the electrode and the reference. As such, reference electrodes are placed in an area with little or no electrical activity. Reference electrodes are not normally placed outside of the head region because electrodes placed at a distance from the head are extremely susceptible to extraneous electrical noise often introduced by the electrocardiogram. The places that are most commonly used as reference points are the earlobes, mastoids, and the tip of the nose. Usually, a ground electrode is also added, and normally it is attached between F_{p1} and F_{p2} in the middle of the subject's forehead. It is extremely important to place the electrodes accurately over the specific regions of the cerebral cortex because errors in symmetrical placement of electrodes over the right and left hemispheres can result in EEG tracings, which may be erroneously interpreted as being asymmetrical.

After each electrode site is measured and marked, an electrolyte gel or paste is rubbed into the electrode to increase conductivity, reduce resistance of the skin, and to help secure the disk to the scalp. Once electrode placement is completed, the impedance of each electrode needs to be checked. This is done by connecting each electrode cable to an impedance meter, which applies a small external voltage to the electrodes and measures the amount of current flowing through the circuit. Because the currents applied to the circuit when measuring impedances are so small (only a few microamperes), the current is usually not even noticed by the subject and poses no danger whatsoever. It is generally agreed that an impedance reading of 5 kΩ or less is necessary for optimal recordings.

Although it is important to know how to measure the location of each electrode site, the majority of laboratories using EEG recordings for research purposes today use special caps that are fitted with recessed electrodes already placed at the specific locations (Electro-cap International, Eaton, OH). The use of electrode caps significantly reduces the time spent measuring for electrode placement, the potential for errors owing to measuring inaccuracy, and the likelihood of electrode shifts. The caps are available in different sizes, and their placement is determined by the subject's head circumference and the distance between the subject's inion and nasion. Electrode caps also require the use of some type of conductive gel as well as low-impedance readings.

EEG Amplifiers

The electrical activity generated by the brain contains fluctuations in voltage that are extremely small. To obtain signals that are large enough to produce deflections in the pens of EEG machines, devices that increase the magnitude of the waves are necessary. These devices are known as amplifiers, and they increase the amplitude of the waves without introducing distortion. This is done by controlling the ability of the amplifiers to accommodate the wide range of voltage fluctuations in the EEG. Specifically, amplifiers in EEG machines are provided with a means of changing amplification or "gain" such that when confronted with fluctuations that are outside of the expected range, the total amplification available is changed. Increasing the gain of a channel in an EEG machine increases the total amplification available and results in larger voltage fluctuations in the tracing. Gain is usually referred to as sensitivity in EEG machines and is expressed as microvolts per millimeter deflection (μV/mm). Thus, as sensitivity increases, a millimeter represents fewer microvolts, and as sensitivity decreases, a millimeter represents more microvolts.

Because activity recorded in the EEG encompasses a wide range of voltage fluctuations, most EEG machines have the option of a maximum gain of 1 μV/mm and a minimum gain of 70 μV/mm. The decision of what sensitivity setting to use depends on the EEG data being recorded. For instance, when dealing with voltages at the low-amplitude end of the scale, as in brain death recordings, voltages as small as 2 μV need to be recorded, requiring the use of more amplification. On the other hand, when dealing with voltages at the high end of the scale, as in hypsarrhythmia, voltages as large as 2000 μV are encountered and less amplification is needed. For EEG recordings within the normal range, the standard sensitivity setting is 7 μV/mm.

EEG Filters

Recordings from electrodes on the scalp are susceptible to contamination from other sources of electrical activity, such as the heart, muscles, and even activity from extrinsic sources, such as electric power lines. These types of electrical activity present in the EEG tracing are known as artifacts and need to be eliminated because they contaminate the recordings. Since it is not always possible to eliminate completely the actual sources of contaminating activity, instruments known as filters are routinely used in EEG recordings. EEG filters are devices that selectively allow activity within specific frequencies to be transmitted while removing or diminishing activity outside the specified frequency ranges.

There are usually three different types of filters in EEG machines: low-frequency, high-frequency, and notch filters. The low-frequency filter, also known as the high-pass filter, attenuates frequencies at the low end of the frequency spectrum while allowing frequencies at the high end to be amplified. The high-frequency filter, also known as the low-pass filter, attenuates frequencies at the high end while allowing frequencies at the low end to be amplified. The notch filter, by contrast, specifically filters out 60 Hz activity, which is usually introduced by power lines or electrical cables in the area.

The settings for the low- and high-frequency filters are determined by the experimenter and depend on the electrical activity of interest. By independently adjusting the filter settings, the experimenter determines the "bandwidth" of the amplifier, and only activity within the desired frequencies is recorded. For instance, recordings of event-related potentials require lower frequency bandwidths (e.g., 0.045–30 Hz) than straight EEG recordings (e.g., 1.5–70 Hz). It is important to note, however, that even though filters eliminate most of the activity in unwanted frequencies, artifacts that occur within the frequencies of interest are not eliminated by the filters and are passed on to the EEG record. Methods for avoiding these types of artifacts are described in detail later on in the chapter.

EEG Montages

A montage refers to a specific arrangement by which a number of electrode pairs is displayed simultaneously in an EEG record. Because the purpose of montages is to make EEG interpretation as easy and accurate as possible, some guidelines should be

Table 1
Commonly Used EEG Montages

Referential with linked earlobes		Bipolar longitudinal		Bipolar transverse	
F7 – A1+A2	F	Fp1 – F7	L	F7 – Fp1	Fp
F3 – A1+A2		F7 – T3		Fp2 – F8	
F4 – A1+A2		T3 – T5		F7 – F3	F
F8 – A1+A2		T5 – O1		F3 – Fz	
C3 – A1+A2	C	Fp2 – F8	R	Fz – F4	
Cz – A1+A2		F8 – T4		F4 – F8	
C4 – A1+A2		T4 – T6		T3 – C3	C
T3 – A1+A2	T	T6 – O2		C3 – Cz	
T4 – A1+A2		FP1 – F3	L	Cz – C4	
T5 – A1+A2		F3 – C3		C4 – T4	
T6 – A1+A2		C3 – P3		T5 – P3	P
P3 – A1+A2	P	P3 – 01		P3 – Pz	
Pz – A1+A2		Fp2 – F4	R	Pz – P4	
P4 – A1+A2		F4 – C4		P4 – T6	
O1 – A1+A2	O	C4 – P4		T5 – 01	O
O2 – A1+A2		P4 – O2		O2 – T6	

used in developing montages. First, montages should follow some kind of anatomic order. For instance, EEG channels representing more anterior electrodes should be presented on the chart above channels representing more posterior electrodes. Second, electrode combinations from the left side of the scalp should be located on the chart above those from the right side of the scalp.

There are two basic types of EEG montages: referential and bipolar. The principle behind referential montages is that electrical activity at different electrode sites can be measured simultaneously against a reference electrode with no cerebral electrical activity. An advantage of this type of montage is that the common reference allows for multiple comparisons of the activity at the various scalp electrodes. The major disadvantage of this type of montage is that there is no perfect reference electrode. For instance, the earlobes, which are one of the most commonly used sites of reference, are close to the temporal lobes and the heart and can sometimes pick up electrical activity from those sources. One way in which these artifacts can be reduced is by using both earlobes together as a reference. This method is called linked-earlobe reference and is commonly used in research and clinical practice. Most EEG machines have the option of linked earlobes (A1 + A2) as a reference for montages.

In contrast to referential montages, in bipolar montages, both electrodes in the pair are considered to be active, and the difference in potential between the two electrodes on the scalp is displayed on the tracing. Bipolar montages link electrodes in a sequential manner that resembles chains in a longitudinal (anterior to posterior) or transverse (coronal) array. The advantage of bipolar montages is that localization of

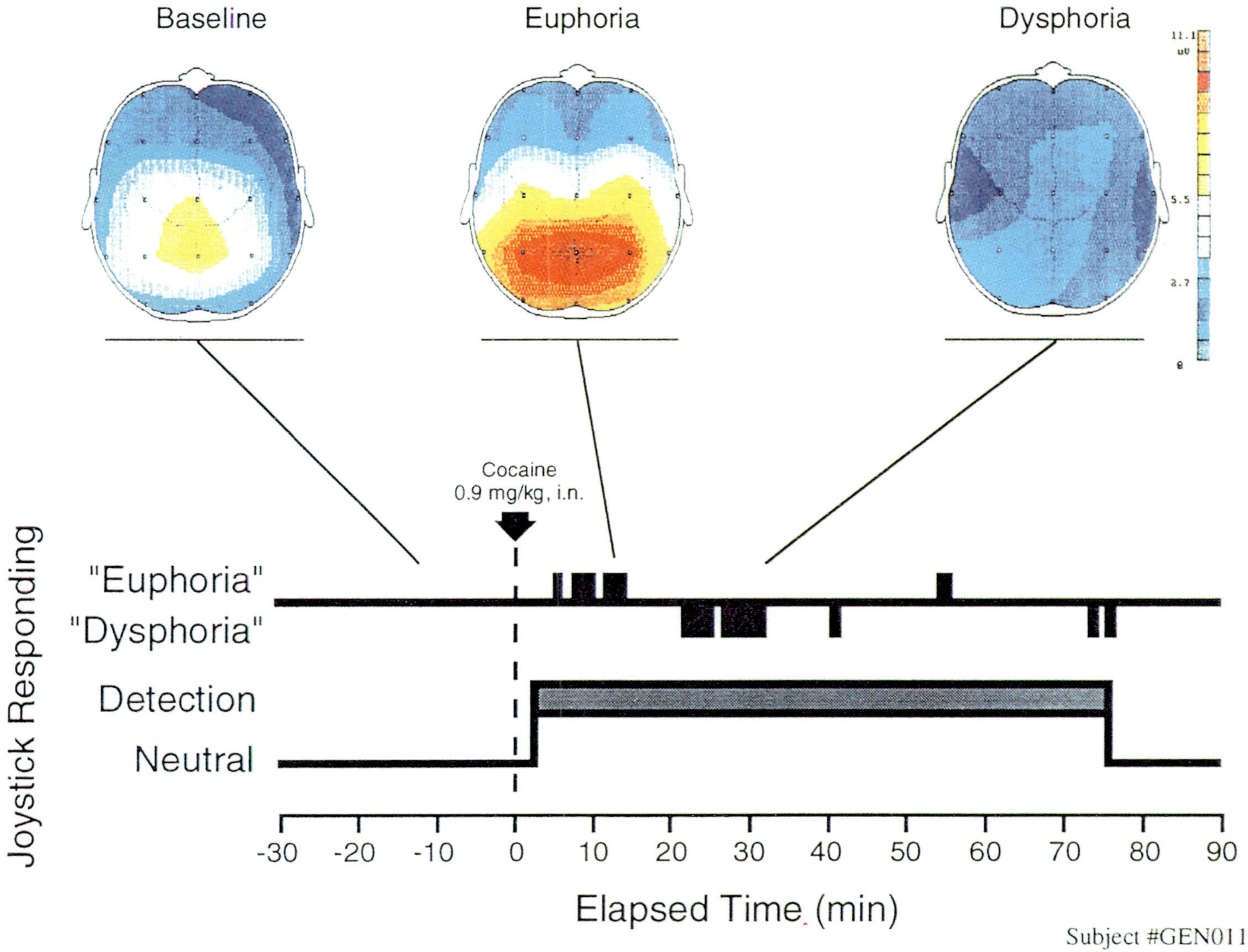

Plate 1. Behavioral and EEG profile of a typical subject after receiving an acute dose of cocaine (0.9 mg/kg, i.n.). *See Chapter 1, Figure 7, p. 14.*

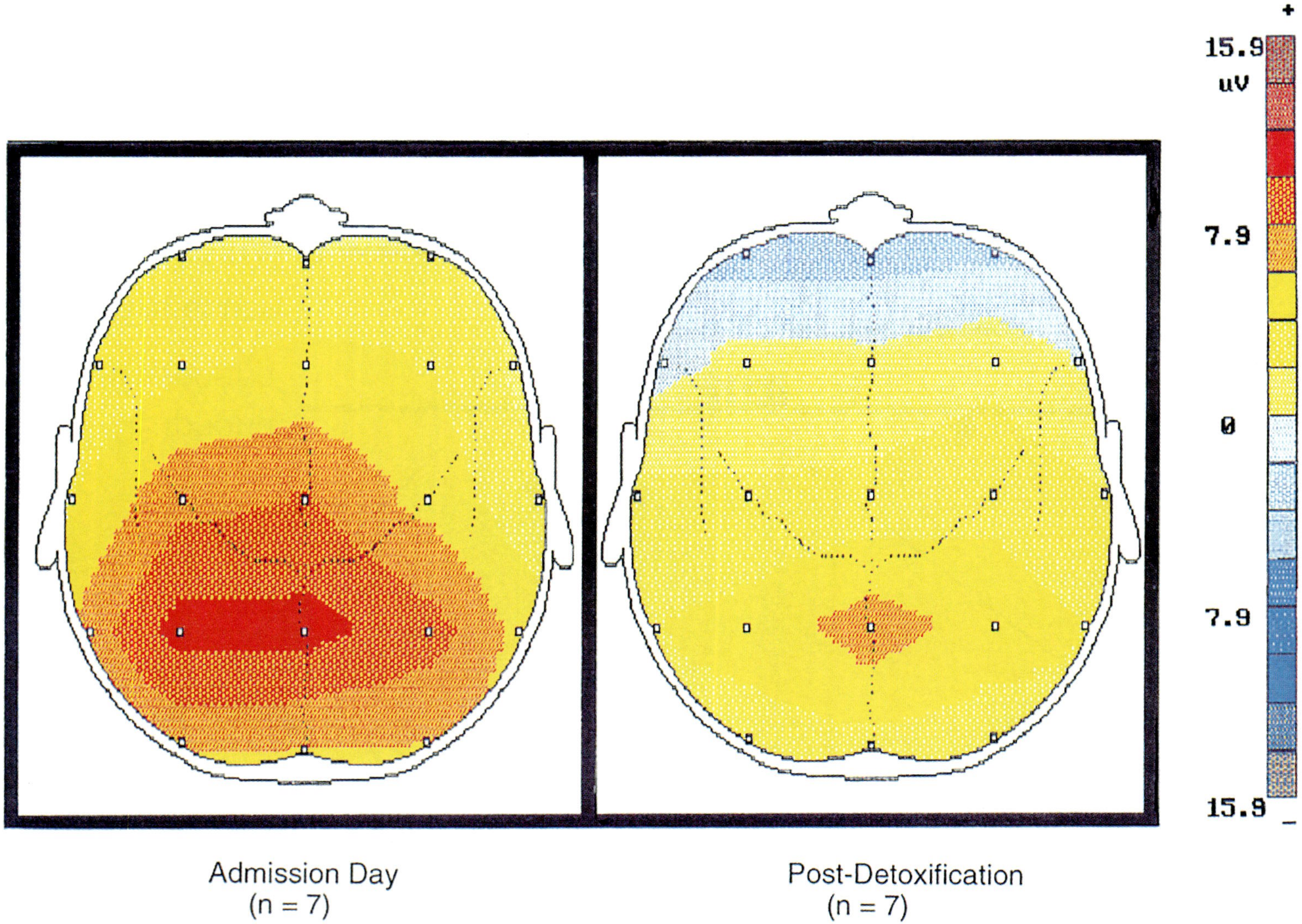

Plate 2. Topographic map of the P300 event-related potential in cocaine- and heroin-dependent subjects on admission (intoxicated state) and following a 12-d detoxification period. *See Chapter 1, Fig. 9, p. 18.*

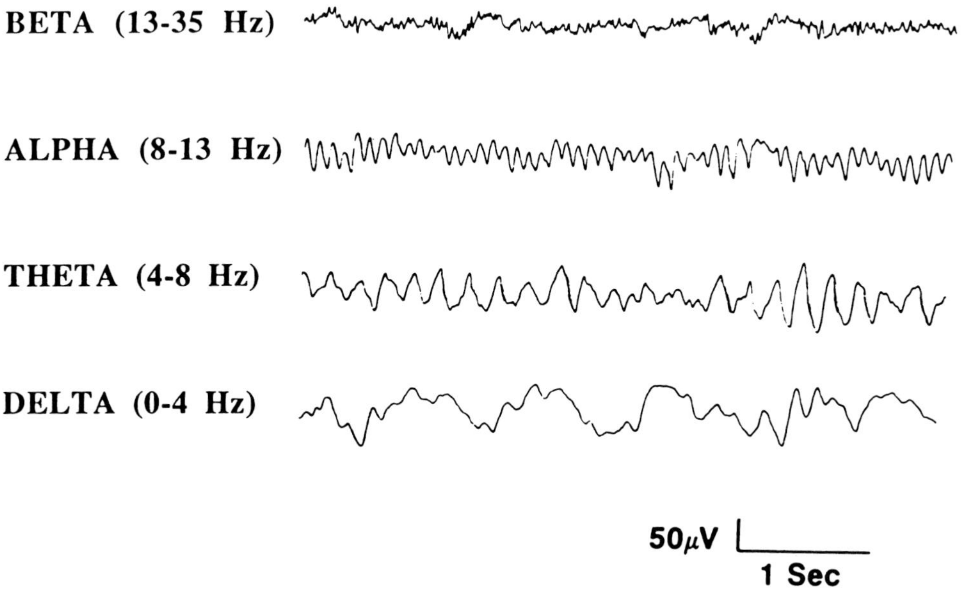

Fig. 3. Sample tracing of the four basic categories of the EEG frequency spectrum.

activity can be easily made by visual inspection of the tracing. However, a disadvantage of these montages is that they do not provide an accurate measure of the amplitude of the waveform of a particular event since the activity of a particular pair of electrodes can be canceled out or summed depending on the magnitude of the voltages of each individual electrode in the pair. Table 1 illustrates some commonly used montages. For more information on the advantages and disadvantages of different types of montages, the reader should refer to Duffy et al. (1989).

Analysis of the EEG

The EEG is a measure of the electrical activity of neurons located in both the cerebral cortex and subcortical nuclei. It is analyzed in terms of its frequency, which represents how many oscillations or cycles occur per second (hertz, Hz), and its amplitude, which represents the magnitude of the waves (measured in microvolts, mV). The amplitude of the EEG provides a quantitative measure of the size of a specific waveform, which depends on the following:

1. The number of neurons firing synchronously
2. The distance between these neurons and the recording electrode
3. The source of the activity being measured.

The frequency spectrum of the EEG ranges from 1 to 70 Hz, and usually separates into four basic categories known as alpha, beta, theta, and delta. The alpha band comprises electrical activity in the range of 8–13 Hz. Alpha activity is normally seen when the subject is awake, relaxed, and with the eyes closed. Its amplitude is usually below 50 μV, but it can range from 5 to 100 μV. These waves are also referred to as

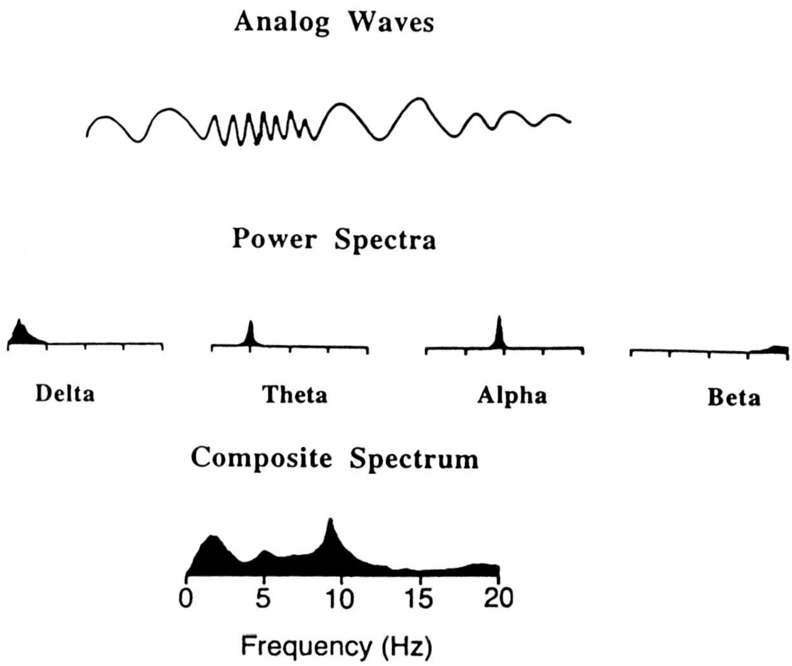

Fig. 4. Diagrammatic representation of the generation of power spectra from analog EEG waveforms.

the posterior-dominant rhythm because they are most pronounced over the occipital region of the scalp. The beta band comprises frequencies over 13 Hz and sometimes as high as 35 Hz. The amplitude of the beta waves is mostly below 30 μV, although it can be variable. Both the alpha and beta bands are further subdivided into slow (8–10 Hz) and fast (11–13 Hz) alpha and slow (13.5–19.5 Hz) and fast (20–26 Hz) beta. The theta band includes electrical activity in the range of 4–8 Hz and is normally seen during drowsiness and during the light stages of sleep. The delta band consists of frequencies under 4 Hz and is normally seen in the deeper stages of sleep. Delta waves have the highest amplitude of all other EEG waves. Figure 3 depicts a sample tracing of the four categories of the EEG frequency spectrum. The horizontal axis in the tracing represents time, and the vertical axis represents amplitude of the electrical signal.

Although visual inspection of the EEG can be an important initial step in identifying the various types of brain waves in a tracing, it is not an objective or reliable method for analyzing EEG activity, and the observed changes are impossible to quantify accurately. One of the first attempts to quantify the EEG involved the use of an ordinary desk ruler as a means of measuring the amplitude of successive waves (Goldstein and Beck, 1965). However, because this method used an arbitrary baseline for the measurements, comparisons with different recordings were extremely difficult. Currently, analysis of EEG activity involves the use of high-speed computers to separate a waveform into its different frequency components. This type of frequency or spectral analysis is known as a fast Fourier transform (FFT) and is a method for

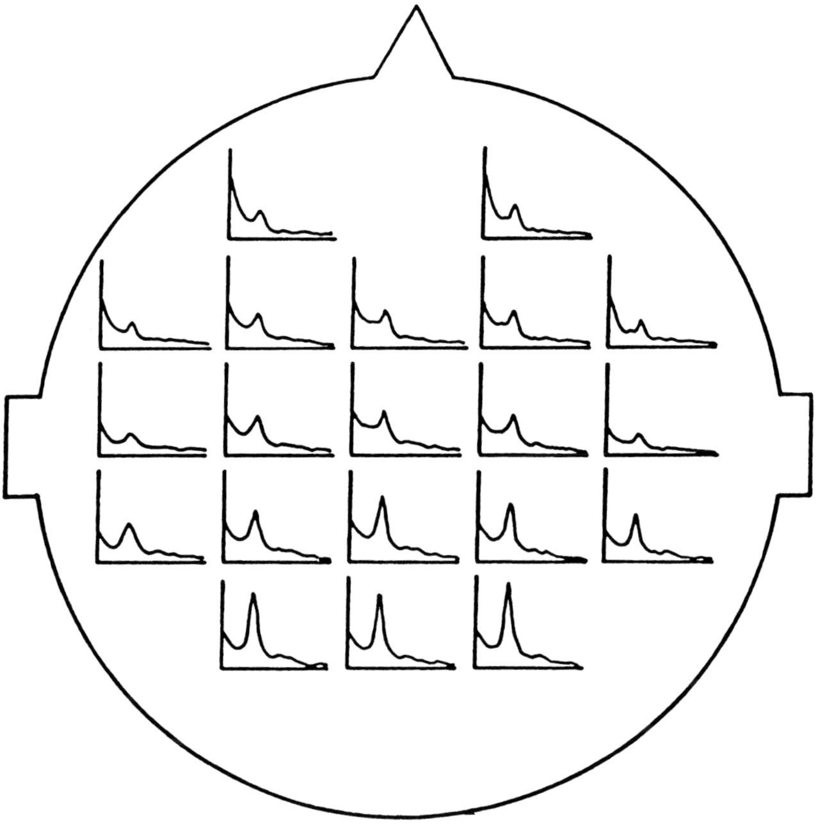

Fig. 5. Schematic diagram of the method employed in generating topographic brain maps. Power spectra are generated for electrical activity recorded in each of the individual scalp electrodes. (From Lukas, 1997, with permission.)

expressing the EEG in terms of its amplitude vs frequency instead of amplitude vs time components (Walter, 1963; Cooley and Tukey, 1965). The FFT is an algorithm that can be used to analyze any continuous waveform into a sum of sine and cosine waves of different amplitudes and frequencies.

The output of the FFT analysis is called a power spectrum, with frequency on the horizontal axis and amplitude on the vertical axis (Fig. 4). The power spectrum represents a summary of the frequency components calculated from sections of EEG called epochs. These EEG epochs usually last 2 s or less. To obtain a representation of the power spectrum over longer periods of time, a method known as the compressed spectral array has been developed. This method involves plotting together a large number of comparable power spectra in close proximity to each other on the same graph in order to obtain a continuous summary of the amplitude/frequency components of the recording. Spectral analysis is a valuable tool for quantifying the effects of drugs of abuse on the brain and serves the basis of the analysis used in topographic mapping of brain electrical activity.

Topographic Mapping

Topographic mapping is a technique that provides a complete view of the distribution of brain electrical activity over the scalp at any point in time. This technique uses high-speed digital computing and mathematical algorithms to interpolate the activity of the scalp area between the EEG electrodes. Essentially, a power spectrum is generated for the electrical activity that has been recorded at each electrode site (Fig. 5). The calculated voltages are then color-coded to quantify the distribution of brain electrical activity over the entire scalp and to aid in the identification of patterns over the scalp. The selection of colors used to portray the different voltages is often arbitrary and is typically used to highlight the areas of interest rather than to provide any real physiologic significance. This technique was first used in 1971 (Duffy 1986) to intermix EEG activity from numerous scalp sites into a single display of electrical activity at a single time-point.

A number of different algorithms are currently used by practitioners for interpolating values between electrode sites (e.g., *see* Duffy, 1986). Even though there is no optimal paradigm that has been agreed on, a commonly used technique is the three-point, three-dimensional linear interpolation. This technique creates values for unknown locations based on the three nearest electrode sites, resulting in images that are smooth in appearance. The reliability of a given interpolation algorithm can be tested by comparing interpolated values with values that are measured at the specific site.

Topographic maps of brain electrical activity are particularly useful as hypothesis-generating tools in that they provide a quantifiable measure of drug-related changes in activity across the entire scalp. By carefully examining and identifying new patterns of activity, new hypotheses and avenues of research can be developed. For example, recent findings of increased alpha activity in the frontal and frontal-central scalp regions of daily marijuana users (Struve et al., 1994, 1998) would have been missed if such studies exclusively investigated alpha activity in the occipital regions of the scalp, where alpha is normally most pronounced.

Artifact Avoidance

When designing experiments involving the use of electrophysiological measures, a number of precautions need to be taken to avoid artifacts that can seriously compromise the quality of the data. For example, because the EEG is extremely sensitive to movement artifacts, subjects need to be provided with an environment that minimizes movement requirements during the experiment. These include:

1. A comfortable chair that allows the subject to remain in a relatively constant position during the conduct of the experiment;
2. Easy access to experimental instruments with minimal movement requirements, such as joystick devices to respond to experimental questionnaires without the need to write and/or respond verbally;
3. Drug-administration systems that deliver the drug in a controlled, systematic manner with minimum disruptions to and requirements from the subject;
4. Physiologic measurements that interfere minimally with the subject; and
5. Blood withdrawal systems that do not involve repeated interruptions to the subject, such as continuous sampling from a long catheter attached to a slow

withdrawal pump in a way that is unobtrusive to the subject, as opposed to discrete blood sampling requiring constant interaction with the subject.

Another issue in conducting drug-related electrophysiologic studies is the variability inherent to the EEG. To minimize the potential of artifact confounds, it is extremely important to:

1. Collect a stable baseline;
2. Consistently record data with the subject's eyes either open or closed; and
3. Conduct studies during the same time of the day so that the subjects' state of alertness is not significantly different across study visits.

In addition, the use of placebo controls and, whenever possible, within-subject comparisons is extremely important. These precautions are necessary to ensure that the observed drug-induced changes in brain electrical activity are owing exclusively to the effects of the drug and not to intersubject variability in EEG parameters unrelated to the study.

Utility of Electroencephalographic Techniques in Substance Abuse Research

An advantage of using EEG tracings to investigate drug-related changes in mood state is that the EEG is available for measurement on a continual basis without the subject being required to perform any task. Thus, the measurements obtained are free of confounds associated with techniques that require a response.

Even though EEG and topographic mapping have been used in neurology for some time, their utility in psychopharmacology has been primarily to classify drugs on the basis of their pharmacological properties according to their effects on the different frequency bands. For many years, attempts to demonstrate direct correlations between drug-induced changes in brain electrical activity and corresponding changes in mood states were generally unsuccessful. These difficulties were most often associated with the use of methods to assess behavioral changes which interfered with the electrophysiological recordings of brain electrical activity. More recently, however, EEG analysis and topographic mapping have been used successfully to assess the effects of drugs of abuse on brain and behavior (e.g., Martin and Kay, 1977; Porjesz and Begleiter, 1985; Lukas et al., 1988, 1989, 1990, 1993).

Measures of Acute Drug Effects

The EEG is a reliable and sensitive measure of the acute effects of drugs on the brain in both animals and humans (Fink et al., 1971; Winters, 1975; Lukas et al., 1980, 1983, 1986, 1988, 1989, 1990). The effects of drugs on the EEG can be measured as specific types of alterations that are usually described as a change from a control or baseline state typically obtained from either a placebo-treated group or from the same subject during a pre-drug recording condition. Several types of specific EEG alterations can be observed. One type of alteration is the emergence of a new waveform with a predominant frequency different from that present during control states or the emergence of new electrophysiological events such as spikes, seizure-like activity or spindles (slow wave/high amplitude bursts of activity). Examples of these types of drug effects are morphine-induced slow-wave bursts (Khazan et al., 1967) or pentylenetetrazol (Metrazol)-induced spikes (Ziskind et al., 1946).

Another type of acute drug effect on the EEG is a dissociation between EEG activity and behavior. During normal control states, behavioral alertness is usually accompanied by EEG desynchrony whereas behavioral sedation is usually accompanied by EEG synchrony. Examples of drug-induced dissociation are atropine-induced EEG synchrony accompanied with behavioral alertness (Longo, 1966) and reserpine-induced behavioral sedation accompanied by EEG desynchrony (Pscheidt et al., 1963). A third type of a drug-induced EEG change is an attenuation or stabilization of the normal fluctuations between the various stages of wakefulness such as phenobarbital-induced (Vastola and Rosen, 1960) and benzodiazepine-induced (Requin et al., 1963) stabilization of spontaneous EEG spikes.

Identifying the specific type of drug-induced alterations in brain electrical activity is useful for a number of applications including characterizing drugs on the basis of their effects on brain electrical activity, determining pharmacological equivalence between an "unknown" drug and a standard, and identifying dose-related differences of compounds belonging to the same chemical class. The review by Fink (1969) of drug-induced EEG alterations further illustrates the utility of EEG techniques for classifying psychoactive drugs into distinct subclasses based on their effects on EEG amplitude and frequency.

Another way in which EEG measures are useful in the study of the acute effects of psychoactive drugs is that they allow for the characterization of the relationship between drug-induced electrophysiological and behavioral changes. Historically, while it has been relatively easy to characterize differences in EEG profiles during distinct overt behavioral states such as wakefulness and sleep, it has been more difficult to detect EEG correlates of drug-induced behavioral states. This latter task of quantifying EEG changes along with changes in degrees of "alertness" is particularly important when studying the effects of psychoactive drugs because the most obvious effect of drugs is reflected in the individual's behavior.

To obtain an assessment of electrophysiologic alterations during drug-induced changes in mood, it is necessary to employ a system for reporting mood effects that does not interfere with the EEG. For instance, the use of questionnaires or verbal reports is not optimal because it would introduce movement artifact into the EEG recording, which would make it difficult to measure the brain activity that is associated with a specific change in mood state. Therefore, to accurately measure changes in brain wave activity during specific drug-induced behavioral states, the subject must be provided with a method for communicating when such specific changes have occurred. Some form of an instrumental joystick or switch closure device has been most frequently used by researchers in this field (Volavka et al., 1973; Koukkou and Lehmann, 1976; Lukas et al., 1986, 1990, 1995; Lukas and Mendelson, 1988; McEachern et al., 1988). The basis for using an instrumental device to report subjective drug effects is that the subject is not required to verbally report changes in mood state, which significantly reduces the potential for artifact in the EEG recordings. In addition, the use of a joystick device allows the investigator to measure only selective behaviors of interest (e.g., euphoria, intoxication, dysphoria) depending on the medication being tested and to keep the instructional set relatively simple.

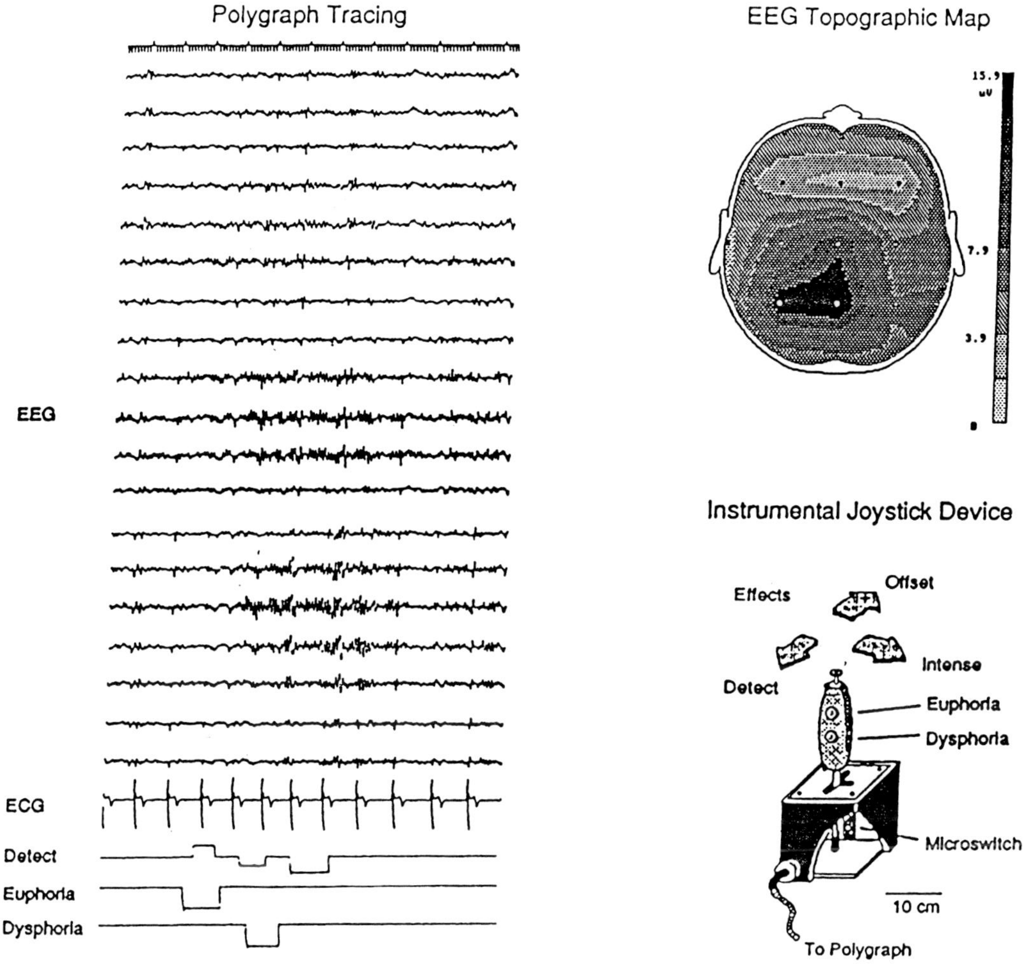

Fig. 6. A sample 19-channel polygraphic tracing and corresponding EEG topographic map. Electrocardiographic (ECG) activity is also shown. The bottom three tracings correspond to movements of the instrumental joystick device (lower right) which the subject moves to communicate changes in behavioral state following drug administration. (From Lukas et al., 1990, with permission.)

We have developed a system in our laboratory that records drug-induced behavioral changes via a joystick device while at the same time causing a deflection in a pen on the EEG machine such that the brain wave patterns being generated at exactly the same time as the behavioral effects are occurring can be identified and analyzed (Fig. 6). This methodology provides a quantifiable real time measure of the changes in mood states and physiological parameters with the corresponding changes in brain electrical activity.

Another important benefit of using a joystick device together with continuous EEG monitoring is that qualitative differences in dose-related effects in mood can be further characterized by dose-related changes in EEG activity. For instance, by analyzing the brain electrical activity that was occurring at the time when subjects in

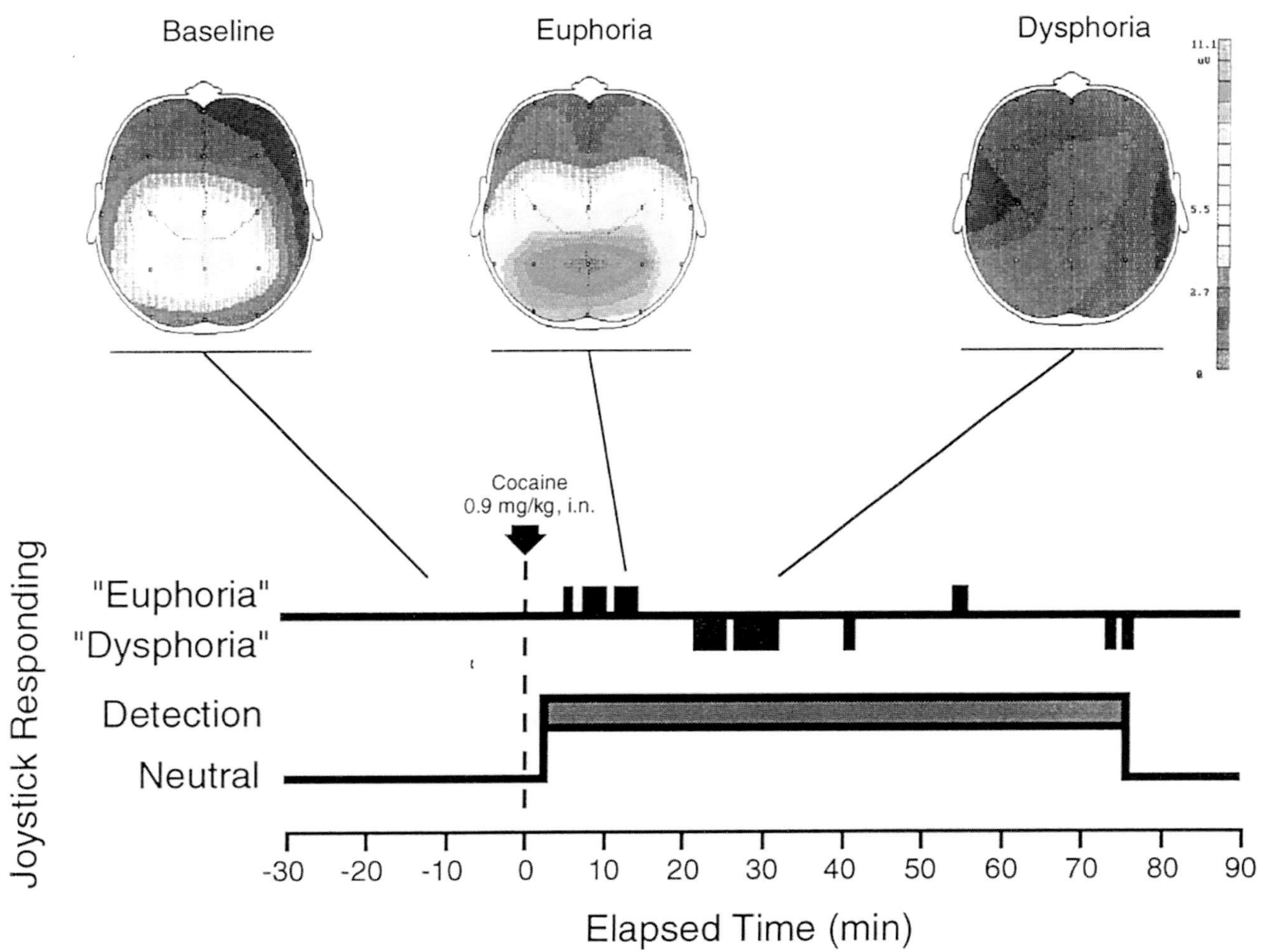

Fig. 7. Behavioral profile of a typical subject after receiving an acute dose of cocaine (0.9 mg/kg, i.n.). The subject had continuous access to the joystick device. Topographic maps of EEG alpha activity are plotted along the same time axis to permit direct comparisons of brain function during baseline, cocaine-induced euphoria and dysphoria. The scale is in microvolts. (*See* color plate 1 appearing after p. 6.)

our laboratory were reporting intense feeling of well-being or euphoria, we were able to electrophysiologically characterize behavioral changes associated with a high dose of cocaine (0.9 mg/kg, i.n.). Specifically, power spectral analysis of the brain electrical activity occurring during cocaine-induced euphoria revealed that it was characterized by pronounced increases in alpha activity over the parietal and occipital areas of the scalp (Fig. 7) (Lukas, 1991). This finding indicates that a qualitatively different electrophysiological phenomenon occurs during cocaine-induced euphoria which is not characteristic of cocaine detection. We have noted similar increases in EEG alpha activity during subjective reports of euphoria following acute administration of ethanol (Lukas et al., 1986, 1989), marihuana (Lukas et al., 1995), as well as marihuana and cocaine together (Lukas, 1991). This example illustrates the importance of using EEG and behavioral measures of drug effects concurrently.

Measures of Tolerance and Dependence

Tolerance can be described as a diminished response to a drug with repeated exposure. It can be quantified electrophysiologically by measuring the degree to which EEG changes seen after acute administration are attenuated with repeated exposure. Power spectral analyses are usually employed to quantify the drug-induced changes in amplitude and/or frequency seen after chronic administration. The specific changes in EEG power are then used to assess tolerance to the particular drug and also to assess cross-tolerance to other compounds. An example of an electrophysiological measure of tolerance is the finding that daily administration of marihuana (1 g/d) for 21 d results in a gradual elimination of the increases in alpha activity normally seen after acute administration (Dornbush et al., 1972).

Dependence is characterized by the presence of withdrawal symptoms following termination of a drug after chronic exposure. Traditionally, studies of dependence have involved multiple evaluations of somatic complaints and autonomic signs that, when taken together, constitute a withdrawal syndrome. The use of checklists measuring physical and psychological symptoms can be extremely sensitive and has been shown to provide reproducible results with drug classes with relatively high dependence potential, such as opiates and barbiturates (e.g., Jasinski, 1977; Brady and Lukas, 1984). However, with other drugs such as marihuana, tobacco and caffeine, measures of somatic complaints and autonomic signs are less intense and might be confused with other behavioral states such as anxiety. It is with these drugs that EEG measures are most valuable in providing useful information on dependence and withdrawal. For example, quantitative EEG measures havc been used to provide electrophysiological correlates of withdrawal during tobacco abstinence and have shown that that after 10–24 h of smoking deprivation, spontaneous alpha activity shifts to a slower predominant frequency and theta and alpha power increase (Ulett and Itil, 1969; Knott and Venables, 1977; Herning et al., 1983). The increases in theta power during withdrawal are consistent with reports of fatigue and drowsiness during tobacco abstinence (Williams, 1979). Readministration of tobacco results in an immediate restoration of alpha frequency to control levels, thus validating the utility of electrophysiological measures as correlates of nicotine dependence.

Electrophysiological measures of both tolerance and dependence can be combined with physiological (e.g., heart rate, skin temperature), behavioral (e.g., subjective reports of intoxication) and cognitive (e.g., attention, reaction time) measures to obtain a more comprehensive assessment of a particular drug's profile. An important advantage of EEG measures is that both tolerance and dependence can be expressed as a percent change in the amount of energy contained in the EEG, thus providing a quantitative method for studying the onset and time course the central nervous system changes.

Correlates of Vulnerabilities to Drug Abuse

Electrophysiological measures are also useful in identifying differences in genetic vulnerabilities or predispositions to developing drug or alcohol abuse problems. Most of this research has been conducted in the area of genetic predisposition to alcoholism and of all the drug classes, only alcohol has been studied systematically enough to permit claims that genetic components influence risk for development of alcohol-related problems (Cadoret and Gath, 1978; Cadoret et al., 1979; Cloninger et al., 1981; Hrubec and Omenn, 1981).

Specifically, the use of electrophysiological techniques has helped identify differences in responses to alcohol in individuals with a family history of alcoholism (FHP) compared to individuals without such a history (FHN). For instance, FHP individuals experience significantly larger increases in alpha power and greater slowing of alpha frequency following the same acute dose of ethanol than FHN individuals, despite similarities in plasma ethanol levels, prior ethanol consumption and current drinking practices (Pollock et al., 1983). This example demonstrates the usefulness of electrophysiological measures as sensitive indicators of neurophysiological function determined at the genetic level and also suggests that EEG measures might be used to discriminate subjects at risk for alcoholism from subjects without such a risk. A more detailed illustration of the utility of electrophysiological techniques in identifying predispositions for alcohol abuse is presented in the ERP section.

Event-Related Potentials

Event-related potentials (ERPs) are a series of positive and negative voltage deflections in the ongoing EEG that are time-locked to sensory, motor, or cognitive events (Hillyard and Picton, 1987). These electrical potentials represent the summation of electrical activity of large numbers of neuronal elements acting in synchrony during information processing (Kutas and Hillyard, 1980; Wood and Allison, 1981). The technique of measuring ERPs involves recording the electrical response of the brain immediately following the presentation of a physical stimulus such as a light flash, a tone, or a mild electric shock. A high speed digital computer is used together with signal averaging techniques to extract the time-locked activity elicited in response to the stimulus and to cancel out the signal produced by the random background EEG "noise." Extracting the ERP "signal" from the background EEG "noise" results in a characteristic, highly reproducible waveform that lasts between 10 and 2000 ms after stimulus onset depending on the experimental paradigm.

ERPs recorded from the scalp have waveforms that can be divided into positive and negative components which occur at a specific time after stimulus onset. The short latency components (<90 ms) are sensitive to variations in the physical parameters of the stimulus and show little change as a function of processing demands or

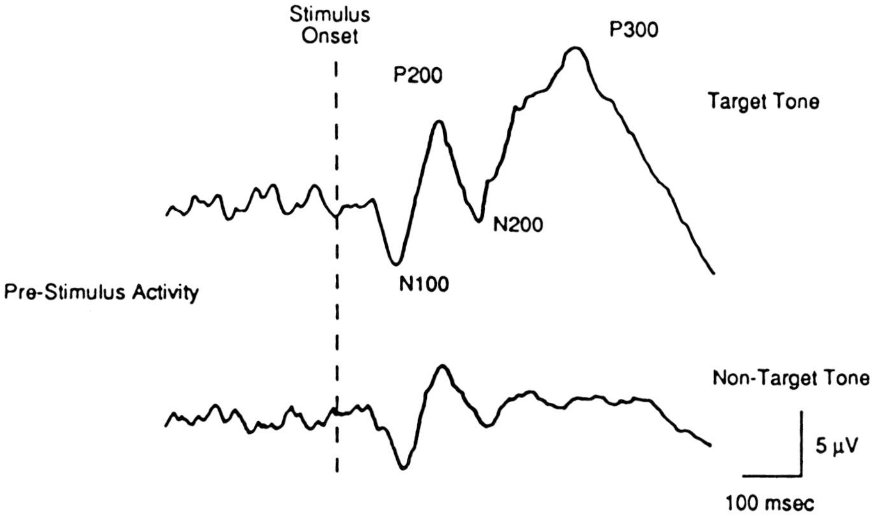

Fig. 8. Sample auditory event-related potential in response to a target (1000 Hz) and nontarget (400 Hz) tone. The P300 wave is clearly seen only after presentation of the target tone.

the psychological state of the subject. These short-latency components are often referred to as "exogenous" because their topography is governed by events outside the subject's control (Donchin et al., 1978). By contrast, the majority of the longer-latency components (occurring after 90 ms) are very sensitive to changes in the state of the subject, the relevance and meaning of the stimulus, and the information demands of the task. These longer-latency components are usually referred to as "endogenous" and are useful indices of the physiological bases of perception and cognition (Hillyard et al., 1978).

One of the most commonly used ERPs in the study of the effects of drugs of abuse on cognitive processing is the P300 (Fig. 8). The P300 is a positive ERP component peaking at about 250–500 ms after stimulus onset, with maximal amplitudes at parietal and central midline electrode sites (Sutton, 1965; Pritchard, 1981; Karniski and Blair, 1989). The P300 is normally elicited after the presentation of a novel or unexpected event to which a subject is told to attend (Johnson and Donchin, 1978; Donchin, 1981). Almost any element of surprise within an experimental setting elicits a P300, independent of the modality of thc eliciting stimulus (Simson et al., 1977; Snyder et al., 1980).

The applications of the P300 ERP component to experimental and clinical studies typically involve the "oddball" paradigm. In this paradigm, the subject is presented with two stimuli that differ from one another on some dimension such as intensity or frequency. One of the stimuli has a low probability of occurring (e.g., 20%) and is presented against a background of a high-probability stimulus (e.g., 80%) to which the subject has been instructed to ignore. The subject is required to discriminate between the low-probability target and the high-probability stimulus by either counting or pressing a button whenever the rare stimuli are encountered (Picton et al., 1974; Duncan-Johnson and Donchin, 1977; Snyder et al., 1980; Polich, 1989). The oddball

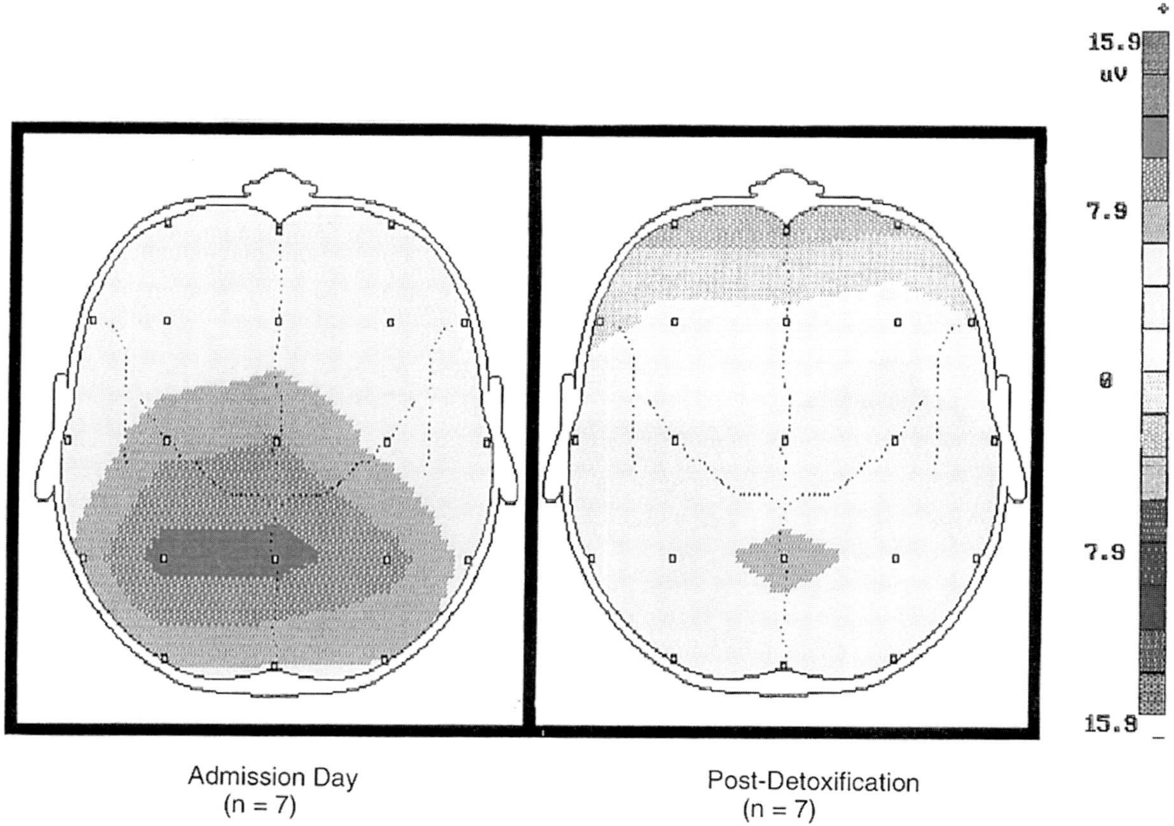

Fig. 9. Topographic map of the P300 event-related potential in a group of cocaine- and heroin-dependent subjects on admission (intoxicated state) and following a 12-d detoxification period. The P300 was generated with an auditory oddball task involving frequency discriminations between a target (1000 Hz) and a non-target (400 Hz) tone at 60 dB sound pressure level. (*See* color plate 2 appearing after p. 6.)

task can be used with auditory (e.g., beeps of different frequencies), visual (e.g., light flashes of different intensities) and somatosensory stimuli (e.g., electrical stimulation of different intensities). The majority of clinical studies have used the auditory modality to generate P300 responses because it is the easiest to reproduce and is less susceptible to eye movement artifact as it can be recorded with eyes closed. However, it is important to note that ERPs generated via the visual modality have been shown to be more sensitive to the effects of family history of alcoholism than ERPs generated via the auditory modality (Polich et al., 1994).

Two parameters are normally used to analyze the P300 event-related potential: amplitude and latency. The amplitude refers to how much energy is being generated and P300 amplitude is indicative of the amount of mental resources allocated to process relevant stimulus, with decreases in P300 amplitude reflecting impairments in the subject's ability to devote cognitive resources to the task (Donchin and Israel, 1980; Donchin, 1981; Polich et al., 1983, 1987). The latency of the P300, on the other hand, refers to how long it takes for the P300 to be generated after the stimulus is presented. P300 latency is an index of the time required for stimulus evaluation and categorization, with longer P300 latencies reflecting increased time needed to process the stimulus (Donchin, 1979; McCarthy and Donchin, 1981; Magliero et al., 1984; Johnson and Donchin, 1985).

Utility of Event-Related Potentials in Substance Abuse Research

The non-invasive and objective quality of ERPs makes this electrophysiological technique a promising method for investigating drug-induced changes in cognitive function. Because ERPs are sensitive to both biological and psychological manipulations, and they permit a simultaneous observation of electrophysiology and cognition, they can provide useful information about the neurophysiological basis of altered states of consciousness (Roth, 1977; Shagass, 1980). Furthermore, because ERP latency and amplitude represent different aspects of cognitive processing and because psychoactive drugs can affect ERP amplitude and latency differentially, drug-induced ERP changes can provide considerable information on the nature and time course of a drug's effects on cognition. Increased recognition of the potential of ERP measures as indices of subtle functional brain deficits associated with drugs of abuse is evidenced by the growing number of laboratories that have incorporated ERP measures into protocols investigating the effects of drugs of abuse on the CNS.

Measures of Acute Drug Effects

One of the most common applications of event-related potentials in substance abuse research is to study the acute effects of psychoactive drugs on information processing capabilities. ERPs have been used to investigate the acute effects of drugs in almost every class (e.g., Roth et al., 1977; Herning et al., 1979; Porjesz and Begleiter, 1981; Velasco et al., 1984; Lukas et al., 1985; Herning et al., 1987; Lukas et al., 1990) and analyses of the specific drug-induced ERP changes are very useful in that they provide information on the vulnerability of various aspects of cognitive function to specific drug effects. Since ERP measures can sometimes be more sensitive than conventional behavioral or neuropsychological measures (Ciesielski et al., 1985;

Herning et al., 1990), they can provide additional information on subtle cognitive impairments during acute intoxication that may not be severe enough to be identified by these other measures. Also, repeated ERP testing after drug administration can provide important information on the duration of the drug's effects on cognition. For instance, we have found that acute administration of cocaine (0.9 mg/kg) results in a significant reduction in P300 amplitude as early as 10 min post-cocaine administration. These impairments persist for about 40 min and are still present when most of the subjects no longer report feeling intoxicated. This example illustrates the utility of ERPs when studying the acute effects of drugs of abuse and highlights the importance of combining electrophysiological measures with behavioral and subjective tests.

Measures of Tolerance and Dependence

Because ERPs are sensitive indices of the functional integrity of the brain (Hillyard et al., 1978; Donchin, 1979), they are also useful measures of tolerance and dependence. In addition, investigating the ERP changes associated with tolerance and dependence can be important in understanding the neuronal mechanisms underlying the development and behavioral display of these phenomena. For instance, ERP measures can be useful in determining the degree of tolerance to a drug's effects on cognition. An example of this is the finding that intoxicated heroin- and cocaine-dependent individuals display P300 responses similar to those of nondependent matched controls (Kouri et al., 1996), suggesting that neurophysiological adaptation to the drugs has occurred. When these individuals are detoxified, however, their dependence is manifested by significant reductions in P300 amplitude, in spite of normal responses on the Digit Span test of the Weschler Memory Scale and minimal physiological and subjective complaints of withdrawal (Kouri et al., 1996) (Fig. 9). This example demonstrates that ERP measures may be more sensitive to subtle changes in functional aspects of CNS that are not detected using other measures.

Correlates of Vulnerabilities to Drug Abuse

Because many of the illnesses believed to have genetic components are characterized by some type of abnormal brain function, it has been postulated that abnormalities in latency, amplitude or topography of ERP components could serve as markers of genetic vulnerabilities. To date, most of the data supporting this notion in substance abuse is in the area of alcoholism. The P300 is a good candidate as a biological marker because there is ample evidence to indicate that its generation is genetically determined (Begleiter et al., 1998) and a number of studies have found that young children with a family history of alcoholism have significantly reduced P300 amplitudes before ever being exposed to alcohol compared with children without such a history (Begleiter et al., 1984, 1987; Porjesz and Begleiter, 1990). In addition, findings of reduced P300 amplitudes in chronic (Porjesz et al., 1980) and recovering (Porjesz et al., 1987) alcoholics further support the notion that that P300 amplitude is a phenotypic marker for predisposition to developing alcoholism (Polich et al., 1994; Porjesz et al., 1998). The usefulness of the P300 as a biological marker of genetic predispositions is not only important for identifying individuals at risk before the onset of the disease but can also provide crucial information on the etiology of the illness. To date, data supporting the role of the P300 as a marker for vulnerabilities to other substance abuse problems is not yet conclusive, however, because of the implication of P300 impairments in a number of other psychiatric disorders (e.g., Roth et al., 1980; Pfefferbaum et al., 1984; Diner et al., 1985; Kutcher et al., 1987) it remains an excellent candidate for a biological marker of genetic vulnerabilities.

Caveats in Interpreting Electrophysiologic Data in Substance Abuse Research

The usefulness of any measure of neurophysiologic activity depends on the reliability, validity, and specificity of the test procedure. The issue of reliability is related to whether the spontaneous changes over time are greater than the observed drug-induced changes. For a method to have clinical value, the variability observed between testing conditions or subjects needs to be smaller than during experimental conditions. Both EEG and ERP measures have good reliability when the testing conditions are kept constant. This is extremely important because several factors including time of day (Geisler and Polich, 1990), season of the year (Polich and Geisler, 1991), recency of food intake (Geisler and Polich, 1990; 1992), and age (Goodin et al., 1978), have been shown to affect certain electrophysiologic parameters. Therefore, even though EEG and ERP measures can provide insight into the effects of drugs of abuse on the brain, their clinical value depends on how well extraneous variability is controlled. One way in which to decrease variability is to use within-subject comparisons whenever possible. In cases when it is not feasible to test the same subject under different conditions or maintain the experimental environment constant between test sessions, it is extremely important to consider the potential influence of confounding variables when interpreting the results and control for these variables statistically.

A second issue that determines the usefulness of electrophysiological measures in substance abuse research is that of external validity. External validity is related to how the impairments observed with a specific method correlate with impairments observed with other measures that test similar neurophysiological or cognitive functions. Even though both EEG and ERPs have good external validity, the clinical utility of the findings obtained with these methods is always enhanced when combined with other measures. Therefore, incorporating the use of measures like neuropsychological tests, physiological recordings and behavioral responses is strongly recommended.

Perhaps the most important aspect regarding the usefulness of EEG and ERP measures in substance abuse research is the issue of specificity. Namely, whether the electrophysiological changes observed are unique to the specific drug or condition tested. Most of the data available to date suggests that EEG and ERP measures have limited diagnostic specificity. For instance, acute administration of either ethanol, cocaine or marihuana all result in significant increases in alpha activity (Lukas et al., 1986, 1990, 1991, 1995), these increases are not only indistinguishable from each other but are also similar to those observed during transcendental meditation (Lindsley, 1952; Brown, 1970; Wallace, 1970). Given the association between alpha activity and pleasurable states, these findings suggest that the drug-induced increases in alpha activity represent a neurophysiologic response associated with reinforcement in general. Even though electrophysiological measures are not always specific enough to discriminate drug effects, this finding has allowed for subtle similarities among drugs of different classes to be identified.

Similarly, even though the reductions in P300 amplitude observed during withdrawal from either heroin, cocaine or ethanol (Porjesz et al., 1987; Kouri et al., 1996; Bauer, 1997; Noldy and Carlen, 1997) are very similar to those observed in a number of psychiatric disorders including dementia (Pfefferbaum et al., 1984) schizophrenia (Roth et al., 1980), depression (Diner et al., 1985) and borderline personality disorder (Kutcher et al., 1987), this lack of diagnostic specificity of the P300 has provided important information on the similarities between acute withdrawal from drugs of abuse and these other psychiatric disorders.

In summary, EEG and ERP measures have high reliability and validity when the experimental conditions (e.g., task demands, patient samples, recording techniques) are kept constant. Even though the diagnostic specificity of these measures is limited, when the findings are interpreted in the context of the specific drug-induced behavioral states being investigated, they can provide important information on the neurophysiological similarities between these and other psychiatric states.

Future Directions

Technological advances together with an integrated approach to brain imaging combining technologies such as EEG, ERP, MRI, fMRI, and PET will dramatically increase the applications of electrophysiological techniques and provide a more comprehensive assessment of the effects of drugs of abuse on brain function. This will prove to be particularly important because the advent of electrode caps, commercially available EEG imaging systems, and mapping software has already increased the availability of electrophysiological techniques to many more research laboratories, especially those not affiliated with neurology departments. However, it is important to note that such ease of computer-assisted recording and analysis of complex EEG waveforms is no substitute for trained personnel in electrophysiology, as paper recording parameters, artifact detection removal and proper analysis must be done or the data will have little relevance to neurophysiological processes. In the hands of trained researchers, however, EEG techniques can be added to enhance existing research and treatment programs. This will provide a new dimension upon which new vistas in vulnerability to drug abuse, measures of tolerance and dependence, and neurobiological correlates of drug craving and drug-induced euphoria can be assessed with greater confidence.

Acknowledgments

This work was supported by grants DA03994 and K05DA00343 from the National Institute on Drug Abuse.

References

Adrian, E. D. and Matthews, B. H. C., The Berger rhythm: potential changes from the occipital lobes in man. Brain 57:355–385, 1934.

Bauer, L. O., Frontal P300 decrements, childhood conduct disorder, family history, and the prediction of relapse among abstinent cocaine abusers. Drug Alcohol Depend. 44:1–10, 1997.

Begleiter, H., Porjesz, B., Bihari, B. and Kissin, B., Event-related brain potentials in boys at risk for alcoholism. Science 225:1493–1496, 1984.

Begleiter, H., Porjesz, B., Rawlings, R. and Eckardt, M., Auditory recovery function and P3 in boys at high risk for alcoholism. Alcohol 4:315–321, 1987.

Begleiter, H., Porjesz, B., Reich, T., Edenberg, H. J., Goate, A., Blangero, J., Almasy, L., Foroud, T., Van Eerdewegh, P., Polich, J., Rohrbaugh, J., Kuperman, S., Bauer, L. O., O'Connor, S. J., Chorlian, D. B., Li, T. K., Conneally, P. M., Hesselbrock, V., Rice, J. P., Schuckit, M. A., Cloninger, R., Nurnberger, J., Jr., Crowe, R. and Bloom, F. E., Quantitative trait loci analysis of human event-related brain potentials: P3 voltage. Electroencephalogr. Clin. Neurophysiol. 108:244–250, 1998.

Berger, H., Über das Elektrenkephalogramm des Menschen. Arch. Psychiatr. Nervenkr. 87:527–570, 1929.

Brady, J. V. and Lukas, S. E., Testing drugs for physical dependence potential and abuse liability, NIDA Res. Monogr. 52: DHHS Publication No. (ADM) 84-1332, 1984.

Brown, B. B., Recognition of aspects of consciousness through association with EEG alpha activity represented by a light signal. Psychophysiology 6:442–452, 1970.

Cadoret, R. and Gath, A., Inheritance of alcoholism in adoptees. Br. J. Psychiatry 132:252–258, 1978.

Cadoret, R. J., Cain, C. A. and Grove, W. M., Development of alcoholism in adoptees raised apart from alcoholic biological relatives. Arch. Gen. Psychiatry 37:561–563, 1980.

Ciesielski, K. T., Madden, J. S., Bligh, J. G. and Schopflocher, D., Long-term brain impairment in chronic alcoholics: N2-P3 cognitive potentials in a template-matching memory task. Alcohol Alcohol. 20:403–408, 1985.

Cloninger, C. R., Bohman, M. and Sigvardsson, S., Inheritance of alcohol abuse: cross-fostering analysis of adopted men. Arch. Gen. Psychiatry 38:861–868, 1981.

Cooley, J. W. and Tukey, J., An algorithm for the machine calculation of complex Fourier series. Math. Computat. 19:297–301, 1965.

Diner, B. C., Holcomb, P. J. and Dykman, R. A., P300 in major depressive disorder. Psychiatry Res. 15:175–184, 1985.

Donchin, E., Event-related potentials: a tool in the study of human information processing. In: Begleiter, H. (ed.) Evoked Brain Potentials and Behavior. New York, Plenum Press, 1979.

Donchin, E., Presidential address, 1980. Surprise!... Surprise? Psychophysiology 18:493–513, 1981.

Donchin, E. and Isreal, J. B., Event related potentials and psychological theory. Prog. Brain Res. 54:697–715, 1980.

Donchin, E., Ritter, W. and McCallum, W. C., Cognitive psychophysiology: the endogenous components of the ERP. In: Callaway, E., Tueting, P. and Koslow, S.H. (eds.) Event Related Potentials in Man. New York, Academic Press, 1978.

Dornbush, R., Clare, G., Zaks, A., Crown, P., Volavka, J. and Fink, M., Twenty-one-day administration of marijuana in male volunteers. In: Lewis, M. F. (ed.) Current Research in Marijuana. New York, Academic Press, pp. 115–128, 1972.

Duffy, F. H., Topographic Mapping of Brain Electrical Activity. Boston, Butterworths, 1986.

Duffy, F. H., Burchfiel, J. L. and Lombroso, C. T., Brain electrical activity mapping (BEAM): a method for extending the clinical utility of EEG and evoked potential data. Ann. Neurol. 5:309–321, 1979.

Duffy, F. H., Iyer, V. G. and Surwillo, W. W., Clinical Electroencephalography and Topographic Mapping. New York, Springer-Verlag, 1989.

Duncan-Johnson, C. C. and Donchin, E., On quantifying surprise: the variation of event-related potentials with subjective probability. Psychophysiology 14:456–467, 1977.

Fink, M., EEG and human psychopharmacology. Annu. Rev. Pharmacol. 9:241–258, 1969.

Fink, M., Shapiro, D. M. and Itil, T. M., EEG profiles of fenfluramine, amobarbital and dextroamphetamine in normal volunteers. Psychopharmacologia 22:369–383, 1971.

Geisler, M. W. and Polich, J., P300 and time of day: circadian rhythms, food intake, and body temperature. Biol. Psychol. 31:117–136, 1990.

Geisler, M. W. and Polich, J., P300, food consumption, and memory performance. Psychophysiology 29:76–85, 1992.

Goldstein, L. and Beck, R. A., Amplitude analysis of the electroencephalogram. Review of the information obtained with the integrative method. Int. Rev. Neurobiol. 8:265–312, 1965.

Goodin, D. S., Squires, K. C., Henderson, B. H. and Starr, A., Age-related variations in evoked potentials to auditory stimuli in normal human subjects. Electroencephalogr. Clin. Neurophysiol. 44:447–458, 1978.

Herning, R. I., Jones, R. T. and Peltzman, D. J., Changes in human event related potentials with prolonged D-9-tetrahydrocannabinol (THC) use. Electroencephalogr. Clin. Neurophysiol. 47:556–570, 1979.

Herning, R. I., Jones, R. T. and Bachman, J., EEG changes during tobacco withdrawal. Psychophysiology 20:507–512, 1983.

Herning, R. I., Hooker, W. D. and Jones, R. T., Cocaine effects on electroencephalographic cognitive event-related potentials and performance. Electroencephalogr. Clin. Neurophysiol. 66:34–42, 1987.

Herning, R. I., Glover, B. J., Koeppl, B., Weddington, W. and Jaffe, J. H., Cognitive deficits in abstaining cocaine abusers. NIDA Res. Monogr. 101:167–178, 1990.

Hillyard, S. A. and Picton, T. W., Electrophysiology of cognition. Handbook of Physiology. Section 1: The Nervous System. Part 2., American Physiology Society, pp. 519–584, 1987.

Hillyard, S. A., Picton, T. W. and Regan, D. M., Sensation, perception and attention: analysis using ERPs. In: Callaway, E., Tueting, P. and Koslow, S.H. (eds.) Event-Related Brain Potentials in Man. New York, Academic Press, 1978.

Hrubec, Z. and Omenn, G. S., Evidence of genetic predisposition to alcoholic cirrhosis and psychosis: twin concordances for alcoholism and its biological end points by zygosity among male veterans. Alcohol. Clin. Exp. Res. 5:207–215, 1981.

Jasinski, D. R., Assessment of the abuse potentiality of morphine like drugs (methods used in man). Hand. Exp. Pharmacol. 45:197–258, 1977.

Jasper, H. H., The ten-twenty electrode system of the International Federation. Electroenceph. Clin. Neurophysiol. 10:371–373, 1958.

Johnson, R., Jr., A triarchic model of P300 amplitude. Psychophysiology 23:367–384, 1986.

Johnson, R., Jr. and Donchin, E., On how P300 amplitude varies with the utility of the eliciting stimuli. Electroencephalogr. Clin. Neurophysiol. 44:424–437, 1978.

Johnson, R., Jr. and Donchin, E., Second thoughts: multiple P300s elicited by a single stimulus. Psychophysiology 22:182–194, 1985.

Karniski, W. and Blair, R. C., Topographical and temporal stability of the P300. Electroencephalogr. Clin. Neurophysiol. 72:373–383, 1989.

Khazan, K., Weeks, J. R. and Schroeder, L. A., Electroencephalographic, electromyographic and behavioral correlates during a cycle of self-maintained morphine addiction in the rat. J. Pharmacol. Exp. Ther. 155:521–531, 1967.

Knott, V. J. and Venables, P. H., EEG alpha correlates of non-smokers, smokers, smoking, and smoking deprivation. Psychophysiology 14:150–156, 1977.

Koukkou, M. and Lehmann, D., Human EEG spectra before and during cannabis hallucinations. Biol. Psychiatry 11:663–677, 1976.

Kouri, E. M., Lukas, S. E. and Mendelson, J. H., P300 assessment of opiate and cocaine users: effects of detoxification and buprenorphine treatment. Biol. Psychiatry 40:617–628, 1996.

Kutas, M. and Hillyard, S. A., Reading senseless sentences: brain potentials reflect semantic incongruity. Science 207:203–205, 1980.

Kutcher, S. P., Blackwood, D. H., St Clair, D., Gaskell, D. F. and Muir, W. J., Auditory P300 in borderline personality disorder and schizophrenia. Arch. Gen. Psychiatry 44:645–650, 1987.

Lindsley, D. B., Psychological phenomena and the electroencephalogram. Electroencephalogr. Clin. Neurophysiol. 4:443–456, 1952.

Longo, V. G., Behavioral and electroencephalographic effects of atropine and related compounds. Pharmacol. Rev. 18:965–996, 1966.

Lukas, S. E., Topographic brain mapping during cocaine-induced intoxication and self-administration. In: Racgani, G., Brunello, N. and Fukuda, T. (eds.) Biological Psychiatry vol. 2. New York, Excerpta Medica, pp. 25–29, 1991.

Lukas, S. E., Advanced electrophysiological imaging techniques for studying drug effects. In: London, E. D. (ed.) Imaging Drug Action in the Brain. Boca Raton, FL, CRC Press, pp. 389–404, 1993.

Lukas, S. E. and Jasinski, D. R., EEG power spectral effects of intravenous nicotine administration in humans. Fed. Proc. 42:1018, 1983.

Lukas, S. E. and Mendelson, J. H., Electroencephalographic activity and plasma ACTH during ethanol-induced euphoria. Biol. Psychiatry 23:141–148, 1988.

Lukas, S. E., Moreton, J. E. and Khazan, N., Comparative study of the electroencephalographic and behavioral effects of l-a-acetylmethadol (LAAM), two of its metabolites and morphine and methadone in the rat. J. Pharmacol. Exp. Ther. 215:382–389, 1980.

Lukas, S. E., Mendelson, J. H., Benedikt, R. A. and Jones, B., Marihuana-induced changes in EEG and P300 evoked responses in male volunteers. Pharmacologist 27:235, 1985.

Lukas, S. E., Mendelson, J. H., Benedikt, R. A. and Jones, B., EEG alpha activity increases during transient episodes of ethanol-induced euphoria. Pharmacol. Biochem. Behav. 25:889–895, 1986.

Lukas, S. E., Mendelson, J. H., Woods, B. T., Mello, N. K. and Teoh, S. K., Topographic distribution of EEG alpha activity during ethanol-induced intoxication in women. J. Stud. Alcohol 50:176–185, 1989.

Lukas, S. E., Mendelson, J. H., Kouri, E., Bolduc, M. and Amass, L., Ethanol-induced alterations in EEG alpha activity and apparent source of the auditory P300 evoked response potential. Alcohol 7:471–477, 1990.

Lukas, S. E., Mendelson, J. H. and Benedikt, R., Electroencephalographic correlates of marihuana-induced euphoria. Drug Alcohol Depend. 37:131–140, 1995.

Magliero, A., Bashore, T. R., Coles, M. G. and Donchin, E., On the dependence of P300 latency on stimulus evaluation processes. Psychophysiology 21:171–186, 1984.

Martin, W. R. and Kay, D. C., Effects of opioid analgesics and antagonists on the EEG. Int. Handb. EEG Clin. Neurophysiol., 7 Part C: 97–109, 1977.

McCarthy, G. and Donchin, E., A metric for thought: a comparison of P300 latency and reaction time. Science 211:77–80, 1981.

McEachern, J., Friedman, L., Bird, M., Lukas, S. E., Orzack, M. H., Katz, D. L., Dessain, E. C., Beake, B. and Cole, J. O., Self-report vs. instrumental measure in the assessment of the subjective effects of *d*-amphetamine. Psychopharmacol. Bull. 24:463–465, 1988.

Noldy, N. E. and Carlen, P. L., Event-related potential changes in cocaine withdrawal: evidence for long-term cognitive effects. Neuropsychobiology 36:53–56, 1997.

Pfefferbaum, A., Wenegrat, B. G., Ford, J. M., Roth, W. T. and Kopell, B. S., Clinical application of the P3 component of event-related potentials. II. Dementia, depression and schizophrenia. Electroencephalogr. Clin. Neurophysiol. 59:104–124, 1984.

Picton, T. W., Hillyard, S. A., Krausz, H. I. and Galambos, R., Human auditory evoked potentials. I. Evaluation of components. Electroencephalogr. Clin. Neurophysiol. 36:179–190, 1974.
Polich, J., Task difficulty, probability, and inter-stimulus interval as determinants of P300 from auditory stimuli. Electroencephalogr. Clin. Neurophysiol. 68:311–320, 1987.
Polich, J., Frequency, intensity, and duration as determinants of P300 from auditory stimuli. J. Clin. Neurophysiol. 6:277–286, 1989.
Polich, J. and Geisler, M. W., P300 seasonal variation. Biol. Psychol. 32:173–179, 1991.
Polich, J., Howard, L. and Starr, A., P300 latency correlates with digit span. Psychophysiology 20:665–669, 1983.
Polich, J., Pollock, V. E. and Bloom, F. E., Meta-analysis of P300 amplitude from males at risk for alcoholism. Psychol. Bull. 115:55–73, 1994.
Pollock, V. E., Volavka, J., Goodwin, D. W., Mednick, S. A., Gabrielli, W. F., Knop, J. and Schulsinger, F., The EEG after alcohol administration in men at risk for alcoholism. Arch. Gen. Psychiatry 40:857–861, 1983.
Porjesz, B. and Begleiter, H., Human evoked brain potentials and alcohol. Alcohol. Clin. Exp. Res. 5:304–317, 1981.
Porjesz, B. and Begleiter, H., Human brain electrophysiology and alcoholism. In: Tarter, R.E. and Van Thiel, D.G. (eds.) Alcohol and the Brain: Chronic Effects. New York, Plenum Press, pp. 603–623, 1985.
Porjesz, B. and Begleiter, H., Event-related potentials in individuals at risk for alcoholism. Alcohol 7:465–469, 1990.
Porjesz, B., Begleiter, H. and Samuelly, I., Cognitive deficits in chronic alcoholics and elderly subjects assessed by evoked brain potentials. Acta Psychiatr. Scand. 62:15–29, 1980.
Porjesz, B., Begleiter, H., Bihari, B. and Kissin, B., Event-related brain potentials to high incentive stimuli in abstinent alcoholics. Alcohol 4:283–287, 1987.
Porjesz, B., Begleiter, H., Reich, T., Van Eerdewegh, P., Edenberg, H. J., Foroud, T., Goate, A., Litke, A., Chorlian, D. B., Stimus, A., Rice, J., Blangero, J., Almasy, L., Sorbell, J., Bauer, L. O., Kuperman, S., O'Connor, S. J. and Rohrbaugh, J., Amplitude of visual P3 event-related potential as a phenotypic marker for a predisposition to alcoholism: preliminary results from the COGA Project. Collaborative Study on the Genetics of Alcoholism. Alcohol. Clin. Exp. Res. 22:1317–1323, 1998.
Pritchard, W. S., Psychophysiology of P300. Psychol. Bull. 89:506–540, 1981.
Pscheidt, G. R., Steiner, W. G. and Himwich, H. E., An electroencephalographic and chemical re-evaluation of the central action of reserpine in the rabbit. J. Pharmacol. Exp. Ther. 144:37–44, 1963.
Requin, S., Lanoir, J., Plas, R. and Naquet, R., Etude comparatrive des effets neurophysiologiques du Librium et du Valium. Cl. Soc. Biol. (Paris). 157:2015–2019, 1963.
Roth, W. T., Late event-related potentials and psychopathology. Schizophrenia Bull. 3:105–120, 1977.
Roth, W. T., Tinklenberg, J. R. and Kopell, B. S., Ethanol and marihuana effects on event-related potentials in a memory retrieval paradigm. Electroencephalogr. Clin. Neurophysiol. 42:381–388, 1977.
Roth, W. T., Horvath, T. B., Pfefferbaum, A. and Kopell, B. S., Event-related potentials in schizophrenics. Electroencephalogr. Clin. Neurophysiol. 48:127–139, 1980.
Shagass, C., Brain potential studies of psychopathology. Compr. Psychiatry 21:483–491, 1980.
Simson, R., Vaughan, H. G., Jr. and Ritter, W., The scalp topography of potentials in auditory and visual Go/NoGo tasks. Electroencephalogr. Clin. Neurophysiol. 43:864–875, 1977.
Snyder, E., Hillyard, S. A. and Galambos, R., Similarities and differences among the P3 waves to detected signals in three modalities. Psychophysiology 17:112–122, 1980.
Struve, F. A., Straumanis, J. J. and Patrick, G., Persistent topographic quantitative EEG sequelae of chronic marihuana use: a replication study and initial discriminant function analysis. Clin. Electroencephalogr. 25:63–75, 1994.

Struve, F. A., Patrick, G., Straumanis, J. J., Fitz-Gerald, M. J. and Manno, J., Possible EEG sequelae of very long duration marihuana use: pilot findings from topographic quantitative EEG analyses of subjects with 15 to 24 years of cumulative daily exposure to THC. Clin. Electroencephalogr. 29:31–36, 1998.

Sutton, S., Braren, M., Zubin, J. and John, E. R., Evoked-potential correlates of stimulus uncertainty. Science 150:1187–1188, 1965.

Ulett, J. A. and Itil, T. M., Quantitative electroencephalogram in smoking and smoking deprivation. Science 164:969–970, 1969.

Vastola, E. F. and Rosen, S., Supression by anticonvulsants of focal electrical seizures in the neocortex. Electroencephalogr. Clin. Neurophysiol. 12:327–332, 1960.

Velasco, M., Velasco, F., Castaneda, R. and Lee, M., Effect of fentanyl and naloxone on the P300 auditory potential. Neuropharmacology 23:931–938, 1984.

Volavka, J., Crown, P., Dornbush, R., Feldstein, S. and Fink, M., EEG, heart rate and mood change ("high") after cannabis. Psychopharmacologia 32:11–25, 1973.

Wallace, R. K., Physiological effects of transcendental meditation. Science 167:1751–1754, 1970.

Walter, D. L., Spectral analysis for electroencephalogram: mathematical determination of neurophysiological relationships from records of limited duration. Exp. Neurol. 8:155–181, 1963.

Williams, D. G., Different cigarette-smoker classification factors and subjective state in acute abstinence. Psychopharmacology (Berl.) 64:231–235, 1979.

Winters, W. D., The coninuum of CNS excitatory states and hallucinosis. In: Siegel, R. K. and West, L. J. (eds.) Hallucinations: Behavior, Experience and Theory. New York, Wiley, pp. 53–75, 1975.

Wood, C. C. and Allison, T., Evaluation of evoked potentials: A neurophysiological perspective. Can. J. Psychol. 35:113–135, 1981.

Ziskind, D. H., Sjaardema, H. and Bercel, N., Minimal electroencephalographic response to Metrazol as a method for measuring convulsive threshold for use in human beings. Science 104:462–463, 1946.

Chapter 2

Positron Emission Tomography and Single-Photon Emission Computed Tomography

Methods and Applications in Substance Abuse Research

Robert T. Malison, MD

INTRODUCTION

Advances in noninvasive neuroimaging methods have created unprecedented inroads into the study of central nervous system (CNS) function in vivo. In particular, positron emission tomography (PET) and single-photon emission computed tomography (SPECT) offer numerous opportunities to advance the field of substance abuse research. Clinical cousins to more basic science techniques (e.g., homogenate receptor binding, in vitro autoradiography, and radioimmunoassay), PET and SPECT permit measurements of local neuronal activity, neurochemistry, and pharmacology in the living human brain. The power of such methods, however, comes at the cost of considerable technological complexities that may hinder their appropriate application and interpretation. This chapter summarizes underlying principles, basic limitations, and varied applications of PET and SPECT as they apply to the field of substance abuse research.

From: *Brain Imaging in Substance Abuse: Research, Clinical, and Forensic Applications*
M. J. Kaufman, ed. © Humana Press Inc., Totowa, New Jersey

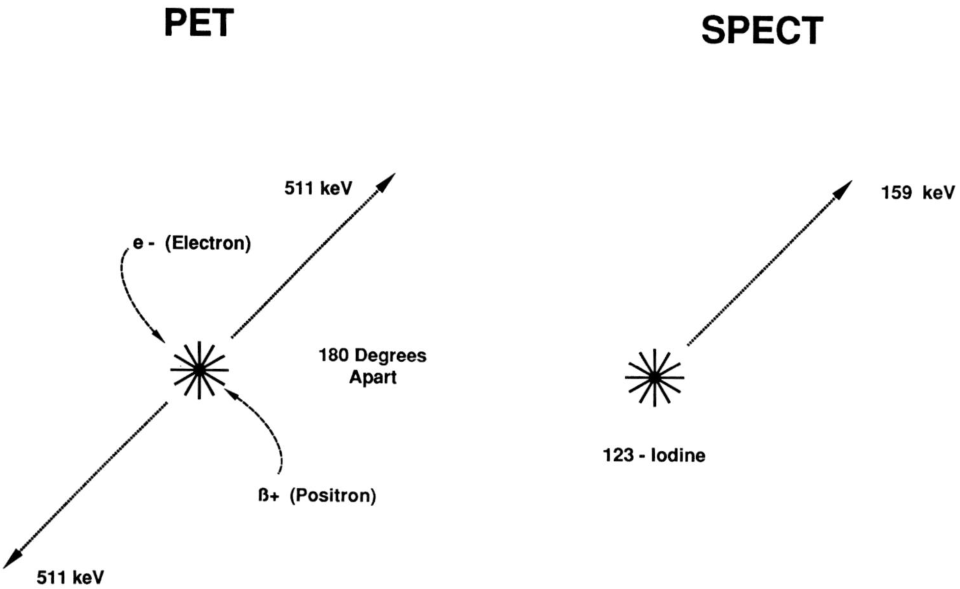

Fig. 1. (Left) In PET, radionuclidic decay produces a positively charged electron called a positron (denoted β+) that travels a finite distance from its site of origin before encountering an electron. The ensuing collision results in annihilation of both particles and the generation of two high-energy photons (i.e., γ-rays) that are emitted in exactly opposite directions. **(Right)** By contrast, SPECT radionuclides give direct rise to a single γ-ray after isotopic decay.

Principles Underlying Positron Emission Tomography and Single-Photon Emission Computed Tomography

PET and SPECT are radiotracer techniques. Specifically, a molecule of biologic interest is radioactively labeled, administered to a patient, and the resulting three-dimensional distribution of radioactivity inferred from the trajectories of escaping high-energy γ-rays. Because radioactive signals arise from within the subject, PET and SPECT are said to be emission techniques (e.g., in contrast to transmission techniques such as an X-ray). Because the resulting images depict the structures of the brain in three dimensions (e.g., in contrast to the planar rendering of spatial features in an X-ray), they are said to be *tomographic*. While PET and SPECT share these core characteristics, differences in their instrumentation and experimental applications arise from differences in their physics of photon generation.

Positron and Single-Photon Generation

Radionuclides, by definition, are intrinsically unstable owing to a net nuclear excess of protons. This quantum imbalance is typically resolved by either of two spontaneous decay schemes: 1) conversion of a nuclear proton into a neutron, which produces a positively charged electron known as a "positron" (i.e., denoted e^+ or β^+), or 2) nuclear capture of an orbiting electron, which results in a metastable daughter nucleus (Hoffman and Phelps, 1986; Sorenson and Phelps, 1987). These outcomes are

Table 1
PET and SPECT Radionuclides, Half-Lives, Energies, and Representative Tracers/Applications

Radionuclide	Decay rate (half-life)	Photon energy	Representative radiotracers	Applications
PET				
^{15}Oxygen	2 min	511 keV	[^{15}O]H_2O	Cerebral blood flow
^{11}Carbon	20 min	511 keV	[^{11}C]cocaine [^{11}C]heroin [^{11}C]raclopride	Neuroreceptor imaging
^{18}Fluorine	2 h	511 keV	[^{18}F]FDG	Cerebral glucose metabolism
SPECT				
^{99m}Technetium	6 h	140 keV	[^{99m}Tc]HMPAO	Cerebral blood flow
^{123}Iodine	13 h	159 keV	[^{123}I]β-CIT [^{123}I]iomazenil [^{123}I]IBZM	Neuroreceptor imaging
^{133}Xenon	5 d	80 keV	[^{133}Xe]	Cerebral blood flow

energetically transient, however, and both result in the release of characteristic high-energy γ-rays. In PET, emitted positrons eventually find their "antimatter" equivalent in an electron, and the ensuing collision produces two very high energy (511 keV) γ-rays of opposite trajectories (i.e., 180° apart) (Fig. 1). In SPECT, metastable daughter nuclei eventually find rest in a more stable ground state, which is accompanied by the release of a single γ-ray of radionuclide-specific energy (typically 80–160 keV) (Fig. 1). A list of the most commonly used positron- and single photon-emitting isotopes is shown in Table 1.

PET and SPECT Cameras

Differences in the design of PET and SPECT cameras derive specifically from their respective patterns of photon emission (i.e., dual vs single photons). Specifically, PET cameras infer the site of an annihilation event from the characteristic "back-to-back" paths and principles of *coincidence detection* of photons (Fig. 2) (Hoffman and Phelps, 1986; Links, 1990). In its simplest conceptual form, a PET camera is a ring of radiation detectors. Each radiation detector comprises two parts: 1) a dense crystalline element (e.g., bismuth germanium oxide, sodium iodide, or cesium fluoride) that captures the invisible, high-energy γ-rays and converts them to visible light, and 2) an adjacent photomultiplier tube that converts this brief flash of light into an electrical pulse. Because opposing detectors are electronically connected, a PET camera infers annihilation along an imaginary line between detectors when "coincident" (to within 3–10 ns) scintillation events are detected in the circuit. While single events are ignored, random coincidences (i.e., coincident scintillations resulting from two different annihilation events) can introduce background noise into PET images (Hoffman et al., 1981). Nonetheless, coincidence detection is overall a very efficient technique and accounts for the exceptional sensitivity of PET.

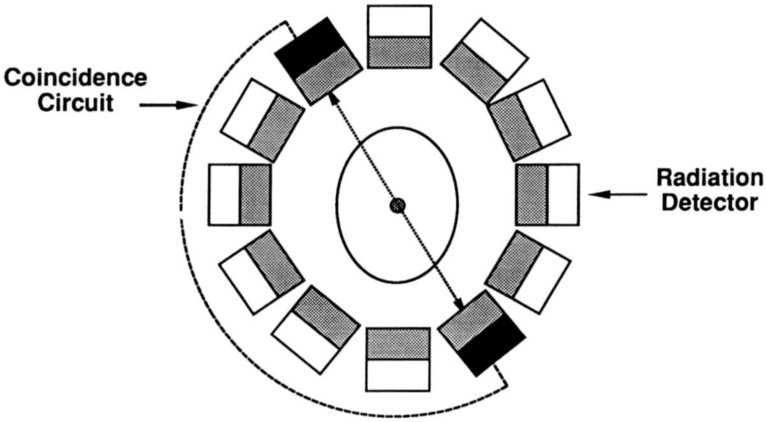

Fig. 2. PET cameras rely upon a series of electronically connected radiation detectors. When two photons reach two different (in this case opposing) detectors simultaneously, producing two coincident scintillations, the camera assumes an annihilation event to have occurred somewhere along the line between the two.

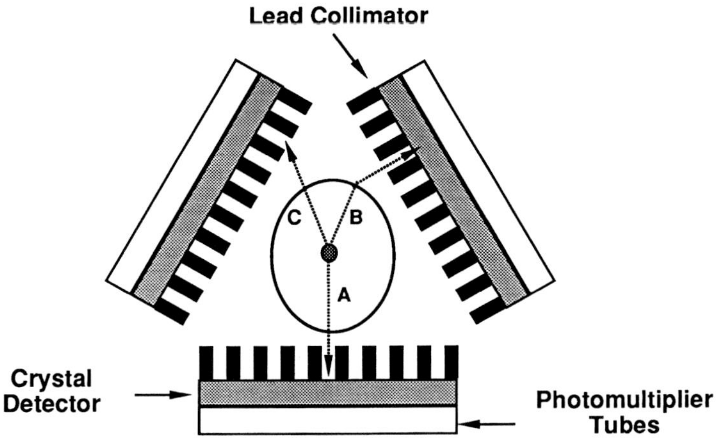

Fig. 3. (A) In SPECT, photon paths are inferred from their ability to pass through the long narrow holes of the instrument's lead collimators. **(B)** In some instances, tissue interactions with photons result in "scatter" and the detection of a photon deviating from its original or true trajectory. This is one source of noise in SPECT images. **(C)** Photons whose trajectories are not parallel to these holes are absorbed by the lead and go undetected.

Instead of coincidence detection, SPECT cameras are based on the technique of *collimation* (Fig. 3) (Jaszczak, 1991), in which a lead block, containing many tiny holes, is interposed between the radiation source and detector. Since the holes in the collimator are sufficiently long and narrow, only photons of essentially parallel trajectory reach the detector. Thus, the linear paths of photons are extrapolated, given knowledge of the orientation of the collimator's holes. Because nonparallel γ-rays are absorbed by the lead and go undetected (Fig. 3), collimation is less efficient than coincidence detection (Budinger, 1980). Nevertheless, advances in collimator design and radiation detection make SPECT sufficiently sensitive for routine use in nearly all of the same applications (Devous, 1989; Jaszczak, 1991).

Computed Tomography

Despite the above-mentioned differences, PET and SPECT rely on the same principles to translate information on individual photon paths into three-dimensional brain images (Parker, 1990). Just as depth perception requires more than a single eye, an inference beyond a photon path to that of the depth of a photon's origin in tissue requires more than a single view. In PET, numerous views or *projections* result from a ring of essentially contiguous radiation detectors (Fig. 2), whereas SPECT cameras more commonly employ several rotating detector "heads" to collect data over an entire 360° (Fig. 3). Once many thousands of photon trajectories have been recorded from multiple vantage points (typically approx 120), a variety of techniques and mathematical algorithms are used to reconstruct an image. Among the simpler and more commonly employed is a technique known as *filtered backprojection*, in which the algorithm retraces a photon's path, assuming an equal probability of decay at all points along the line in the image (Hoffman and Phelps, 1986; Jaszczak, 1991). As retracings from multiple decay events from multiple projections intersect, brain areas having high levels of radioactivity begin to stand out as individual probability values are summed. Since some areas without activity will be assigned radiation values by virtue of the algorithm's statistical guess, a filter is required to subtract spurious values from the images. Choice of filter type (e.g., Ramp, Butterworth, Hanning) (Parker, 1990) is beyond the scope of this chapter; however, tradeoffs between spatial resolution and noise amplification exist and are among the factors considered.

Basic Limitations of Positron Emission Tomography and Single-Photon Emission Computed Tomography

While PET and SPECT offer an unprecedented and, in many instances, unique ability to quantitatively assess physiologic processes in vivo, important limits exist with respect to their quantitative accuracy. Specifically, issues related to radioactive decay, attenuation, scatter, limited spatial resolution/partial volume effects, and in vivo modeling all strongly influence PET and SPECT data (Hoffman and Phelps, 1986; Sorenson and Phelps, 1987; Links, 1990).

Radioactive Decay

The process of radioactive decay introduces potential biases into image accuracy based on both spatial and statistical effects. The former is mostly a theoretical issue for PET and derives from 1) the spatial separation of radioactive decay (i.e., positron emission) and positron annihilation (i.e., γ-ray emission) (Phelps et al., 1975), and 2) the noncolinearity of photons (i.e., those emitted at an angle slightly different from 180°). Thus, quantitative biases arise from isotope-specific limits on spatial resolution (2–3 mm; *see below*). Neither of these factors places such a theoretical limit on SPECT.

By contrast, both techniques are impacted by the fundamentally statistical nature of radioactive decay. Radioactive decay is well described mathematically by an exponential function (Sorenson and Phelps, 1987), and the so-called radioactive "half-life" is a physical constant that describes this rate of decay. Despite the physical constancy of this parameter for a given isotope (Table 1), radioactive decay occurs with a predictable, probabilistic fluctuation (as described by the Poisson distribution) as the rate of individual decay events varies slightly from moment to moment over time. If a curve were graphically fit to such values, the appropriate exponential decay rate (i.e., half-life) would always be derived, but individual measurements would fall slightly above or below the line. The brain-imaging equivalent of this phenomenon is a "Swiss-cheese" appearance to images of an object containing a uniform concentration of radioactivity. Since this "noise" is truly statistical, it may be overcome in PET and SPECT experiments by simply collecting more counts, a goal achievable through either longer sampling times or greater instrument sensitivity. Depending on which approach is taken, however, either temporal or spatial resolution is sacrificed (e.g., a collimator with larger holes will allow more photons through, but will include those with slightly less than parallel trajectories).

Photon Attenuation

Despite their high energies, some photons lose sufficient energy and fail to escape the body (and hence detection) by virtue of their scattering (Compton effects) or absorption (photoelectric effects) in tissue (Sorenson and Phelps, 1987). The physical basis of these effects results from interactions of γ-rays with atomic electrons. The chances of being scattered and absorbed (i.e., attenuated) increase as a function of both distance traveled and tissue density. Thus, radioactive signals are weakest from the center of the brain as compared to its periphery (roughly 4- to 5-fold) and less for photons passing through bone and water as compared to water and air, respectively (Links, 1990; Jaszczak, 1991). Thus, to compare levels of radioactivity in different brain regions, correcting for the effects of photon attenuation is essential (Huang et al., 1979). Although methods exist that take only distance into account ("uniform" attenuation correction), newer PET and SPECT cameras are routinely equipped with transmission scanning capabilities (similar to computed tomography), enabling the clinician to incorporate information on tissue density as well. The latter, "nonuniform," approach is generally optimal because heads vary in size and shape, and the attenuation properties of bone, tissue, fluid, and air differ (Rajeevan et al., 1998). In general, photon attenuation is less problematic for PET than for SPECT, since dual photons have higher energies and, because of coincidence detection, their attenuation is depth-independent.

Photon Scatter

Under circumstances when scatter does not prevent a photon from being detected by a PET/SPECT camera, an additional artifact is introduced into PET/SPECT images as a result of the deviation from its original trajectory (i.e., an incorrect trajectory is assumed by the camera). The net effect of such errors is similar to that of random coincidences, namely, an increase in background noise and a compromise of image contrast. In addition to recording the number of photons detected, PET and SPECT cameras are also equipped to measure photon energy, which allows discrimination between scattered and nonscattered events—since a fraction of the scattered photon's

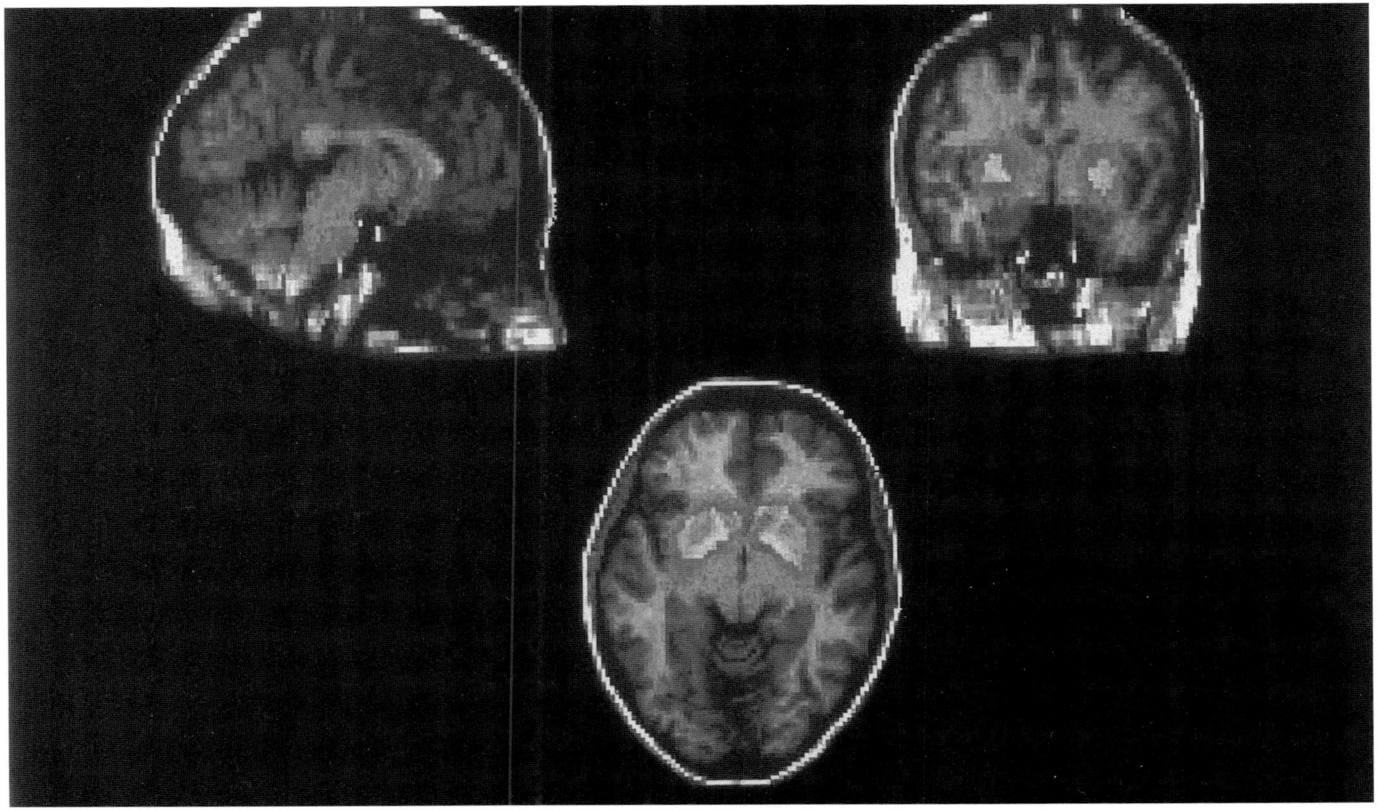

Fig. 4. Sagittal (top left), coronal (top right), and transaxial (bottom), views of the in vivo distribution of the cocaine analog [^{123}I]β-CIT as imaged by SPECT and coregistered with MRI. The highest numbers of cocaine binding sites are seen in the striata (i.e., caudate and putamen) bilaterally, and the brainstem, brain regions rich in dopamine and serotonin transporters, respectively. (*See* color plate 3 appearing after p. 134.)

energy is lost to the interacting atomic electron. Such approaches are imperfect, however, because the energy spectra of scattered and nonscattered photons frequently overlap, and scatter is both depth-dependent and proportional to the electron density of the tissue. Thus, the development of more sophisticated scatter correction methods is an area of active research in image reconstruction (Jaszczak, 1991).

Limited Spatial Resolution

In contrast to magnetic resonance images, PET and SPECT images appear "blurry" (Fig. 4). While the effects of lower resolution on our subjective visual perception is obvious, the consequences of lower spatial resolution on image quantitation are less intuitive and warrant some elaboration (Hoffman et al., 1981; Links, 1990).

When imaged in a PET or SPECT camera, a single point of radioactivity appears not as a point, but rather as a fuzzy circle with an activity profile that approximates a gaussian curve (or a function of several such curves). The degree of "spread" in this curve is used to measure the resolving capacity of a camera. Specifically, the width of the curve at its half-maximal intensity, the "full-width-at-half-maximum" (FWHM), is the parameter most commonly used to define the resolution of a camera. More practically, the FWHM is also the distance by which two points must be separated to be perceived as spatially distinct. The FWHM varies according to the imaging device and is determined by instrumentation and physical factors, including the precision of collimation, the number and size of detectors, and the accuracy in localizing a scintillation event within a crystalline element.

The impact of limited spatial resolution on measured radioactivity, called *partial volume errors*, takes two different, albeit related, forms. As intuitively conveyed from the description above, radioactivity from a relatively "hot" brain region can spill over into an area of lesser or no activity. Conversely (and less intuitively), for objects smaller than two to three times the FWHM resolution of a camera, the radioactive signal is effectively diluted, as averaging with "colder" brain areas occurs. In the latter situation, image intensity becomes increasingly a function of object size and less of radioactive density (Kessler et al., 1984). Thus, for researchers focusing on smaller brain structures and/or conditions in which changes in brain anatomy may exist (e.g., cortical atrophy accompanying alcoholism), several approaches may be adopted. In one approach, errors are simulated in a plastic model that contain cavities filled with radioactivity that approximate the actual distribution of tracer in the brain. By imaging such phantoms, regionally specific correction factors, or recovery coefficients, are derived that may be applied when imaging human subjects. Alternatively, investigators are increasingly incorporating structural (e.g., MRI), a priori functional (e.g., relative blood flow ratios in gray and white matter), and physical (e.g., the three-dimensional point spread function of a PET or SPECT camera) information to mathematically correct for such effects (Müller-Gärtner et al., 1992).

Tracer Modeling

Since a number of physiologic processes may influence the in vivo distribution of a tracer (e.g., peripheral metabolism/clearance, regional cerebral blood flow, protein binding), model-based methods are required for extracting from the mixture information specific to the process of interest. The complexity of modeling principles precludes a

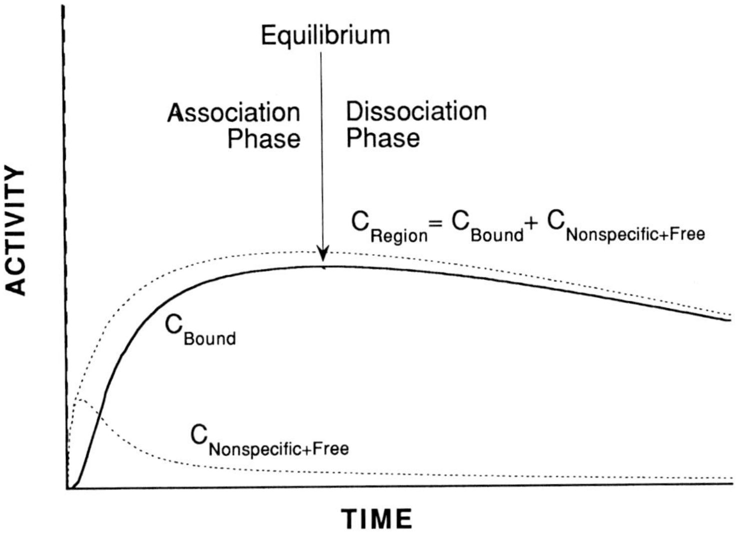

Fig. 5. Hypothetical time–activity curves depicting changes in regional uptake of a reversible radiotracer in vivo. Total radioactivity in a given region of interest (C_{region}) is shown to consist of specifically bound radioactivity (C_{bound}) and radioactivity nonspecifically bound or free ($C_{nonspecfic+free}$). The latter concentrations are typically inferred from a brain region lacking the physiological process of interest (e.g., a brain region devoid of neuroreceptors) while the former is calculated from the difference between C_{region} and $C_{nonspecfic+free}$.

detailed discussion in the current chapter. Nevertheless, enumeration of several basic concepts will provide the reader with a framework for appreciating the variety of methods employed, including kinetic, graphical, and equilibrium techniques.

The ultimate goal of most PET or SPECT imaging experiments is a numerical outcome measure that reflects a physiologic parameter of interest (e.g., rate of glucose synthesis, receptor density, rate of cerebral blood flow, and so forth). While the latter information may be depicted as a so-called "parametric" image (Friston, 1995), more commonly, PET/SPECT data take the form of time–activity curves, in which images of brain radioactivity are acquired for a period of time following tracer administration (Fig. 5).

Several model-based methods are used in quantitating physiologic process from such time–activity data, including kinetic (Mintun et al., 1984), graphical (Patlak et al., 1983; Logan et al., 1990), and equilibrium (Farde et al., 1986; Carson et al., 1993) approaches. The approach of choice depends on a radiotracer's in vivo kinetics (i.e., its reversibility or irreversibility) and the imaging context, with the ultimate goal of employing the simplest method for achieving a reliable outcome measure. From an imaging perspective (one occasionally at odds with pharmacologic definitions), a tracer is defined as *reversible* if phases of association (i.e., tracer uptake), dissociation (i.e., tracer washout), and hence equilibrium (a point or period during which net rates of association and dissociation are equal) exist (Fig. 5). Conversely, a tracer is said to be *irreversible* if equilibrium is never achieved or occurs outside of the time frame of the imaging experiment (i.e., only association is observed). Kinetic and graphical

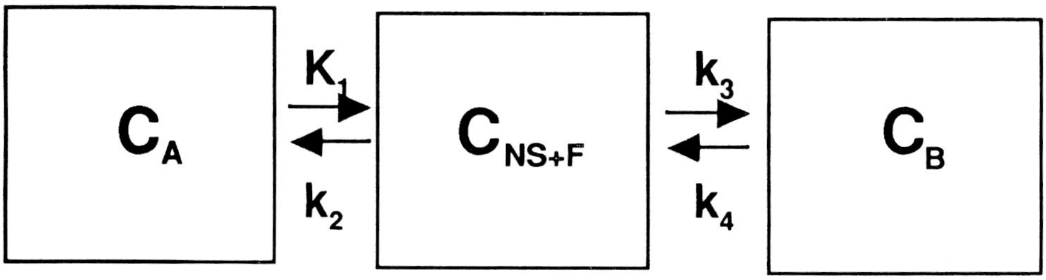

Fig. 6. A typical, so-called "three-compartment model" is depicted, including arterial (C_A), nonspecific/free (C_{NS+F}), and specifically bound (C_B) concentrations of radioactivity for a reversible radiotracer. A series of fractional rate constants (i.e., K_1–k_4) connect compartments and describe tracer exchange between compartments over time (e.g., as depicted in Fig. 5). In the case of an irreversible tracer, where no dissociation is detected, k_4 is eliminated from the model.

methods can be applied to both reversible and irreversible ligands, while equilibrium methods apply only to reversible ones.

All model-based methods rely on the concept of a *compartment*, a physiologic or biochemical "space" in which a tracer's concentration is assumed to be homogeneous. A model consists of a configuration of a series of compartments (e.g., arterial/capillary, specific binding, nonspecific binding, free radiotracer, and so forth) and forms the basis for a mathematical description of a tracer's behavior in a biologic system. Connecting compartments are a series of fractional rate constants that are used to describe the rate and direction of tracer transfer (Fig. 6). Thus, changes in tracer concentration in any given compartment can be expressed in mathematical terms as the amount of tracer entering and leaving per unit time. In the kinetic approach, rate constants are typically estimated by a nonlinear, least squares, curve-fitting procedure that minimizes differences between the experimental time–activity curves and the modeled values of activity (Mintun et al., 1984). By contrast, graphical approaches seek to linearize the relationship between brain and blood activity by various techniques (e.g., by expressing time–activity data as integrals or functions of areas under the time–activity curves), and the rate constants are determined by simple linear regression (Patlak et al., 1983; Logan et al., 1990). In both instances, rate constants or their ratios define in a model-specific fashion the physiologic process of interest (i.e., rate of glucose synthesis, receptor density, rate of cerebral blood flow).

In contrast to kinetic and graphical approaches, where physiologic information is gleaned from changes in compartmental radioactivity over time, equilibrium approaches seek to identify situations when net compartmental radioactivity is unchanging—that is, when equilibrium exists. As alluded to above, a single moment of equilibrium binding exists following the bolus administration of a reversible radiotracer and occurs precisely at the time of peak specific brain activity (i.e., when net uptake and washout are equal) (Farde et al., 1986). Alternatively, a prolonged state of in vivo equilibrium may be achieved by a bolus followed by a constant infusion of a tracer (Carson et al., 1993; Laruelle et al., 1993). Under such equilibrium conditions, physiological variables of interest (e.g., volumes of distribution, binding potential) are obtained from a simple ratio of brain and plasma activities. While the equilibrium approach is distinct from kinetic and graphical methods, several of these approaches may be used in conjunction to aid in the development and/or validation of the simplest and most accurate method of quantitation. For example, kinetic studies may be used to assist in the development of experimental parameters used in a bolus plus constant infusion paradigm, from which a simple ratio from a single brain scan may ultimately prove to be as accurate as much longer, more sampling intensive, and more mathematically complex ones (Laruelle et al., 1994).

Applications in Substance Abuse Research

Perhaps the greatest advantage of PET and SPECT lies in their tremendous flexibility for studying a variety of brain functions, an attribute based on the virtually unlimited number of biologically relevant compounds that lend themselves to radiolabeling. To date, studies in substance abuse disorders have taken advantage of these techniques to study the in vivo pharmacology of drugs of abuse as well as the effects of abused drugs and/or drug addiction on neuronal activity/metabolism and brain chemistry. A majority of substance abuse studies have focused on cocaine addiction, and this disorder will be emphasized to illustrate the types of applications.

In Vivo Pharmacology

PET and SPECT have been used to understand various aspects of the pharmacology of abused substances, including their pharmacokinetics, their occupancy of molecular targets in the brain (i.e., receptors, transporters), and their competition with pharmacologic antagonists and/or known pharmacotherapies.

Since all drugs of abuse are fundamentally organic (i.e., carbon containing) molecules, [^{11}C] radiochemistry makes PET uniquely suited to the study of their pharmacokinetics (i.e., since insertion of the radiolabel does not alter the native pharmacology of the parent drug). In fact, PET radiotracers currently exist for [^{11}C]cocaine, [^{11}C]heroin, [^{11}C]morphine, and [^{11}C]nicotine (Hartvig et al., 1984; Fowler et al., 1989; Halldin et al., 1992), and tracer doses of these compounds have been used to study the pharmacokinetics of each in vivo. Among the earliest applications is work by Fowler and colleagues (Fowler et al., 1989). Their pioneering work with [^{11}C]cocaine in humans demonstrated extremely high levels of brain uptake (8–10% of the injected dose) into basal ganglia (a brain region containing the highest concentrations of dopamine transporters) that occurred rapidly (peaking within 4–6 min) and cleared quickly (with an initial brain half-life of approx 20 min). These studies were consistent with the known kinetics of cocaine's behavioral euphoria.

In addition to studies of pharmacokinetics, PET and SPECT have been used to assess the degree to which drugs of abuse occupy the molecular targets of their action. Again, studies of cocaine and the dopamine transporter are illustrative. The first such study by Malison and colleagues (Malison et al., 1995) used SPECT and the radioiodinated cocaine analog [^{123}I]β-CIT (also known as [^{123}I]RTI-55). Using sequential cocaine displacements, behaviorally relevant (i.e., euphorigenic) doses of cocaine were shown to occupy measurable (conservatively, ≥15%) levels of the DAT in vivo. Although differences in the relative kinetics of the radiotracer (i.e., [^{123}I]β-CIT) and displacer (i.e., cocaine) precluded exact occupancy measures (Malison et al., 1986), subsequent studies by Logan and colleagues (Logan et al., 1997) have more definitively established occupancy values in excess of 60–70% for subjects experiencing a drug-induced "high" (Volkow et al., 1997a). Such high levels of occupancy are not necessarily characteristic of all abused drugs as suggested by work with benzodiazepines. Specifically, SPECT displacement studies with [^{123}I]iomazenil indicate that pharmacologically active doses of lorazepam occupy fewer than 5% of benzodiazepine receptors (Sybirska et al., 1993), data consistent with the existence of a large receptor reserve in humans.

Neuronal Activity/Metabolism

Regional changes in neuronal activity are associated with changes in energy utilization that can be assessed with radiotracer techniques in one of two ways: 1) through measures of the regional cerebral rates of glucose metabolism (rCGM), or 2) through measures of regional cerebral blood (rCBF), which under most physiological conditions is positively coupled to glucose metabolism. In the case of PET, techniques involving radiolabeled analogs of glucose (i.e., [^{18}F]fluorodeoxyglucose or [^{18}F]FDG) and radiolabeled water (i.e., [^{15}O]H_2O) are used to measure rCGM and rCBF, respectively. Although no comparable SPECT analog of [^{18}F]FDG exists, several tracers exist for measuring rCBF, including ^{99m}Tc-HMPAO, ^{123}I-iodoamphetamine, and ^{133}Xe.

Using such techniques, investigations haven fallen broadly into two areas as relates to substance abuse, including both the acute effects of drug administration and the long-term consequences of addiction on neuronal activity (e.g., during states of drug abstinence and/or treatment). Among the first to exploit such techniques for studies of human drug abusers, London and colleagues (London et al., 1990) examined the effects of intravenous cocaine (30 mg) on rCGM using [^{18}F]FDG and PET. Cocaine induced global reductions in brain metabolism that were inversely correlated with ventricular size. These investigators posited that reductions in brain metabolism may be one mechanism whereby drugs are reinforcing/rewarding. In addition, Volkow and colleagues have attempted to understand the metabolic correlates of both acute (i.e., ≤1 wk) and sustained (i.e., 1–4 mo) drug abstinence in chronic cocaine abusers (Volkow et al., 1991, 1993). The latter studies have indicated patterns of abnormally high metabolic rates in orbitofrontal cortex and striatum upon initial detoxification that change to reductions in metabolic activity in prefrontal cortex, orbitofrontal cortex, temporal cortex and cingulate gyrus as compared to non-drug-dependent controls. These studies suggest a temporally dynamic and regionally complex circuitry of abnormalities in brain function that are associated with cocaine addiction and its clinical manifestations.

Most recently, PET researchers have applied [^{15}O]H_2O and [^{18}F]FDG techniques to studies of cognitive activation in an attempt to understand more transient psychological states, including cue-induced drug craving (Grant et al., 1996; Childress et al., 1999). In both instances, investigators have started to highlight the importance of brain structures like the amygdala and medial temporal lobe in mediating the learned/conditioned aspects of addiction. While such activation paradigms are extremely exciting and have tremendous potential, this area of research is likely to give way to functional magnetic resonance imaging (fMRI) techniques given the latter's superior temporal and spatial resolution and lack of radiation exposure (Breiter et al., 1997).

Brain Chemistry

Two major attributes of PET and SPECT, high sensitivity and biochemical selectivity, make these methods the technique of choice for the majority of in vivo neurochemical measurements. Their sensitivity enables measurement of substrates at concentrations $10^{-12}M$, several orders of magnitude lower than magnetic resonance spectroscopy capabilities (10^{-3} to $10^{-5}M$). Thus, PET and SPECT are capable of measuring various facets of neurochemical function in the brain, including synthesis and release of transmitters, receptors, transporters, and metabolic enzymes, with active developmental research aimed at probes of second messenger systems and gene expression.

Neurotransmitter Synthesis

Analogous to [^{18}F]FDG techniques for measuring glucose metabolic rates, radiolabeled substrates of specific synthetic enzymes make possible in vivo measurements of neurotransmitter synthesis rates in the living brain. Two examples include 6-[^{18}F]fluoro-L-3,4-dihydroxyphenylalanine ([^{18}F]FDOPA) (Garnett et al., 1983) and [^{11}C]alpha-methyl-tryptophan ([^{11}C]α-Me-TRP) (Diksic and Grdisa, 1995), probes of dopamine (aromatic L-amino acid decarboxylase) and serotonin (tryptophan hydroxylase) synthesis rates, respectively. Using the former tracer, Baxter and colleagues (1988), documented reduced rates of dopamine synthesis in cocaine abusers as compared to controls. In addition, [^{18}F]FDOPA has been successfully used in animal studies as a measure of psychostimulant- (i.e., methamphetamine-) induced neurotoxicity in striatum (Melega et al., 1996).

Receptors and Transporters

Currently, neurotransmitter receptors and transporters are the neurochemical targets receiving greatest attention in PET and SPECT imaging. Focus on these molecules has been based on the notion that alterations in the drug's binding site and/or neurotransmitter system may provide insights into neurochemical lesions and/or adaptations in the addicted brain. In cocaine addiction, initial studies focused on regulation on the D_2 receptor. Using [^{18}F]N-methylspiperone and PET, Volkow and colleagues (Volkow et al., 1990) reported reductions in striatal D_2 receptors in recently detoxified cocainc abusers. Subsequent work has suggested persistence of these reductions for abstinence intervals up to 3–4 mo (Volkow et al., 1993). Complementing this work of post-synaptic dopamine function have been analogous studies of the presynaptic dopamine transporter. Although an initial study failed to find differences in DAT between cocaine abusers and controls (Volkow et al., 1996), work by Malison and colleagues (Malison et al., 1998a) revealed moderate (~25%) elevations in striatal cocaine binding sites in acutely (i.e., $\leq$ 96 h) abstinent cocaine abusers as measured by [^{123}I]β-CIT and SPECT. The latter findings were consistent with previous post-mortem reports in cocaine-related deaths (Little et al., 1993; Staley et al., 1994). Although these elevations appeared to persist within the same cohort of subjects after 1 month of cocaine abstinence, subsequent studies in formerly cocaine dependent subjects in residential drug treatment (mean abstinence interval 9 mo) indicates an apparent normalization in DAT (Malison et al., 1996). While definitive studies of the causes of such neurochemical alterations in dopaminergic markers remain to be done, such studies are consistent with enduring (or perhaps premorbid) changes in brain neurochemistry that characterize the addicted brain.

Neurotransmitter Release

Among the early criticisms of in vivo measurements of neuroreceptors were the potentially confounding influences created by competitive binding between the endogenous (i.e., neurotransmitter) and exogenous (i.e., radiotracer) ligands. However, this perceived liability has been exploited in recent studies that aim primarily to measure neurotransmitter release instead of the receptors themselves. Several PET and SPECT dopamine D_2 receptor imaging studies in humans and monkeys now provide good evidence that both the resting levels of synaptic dopamine and the levels of stimulant-induced dopamine release may be inferred from corresponding reciprocal changes in the occupancy by the radiotracer (Dewey et al., 1991; Laruelle et al., 1997). For example, psychostimulant administration has been shown to produce displacement in radioligand binding, an effect mediated indirectly through the release of endogenous dopamine. Using such techniques (i.e., methylphenidate administration in conjunction with [^{11}C]raclopride PET imaging), Volkow and colleagues (Volkow et al., 1997b) tested hypotheses of neurochemical sensitization in living cocaine abusers. Contrary to expectations, cocaine abusers were found to have reduced levels of stimulant-induced dopamine release (as reflected by smaller reductions in [^{11}C]raclopride uptake) as compared to controls. A recent abstract by Malison and colleagues using the SPECT D_2 receptor imaging agent [^{123}I]IBZM and amphetamine provides preliminary replication of this finding (Malison et al., 1999). These latter studies emphasize the importance of using in vivo neuroimaging techniques to validate preclinical models of addiction, and they illustrate the potential of these techniques for feeding back and informing basic science research into substance abuse.

Conclusions

PET and SPECT imaging are radiotracer techniques whose high sensitivity and specificity allow for studies of in vivo pharmacology, local neuronal activity, and in vivo neurochemistry in substance abuse disorders. Such methods have particular relevance to the clinical study of addiction insofar as they can be applied to the living human brain. Despite the tremendous view into brain function they afford, the technical complexity of these methods currently limit extensive application within the field of substance abuse. For the time being, PET and SPECT continue to require a large multidisciplinary group of collaborators in areas of drug development, radiochemistry, instrumentation physics, pharmacology, compartmental modeling, radiation health physics, and the basic and clinical neurosciences. As such, these techniques remain research tools first and foremost. However, for the field of addiction psychiatry to fully benefit from the revelations afforded by PET and SPECT, an appreciation of their basic principles and applications will be required of all members of the substance abuse research community. This chapter has reviewed several of the important methodological aspects of functional imaging that will hopefully be useful to those working in this exciting research field.

References

Baxter, L. R., Jr., Schwartz, J. M., Phelps, M. E., Mazziotta, J. C., Barrio, J., Rawson, R. A., Engel, J., Guze, B. H., Selin, C. and Sumida, R., Localization of neurochemical effects of cocaine and other stimulants in the human brain. J. Clin. Psychiatry 49(Suppl.):23–26, 1988.

Breiter, H. C., Gollub, R. L., Weisskoff, R. M., Kennedy, D. N., Makris, N., Berke, J. D., Goodman, J. M., Kantor, H. L., Gastfriend, D. R., Riorden, J. P., Mathew, R. T., Makris, N., Rosen, B. R. and Hyman, S. E., Acute effects of cocaine on human brain activity and emotion. Neuron 19:591–611, 1997.

Budinger, T. F., Physical attributes of single-photon tomography. J. Nucl. Med. 21:579–592, 1980.

Carson, R. E., Channing, M. A., Blasberg, R. G., Dunn, B. B., Cohen, R. M., Rice, K. C. and Herscovitch, P., Comparison of bolus and infusion methods for receptor quantitation: application to [^{18}F]cyclofoxy and positron emission tomography. J. Cereb. Blood Flow Metab. 13:24–42, 1993.

Childress, A. R., Mozley, P. D., McElgin, W., Fitzgerald, J., Reivich, M. and O'Brien, C. P., Limbic activation during cue-induced cocaine craving. Am. J. Psychiatry 156:11–18, 1999.

Devous, M., Imaging brain function by single-photon emission computer tomography, in Andreasen, N. C. (ed.), Brain Imaging: Applications in Psychiatry. Washington, D.C.: American Psychiatric Press, pp. 147–234, 1989.

Dewey, S. L., Logan, J., Wolf, A. P., Brodie, J. D., Angrist, B., Fowler, J. S. and Volkow, N. D., Amphetamine induced decreases in (^{18}F)-N-methylspiroperidol binding in the baboon brain using positron emission tomography (PET). Synapse 7:324–327, 1991.

Diksic, M. and Grdisa, M., Alpha-methyl-L-tryptophan as a tracer to study brain serotonergic system. Neurochem. Res. 20:1353–1360, 1995.

Farde, L., Hall, H., Ehrin, E. and Sedvall, G., Quantitative analysis of D_2 dopamine receptor binding in the living human brain by PET. Science 231:258–261, 1986.

Fowler, J. S., Volkow, N. D., Wolf, A. P., Dewey, S. L., Schlyer, D. J., Macgregor, R. R., Hitzemann, R., Logan, J., Bendriem, B., Gatley, S. J. and Christman, D., Mapping cocaine binding sites in human and baboon brain in vivo. Synapse 4:371–377, 1989.

Friston, K. J., Commentary and opinion: II. Statistical parametric mapping: ontology and current issues. J. Cereb. Blood Flow Metab. 15:361–370, 1995.

Garnett, E. S., Firnau, G. and Nahmias, C., Dopamine visualized in the basal ganglia of living man. Nature 305:137–138, 1983.

Grant, S., London, E. D., Newlin, D. B., Villemagne, V. L., Liu, X., Contoreggi, C., Phillips, R. L., Kimes, A. S. and Margolin, A., Activation of memory circuits during cue-elicited cocaine craving. Proc. Natl. Acad. Sci. USA 93:12040–12045, 1996.

Halldin, C., Nagren, K., Swahn, C. G., Langstrom, B. and Nyback, H., (S)- and (R)-[^{11}C]nicotine and the metabolite (R/S)-[^{11}C]cotinine. Preparation, metabolite studies and in vivo distribution in the human brain using PET. Int. J. Rad. Appl. Instrum. [B] 19:871–880, 1992.

Hartvig, P., Bergstrom, K., Lindberg, B., Lundberg, P. O., Lundqvist, H., Langstrom, B., Svard, H. and Rane, A., Kinetics of ^{11}C-labeled opiates in the brain of rhesus monkeys. J. Pharmacol. Exp. Ther. 230:250–255, 1984.

Hoffman, E. and Phelps, M., Positron emission tomography: principles and quantitation. In: Phelps, M., Mazziotta, J. and Schelbert, H. (eds.) Positron emission tomography and autoradiography: principles and applications for the brain and heart. New York: Raven, pp. 237–286, 1986.

Hoffman, E. J., Huang, S. C., Phelps, M. E. and Kuhl, D. E., Quantitation in positron emission computed tomography: 4. Effect of accidental coincidences. J. Comput. Assist. Tomogr. 5:391–400, 1981.

Huang, S. C., Hoffman, E. J., Phelps, M. E. and Kuhl, D. E., Quantitation in positron emission computed tomography: 2. Effects of inaccurate attenuation correction. J. Comput. Assist. Tomogr. 3:804–814, 1979.

Jaszczak, R., SPECT: state-of-the-art scanners and reconstruction strategies, in Diksic, M. and Reba, R. (eds.) Radiopharmaceuticals and brain pathology studied with PET and SPECT. Boca Raton: CRC Press, pp. 93–118, 1991.

Kessler, R. M., Ellis, J. R. Jr. and Eden, M., Analysis of emission tomographic scan data: limitations imposed by resolution and background. J. Comput. Assist. Tomogr. 8:514–522, 1984.

Laruelle, M., Abi-Dargham, A., Rattner, Z., al-Tikriti, M. S., Zea-Ponce, Y., Zoghbi, S. S., Charney, D. S., Price, J., Frost, J. J., Hoffer, P. B., Baldwin, R. and Innis, R., Single photon emission tomography measurement of benzodiazepine receptor number and affinity in primate brain: a constant infusion paradigm with [^{123}I]iomazenil. Eur. J. Pharmacol. 230:119–123, 1993.

Laruelle, M., Wallace, E., Seibyl, J. P., Baldwin, R. M., Zea-Ponce, Y., Zoghbi, S. S., Neumeyer, J. L., Charney, D. S., Hoffer, P. B. and Innis, R. B., Graphical, kinetic, and equilibrium analyses of in vivo [^{123}I] β-CIT binding to dopamine transporters in healthy human subjects. J. Cereb. Blood Flow Metab. 14:982–994, 1994.

Laruelle, M., Iyer, R. N., al-Tikriti, M. S., Zea-Ponce, Y., Malison, R., Zoghbi, S. S., Baldwin, R. M., Kung, H. F., Charney, D. S., Hoffer, P. B., Innis, R. B. and Bradberry, C. W., Microdialysis and SPECT measurements of amphetamine-induced dopamine release in nonhuman primates. Synapse 25:1–14, 1997.

Links, J., Physics and instrumentation of positron emission tomography, in Frost, J. and Wagner, H. N. Jr. (eds.) Quantitative imaging: neuroreceptors, neurotransmitters, and enzymes. New York: Raven Press, pp. 37–50, 1990.

Little, K. Y., Kirkman, J. A., Carroll, F. I., Clark, T. B. and Duncan, G. E., Cocaine use increases [^{3}H]WIN 35428 binding sites in human striatum. Brain Res. 628:17–25, 1993.

Logan, J., Fowler, J. S., Volkow, N. D., Wolf, A. P., Dewey, S. L., Schlyer, D. J., MacGregor, R. R., Hitzemann, R., Bendriem, B., Gatley, S. J. and Christman, D., Graphical analysis of reversible radioligand binding from time-activity measurements applied to [N-^{11}C-methyl]-(–)-cocaine PET studies in human subjects. J. Cereb. Blood Flow Metab. 10:740–747, 1990.

Logan, J., Volkow, N. D., Fowler, J. S., Wang, G. J., Fischman, M. W., Foltin, R. W., Abumrad, N. N., Vitkun, S., Gatley, S. J., Pappas, N., Hitzemann, R. and Shea, C. E., Concentration and occupancy of dopamine transporters in cocaine abusers with [^{11}C]cocaine and PET. Synapse 27:347–356, 1997.

London, E. D., Cascella, N. G., Wong, D. F., Phillips, R. L., Dannals, R. F., Links, J. M., Herning, R., Grayson, R., Jaffe, J. H. and Wagner, H. N. Jr., Cocaine-induced reduction of glucose utilization in human brain: a study using positron emission tomography and [fluorine 18]-fluorodeoxyglucose. Arch. Gen. Psychiatry 47:567–574, 1990.

Malison, R. T., Best, S. E., Wallace, E. A., McCance, E., Laruelle, M., Zoghbi, S. S., Baldwin, R. M., Seibyl, J. S., Hoffer, P. B., Price, L. H., Kosten, T. R. and Innis, R. B., Euphorigenic doses of cocaine reduce [^{123}I]β-CIT SPECT measures of dopamine transporter availability in human cocaine addicts. Psychopharmacology (Berl.) 122:358–362, 1995.

Malison, R. T., Best, S. E., Zoghbi, S., Zea-Ponce, Y., Baldwin, R. M., Charney, D., Hoffer, P., Seibyl, J. P., Price, L. H., Kosten, T. R. and Innis, R. B., SPECT imaging of dopamine transporters during sustained cocaine abstinence with [^{123}I]β-CIT. J. Nucl. Med. 37:44P, 1996.

Malison, R. T., Best, S. E., van Dyck, C. H., McCance, E. F., Wallace, E. A., Laruelle, M., Baldwin, R. M., Seibyl, J. P., Price, L. H., Kosten, T. R. and Innis, R. B., Elevated striatal dopamine transporters during acute cocaine abstinence as measured by [^{123}I]β-CIT SPECT. Am. J. Psychiatry 155:832–834, 1998a.

Malison, R. T., Innis, R. B. and Laruelle, M., RE: Logan et al., 1997. [Letter]. Synapse 30:236–237, 1998b.

Malison, R., Mechanic, K., Klumpp, H., Baldwin, R., Kosten, T., Seibyl, J. and Innis, R., Reduced amphetamine-stimulated dopamine release in cocaine addicts as measured by [^{123}I]IBZM SPECT. J. Nucl. Med. 40:110P, 1999.

Melega, W. P., Quintana, J., Raleigh, M. J., Stout, D. B., Yu, D. C., Lin, K. P., Huang, S. C. and Phelps, M. E., 6-[^{18}F]fluoro-L-DOPA-PET studies show partial reversibility of long-term effects of chronic amphetamine in monkeys. Synapse 22:63–69, 1996.

Mintun, M. A., Raichle, M. E., Kilbourn, M. R., Wooten, G. F. and Welch, M. J., A quantitative model for the in vivo assessment of drug binding sites with positron emission tomography. Ann. Neurol. 15:217–227, 1984.

Müller-Gärtner, H. W., Links, J. M., Prince, J. L., Bryan, R. N., McVeigh, E., Leal, J. P., Davatzikos, C. and Frost, J. J., Measurement of radiotracer concentration in brain gray matter using positron emission tomography: MRI-based correction for partial volume effects. J. Cereb. Blood Flow Metab. 12:571–583, 1992.

Parker, J., Physics and Instrumentation of Positron Emission Tomography. Boca Raton, CRC Press, 1990.

Patlak, C. S., Blasberg, R. G. and Fenstermacher, J. D., Graphical evaluation of blood-to-brain transfer constants from multiple-time uptake data. J. Cereb. Blood Flow Metab. 3:1–7, 1983.

Phelps, M. E., Hoffman, E. J., Huang, S. C. and Ter-Pogossian, M. M., Effect of positron range on spatial resolution. J. Nucl. Med. 16:649–652, 1975.

Rajeevan, N., Zubal, I. G., Ramsby, S. Q., Zoghbi, S. S., Seibyl, J. and Innis, R. B., Significance of nonuniform attenuation correction in quantitative brain SPECT imaging. J. Nucl. Med. 39:1719–1726, 1998.

Sorenson, J. and Phelps, M., Physics in Nuclear Medicine. Philadelphia: W. B. Saunders, 1987.

Staley, J. K., Hearn, W. L., Ruttenber, A. J., Wetli, C. V. and Mash, D. C., High affinity cocaine recognition sites on the dopamine transporter are elevated in fatal cocaine overdose victims. J. Pharmacol. Exp. Ther. 271:1678–1685, 1994.

Sybirska, E., Seibyl, J. P., Bremner, J. D., Baldwin, R. M., al-Tikriti, M. S., Bradberry, C., Malison, R. T., Zea-Ponce, Y., Zoghbi, S., During, M., Woods, S., Hoffer, P., Charney, D. and Innis, R., [^{123}I]iomazenil SPECT imaging demonstrates significant benzodiazepine receptor reserve in human and nonhuman primate brain. Neuropharmacology 32:671–680, 1993.

Volkow, N. D., Fowler, J. S., Wolf, A. P., Schlyer, D., Shiue, C. Y., Alpert, R., Dewey, S. L., Logan, J., Bendriem, B., Christman, D., Hitzemann, R. and Henn, F., Effects of chronic cocaine abuse on postsynaptic dopamine receptors. Am. J. Psychiatry 147:719–724, 1990.

Volkow, N., Fowler, J., Wolf, A., Hitzemann, R., Dewey, S., Bendriem, B., Alpert, R. and Hoff, A., Changes in brain glucose metabolism in cocaine dependence and withdrawal. Am. J. Psychiatry 148:621–626, 1991.

Volkow, N. D., Fowler, J. S., Wang, G. J., Hitzemann, R., Logan, J., Schlyer, D. J., Dewey, S. L. and Wolf, A. P., Decreased dopamine D_2 receptor availability is associated with reduced frontal metabolism in cocaine abusers. Synapse 14:169–177, 1993.

Volkow, N. D., Wang, G. J., Fowler, J. S., Logan, J., Hitzemannn, R., Gatley, S. J., MacGregor, R. R. and Wolf, A. P., Cocaine uptake is decreased in the brain of detoxified cocaine abusers. Neuropsychopharmacology 14:159–168, 1996.

Volkow, N. D., Wang, G. J., Fischman, M. W., Foltin, R. W., Fowler, J. S., Abumrad, N. N., Vitkun, S., Logan, J., Gatley, S. J., Pappas, N., Hitzemann, R. and Shea, C. E., Relationship between subjective effects of cocaine and dopamine transporter occupancy. Nature 386:827–830, 1997a.

Volkow, N. D., Wang, G. J., Fowler, J. S., Logan, J., Gatley, S. J., Hitzemann, R., Chen, A. D., Dewey, S. L. and Pappas, N., Decreased striatal dopaminergic responsiveness in detoxified cocaine-dependent subjects. Nature 386:830–833, 1997b.

Chapter 3

Fundamentals of Magnetic Resonance

Perry F. Renshaw, MD, PhD, *Blaise deB. Frederick,* PhD, *and Luis C. Maas III,* MD, PhD

Introduction

Magnetic resonance methods currently in use for the assessment of human subjects include magnetic resonance imaging (MRI), magnetic resonance spectroscopy (MRS), and functional magnetic resonance imaging (fMRI). MRI provides detailed information regarding brain anatomy, with spatial resolution on the order of 1 mm^3, and is widely used to characterize neuropathological conditions in clinical practice. MRS allows the detection of signals from certain drugs and from a limited number of endogenous neurochemicals, with spatial resolution on the order of 1 cm^3, depending upon the compound under investigation. fMRI refers to a family of methods for obtaining brain images which are sensitive to changes in cerebral metabolism with spatial resolution on the order of a few millimeters and temporal resolution of a few seconds. MRI, MRS, and fMRI rely on the same basic principles and, at least for human studies, generally use the same hardware. Although the technology is evolving rapidly, there are currently more than 1000 installed 1.5 Tesla (T) MR scanners in the United States which are capable of performing some or all of these methodologies. Thus, this technology is widely disseminated and available to investigators at a number of clinical research sites. This review will describe the basic principles of MRI, MRS, and fMRI. With this information as background, the literature on the use of MR in substance abuse research is reviewed in Chapter 6.

From: *Brain Imaging in Substance Abuse: Research, Clinical, and Forensic Applications*
M. J. Kaufman, ed. © Humana Press Inc., Totowa, New Jersey

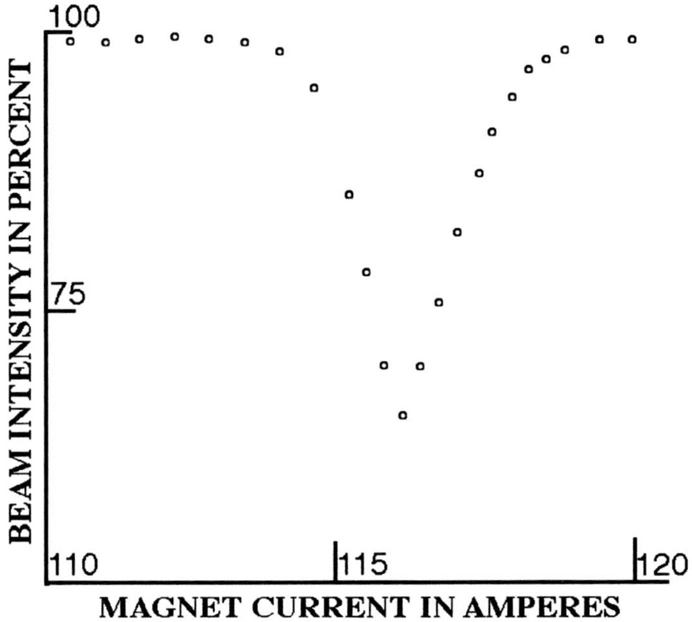

Fig. 1. Initial report of nuclear magnetic resonance. The signal represents the intensity of a lithium chloride (LiCl) molecular beam. The minimum intensity was achieved (~116 amps) when the applied current produced a magnetic field at the Larmor frequency, which reoriented the nuclear spins. (From Rabi et al., 1938, with permission.)

General Principles

The first report of an experiment designed to exploit the nuclear magnetic resonance (MR) phenomenon was made in 1938 (Rabi et al., 1938) (Fig. 1). In this study, magnetic resonance signals were detected from a molecular beam of lithium chloride. Several years later, techniques designed for the MR assessment of bulk matter were developed and reported by two independent research groups (Bloch et al., 1946; Purcell et al., 1946). These experiments were designed to take advantage of the fact that every atomic nucleus has a spin angular momentum quantum number, I, which can take on half-integer values, 0, 1/2, 1, 3/2, …. (reviewed in Farrar, 1989). Within a magnetic field (B_0), nuclei with nonzero quantum numbers will have $2I + 1$ equally spaced energy levels, which are separated by an amount of energy (ΔE) given by

$$\Delta E = \mu B_0 / I \quad (1)$$

where μ is the nuclear magnetic moment. In the MR experiment, energy at an appropriate frequency is applied to the nucleus to induce a transition between energy levels. The frequency of energy needed to induce this transition, or the resonance frequency, ν_0, may be expressed as

$$\nu_0 = \Delta E / h \quad (2)$$

where h is Planck's constant.

Several points can be made regarding these relationships by considering the case of a specific nucleus. For example, the most widely studied nucleus is the hydrogen

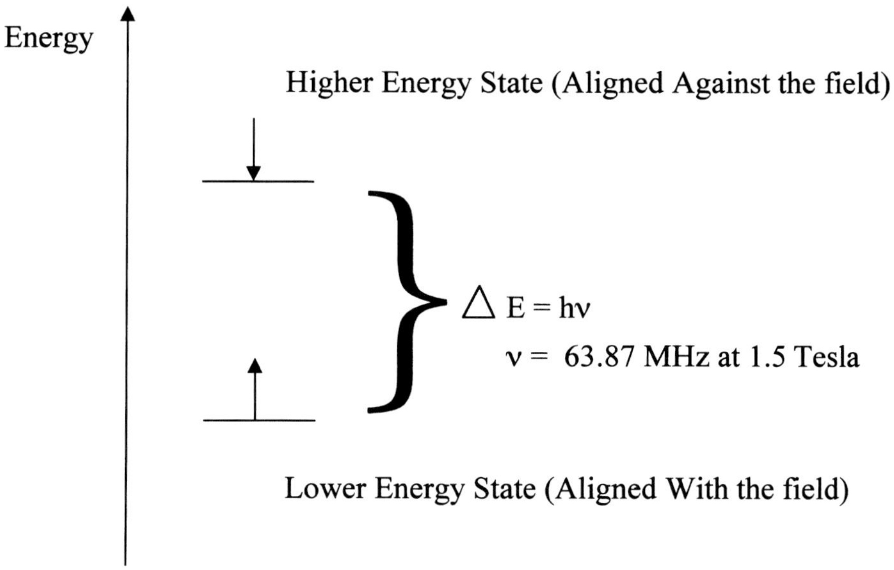

Fig. 2. Behavior of a hydrogen nucleus within a magnetic field. Irradiation at the resonance frequency allows nuclei aligned with the field (lower energy level) to absorb energy and become aligned against the field.

atom, which may be designated ^{1}H and which has a spin quantum number $I = 1/2$. Thus, in a magnetic field, we expect that the ^{1}H nucleus will have two energy levels. At 1.5 T, which is currently the most common field strength for magnetic resonance studies of the human brain, Equations (1) and (2) may be used to calculate that radiofrequency irradiation (RF) at 63.87 MHz, the resonance or Larmor frequency, that may be used to induce transitions between the two energy levels. Physically, the lower energy level corresponds to the magnetic moment of the ^{1}H nucleus being aligned with B_0, whereas the higher energy level is characterized by the magnetic moment being aligned against B_0 (Fig. 2).

It is also useful to consider how a collection of hydrogen nuclei might behave. In the absence of an applied magnetic field, the nuclear spins are aligned randomly (i.e., there are no energy levels). As a magnetic field is applied, the nuclei distribute themselves between the parallel and anti-parallel orientations, preferentially in the lower energy state, according to what is known as a Boltzmann distribution (reviewed in Farrar, 1989). For field strengths which are used in human studies, the difference in the number of spins aligned with, as opposed to against, the field is a very small fraction of the total number of nuclei in the collection (e.g., 10 of every million nuclei at 1.5 T and 37°C). Thus, it is a common convention in nuclear magnetic resonance to consider the net magnetic moment, M, of a sample, which reflects this net difference in the number of nuclei in the two energy levels.

In MR experiments, nuclei under investigation have angular momentum and tend to precess, or spin, around the magnetic field like a gyroscope. A common notation which is often used to describe this behavior invokes a "rotating frame." In this convention, the net magnetic moment M is represented as a motionless vector along the z axis (Fig. 3). Application of RF energy at the resonance frequency has the net effect

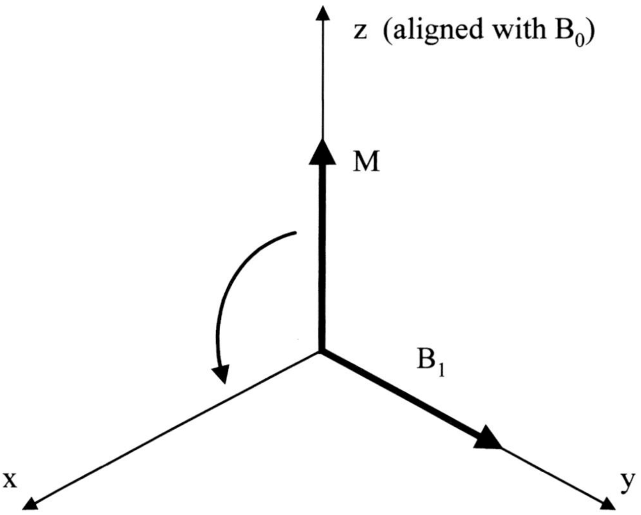

Fig. 3. The rotating frame. Application of RF irradiation at the resonance frequency has the effect of moving the net magnetic moment off of the *z* axis, out of alignment with the main magnetic field B_0, toward the *xy*, or transverse plane.

of moving the magnetization vector *M* off of the *z* axis, toward the *xy*, or transverse, plane. In this schema, the projection of *M* onto the *xy* plane represents the degree to which signal may observed in an MR experiment. Thus, when *M* lies completely in the transverse plane, there are equal numbers of nuclei in both the upper and lower energy levels, and this is the maximum amount of signal that can be detected. The decay of *M* in the transverse plane is described by the spin-spin relaxation time constant T2, and the recovery of *M* along the *z* axis occurs according to the spin-lattice relaxation time T1. The rotating frame is an especially useful notation to use in describing the amount of energy which is applied to nuclei under investigation in magnetic resonance experiments.

In practice, applications of RF at the resonance frequency are used to move some of the nuclei in the lower energy level to the higher energy level in a NMR experiment. When the RF irradiation is turned off, an RF signal is emitted from the sample at the resonance frequency. The nuclei return to their equilibrium in alignment with B_0 at rates determined by the spin-lattice (T1) relaxation time. In biological samples, the observed RF signal may decay much more rapidly than one might expect on the basis of T1, which generally ranges from 0.1 to 10 s for spin 1/2 nuclei in solvents. This is due to processes which allow the nuclear spins to come to equilibrium with each other, and is characterized by the spin-spin relaxation time, T2.

Magnetic Resonance Spectroscopy

Evolution of Methods

Since similar nuclei in different molecular structures have slightly different resonance frequencies, it was expected that this could be observed as magnetic field strengths increased and became more uniform. This was first demonstrated in 1951,

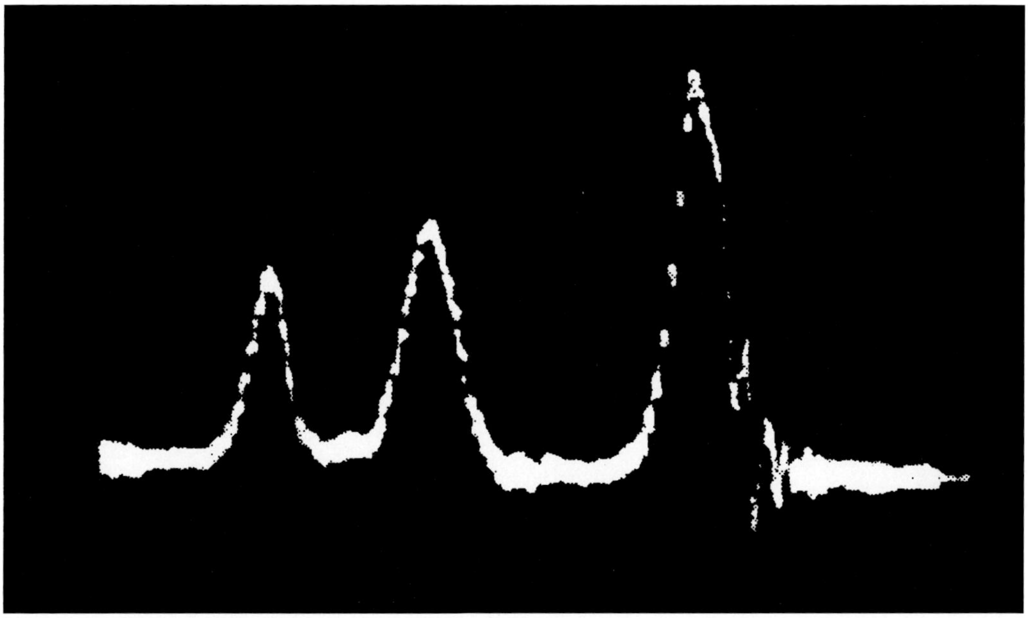

Fig. 4. Oscillograph trace of the nuclear magnetic resonance signal from ethyl alcohol. The peaks from left to right represent the —OH, —CH_2, and —CH_3 groups of alcohol. (From Arnold et al., 1951, with permission.)

when Arnold and colleagues reported that samples of ethanol gave rise to a spectrum with three separate resonance lines (Fig. 4). These lines arose from protons within the methyl (—CH_3), methylene (—CH_2), and hydroxyl (—OH) groups of ethanol. In early experiments, RF signals were detected as the intensity of B_0 was slowly increased in order to create spectra that included signals from nuclei with different resonance frequencies, or chemical shifts, and this type of study was known as a continuous wave (cw) experiment. In 1966, Ernst and Anderson reported that it was possible to use Fourier transform methods in order to construct entire spectra following short pulses of RF irradiation at a single resonance frequency (Fig. 5).

A complete spectrum could be recorded following a single RF pulse. This provided increased sensitivity and made it possible to observe signals from lower concentrations of substances containing hydrogen nuclei, or to observe signals from less sensitive nuclei, such as ^{31}P or ^{13}C (Table 1).

As MR methods became more widely utilized, studies of biological samples were undertaken. One of the first reports on the application of MR spectroscopy to cells and tissues was made in 1955 by Odeblad and Lindstrom, who detected ^{1}H MR signals from yeast, erythrocytes, and animal tissues (Odeblad and Lindstrom, 1955). In these early experiments, MR spectra from tissues were complicated by the enormous intensity of the water (H_2O) resonance (~80 *M* in hydrogen) in comparison to other resonance lines (~10 m*M*). Ultimately, water suppresion methods would be developed *(see below)*. With the development of pulse MR methods, it became possible to evaluate phosphorus (^{31}P) resonances and, in 1973, Moon and Richards recorded ^{31}P spectra

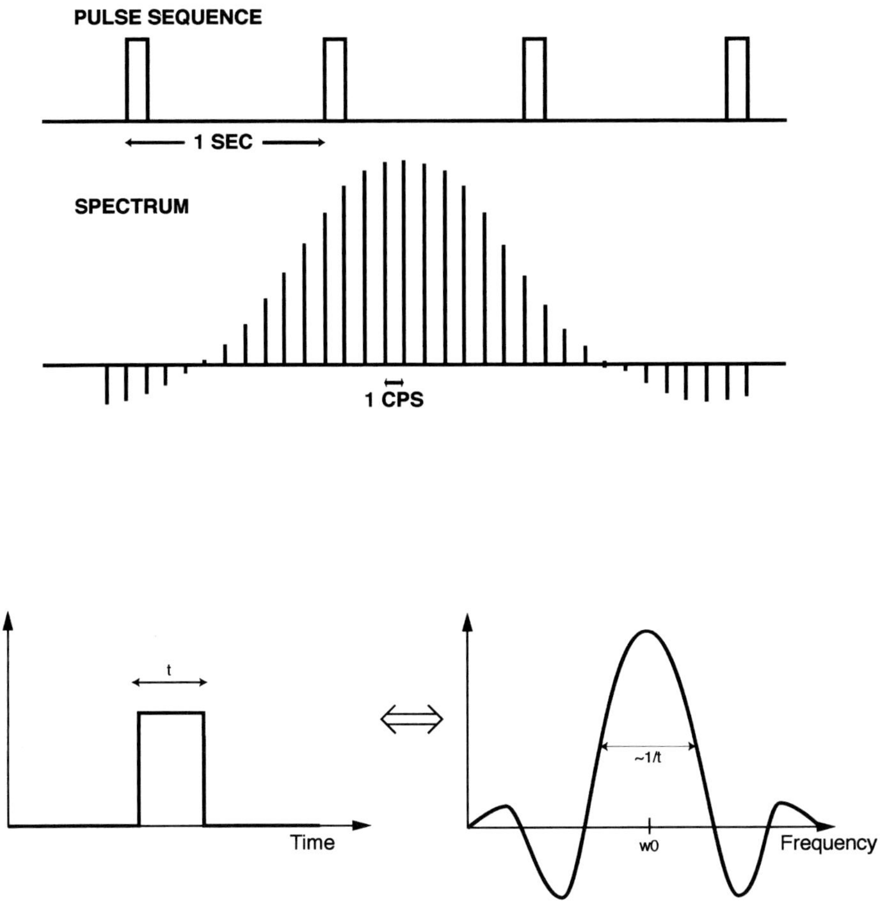

Fig. 5. Top: Initial description of the use of repeated radiofrequency pulses to generate spectra. (Adapted from Ernst and Anderson, 1966, with permission.) **Bottom:** A short pulse in time excites a range of frequencies proportional to the reciprocal of the pulse width. This is the fundamental relationship between time and frequency described by Fourier transformation (Bracewell, 1986). Pulse sequence and Fourier transform methods revolutionized the field of nuclear magnetic resonance.

from erythrocytes (Moon and Richards, 1973). The next year, Hoult and colleagues reported results from ^{31}P MR studies of excised muscle (Hoult et al., 1974). Phosphorus MR spectra provide information on the concentration of high energy phosphate compounds as well as phospholipid metabolites. Improvements in magnet design, which allowed the construction of larger, horizontal bore magnets, and the development of the surface coil (Ackerman et al., 1980) made it possible to conduct in vivo studies. A surface coil is an RF transmitter/receiver (i.e., an antenna) which may be placed adjacent to, rather than around, the tissue of interest. By 1986, the scientific literature included reports of in vivo ^{31}P MR studies of brain, kidney, liver, heart, skeletal muscle, and bowel (reviewed in Radda, 1986).

Table 1
Relative NMR Sensitivities of Biologically Relevant Nuclei

Nucleus	Spin quantum number (I)	NMR frequency at 1.5 T	Relative sensitivity at constant field	% Natural abundance
^{1}H	1/2	63.87	1.00	99.8
^{19}F	1/2	60.08	0.83	100
^{7}Li	3/2	24.83	0.29	92.58
^{23}Na	3/2	16.89	0.09	100
^{31}P	1/2	25.88	0.06	100
^{13}C	1/2	16.07	0.02	1.1
^{39}K	3/2	2.99	0.0005	93.2

With the successful demonstration that ^{31}P MR spectroscopy was feasible, studies of other, even less sensitive nuclei began to appear. Metabolic studies involving both natural abundance and enhanced ^{13}C MR spectroscopy were published (Cohen et al., 1979; Alger et al., 1984). As ^{13}C has a low natural abundance (Table 1), the administration of ^{13}C-enriched biochemical precursors provided an important new window on cerebral metabolism (Mason et al., 1996). ^{23}Na gives rise to a single distinct resonance. However, the use of paramagnetic shift reagents, which alter the resonance frequency of ions in their vicinity and which do not penetrate cells, makes it possible to detect separate resonances from intracellular and extracellular spaces (Balschi et al., 1982; Gupta and Gupta, 1982). Thus, ^{23}Na MR spectroscopy permits the study of ionic fluxes across membranes, which may be altered during cerebral ischemia or by a range of drugs (Boada et al., 1997). MR spectroscopy may also be used to noninvasively measure human brain levels of a number of psychotropic medications, including lithium (^{7}Li MRS) (Renshaw and Wicklund, 1988) (Fig. 6) and some fluorinated polycyclic drugs (^{19}F MRS) (Komoroski et al., 1991; Renshaw et al., 1992). These studies are motivated, in part, by the fact that brain drug levels are often substantially different from serum levels. These studies have generally reported whole-brain drug concentrations, due to the relatively low brain concentrations of the therapeutic agents (0.1–1.0 m*M* for lithium and 1–10 μ*M* for fluorinated drugs).

The utility of ^{19}F MRS as a means for assessing brain drug levels has been validated using a nonhuman primate model (Christensen et al., 1998). In this study, brain concentrations of the anorectic drug, dexfenfluramine, as well as its active metabolite, dex-norfenfluramine, were measured in three rhesus monkeys using ^{19}F MRS. In vivo estimates of brain drug levels were in very good agreement with those determined subsequently using in vitro analytical methods. These studies set the stage for human ^{19}F MRS studies of individuals taking dexfenfluramine as a treatment for obesity. Dexfenfluramine is structurally related to amphetamine, and preclinical studies had suggested that administration of the drug to a number of animal species resulted in both serotonin depletion and damage to serotonergic neurons (McCann et al., 1994, 1997). These human studies provided direct evidence that human brain dexfenfluramine levels were substantially below those which had been shown to deplete brain serotonin levels in humans (Fig. 7) (Christensen et al., 1999).

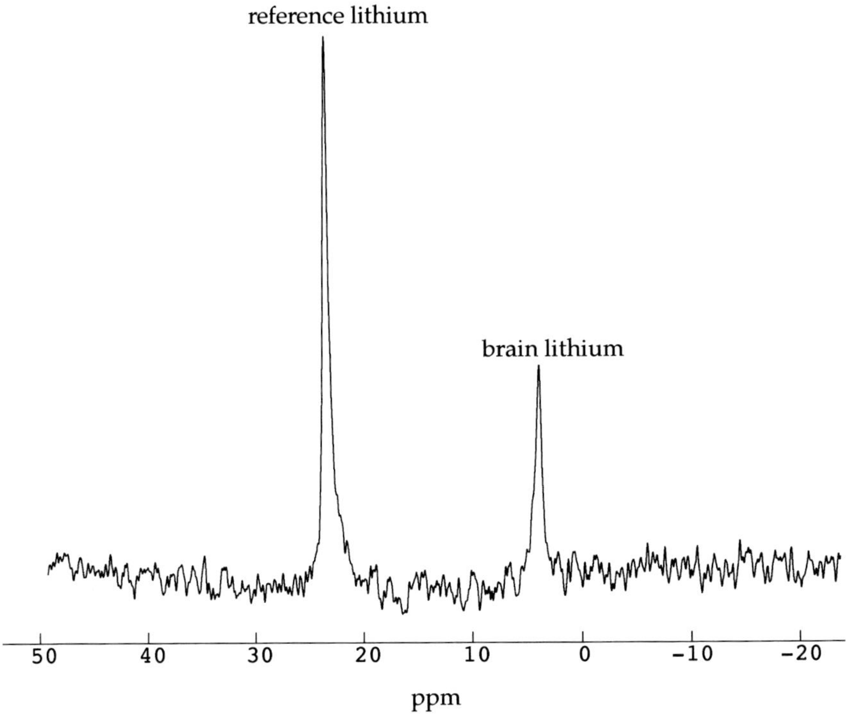

Fig. 6. Brain lithium-7 MR spectrum from a 31-yr-old man taking lithium carbonate, 1500 mg/d. Brain lithium levels are calculated by comparison of the intensity of the brain lithium reference with the intensity of both internal and external standards (Gonzalez et al., 1993). For this spectrum, brain lithium level was 0.49 m*M* with a corresponding serum level of 0.70 m*M*.

Current Status of Research

At the present time, brain MRS studies of human subjects are generally performed using 1.5 T clinical MR scanners. The implementation of MRS methods on these clinical instruments has not been a high priority of medical instrument vendors, in largest measure because there are relatively few clinical indications for MRS. Thus, the majority of MRS studies are conducted at only a few clinical research sites. Two different MRS-visible nuclei are evaluated in most studies of brain biochemistry: phosphorus (^{31}P) and hydrogen (^{1}H or proton). Unlike ^{7}Li or ^{19}F MR spectra, ^{31}P MR and ^{1}H spectra include several resonance lines which arise from well-defined metabolite pools. ^{31}P MR spectra provide information on the concentration of high-energy phosphate compounds (e.g., phosphocreatine (PCr) and nucleoside triphosphate (NTP, primarily reflecting adenosine triphosphate in the brain), phospholipid metabolites (phosphomonoesters [PME] and phosphodiesters [PDE]), and inorganic phosphate (Pi). Information on alterations in brain energy metabolism may be gained by measuring the relative levels of PCr (~2.9 m*M*/L), NTP (2.9 m*M*/L), and Pi (1.0 m*M*/L) (Buchli et al., 1994). The brain PME resonance, which arises primarily from the phospholipid precursors phosphoethanolamine (PEt) and phosphocholine (PCh), as well as from sugar phosphates, derives from a total metabolite pool of approx 3.0 m*M* (Pettegrew et

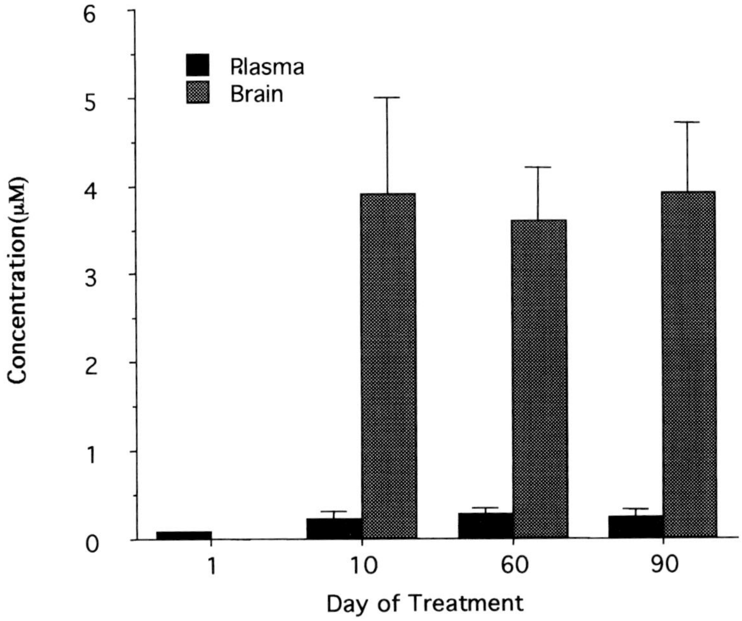

Fig. 7. Concurrent measurements of plasma and brain dexfenfluramine + dex-norfenfluramine levels in obese, but otherwise healthy, volunteers. Subjects were treated with 15 mg bid dexfenfluramine for a total of 90 d.

al., 1991). The in vivo PDE resonance has a broad component, arising from membrane bilayers, and a narrow component, which is derived from the phospholipid catabolites glycerophosphocholine (GPC) and glycerophosphoethanolamine (GPE).

At 1.5 T, metabolite information can usually be obtained from brain regions as small as 25–50 cm^3. ^{31}P MRS data are typically acquired either from single volumes (voxels) using spatial localization, such as DRESS (Bottomley et al., 1984); ISIS (Ordidge, 1986) or from low resolution, two- or three-dimensional spectroscopic images (Brown et al., 1982). The sensitivity of phosphorus spectroscopy can be increased by the proton decoupling technique which reduces the magnetic interactions between protons and phosphorus containing nuclei that result in peak splittings (Luyten et al., 1989; Murphy-Boesch et al., 1993). The line narrowing effect of proton decoupling allows the resolution of the phospholipid precursors, phosphocholine (PC) and phosphoethanolamine (PE), in the PME peak and the phospholipid breakdown products, glycerophosphocholine (GPC) and glycerophosphoethanolamine (GPE), in the PDE peak (Fig. 8).

In vivo proton (^{1}H) MR spectroscopy provides a means to detect and quantify a number of cerebral metabolites, including *N*-acetylaspartate (NAA), creatine/phosphocreatine (Cre), cytosolic choline compounds (Cho), and myoinositol (mI). Approximate gray matter concentrations of these metabolites are: NAA, 8–11 m*M*; Cre, 6–7 m*M*; Cho, 0.9–1.4 m*M*; and mI 4–5 m*M* (Pouwels and Frahm, 1998). NAA contributes the largest signal to water-suppressed cerebral spectra and is found primarily in neurons (Birken and Oldendorf, 1989; Tsai and Coyle, 1995). Consequently, the NAA resonance has been viewed as a neuronal marker by a number of investigators.

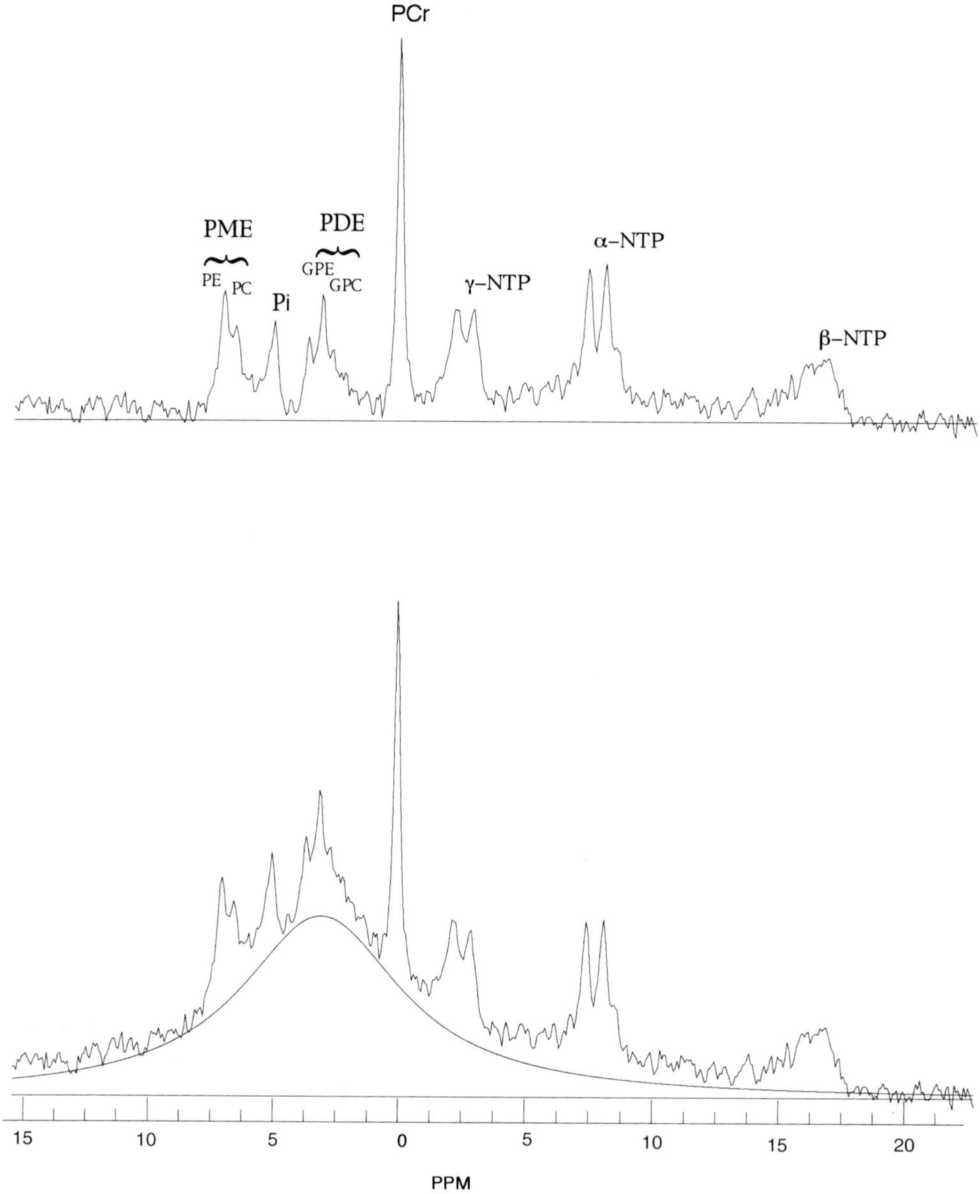

Fig. 8. Proton-decoupled, ^{31}P MR spectrum from a 5-cm thick axial brain slice. Data were acquired from a healthy 32-yr-old volunteer. **Top:** Metabolite resonances arising from relatively mobile compounds. **Bottom:** Subtraction of a broad resonance that derives from phospholipids.

Phosphocreatine is a high-energy phosphate and the Cre resonance has been used as a reference standard, reflecting the fact that the total concentration of creatine and phosphocreatine is similar in many brain regions, although it is slightly higher in cerebral cortex than in white matter (Petroff et al., 1989). Most of the choline in the brain is incorporated in the membrane lipid phosphatidylcholine, which undergoes a restricted

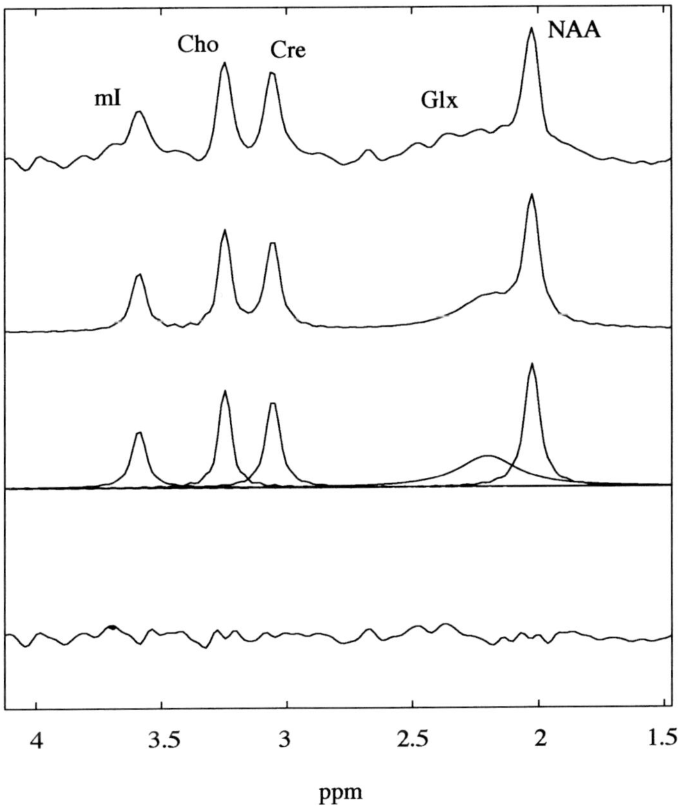

Fig. 9. Proton MR spectrum from a 2 cm^3 volume centered on the left anterior cingulate cortex. The top line displays the actual spectrum, the middle two lines demonstrate fit spectrum and individual resonance lines, and the bottom trace displays residual signal after fit. Data were obtained from a healthy 22-yr-old volunteer.

range of motion and, therefore, is largely invisible to in vivo MRS (Miller, 1991). The major contributors to the Cho peak are phosphocholine and glycerophosphocholine (Barker et al., 1994). Myoinositol is involved in phospholipid metabolism as well as in the maintenance of osmotic equilibrium (Moore et al., 1999).

Proton MRS is complicated by the fact that the signals from most metabolites of interest are five orders of magnitude smaller than the signals arising from tissue water and lipid. However, effective methods for the routine suppression of water signals have been reduced to practice (e.g., Haase et al., 1985; Doddrell et al., 1986). Using a 1.5 T MR scanner, metabolite information can be obtained from brain volumes on the order of 1–10 cm^3. The relatively high spatial resolution of proton MRS makes it possible to distinguish metabolite differences in gray and white matter (Pouwels and Frahm, 1998), although relatively few studies to date have reported segmented imaging data in conjunction with metabolite information (Renshaw et al., 1997; Lim et al., 1998) (Fig. 9).

Some metabolites, such as glutamine, glutamate, and GABA, are present at relatively high concentrations in brain but give rise to a broad, complex ^1H MRS resonance with multiple overlapping peaks. This composite resonance has sometimes

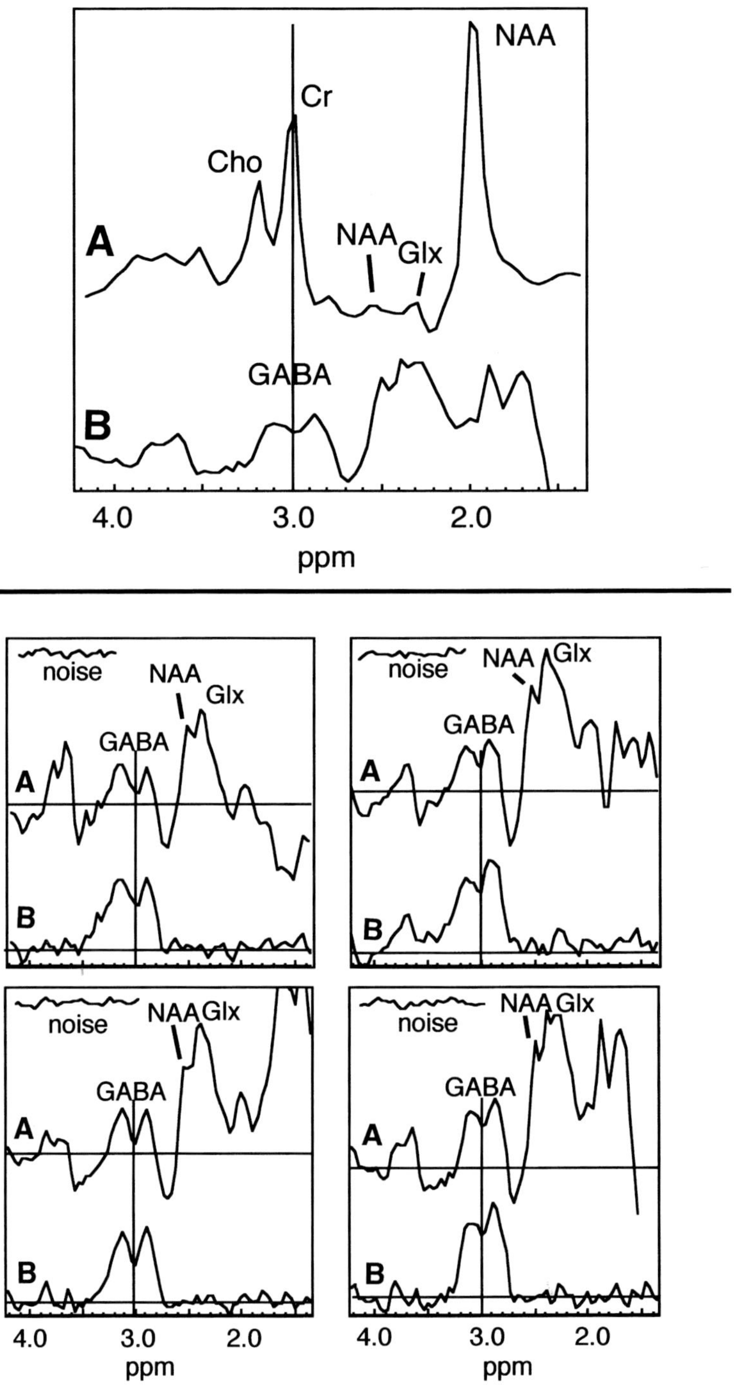

Fig. 10. The selective detection of MRS signals is facilitated by the use a double quantum filter, a spectral editing technique (Keltner et al., 1997). **Top:** A typical, single quantum MRS spectrum **(A)** and double quantum MR spectrum **(B)** with vertical scale expanded 12.5×. **Bottom:** Double quantum MR spectra before **(A)** and after **(B)** singular value decomposition to improve spectral analysis from each of 4 healthy volunteers. All spectra were obtained from a 42 cm^3 occipital cortex volume.

Fig. 11. First published magnetic resonance image showing two tubes of water. (From Lauterbur, 1973, with permission.)

been referred to as the "Glx" resonance (e.g., Prost et al., 1997; Thomas et al., 1998). However, it is possible to deconvolve these resonance lines using methods which allow the selective excitation of specific molecules, such as GABA (e.g., Keltner et al., 1996; Keltner et al., 1997) (Fig. 10). These methods are generally characterized by limited sensitivity, as the available MRS signal is not fully detected. Therefore, measurements of brain GABA levels are likely to be more reliable at higher field strengths.

Magnetic Resonance Imaging

Methods

In 1973, Lauterbur published the first magnetic resonance image (Lauterbur, 1973). In this experiment, systematic variation of magnetic field gradients was employed to allow the localization of two capillary tubes of water in a phantom (Fig. 11). In one dimension, the application of a magnetic field gradient across a sample prior to the application of an RF pulse provides a means to localize signals that come from different locations across the gradient (Fig. 12). In this case, the resonance frequency of a nuclear spin indicates its position along the gradient (this is known as frequency encoding).

In principle, one could imagine constructing a three dimensional image by applying combinations of linear gradients in each of three perpendicular planes sequentially. However, this is not efficient in terms of sampling times. A commonly used method is slice selective, spin echo imaging. In this technique, a gradient is applied during a RF excitation. As a result, only a slice of tissue is excited, rather than the entire volume. This reduces the imaging problem from three to two dimensions. Within this slice, a gradient is still applied during acquisition. Further spatial encoding is achieved through the application of a magnetic field gradient after the RF pulse but

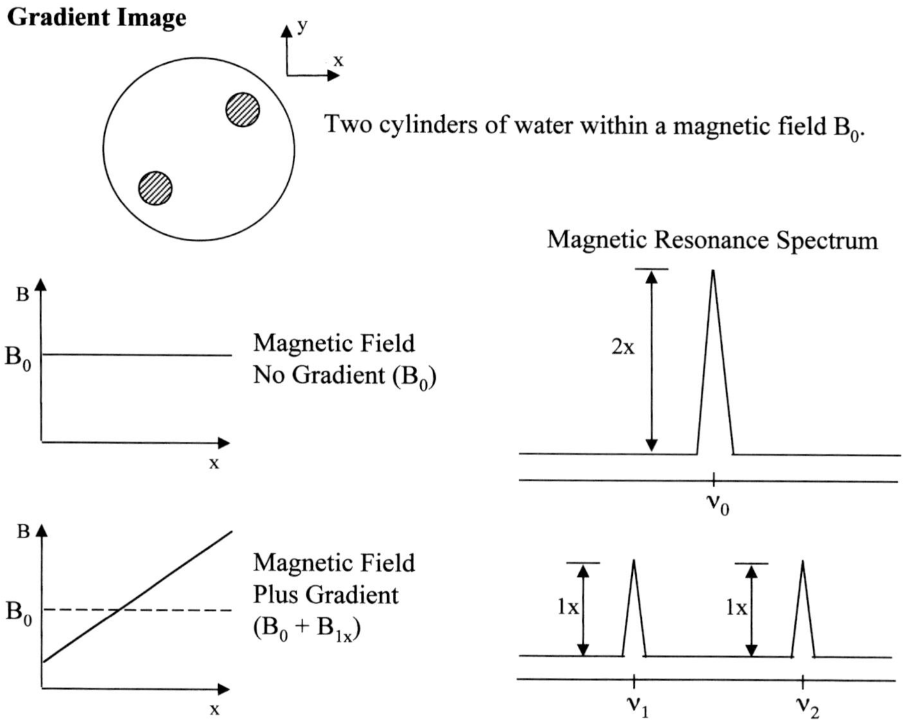

Fig. 12. Use of magnetic field gradients to provide spatial localization. The sample consists of two cylinders of water. When no gradient is applied, a simple spectrum containing a single water peak at resonance frequency ν_0 is observed. The application of a magnetic field gradient along the sample gives the water in each tube a separate resonance frequency which may be directly related to the total magnetic field at the location of each tube.

before the collection of the magnetic resonance signal on subsequent acquistions. In this instance, the excited spins at different points along the field gradient acquire a slightly different phase (this is known as phase encoding). By careful application of magnetic field gradients to allow both frequency and phase encoding, two-dimensional images may be constructed.

MRI produces images with excellent soft-tissue contrast, as well as excellent spatial resolution. MRI is especially sensitive to white matter lesions and provides excellent visualization of posterior fossa contents. Moreover, MRI data can be resliced in any plane without substantial loss of spatial resolution. Bone and other mineral deposits produce an MRI signal void, because the nuclei trapped in a solid matrix cannot be perturbed by the RF pulse. Fresh blood from an acute bleed (< 48–72 h) is not easily distinguished from gray matter, although subacute bleeding (< 48–72 h) or chronic hematomas can be reliably identified.

Image Contrast

It is also possible to vary the rate at which RF pulses are presented (TR, or repetition time) as well as the time that signals are collected (TE, or echo time). Thus,

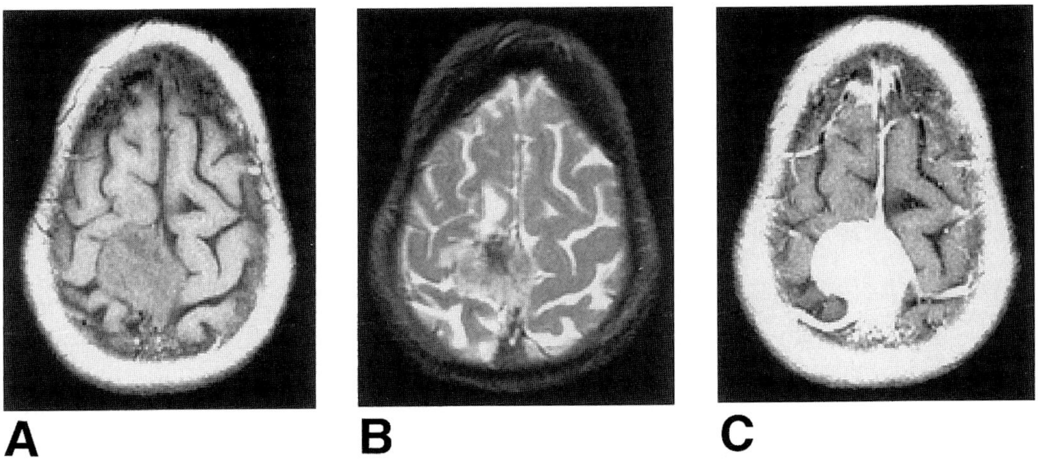

Fig. 13. T1-weighted **(A)**, T2-weighted **(B)**, and T1-weighted, postcontrast **(C)** images. These images were acquired from a 70-yr-old woman with a recent history of declining memory. An unsuspected meningioma was detected and is most visible in the contrast-enhanced images **(C)** as a very intense (white) area.

images may be obtained using different acquisition parameters and, in clinical practice, image sets are often referred to as being T1-weighted or T2-weighted. T1-weighted images appear to represent neuroanatomy with great clarity; gray matter is dark, white matter is light, and CSF is very dark. T2-weighted images look very different and are designed to highlight areas of pathology; regions which contain extravasated blood appear dark because of the paramagnetic effects of iron and regions containing tumor or edema appear light because of a relatively increased water content.

Contrast Agents

Contrast agents may be used to enhance MRI images (Bradley et al., 1993). Agents which have been approved for clinical use are strongly paramagnetic and contain chelated gadolinium. These agents work by altering the local magnetic environment and, by extension, tissue relaxation times. Contrast agents will diffuse from the intravascular to the extracellular space when there is some compromise of the blood brain barrier (e.g., in the case of cerebral neoplasm or inflammation, Fig. 13). MR contrast is well tolerated and the most common severe reaction is the induction of an asthma attack in patients with pre-existing reactive airway disease.

Contraindications

MRI does not require exposure to ionizing radiation. Thus, patients can safely have multiple serial scans without concerns about aggregate radiation dose. MRI, although probably quite safe, is still deemed relatively contraindicated during early pregnancy (Magin et al., 1992), but is preferable to ionizing radiation exposure. Because of the strong magnetic field associated with MRI, the presence of metallic implants of any kind are relative contraindications to MRI (Kanal and Shellock, 1994). Specifically, metal aneurysm clips can be twisted off, shrapnel remnants can be drawn through tissue and heated to scalding temperatures, and cardiac pacemakers can be deprogrammed or stimulated to misfire, all due to the force of the magnetic field. Metallic orthopedic pins, which are typically nonmagnetic, may be permissible as long as they are far from the site to be imaged, since although they will not pose substantial risk, they produce local image artifacts. Other equipment with metallic components is also prohibited from the scanner suite. Therefore, MRI may also be contraindicated for medical inpatients connected to ancillary devices (e.g., intravenous pumps, cardiac monitors, or respirators).

Claustrophobia

MRI scanner bores are usually 2–3 ft wide and several feet deep, thereby producing a considerable sense of confinement for many patients. This factor, coupled with the loud clanking noise of the scanner and scanning times from 20–40 min or more, cause ~10% of patients to report significant discomfort or anxiety, with up to 1% experiencing frank claustrophobic or panic reactions (Melendez and McCrank, 1993). Oral administration of a benzodiazepine or other sedative agent (i.e., alprazolam 0.5–1.0 mg or chloral hydrate 500–1000 mg) 30 min prior to beginning the scanning procedure is effective as prophylaxis against such anxiety reactions (Klein, 1991; Greenberg et al., 1993).

Functional Magnetic Resonance Imaging

Functional brain imaging studies have historically been limited both by the need to use radioactive tracers as well as by poor temporal resolution. Recent developments in the area of magnetic resonance imaging (MRI) may largely surmount these limitations. First, the development of high-speed, echo planar imaging (EPI) devices (Stehling et al., 1991) has greatly enhanced the temporal resolution of MRI. With EPI, single images can be acquired in 50–100 ms; multiple images can be acquired within one second. However, fMRI, which may be performed with or without a high speed MR scanner, selectively detects image parameters which are proportional to cerebral blood flow or blood volume. This strategy capitalizes on the fact that, in general, focal changes in neuronal activity are closely coupled to changes in cerebral blood flow (Fox et al., 1988) and blood volume (Fox and Raichle, 1986).

fMRI studies may be divided into two separate classes: (1) those that make use of endogenous physiological factors to detect changes in cerebral activation, the "noncontrast" techniques (Ogawa et al., 1990; Kwong et al., 1992), and (2) those that require the intravenous administration of a paramagnetic agent, the "contrast" techniques (Belliveau et al., 1990). Noncontrast techniques make use of either T1-weighted pulse sequences to detect changes in blood flow or, more commonly, T2-weighted pulse sequences to detect changes in the local concentration of paramagnetic deoxyhemoglobin. The latter method has been referred to as "blood oxygen-level-dependent" imaging (or BOLD). In a BOLD experiment, regional brain activation is associated with changes in both blood flow and blood volume, the magnitude of the former exceeding that of the latter (Fig. 14). This leads to a washout of paramagnetic deoxyhemoglobin, resulting in decreased phase dispersion of surrounding tissue proton molecules, and increased local signal intensity (Ogawa et al., 1992). One major drawback to BOLD studies is low sensitivity; at 1.5 T, the magnitude of the observed

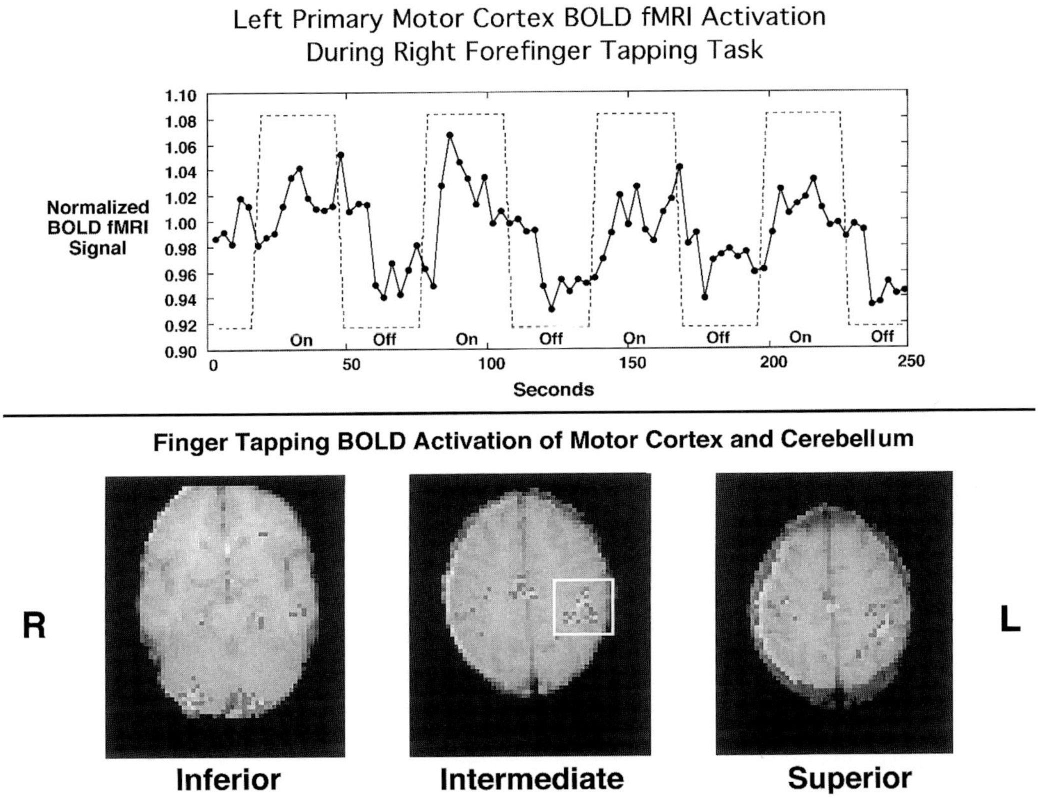

Fig. 14. Example of BOLD fMRI study in a single subject during finger tapping. This volunteer was asked to tap his right thumb and forefinger together for 30 s during "On" periods and then prompted to rest for 30 s during "Off" periods. **Top:** During finger tapping, an increase in image signal intensity occurs in the left primary motor cortex. Note the slight delay between the "On–Off" condition change and the BOLD signal intensity change which results from hemodynamic delay. **Bottom:** Cortical activation is mapped onto the axial MRI images. Activation occurs in the left motor cortex (white box in intermediate brain slice), on the midline in the supplementary motor cortex (intermediate and superior slices), and in both cerebellar hemispheres (bottom of inferior slice). The ipsilateral cerebellum has greater activation (bright or yellow) because cerebellar connections are not crossed. A, anterior; P, posterior; R, right side of head; L, left side of head. (Courtesy of J. M. Levin, M.D., M.P.H., Brain Imaging Center, McLean Hospital.) (*See* color plate 4 [top] appearing after p. 134)

signal intensity changes is relatively small. For instance, photic stimulation, which induces a 70% increase in occipital cortical blood flow, produces a 2–4% MR signal intensity increase on 1.5 T MR scanners (Kwong et al., 1992). However, the magnitude of the BOLD effect increases with field strength (Turner et al., 1993), and this has led to an increasing number of 3 and 4 T MR scanners at clinical research sites.

BOLD fMRI

Principles

The physiologic basis of BOLD is demonstrated in Fig. 15. The degree of BOLD signal intensity change is associated with changes both in cerebral blood flow and

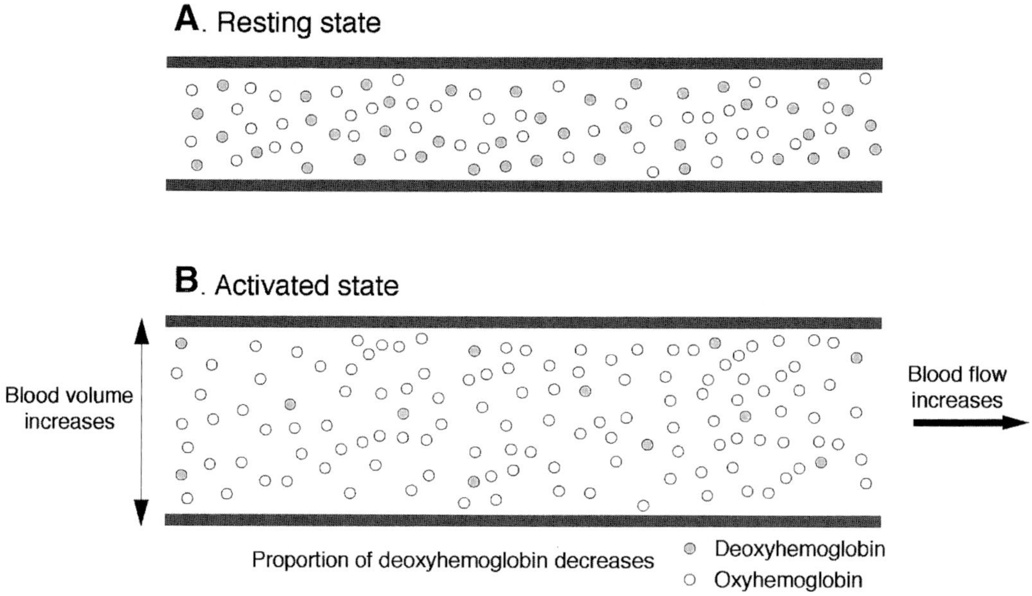

Fig. 15. Schematic of BOLD physiology. Activation of a local brain region, by either a task or a pharmacological challenge, is associated with increases in blood flow and volume which exceed the degree to which oxygen consumption is increased. Thus, there is a net "washout" of deoxyhemoglobin and an increase in image signal intensity.

blood volume, and does not correlate directly with either hemodynamic measure. Further, since BOLD signal intensity changes arise from a decrease in the local deoxyhemoglobin levels, states or disorders associated with altered hemoglobin levels may alter BOLD results. For example, men have greater hematocrits and larger BOLD signal changes in response to photic stimulation than women (Levin et al., 1998c). Similarly, hemodilution by the rapid infusion of intravenous saline is associated with decreased BOLD signal changes (Levin et al., 1998a).

In the context of trying to use fMRI to understand the effects of drugs of abuse on the brain, it is important to consider the fact that some drugs have direct effects on the cerebral vasculature (Iadecola, 1998; Krimer et al., 1998), which will also alter BOLD signals independent of neuronal activity levels. Evidence of such a pharmacological effect is provided by the recent observation that ethanol, a vasodilator, reduces BOLD signal intensity changes in response to photic stimulation after oral administration (Levin et al., 1998b) (Chapter 6, Fig. 4). Pharmacological vasoconstriction, induced by cocaine, has been associated with increased BOLD signal intensity change within 5 min of drug administration (Levin 1999). That finding stands in contrast to the report of unaltered BOLD signal intensity 25 min following cocaine administration (Gollub et al., 1998). These apparently divergent findings are, perhaps, best reconciled by the observation that plasma cocaine levels peak approximately six minutes following slow intravenous infusion (Sholar et al., 1998). Further evidence for the fact that vasoconstrictive drugs alter BOLD fMRI results has recently been reported by Zhang and colleagues (Zhang et al., 1998). These investigators noted that both cocaine methiodide, which does not cross the blood–brain barrier, and cocaine are associated with similar changes in image signal intensity following intravenous administration to rats.

Data Processing Methods

A number of analytic methods have been applied to fMRI data sets. For analyzing all of the information contained at each coordinate (pixel) of an image set ("pixel wise analysis"), three methods have been used most commonly: difference t-test methods, correlation coefficient analysis, and variants of Fourier analysis. In difference t-test methods, an averaged baseline image is subtracted from an averaged stimulus image, to create a pixel-by-pixel difference image between the baseline and activated states. Bright regions in the resulting difference image correspond to areas of activation. In correlation coefficient analysis, a correlation coefficient is computed between the time course of pixel signal intensity and a reference time function (Bandettini et al., 1993). The simplest case involves the use of a "box car" reference function, which models observed activation as a simple on–off phenomenon. In this case, t-test methods and correlation coefficient analyses are equivalent. However, more complicated models, which take into account the temporal relationship between neuronal activation and altered cerebral hemodynamics, may provide a more sensitive analysis. Finally, analytic methods which assess the frequency of stimulus switching (Fourier methods) have also been proposed (Bullmore et al., 1996). At the present time, MR scanners capable of acquiring echo planar images are increasingly common, and packages for processing and analyzing fMRI data from both commercial vendors and academic centers have become available (reviewed by Gold et al., 1998).

Advantages and Limitations

Compared with other functional brain imaging methods, BOLD fMRI is characterized by relatively high spatial resolution, on the order of one millimeter in plane (Raichle, 1998). Consequently, as noted by Hajnal, these data are also very sensitive to motion artifacts which may be correlated with the presentation of stimuli (Hajnal et al., 1994). To correct for small degrees of in plane motion, novel methods for the post processing of motion artifacts have been developed (e.g., Eddy et al., 1996; Maas et al., 1997a). Unfortunately, it is not possible to correct BOLD fMRI time series data for motion which exceeds 1–2 mm in translation or 1–2° in rotation or out of plane motion and, in practice, a fair number of data sets must be excluded from analysis (e.g., Breiter et al., 1997). Additionally, physiologic sources such as respiratory and cardiac effects induce BOLD signal changes of magnitudes similar to those produced by brain activation, and techniques for removing such signals have been reported (e.g., Biswal et al., 1996; Buonocore and Maddock, 1997).

Even with good processing tools, a fundamental limitation to the spatial resolution of BOLD fMRI arises from the fact that changes in signal intensity due to a washout of deoxyhemoglobin are most easily detected in blood vessels, which may be distant from the actual site of brain activation (Ogawa et al., 1998). In addition, magnetic field variations across the brain, which are generally largest in those regions which lie next to air filled sinuses, may lead to distortions in echo planar images (Jezzard and Balaban, 1995). The significance of these limitations in practice is not entirely clear. In studies designed to compare fMRI results with PET measures, relatively good agreement has been reported (Sadato et al., 1997; Ojemann et al., 1998; Xiong et al., 1998). In addition, early efforts to develop "real time" fMRI methods to provide functional information during neurosurgery have been encouraging (Schulder et al., 1997; Gering and Weber, 1998).

Another important advantage of BOLD fMRI, relative to emission tomography, is improved temporal resolution (Ogawa et al., 1998). In practice, the temporal resolution of BOLD fMRI, on the order of seconds, is limited primarily by human physiology, rather than MR scanner hardware. Following the presentation of a target stimulus, detection of relevant image signal intensity changes is complicated by the poorly understood hemodynamic transfer function, which describes the relationship between neuronal activation and the blood flow and volume changes which regulate the activation-induced signal changes (Kim et al., 1997; Frank et al., 1998; Fransson et al., 1998). Lags of 4 to 8 s from the onset or termination of the stimulus to the corresponding change in signal intensity (Fig. 14) are generally observed in fMRI data (Lee et al., 1995; Jezzard and Song, 1996). As the factors which influence the hemodynamic transfer function are more clearly defined, it is likely that further improvements in the temporal resolution of BOLD fMRI will be realized.

Dynamic Susceptibility Contrast MRI

Principles

Dynamic susceptibility contrast MRI (DSC MRI) is a tracer kinetic technique. It utilizes the bolus injection of a paramagnetic contrast agent to produce changes in tissue magnetic susceptibility and MR image intensity (Belliveau et al., 1990). During the first pass of the contrast agent, MR signal intensity may decrease by as much as 20–40%. This method may be used to map the distribution of cerebral blood volume (CBV) at rest (Fig. 16), or to measure changes in response to cerebral activation (Belliveau et al., 1991). Resting CBV maps have been shown to correlate well with PET images of fluorodeoxyglucose uptake (Gonzalez et al., 1995), and early reports suggest that CBV mapping may be useful in assessing persons with central nervous system tumors (Aronen et al., 1995), stroke (Warach et al., 1996), epilepsy (Warach et al., 1994), dementia (Harris et al., 1996; Maas et al., 1997b), and psychotic disorders (Cohen et al., 1995; Loeber et al., 1999).

In 1991, Belliveau and colleagues (Belliveau et al., 1991) produced the first functional MR images of brain activation with photic stimulation using DSC MRI. In that study, DSC MR images were acquired using multiple doses of contrast agent administered both before and during a period of photic stimulation. By comparing the image sets, it was possible to localize the activated primary visual cortex (V1) and to estimate the increase in cerebral blood volume. While the reported location of V1 was in excellent agreement with locations calculated on the basis of prior PET studies, the estimated increase in regional CBV (32 ± 10%) was somewhat larger than that which might have been predicted on the basis of earlier work. However, Runge and colleagues subsequently demonstrated in cats that the use of repeated doses of contrast agent in

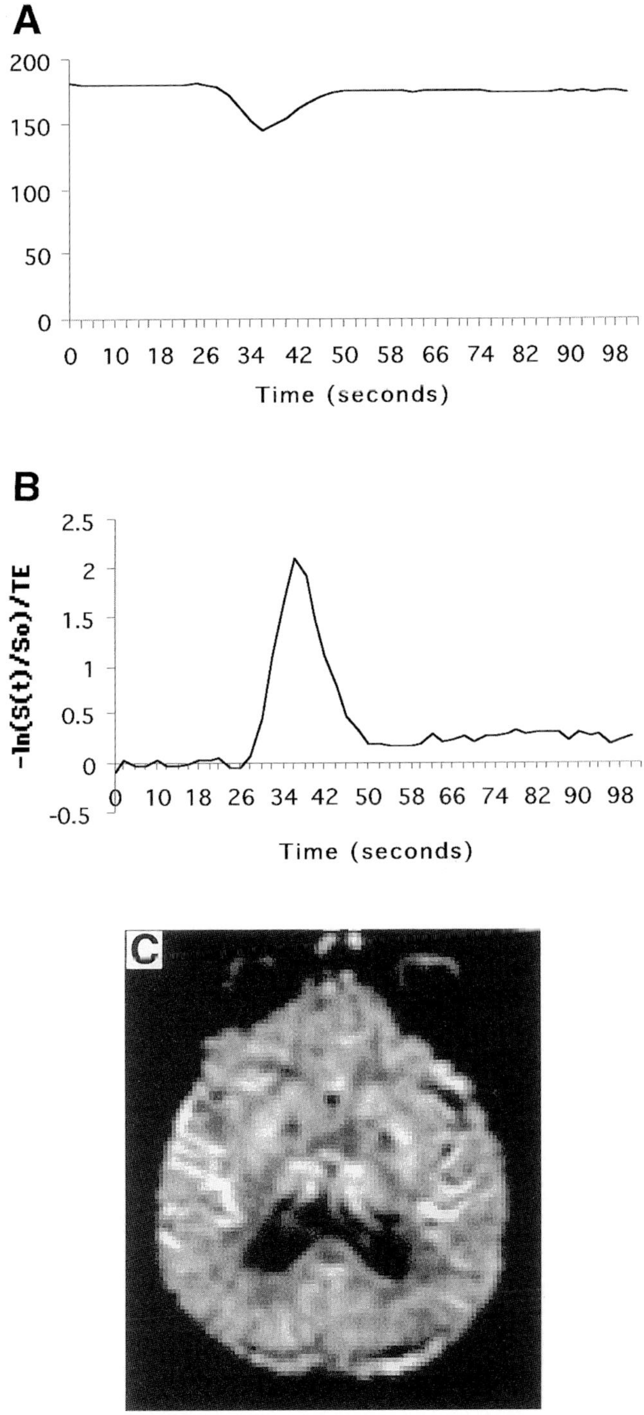

Fig. 16. DSC MRI. **A**: The decrease in image signal intensity associated with the bolus administration and first pass of a paramagnetic contrast agent through the cerebral vasculature. **B**: These data may be transformed to produce a measure that is proportional to cerebral blood volume (CBV) (Belliveau et al., 1990). **C**: The numerical data have been integrated to produce an axial brain map of CBV; the top and bottom represent anterior and posterior portions of brain, respectively. CBV is high in cortical regions and is absent from the centrally located ventricles.

multiple bolus DSC MRI experiments is associated with persistent effects resulting from initial contrast injections on image intensity (Runge et al., 1994).

In order to minimize the artifacts associated with repeated contrast injections, Levin and colleagues investigated the properties of multiple injections of gadoteridol on serial measurements of CBV in man (Levin et al., 1995). By using four injections of gadoteridol (0.075 m*M*/kg), the effects of prior contrast administration, which are pronounced between the first and second injections, are attenuated substantially between the second and third injections and between the third and fourth injections. This multiple bolus method can be used to make measurements of pharmacological activation. Specifically, a 21% increase in relative CBV was calculated following an intravenous injection of the potent vasodilator acetazolamide, a value that agrees well with other, more invasive methods for measuring CBV (Levin et al., 1995). Global decreases and increases in relative CBV, soon after the intravenous administration of cocaine (Kaufman et al., 1998) and alprazolam (Streeter et al., 1998), respectively, have also been reported.

Limitations

As with BOLD fMRI, DSC MRI is also associated with some inherent limitations. For example, the method provides only a relative, as opposed to an absolute, measure of CBV. In principle, quantitative measurements of CBV and cerebral blood flow (CBF) could be made if the arterial input function could be determined (Rempp et al., 1994). However, in practice it is very difficult to measure an input function which is appropriate for distinct brain regions (Weisskoff et al., 1993). A second limitation to DSC MRI arises from the fact that cerebral vascular tone changes in response to factors other than a local increase in neuronal activity, such as hypercapnea or the direct effects of drugs (Levin et al., 1995).

Other Magnetic Resonance Methods

The biomedical application of magnetic resonance methods is continuing to advance at a rapid pace. Therefore, a brief summary of several emerging methodologies is provided.

Diffusion Weighted Imaging

Diffusion weighted imaging (DWI) provides a means to obtain images which are sensitive to the molecular motion of water (Le Bihan et al., 1992). DWI capitalizes on the fact that as water diffuses across magnetic field gradients, MR signals from water molecules tend to dephase and to disappear (relax) more quickly. The rate at which this dephasing occurs is proportional to the strength of the magnetic field gradient as well as the rate of diffusion.

DWI has recently become a popular method to evaluate individuals who are in the early stages of a cerebral infarction (Warach et al., 1992). During episodes of cerebral ischemia, water protons diffuse more slowly and this may be reflected using DWI. Evaluating the extent to which DWI may be used to monitor the evolution of strokes, as well as the effects of putative therapies, is currently an area of active research (Lo et al., 1994).

Magnetic Resonance Angiography

Magnetic resonance angiography (MRA) is a noninvasive technique that uses the magnetic resonance signal from flowing blood to create an image of cerebral vasculature. Several techniques can be used to acquire MRA images, including phase contrast angiography and three-dimensional time of flight (3DTOF) angiography. With the 3DTOF technique, stationary tissue (e.g., brain) has its magnetization saturated and produces minimal signal. Tissue that is in motion at slow velocities (venous blood) also gives off minimal signal. Only blood flowing at high velocity (arterial blood) gives off substantial MR signal. Acquisition parameters can be programmed so that selective images of blood flow in arteries or veins can be made. MRA techniques are highly sensitive to blood flow perturbations which reduce vessel signal intensity. When blood flows past a vessel narrowing (stenotic region), a portion slows down because of local turbulence, while a portion (toward the middle of the vessel) speeds up. The decelerated blood has its magnetization saturated and also loses phase coherence, while the accelerated blood loses phase coherence, and these effects result in lower blood flow signal.

The 3DTOF technique acquires multiple thin slice (~1.5 mm thick) images of brain which are used to reconstruct composite images of the brain vascular system. The composite images are known as maximum intensity projections (MIPs) and include only the brightest pixels from each source image which presumably are from flowing blood. It is possible to produce maximum intensity projection images in many different orientations using 3DTOF data. Angiographic techniques may be particularly useful in characterizing the blood flow abnormalities associated with acute and chronic drug abuse.

Relaxometry

By varying the image acquisition parameters, TR (pulse repetition time) and TE (echo time), it is possible to construct images of the proton relaxation times T1 and T2. The development of methods for echo planar imaging makes it possible to collect images with a large number of TR and/or TE values quite rapidly and, thereby, to estimate localized T1 and T2 values very reliably. This relaxation time mapping is sometimes referred to as relaxometry.

Changes in relaxation times may reflect anomalous cerebral development, as recently demonstrated in schizophrenia (Andreasen et al., 1991; Williamson et al., 1992; Yurgelun-Todd et al., 1995). Alternatively, alterations in cerebral perfusion may lead to small changes in T2 which can be detected using echo planar imaging (Teicher et al., 2000). In the area of substance abuse, relaxation time measurements have also been used to assess brain hydration. In general, as brain water content decreases, relaxation times become shorter.

Magnetization Transfer

Within the brain, water molecules often interact with other, larger molecules due to dipolar effects, such as hydrogen bonding. Water which is "bonded" to a larger molecule will have very different magnetic resonance properties than "free" water. In particular, bonded water tends to have very short relaxation times and, in a magnetic resonance spectrum, a very wide resonance peak. Thus, irradiation at a frequency which is quite different from the resonance frequency of the free water pool can sometimes excite the bonded water pool. This effect is referred to as magnetization transfer (MT). Assessment of MT effects may be used to characterize the interactions of both water and ethanol with brain macromolecules.

Summary

The phenomenon of nuclear magnetic resonance was first demonstrated approximately 60 years ago. A series of remarkable technical advances, all based on a similar set of physical principles, has made it possible to obtain noninvasive measures of brain anatomy, chemistry, and function. While these emerging techniques have not been widely employed by substance abuse researchers, preliminary results have been extremely encouraging (see Chapter 6). Although many aspects of addiction can be modeled in cellular and animal systems, observations derived from human subjects with drug abuse and dependence may be especially important for efforts to improve our understanding of these disorders and to improve treatments.

Acknowledgments

We thank Ms. Rosemond A. Villafuerte and Ms. Jeannette Y. Bang for their assistance in the preparation of this manuscript, and would like to thank the National Institute on Drug Abuse for grant support (DA 09448).

References

Ackerman, J. J. H., Grove, T. H., Wong, G. G., Gadian, D. G. and Radda, G. K., Mapping of metabolites in whole animals by ^{31}P NMR using surface coils. Nature 283:167–170, 1980.

Alger, J. R., Behar, K. L., Rothman, D. L. and Shulman, R. G., Natural-abundance ^{13}C NMR measurement of hepatic glycogen in the living rabbit. J. Magn. Reson. 56:334–337, 1984.

Andreasen, N. C., Ehrhardt, J. C., Swayze, V. W., 2nd., Tyrrell, G., Cohen, G., Ku, J. S. and Arndt, S., T1 and T2 relaxation times in schizophrenia as measured with magnetic resonance imaging. Schizophrenia Res. 5:223–232, 1991.

Arnold, J. T., Dharmatti, S. S. and Packard, M. E., Chemical effects on nuclear induction signals from organic compounds. J. Chem. Phys. 19:507, 1951.

Aronen, H. J., Glass, J., Pardo, F. S., Belliveau, J. W., Gruber, M. L., Buchbinder, B. R., Gazit, I. E., Linggood, R. M., Fischman, A., Rosen, B. R. and Hochberg, F. H., Echo-planar MR cerebral blood volume mapping of gliomas: clinical utility. Acta Radiol. 36:520–528, 1995.

Balschi, J. A., Cirillo, V. P. and Springer, C. S. J., Direct high-resolution nuclear magnetic resonance studies of cation transport in vivo, Na^+ transport in yeast cells. Biophys. J. 38:323–326, 1982.

Bandettini, P. A., Jesmanowicz, A., Wong, E. C. and Hyde, J. S., Processing strategies for time-course data sets in functional MRI of the human brain. Magn. Reson. Med. 30:161–173, 1993.

Barker, P. B., Breiter, S. N., Soher, B. J., Chatham, J. C., Forder, J. R., Samphilipo, M. A., Magee, C. A. and Anderson, J. H., Quantitative proton spectroscopy of canine brain: in vivo and in vitro correlations. Magn. Reson. Med. 32:157–163, 1994.

Belliveau, J. W., Rosen, B. R., Kantor, H. L., Rzedzian, R. R., Kennedy, D. N., McKinstry, R. C., Vevea, J. M., Cohen, M. S., Pykett, I. L. and Brady, T. J., Functional cerebral imaging by susceptibility-contrast NMR. Magn. Reson. Med. 14:538–546, 1990.
Belliveau, J. W., Kennedy, D. N. J., McKinstry, R. C., Buchbinder, B. R., Weisskoff, R. M., Cohen, M. S., Vevea, J. M., Brady, T. J. and Rosen, B. R., Functional mapping of the human visual cortex by magnetic resonance imaging. Science 254:716–719, 1991.
Birken, D. L. and Oldendorf, W. H., N-acetyl-L-aspartic acid: a literature review of a compound prominent in ^{1}H-NMR spectroscopic studies of brain. Neurosci. Biobehav. Rev. 13:23–31, 1989.
Biswal, B., DeYoe, A. E. and Hyde, J. S., Reduction of physiological fluctuations in fMRI using digital filters. Magn. Reson. Med. 35:107–113, 1996.
Bloch, F., Hansen, W. W. and Packard, M., Nuclear induction. Phys. Rev. 69:127, 1946.
Boada, F. E., Gillen, J. S., Shen, G. X., Chang, S. Y. and Thulborn, K. R., Fast three dimensional sodium imaging. Magn. Reson. Med. 37:706–715, 1997.
Bottomley, P. A., Foster, T. B. and Darrow, R. D., Depth-resolved surface coil spectroscopy (DRESS) for in vivo ^{1}H, ^{31}P and ^{13}C NMR. J. Magn. Reson. 59:338–343, 1984.
Bracewell, R. N., The Fourier Transform and Its Applications. Singapore, McGraw-Hill Book Company, 1986.
Bradley, W. G. J., Yuh, W. T. and Bydder, G. M., Use of MR imaging contrast agents in the brain. J. Magn. Reson. Imaging 3:199–218, 1993.
Breiter, H. C., Gollub, R. L., Weisskoff, R. M., Kennedy, D. N., Makris, N., Berke, J. D., Goodman, J. M., Kantor, H. L., Gastfriend, D. R., Riorden, J. P., Mathew, R. T., Rosen, B. R. and Hyman, S. E., Acute effects of cocaine on human brain activity and emotion. Neuron 19:591–611, 1997.
Brown, T. R., Kincaid, B. M. and Ugurbil, K., NMR chemical shift imaging in three dimensions. Proc. Natl. Acad. Sci. USA 79:3523–3526, 1982.
Buchli, R., Duc, C. O., Martin, E. and Boesiger, P., Assessment of absolute metabolite concentrations in human tissue by ^{31}P MRS in vivo. Part I: Cerebrum, cerebellum, cerebral gray and white matter. Magn. Reson. Med. 32:447–452, 1994.
Bullmore, E., Brammer, M., Williams, S. C., Rabe-Hesketh, S., Janot, N., David, A., Mellers, J., Howard, R. and Sham, P., Statistical methods of estimation and inference for functional MR image analysis. Magn. Reson. Med. 35:261–277, 1996.
Buonocore, M. H. and Maddock, R. J., Noise suppression digital filter for functional magnetic resonance imaging based on image reference data. Magn. Reson. Med. 38:56–69, 1997.
Christensen, J. D., Babb, S. M., Cohen, B. M. and Renshaw, P. F., Quantitation of dexfenfluramine/d-norfenfluramine concentration in primate brain using ^{19}F NMR spectroscopy. Magn. Reson. Med. 39:149–154, 1998.
Christensen, J. D., Yurgelun-Todd, D. A., Babb, S. M., Gruber, S., Cohen, B. M. and Renshaw, P. F., Measurement of human brain dexfenfluramine concentration by ^{19}F magnetic resonance spectroscopy. Brain Res. 834:1–5, 1999.
Cohen, B. M., Yurgelun-Todd, D. A., English, C. D. and Renshaw, P. F., Abnormalities of regional distribution of cerebral vasculature in schizophrenia detected by dynamic susceptibility contrast MRI. Am. J. Psychiatry 152:1801–1803, 1995.
Cohen, S. M., Shulman, R. G. and McLaughlin, A. C., Effects of ethanol on alanine metabolism in perfused mouse liver studied by ^{13}C NMR. Proc. Natl. Acad. Sci. USA 76:4808–4812, 1979.
Doddrell, D. M., Galloway, G., Brooks, W., Field, J., Bulsing, J., Irving, M. and Baddeley, H., Water signal elimination in vivo using suppression by mistimed echo and repetitive gradient episodes. J. Magn. Reson. 70:176–180, 1986.
Eddy, W. F., Fitzgerald, M. and Noll, D. C., Improved image registration by using Fourier interpolation. Magn. Reson. Med. 36:923–931, 1996.

Ernst, R. R. and Anderson, W. A., Application of Fourier transform spectroscopy to magnetic resonance. Rev. Sci. Inst. 37:93–102, 1966.

Farrar, T. C., An introduction to pulse NMR spectroscopy. The Farragut Press, Madison, 1989.

Fox, P. T. and Raichle, M. E., Focal physiological uncoupling of cerebral blood flow and oxidative metabolism during somatosensory stimulation in human subjects. Proc. Natl. Acad. Sci. USA 83:1140–1144, 1986.

Fox, P. T., Raichle, M. E., Mintun, M. A. and Dence, C., Nonoxidative glucose consumption during focal physiologic neural activity. Science 241:462–464, 1988.

Frank, L. R., Buxton, R. B. and Wong, E. C., Probabilistic analysis of functional magnetic resonance imaging data. Magn. Reson. Med. 39:132–148, 1998.

Fransson, P., Kruger, G., Merboldt, K. D. and Frahm, J., Temporal characteristics of oxygenation-sensitive MRI responses to visual activation in humans. Magn. Reson. Med. 39:912–919, 1998.

Gering, D. T. and Weber, D. M., Intraoperative, real-time, functional MRI. J. Magn. Reson. Imaging 8:254–257, 1998.

Gold, S., Christian, B., Arndt, S., Zeien, G., Cizadlo, T., Johnson, D. L., Flaum, M. and Andreasen, N. C., Functional MRI statistical software packages: a comparative analysis. Human Brain Mapping 6:73–84, 1998.

Gollub, R. L., Breiter, H. C., Kantor, H., Kennedy, D., Gastfriend, D., Mathew, R. T., Makris, N., Guimaraes, A., Riorden, J., Campbell, T., Foley, M., Hyman, S. E., Rosen, B. and Weisskoff, R., Cocaine decreases cortical cerebral blood flow but does not obscure regional activation in functional magnetic resonance imaging in human subjects. J. Cereb. Blood Flow Metab. 18:724–734, 1998.

Gonzalez, R. G., Guimaraes, A. R., Sachs, G. S., Rosenbaum, J. F., Garwood, M. and Renshaw, P. F., Measurement of human brain lithium in vivo by MR spectroscopy. AJNR Am. J. Neuroradiol. 14:1027–1037, 1993.

Gonzalez, R. G., Fischman, A. J., Guimaraes, A. R., Carr, C. A., Stern, C. E., Halpern, E. F., Growdon, J. H. and Rosen, B. R., Functional MR in the evaluation of dementia: correlation of abnormal dynamic cerebral blood volume measurements with changes in cerebral metabolism on positron emission tomography with fluorodeoxyglucose [F 18]. AJNR Am. J. Neuroradiol. 16:1763–1770, 1995.

Greenberg, S. B., Faerber, E. N., Aspinall, C. L. and Adams, R. C., High-dose chloral hydrate sedation for children undergoing MR imaging: safety and efficacy in relation to age. AJR Am J. Roentgenol. 161:639–641, 1993.

Gupta, R. K. and Gupta, P., Direct observation of resolved resonances from intra- and extracellular sodium-23 ions in NMR studies of intact cells and tissues using dysprosium(III)tripolyphosphate as paramagnetic shift reagent. J. Magn. Reson. 47:344–350, 1982.

Haase, A., Frahm, J., Hanicke, W. and Matthaei, D., ^{1}H NMR chemical shift selective (CHESS) imaging. Physics Med. Biol. 30:341–344, 1985.

Hajnal, J. V., Myers, R., Oatridge, A., Schwieso, J. E., Young, I. R. and Bydder, G. M., Artifacts due to stimulus correlated motion in functional imaging of the brain. Magn. Reson. Med. 31:283–291, 1994.

Harris, G. J., Lewis, R. F., Satlin, A., English, C. D., Scott, T. M., Yurgelun-Todd, D. A. and Renshaw, P. F., Dynamic susceptibility contrast MRI of regional cerebral blood volume in Alzheimer's disease. Am. J. Psychiatry 153:721–724, 1996.

Hoult, D. I., Busby, S. J. W., Gadian, D. G., Radda, G. K., Richards, R. E. and Seeley, P. J., Observation of tissue metabolites using ^{31}P nuclear magnetic resonance. Nature 252:285–287, 1974.

Iadecola, C., Neurogenic control of the cerebral microcirculation: is dopamine minding the store? Nat. Neurosci. 1:263–265, 1998.

Jezzard, P. and Balaban, R. S., Correction for geometric distortion in echo planar images from B_0 field variations. Magn. Reson. Med. 34:65–73, 1995.

Jezzard, P. and Song, A. W., Technical foundations and pitfalls of clinical fMRI. Neuroimage 4:S63–S75, 1996.

Kanal, E. and Shellock, F. G., The value of published data on MR compatibility of metallic implants and devices. AJNR Am. J. Neuroradiol. 15:1394–1396, 1994.

Kaufman, M. J., Levin, J. M., Maas, L. C., Rose, S. L., Lukas, S. E., Mendelson, J. H., Cohen, B. M. and Renshaw, P. F., Cocaine decreases relative cerebral blood volume in humans: a dynamic susceptibility contrast magnetic resonance imaging study. Psychopharmacology (Berl.) 138:76–81, 1998.

Keltner, J. R., Wald, L. L., Christensen, J. D., Maas, L. C., Moore, C. M., Cohen, B. M. and Renshaw, P. F., A technique for detecting GABA in the human brain with PRESS localization and optimized refocusing spectral editing radiofrequency pulses. Magn. Reson. Med. 36:458–461, 1996.

Keltner, J. R., Wald, L. L., Frederick, B. de B. and Renshaw, P. F., In vivo detection of GABA in human brain using a localized double-quantum filter technique. Magn. Reson. Med. 37:366–371, 1997.

Kim, S. G., Richter, W. and Ugurbil, K., Limitations of temporal resolution in functional MRI. Magn. Reson. Med. 37:631–636, 1997.

Klein, D. S., Prevention of claustrophobia induced by MR imaging: use of alprazolam. AJR Am. J. Roentgenol. 156:633, 1991.

Komoroski, R. A., Newton, J. E., Karson, C., Cardwell, D. and Sprigg, J., Detection of psychoactive drugs in vivo in humans using ^{19}F NMR spectroscopy. Biol. Psychiatry 29:711–714, 1991.

Krimer, L. S., Muly, E. C., Williams, G. V. and Goldman-Rakic, P. S., Dopaminergic regulation of cerebral cortical microcirculation. Nat. Neurosci. 1:286–289, 1998.

Kwong, K. K., Belliveau, J. W., Chesler, D. A., Goldberg, I. E., Weisskoff, R. M., Poncelet, B. P., Kennedy, D. N., Hoppel, B. E., Cohen, M. S., Turner, R., Cheng, H.-M., Brady, T J. and Rosen, B. R., Dynamic magnetic resonance imaging of human brain activity during primary sensory stimulation. Proc. Natl. Acad. Sci. USA 89:5675–5679, 1992.

Lauterbur, P. C., Image formation by induced local interactions: examples employing nuclear magnetic resonance. Nature 242:190–191, 1973.

Le Bihan, D., Turner, R., Douek, P. and Patronas, N., Diffusion MR imaging: clinical applications. AJR Am. J. Roentgenol. 159:591–599, 1992.

Lee, A. T., Glover, G. and Meyer, C. H., Discrimination of large venous vessels in time-course spiral blood-oxygen-level-dependent magnetic resonance functional neuroimaging. Magn. Reson. Med. 33:745–754, 1995.

Levin, J. M., Kaufman, M. J., Ross, M. H., Mendelson, J. H., Maas, L. C., Cohen, B. M. and Renshaw, P. F., Sequential dynamic susceptibility contrast MR experiments in human brain: residual contrast agent effect, steady state, and hemodynamic perturbation. Magn. Reson. Med. 34:655–663, 1995.

Levin, J. M., Ross, M. H., Kaufman, M. J., Lange, N., Frederick, B., von Rosenberg, H. L., Mendelson, J. H., Cohen, B. M. and Renshaw, P. F., BOLD fMRI signal depends upon baseline hemoglobin concentration. International Society for Magnetic Resonance in Medicine, Sixth Scientific Meeting and Exhibition.. Sydney, Australia, p. 13, 1998a.

Levin, J. M., Ross, M. H., Mendelson, J. H., Kaufman, M. J., Lange, N., Maas, L. C., Mello, N. K., Cohen, B. M. and Renshaw, P. F., Reduction in BOLD fMRI response to primary visual stimulation following alcohol ingestion. Psychiatry Res. 82:135–146, 1998b.

Levin, J. M., Ross, M. H., Mendelson, J. H., Mello, N. K., Cohen, B. M. and Renshaw, P. F., Sex differences in blood-oxygenation-level-dependent functional MRI with primary visual stimulation. Am. J. Psychiatry 155:434–436, 1998c.

Levin, J. M., Kaufman, M. J., Ross, M. H., Roc, A. C., Maas, L. C., Mendelson, J. H., Cohen, B. M. and Renshaw, P. F., Cocaine Increases BOLD fMRI Response to Photic Stimulation. International Society for Magnetic Resonance in Medicine, Seventh Scientific Meeting and Exhibition. Philadelphia, PA, p. 838, 1999.

Lim, K. O., Adalsteinsson, E., Spielman, D., Sullivan, E. V., Rosenbloom, M. J. and Pfefferbaum, A., Proton magnetic resonance spectroscopic imaging of cortical gray and white matter in schizophrenia. Arch. Gen. Psychiatry 55:346–352, 1998.

Lo, E. H., Matsumoto, K., Pierce, A. R., Garrido, L. and Luttinger, D., Pharmacologic reversal of acute changes in diffusion-weighted magnetic resonance imaging in focal cerebral ischemia. J. Cereb. Blood Flow Metab. 14:597–603, 1994.

Loeber, R. T., Sherwood, A. R., Renshaw, P. F., Cohen, B. M. and Yurgelun-Todd, D. A., Differences in cerebellar blood volume in schizophrenia and bipolar disorder. Schizophrenia Res. 37:81–89, 1999.

Luyten, P. R., Bruntink, G., Sloff, F. M., Vermeulen, J. W. A. H., van der Heijden, J. I., den Hollander, J. A. and Heerschap, A., Broadband proton decoupling in human ^{31}P NMR spectroscopy. NMR Biomed. 1:177–183, 1989.

Maas, L. C., Frederick, B. de B. and Renshaw, P. F., Decoupled automated rotational and translational registration for functional MRI time series data: the DART registration algorithm. Magn. Reson. Med. 37:131–139, 1997a.

Maas, L. C., Harris, G. J., Satlin, A., English, C. D., Lewis, R. F. and Renshaw, P. F., Regional cerebral blood volume measured by dynamic susceptibility contrast MR imaging in Alzheimer's disease: a principal components analysis. J. Magn. Reson. Imaging 7:215–219, 1997b.

Magin, R. L., Liburdy, R. P. and Persson, B. (eds.), Annals of the New York Academy of Science, vol. 649: Biological Effects and Safety Aspects of Nuclear Magnetic Resonance Imaging and Spectroscopy. New York Academy of Science, New York, 1992.

Mason, G. F., Behar, K. L. and Lai, J. C., The ^{13}C isotope and nuclear magnetic resonance: unique tools for the study of brain metabolism. Metab. Brain Dis. 11:283–313, 1996.

McCann, U., Hatzidimitriou, G., Ridenour, A., Fischer, C., Yuan, J., Katz, J. and Ricaurte, G., Dexfenfluramine and serotonin neurotoxicity: further preclinical evidence that clinical caution is indicated. J. Pharmacol. Exp. Ther. 269:792–798, 1994.

McCann, U. D., Seiden, L. S., Rubin, L. J. and Ricaurte, G. A., Brain serotonin neurotoxicity and primary pulmonary hypertension from fenfluramine and dexfenfluramine. A systematic review of the evidence. JAMA 278:666–672, 1997.

Melendez, C. and McCrank, E., Anxiety-related reactions associated with magnetic resonance imaging examinations. JAMA 270:745–747, 1993.

Miller, B. L., A review of chemical issues in ^{1}H NMR spectroscopy: N-acetyl aspartate, creatine, and choline. NMR Biomed. 4:47–54, 1991.

Moon, R. B. and Richards, J. H., Determination of intracellular pH by ^{31}P magnetic resonance. J. Biol. Chem. 248:7276–7278, 1973.

Moore, C. M., Breeze, J. L., Kukes, T. J., Rose, S. L., Dager, S. R., Cohen, B. M. and Renshaw, P. F., Effects of myo-inositol ingestion on human brain myo-inositol levels: a proton magnetic resonance spectroscopic imaging study. Biol. Psychiatry 45:1197–1202, 1999.

Murphy-Boesch, J., Stoyanova, R., Srinivasan, R., Willard, T., Vigneron, D., Nelson, S., Taylor, J. S. and Brown, T. R., Proton-decoupled ^{31}P chemical shift imaging of the human brain in normal volunteers. NMR Biomed. 6:173–180, 1993.

Odeblad, E. and Lindstrom, G., Some preliminary observations on the proton magnetic resonance in biologic samples. Acta Radiol. 43:469–476, 1955.

Ogawa, S., Lee, T. M., Kay, A. R. and Tank, D. W., Brain magnetic resonance imaging with contrast dependent on blood oxygenation. Proc. Natl. Acad. Sci. USA 87:9868–9872, 1990.

Ogawa, S., Tank, D. W., Menon, R., Ellermann, J. M., Kim, S. G., Merkle, H. and Ugurbil, K., Intrinsic signal changes accompanying sensory stimulation: functional brain mapping with magnetic resonance imaging. Proc. Natl. Acad. Sci. USA 89:5951–5955, 1992.

Ogawa, S., Menon, R. S., Kim, S. G. and Ugurbil, K., On the characteristics of functional magnetic resonance imaging of the brain. Ann. Rev. Biophys. Biomolec. Structure 27:447–474, 1998.

Ojemann, J. G., Buckner, R. L., Akbudak, E., Snyder, A. Z., Ollinger, J. M., McKinstry, R. C., Rosen, B. R., Petersen, S. E., Raichle, M. E. and Conturo, T. E., Functional MRI studies of word-stem completion: reliability across laboratories and comparison to blood flow imaging with PET. Human Brain Mapping 6:203–215, 1998.

Ordidge, R. J., Connelly, A. and Lohman, J. A. B., A general approach to selection of multiple cubic volume elements using the ISIS technique. J. Magn. Reson. 66:283–294, 1986.

Petroff, O. A. C., Spencer, D. D., Alger, J. R. and Prichard, J. W., High-field proton magnetic resonance spectrosocpy of human cerbrum obtained during surgery for epilepsy. Neurology 39:1197–1201, 1989.

Pettegrew, J. W., Keshavan, M. S., Panchalingam, K., Strychor, S., Kaplan, D. B., Tretta, M. G. and Allen, M., Alterations in brain high-energy phosphate and membrane phospholipid metabolism in first-episode, drug-naive schizophrenics. A pilot study of the dorsal prefrontal cortex by in vivo phosphorus 31 nuclear magnetic resonance spectroscopy. Arch. Gen. Psychiatry 48:563–568, 1991.

Pouwels, P. J. and Frahm, J., Regional metabolite concentrations in human brain as determined by quantitative localized proton MRS. Magn. Reson. Med. 39:53–60, 1998.

Prost, R. W., Mark, L., Mewissen, M. and Li, S. J., Detection of glutamate/glutamine resonances by ^{1}H magnetic resonance spectroscopy at 0.5 tesla. Magn. Reson. Med. 37:615–618, 1997.

Purcell, E. M., Torrey, H. C. and Pound, R. V., Resonance absorption by nuclear magnetic moments in a solid. Phys. Rev. 69:37–38, 1946.

Rabi, I. I., Zacharias, J. R., Millman, S. and Kusch, P., A new method of measuring nuclear magnetic moment. Phys. Rev. 53:318, 1938.

Radda, G. K., The use of NMR spectroscopy for the understanding of disease. Science 233:640–645, 1986.

Raichle, M. E., Behind the scenes of functional brain imaging: a historical and physiological perspective. Proc. Natl. Acad. Sci. USA 95:765–772, 1998.

Rempp, K. A., Brix, G., Wenz, F., Becker, C. R., Guckel, F. and Lorenz, W. J., Quantification of regional cerebral blood flow and volume with dynamic susceptibility contrast-enhanced MR imaging. Radiology 193:637–641, 1994.

Renshaw, P. F. and Wicklund, S., In vivo measurement of lithium in humans by nuclear magnetic resonance spectroscopy. Biol. Psychiatry 23:465–475, 1988.

Renshaw, P. F., Guimaraes, A. R., Fava, M., Rosenbaum, J. F., Pearlman, J. D., Flood, J. G., Puopolo, P. R., Clancy, K. and Gonzalez, R. G., Accumulation of fluoxetine and norfluoxetine in human brain during therapeutic administration. Am. J. Psychiatry 149:1592–1594, 1992.

Renshaw, P. F., Lafer, B., Babb, S. M., Fava, M., Stoll, A. L., Christensen, J. D., Moore, C. M., Yurgelun-Todd, D. A., Bonello, C. M., Pillay, S. S., Rothschild, A. J., Nierenberg, A. A., Rosenbaum, J. F. and Cohen, B. M., Basal ganglia choline levels in depression and response to fluoxetine treatment: an in vivo proton magnetic resonance spectroscopy study. Biol. Psychiatry 41:837–843, 1997.

Runge, V. M., Kirsch, J. E., Wells, J. W., Dunworth, J. N., Hilaire, L. and Woolfolk, C. E., Repeat cerebral blood volume assessment with first-pass MR imaging. J. Magn. Reson. Imaging 4:457–461, 1994.

Sadato, N., Ibanez, V., Campbell, G., Deiber, M. P., Le Bihan, D. and Hallett, M., Frequency-dependent changes of regional cerebral blood flow during finger movements: functional MRI compared to PET. J. Cereb. Blood Flow Metab. 17:670–679, 1997.

Schulder, M., Maldjian, J. A., Liu, W. C., Mun, I. K. and Carmel, P. W., Functional MRI-guided surgery of intracranial tumors. Stereotactic Funct. Neurosurgery 68:98–105, 1997.

Sholar, M. B., Mendelson, J. H., Mello, N. K., Siegel, A. J., Kaufman, M. J., Levin, J. M., Renshaw, P. F. and Cohen, B. M., Concurrent pharmacokinetic analysis of plasma cocaine and adrenocorticotropic hormone in men. J. Clin. Endocrinol. Metab. 83:966–968, 1998.

Stehling, M. K., Turner, R. and Mansfield, P., Echo-planar imaging: magnetic resonance imaging in a fraction of a second. Science 254:43–50, 1991.

Streeter, C. C., Ciraulo, D. A., Harris, G. J., Kaufman, M. J., Lewis, R. F., Knapp, C. M., Ciraulo, A. M., Maas, L. C., Ungeheuer, M., Szulewski, S. and Renshaw, P. F., Functional magnetic resonance imaging of alprazolam-induced changes in humans with familial alcoholism. Psychiatry Res. 82:69–82, 1998.

Teicher, M. H., Anderson, C. M., Polcari, A., Glod, C. A., Maas, L. C. and Renshaw, P. F., Functional deficits in basal ganglia of children with attention-deficit/hyperactivity disorder revealed using fMRI relaxometry. Nature Med. 6:470–473, 2000.

Thomas, M. A., Ke, Y., Levitt, J., Caplan, R., Curran, J., Asarnow, R. and McCracken, J., Preliminary study of frontal lobe ^{1}H MR spectroscopy in childhood-onset schizophrenia. J. Magn. Reson. Imaging 8:841–846, 1998.

Tsai, G. and Coyle, J. T., N-Acetylaspartate in neuropsychiatric disorders. Prog. Neurobiol. 46:531–569, 1995.

Turner, R., Jezzard, P., Wen, H., Kwong, K. K., Le Bihan, D., Zeffiro, T. and Balaban, R. S., Functional mapping of the human visual cortex at 4 and 1.5 tesla using deoxygenation contrast EPI. Magn. Reson. Med. 29:277–279, 1993.

Warach, S., Chien, D., Li, W., Ronthal, M. and Edelman, R. R., Fast magnetic resonance diffusion-weighted imaging of acute human stroke. Neurology 42:1717–1723, 1992.

Warach, S., Levin, J. M., Schomer, D. L., Holman, B. L. and Edelman, R. R., Hyperperfusion of ictal seizure focus demonstrated by MR perfusion imaging. AJNR Am. J. Neuroradiol. 15:965–968, 1994.

Warach, S., Dashe, J. F. and Edelman, R. R., Clinical outcome in ischemic stroke predicted by early diffusion-weighted and perfusion magnetic resonance imaging: a preliminary analysis. J. Cereb. Blood Flow Metab. 16:53–59, 1996.

Weisskoff, R. M., Chesler, D., Boxerman, J. L. and Rosen, B. R., Pitfalls in MR measurement of tissue blood flow with intravascular tracers: which mean transit time? Magn. Reson. Med. 29:553–558, 1993.

Williamson, P., Pelz, D., Merskey, H., Morrison, S., Karlik, S., Drost, D., Carr, T. and Conolon, P., Frontal, temporal, and striatal proton relaxation times in schizophrenic patients and normal comparison subjects. Am. J. Psychiatry 159:549–551, 1992.

Xiong, J., Rao, S., Gao, J. H., Woldorff, M. and Fox, P. T., Evaluation of hemispheric dominance for language using functional MRI: a comparison with positron emission tomography. Human Brain Mapping 6:42–58, 1998.

Yurgelun-Todd, D. A., English, C. D. and Cohen, B. M., Abnormal proton relaxation times in schizophrenia: an echo-planar study. Society of Magnetic Resonance, Third Scientific Meeting and Exhibition. Nice, France, p. 1239, 1995.

Zhang, M., Booze, R. M., Nicholls, M. A., Andersen, A. H., Welch, M. A., Strupp, B. J., Mactutus, C. F. and Avison, M. J., Cerebral response to cocaine and cocaine methiodide in the adult rat studied by fMRI. International Society for Magnetic Resonance in Medicine, Sixth Scientific Meeting and Exhibition. Sydney, Australia, p. 1580, 1998.

Chapter 4

Electroencephalographic Studies of Substance Use and Abuse

Lance O. Bauer, PHD

INTRODUCTION

This chapter provides an overview of the extant studies focusing on the acute and post-use effects of a selected number of drugs of abuse. This overview is not intended to provide an exhaustive summary of the hundreds of studies of human subjects published in peer-reviewed journals. Rather, the goal is to orient the reader toward the most consistent findings. Current trends in the literature are described and solutions to technical or methodological weaknesses are occasionally suggested.

ELECTROENCEPHALOGRAPHIC STUDIES OF THE ACUTE EFFECTS OF PSYCHOACTIVE DRUGS

Spontaneous EEG Activity

It is relatively obvious that a critical reader should be mindful of the dose(s) of the drug administered in any given EEG study as well as whether the EEG data were collected before, during, or after the attainment of the peak blood level. An important but less obvious consideration in comparing findings across studies is whether the data were collected at-rest or during a task, or during eyes-closed versus eyes-open conditions. Other important methodological differences contributing to variable findings across studies include the filter bandpass settings, the length of the recording period, whether or not sleeping was prevented, the use of objective

From: *Brain Imaging in Substance Abuse: Research, Clinical, and Forensic Applications*
M. J. Kaufman, ed. © Humana Press Inc., Totowa, New Jersey

versus subjective epoch selection methods, and the implementation of appropriate preprocessing techniques, such as baseline-correction and co-sine tapering of individual EEG epochs.

Conventionally, the spontaneous EEG is quantified by computing the power or energy of the signal in discrete frequency bands, viz., delta (1–4 Hz), theta (4–7 Hz), alpha (7–13 Hz), and beta (>13 Hz). Less commonly, researchers have examined the coherence of activity in these bands across electrode sites, regions, or cerebral hemispheres. Unfortunately, the computation of EEG coherence is sensitive to numerous assumptions and artifacts (Biggins et al., 1991; Nunez et al., 1997; Srinivasan et al., 1998). As a consequence, its reliability and validity in studies of the effects of drug use and abuse are not well established.

Alcohol

The literature describing the acute effects of ethyl alcohol on the spontaneous EEG is extensive. Early studies (Davis et al., 1941; Engel and Rosenbaum, 1944; Docter et al., 1966) revealed increases in alpha activity. These increases were detected by an electronic integration of EEG voltage after the application of a 7–13 Hz bandpass filter or by an observer's rating of the percentage of the chart record containing bursts of alpha activity. Modern studies (Ekman et al., 1964; Begleiter and Platz, 1972; Propping et al., 1980; Kaplan et al., 1988; Ehlers et al., 1989; Lukas et al., 1989b, 1990; Bauer and Hesselbrock, 1993; Cohen et al., 1993a,b; Stenberg et al., 1994) have employed more objective mathematical techniques, namely, a fast Fourier Transform or zero-cross analysis, and have replicated the early reports of enhanced alpha power or have, in addition, demonstrated a slowing of the predominant alpha frequency.

Although some studies have detected enhancements in EEG alpha power following alcohol doses as low as 0.32 g/kg (Bauer and Hesselbrock, 1993), the majority of studies have only examined the effects of higher doses, ranging from 0.7 to >1 g/kg. A few studies employing these higher doses found an increase in 4–7 Hz theta power in addition to the increase in alpha (Ehlers et al., 1989; Stenberg et al., 1994). These less common reports of increased theta power may be an artifact of longer recording periods, undetected drowsiness or sleep, and/or a noxious indirect effect of high doses of alcohol (e.g., nausea or vertigo; Pollak et al., 1998). Relatively few studies (Kopun and Propping, 1977) have employed sophisticated pharmacodynamic modeling techniques to elucidate dose-effect and time-effect relationships between alcohol administration and EEG power in either the alpha or theta frequency bands.

Despite strong agreement across studies in showing an enhancement of alpha activity after alcohol administration, it is important to recognize that individual subjects can differ substantially in the magnitude of the enhancement. Studies comparing the EEGs of monozygotic versus dizygotic twins have revealed that one source of variability across individuals is genetic (Propping, 1977; Sorbel et al., 1996). For example, Sorbel and colleagues (1996) recorded EEG activity from 53 monozygotic and 38 same-sex dizygotic twin pairs. All of the subjects were Caucasian. Analyses of EEG data obtained before alcohol administration in these subjects revealed significantly greater within-pair correlations for delta, theta, slow and fast alpha, and slow and fast beta power among monozygotic versus dizygotic twins. This result is not surprising, for the high heritability of the baseline EEG has been recognized for many years

(Propping, 1977; Lykken et al., 1982; Stassen et al., 1987). However, a relatively novel contribution of the Sorbel et al. study was the demonstration that a moderate dose of alcohol was associated with an approximate doubling of the heritability indices for slow and fast alpha power to levels of $H^2 = 0.83$ and $H^2 = 0.82$, respectively. In other words, the effects of alcohol on the EEG are as heritable as the EEG itself. Sorbel and colleagues suggested that alcohol may also act to attenuate the effects of the environment on the EEG and allow the genetic contribution to become more apparent.

A number of studies have identified sources of interindividual variation in the EEG response to alcohol which may be genetic and related to a heightened future risk for alcoholism. For example, Ehlers and colleagues (1998) examined EEG activity before and after alcohol administration in 48 Native American Mission Indian men. These men were assigned to groups based upon two hypothesized risk factors for future alcoholism: (1) the presence versus absence of a family history of alcoholism and (2) a higher versus lower degree of Native American ancestry. The results revealed that men at higher risk due to a higher degree of Native American ancestry exhibited a smaller increase in slow alpha activity following alcohol administration than men with <50% Native American ancestry. In a parallel analysis, high-risk men with a family history of alcoholism were likewise found to exhibit a smaller increase in slow alpha activity following alcohol administration than their lower-risk, family history negative counterparts. Therefore, the EEG effects of Native American Heritage and a family history of alcoholism appear to be similar. Whether the effects of these two risk factors are independent or overlapping remains to be determined.

In 1993, we examined electroencephalographic activity in 78, nonalcoholic men, 21–25 yr old, at higher versus lower risk for future alcoholism based upon the presence versus absence of a family history of alcohol dependence as well as one other risk factor, namely, the presence versus absence of a personal diagnosis of Antisocial Personality Disorder (ASPD) (Bauer and Hesselbrock, 1993). The four groups of subjects were compared at baseline and at multiple time points following the administration of a placebo beer and an alcoholic (0.32 g/kg) beer.

The EEG differences among the groups varied as a function of condition and time. For instance, at baseline, the EEGs of subjects with both risk factors for alcohol/drug abuse contained significantly more fast beta activity than the EEGs of subjects with either one or no risk factors. However, after subjects consumed the placebo beer, the interaction disappeared and was replaced by a main effect of family history (FH-pos > FH-neg) on fast alpha (10.9–12.5 Hz) power. The FH effect remained until blood alcohol concentrations began to rise 10 min after subjects drank the alcoholic beer. At that time, fast alpha activity in the family history positive group declined markedly to the same level as the FH-neg group. These demonstrations of a significant EEG response to a placebo, and enhanced electroencephalographic sensitivity to the effects of a rising blood alcohol level, among high risk, FH-positive subjects agree with findings reported by Pollock and colleagues (Pollock et al., 1983, 1986).

It should be noted that our 1993 demonstration of enhanced EEG sensitivity to alcohol among family history positive subjects disagrees with the effects of a family history of alcoholism reported by Ehlers and colleagues (1998). One important factor to consider in explaining the apparent contradiction is the point along the blood alcohol level (BAL) curve at which group differences were assessed. In our study, FH-positive subjects exhibited enhanced EEG responsiveness along the ascending limb of the BAL curve. In Ehlers and colleagues' study, FH-positive subjects exhibited diminished EEG responsiveness along the descending limb of the curve.

This differing response to alcohol as a function of ascending versus descending blood levels has been recognized as an important variable for organizing and interpreting the literature. Newlin and Thomson (1990) proposed a theory to explain the large number of seemingly contradictory findings regarding the self-reported effects of alcohol. Their theory incorporated the notion that individuals with a family history of alcoholism are genetically endowed with a nervous system which enhances the positive effects of a rising BAL and attenuates the subsequent negative effects of a declining BAL. The combination of enhanced acute sensitivity and enhanced acute tolerance is theorized as providing a particularly powerful reinforcer for future alcohol dependence. In a test of the Newlin and Thomson theory, Cohen and colleagues (1993b) examined the EEG effects of alcohol at multiple time points along both limbs of the BAL curve. Their findings supported the theory and help to explain seemingly contradictory EEG findings (Bauer and Hesselbrock, 1993; Volavka et al., 1996; Ehlers et al., 1998).

Benzodiazepines

An extensive literature documents the significant effects of drugs from the benzodiazepine class on the spontaneous electroencephalogram. Although the benzodiazepines and alcohol are both members of the larger family of sedative-hypnotics, their EEG effects are quite distinct. From this example, as well as others, one should infer that the drugs of abuse do not share a common electroencephalographic effect (see Table 1), and that the predominant electroencephalographic effects of a drug cannot be inferred from knowledge of its behavioral effects, i.e., sedation versus stimulation.

Over a wide range of doses possessing either sub-hypnotic or hypnotic behavioral effects, the benzodiazepines have been shown to enhance the amount of high frequency beta activity in the EEG (Montagu, 1972; Brown et al., 1979; Bond et al., 1983, 1992; Laurian et al., 1984; Merlo and Lion, 1985; Greenblatt et al., 1989; Breimer et al., 1990, 1991; Buhrer et al., 1990; Manmaru and Matsuura, 1990; Mandema et al., 1991; Van Steveninck et al., 1993; Greenblatt et al., 1994; Kinoshita et al., 1994; Fiset et al., 1995; Bauer et al., 1997; Feshchenko et al., 1997). The increase in EEG beta power following benzodiazepine administration is significant regardless of whether the EEG is recorded during eyes-open or eyes-closed conditions, or during a mental arithmetic task or at-rest. The EEG effect is also robust to the varying procedures that have been used for quantifying EEG beta power, including fast Fourier and zero-cross analysis, and absolute versus relative indices of spectral power.

Importantly, EEG beta power has been accepted as a sensitive and reliable dependent metric for modeling the pharmacokinetic and pharmacodynamic properties of the benzodiazepines (Laurijssens and Greenblatt, 1996). The change in EEG beta power over time closely parallels time-related changes in plasma midazolam, alprazolam, and diazepam levels. Changes in EEG beta power can be detected at midazolam doses as low as 10 μg/kg (Bauer et al., 1997) and are sensitive to a broad range of doses. As evidence of the specificity of the EEG response to benzodiazepines,

Table 1
Summary of Acute Quantitative EEG Effects of Alcohol, Benzodiazepines, Marijuana/THC, Opioids, Cocaine, and Several Other Drugs of Abuse

	Delta (< 4 Hz)	Theta (~4–7 Hz)	Alpha (~7–13 Hz)	Beta (13–~30 Hz)
Alcohol			+	
Benzodiazepines				+
Marijuana/THC			+	
Opioids	+	+		
Cocaine			?+?	+
Hallucinogens (1–4)		+		
Barbiturates (5)				+
Amphetamine (6–9)		–	?+?	+
Inhalants (10,11)		+		

"–" = inhibition; "+" = facilitation.

1. Weber et al., 1977; 2. White et al., 1985; 3. Engelhardt et al., 1994; 4. Kochs and Bischoff, 1994; 5. Feshchenko et al., 1997; 6. Hamilton et al., 1983; 7. Saletu et al., 1993; 8. Caldwell et al., 1995; 9. Slattum et al., 1996; 10. Biscaldi et al., 1981; 11. Grasso et al., 1984.

investigators have shown that benzodiazepine enhancement of EEG beta power can be reversed by the administration of the selective benzodiazepine antagonist flumazenil (Engelhardt et al., 1992). Furthermore, anxiolytics that are not members of the benzodiazepine class, such as buspirone, do not increase EEG beta power (Bond et al., 1983; Greenblatt et al., 1994).

Marijuana/THC

Early investigations of the electroencephalographic effects of marijuana/THC by Wikler and colleagues (1946) revealed no specific qualitative changes after subjects smoked 1–4 marijuana cigarettes. Subsequent studies have incorporated many improvements in drug delivery and dosage control and in data collection and analysis. Despite these maneuvers, subsequent studies have likewise failed to detect clinically significant changes in the EEG after acute exposure to marijuana or its active ingredient, THC (Ames, 1958; Hollister et al., 1970; Jones and Stone, 1970; Tassinari et al., 1973, 1974).

Despite the absence of evidence for a clinically significant qualitative change in the EEG, quantitative analysis methods have revealed a reliable pattern of subclinical changes in normal EEG rhythms after THC administration. The typical finding, with relatively few exceptions, is a dose-dependent transient increase in alpha power and a decrease in beta power (Dornbush et al., 1971; Volavka et al., 1971; Fink et al., 1976). Reviews of this literature have been authored by Fink and colleagues (Fink et al., 1976).

A few investigators have attempted to link the increase in EEG alpha power elicited by marijuana/THC administration to mood states or perceptual changes. For example, Lukas and colleagues (1995) focused their EEG analyses on periods of time following THC administration at which subjects reported feelings of euphoria. Their analyses demonstrated a subtle but statistically significant increase in EEG alpha power during these discrete periods. However, Koukkou and Lehmann (1978) found no association between THC-evoked changes in alpha power and self-reported levels of euphoria. Rather, they reported significant positive correlations between alpha power and self-reports of dysphoria, body-image distortion, and attention and thought disturbances. The source of the discrepant findings reported in these studies is presently unclear, but may involve differences across studies in the subjects' level of experience with THC and their expectations regarding its effects.

Opioids

Opioid-induced slowing of the human electroencephalogram was first detected by visual analysis of EEG chart recordings (Berger, 1937). The slowing was defined using various methods. The earliest reports described a decrease in the number of voltage fluctuations emitted over the analysis period. Other reports documented an increase in the number of epochs with slow wave activity or in the duration of these epochs. Objective analysis methods have identified an overall slowing of the average frequency of the EEG, a decrease in alpha power, and a compensatory increase in delta and theta power (Volavka et al., 1974) following the intravenous administration of 25 mg heroin. Also, 30 mg but not 15 mg, intramuscular (i.m.) injections of morphine sulfate have been shown to increase delta and theta power, as well as alpha power (Phillips et al., 1994). The latter study is noteworthy because the EEG was recorded while subjects performed an active stimulus monitoring task. Accordingly, the increase in delta, theta, and alpha power occasioned by the i.m. administration of 30 mg morphine cannot be ascribed to the elicitation of sleep. Given the use of this important control over behavior, one can be more confident in attributing the EEG change to a direct pharmacological effect of morphine.

At doses employed in the practice of anesthesia, there is a lawful relationship between the administered quantity of a variety of opioids, e.g., fentanyl (Scott et al., 1991), sufentanil (Scott et al., 1991), alfentanil (Lemmens et al., 1994), and either EEG delta power or the spectral edge (i.e., the frequency below which 95% of the area of the EEG power spectrum resides). These relationships have been successfully employed in pharmacokinetic-pharmacodynamic modeling of opioidergic activity (Lemmens et al., 1995).

Cocaine

In case reports published shortly after the discovery of the EEG, Hans Berger described the acute effects of subcutaneous cocaine on the human electroencephalogram (Berger, 1931). His initial study revealed an increase in alpha abundance following the subcutaneous administration of a 30 mg dose to two research subjects. In a subsequent study employing amplifiers that allowed him to measure EEG activity at higher frequencies, Berger (1937) observed an increase in beta power, but no increase in alpha power, in a single subject receiving a 20 mg dose.

Since the 1930s, there have been few attempts to replicate Berger's historic work. One exception is a 1985 study by Herning and colleagues which examined the effects of intravenous versus oral cocaine administration in separate groups consisting of 50 and 33 subjects, respectively (Herning et al., 1985a). In their study, both routes of administration were associated with significant increases in delta and beta activity. The unexpected increase in delta activity might be interpreted as a result of increased electromyographic activity and movement artifact in the EEG, rather than a direct pharmacological effect. The increase in beta power was positively correlated with cocaine plasma levels but was unrelated to the dose administered. As in Berger's 1937 study, there was no detectable change in alpha activity occasioned by cocaine administration.

A subsequent study by Herning and colleagues (1994b) demonstrated a significant enhancement of beta power and a more moderate enhancement in alpha power following the intravenous (i.v.) administration of 40 mg cocaine. A lower, 20 mg i.v. dose had no effects on either beta or alpha power relative to the placebo condition. The increase in EEG beta power was linked by the authors to a hypothesized decrease in cortical blood flow. This hypothesis is consistent with the known vasoconstrictive properties of cocaine.

The sporadic reports (Berger, 1931; Lukas et al., 1989a; Herning et al., 1994b) of increased alpha power following the administration of cocaine are difficult to rectify with the view of cocaine as a potent psychostimulant. One possible explanation for the increase pertains to cocaine's short half-life and the rapid decline in its stimulatory effects. In other words, the emergence of slow wave (i.e., alpha) activity following the acute administration of cocaine might be interpreted as a withdrawal or rebound phenomenon, rather than a direct effect of cocaine on the neural generators of EEG alpha. Unfortunately, none of the published manuscripts describing cocaine's acute electroencephalographic effects provide relevant time-line data that would allow discernment of the temporal relationship between the emergence of changes in beta and alpha power.

Evoked Potentials (EP) and Event-Related Potentials (ERP)

Short latency electroencephalographic potentials provide researchers with an opportunity to study the impact of drugs of abuse upon the transmission of neural activity along sensory pathways ascending to the level of primary sensory cortex. The longer latency event-related potentials permit researchers to study the subsequent activation of higher level centers, including those involved in anticipating the stimulus (e.g., via studies of the contingent negative variation or the processing negativity), its encoding (N1 and P2 components), recognition or decision making (mismatch negativity, N2, and P300 components), and response selection and output (bereitschaftspotential, premotor positivity). EPs and ERPs are obtained by recording brief epochs of neural activity at sites overlying peripheral sensory pathways or the brain. Consistent voltage fluctuations are then extracted from the random background noise by constructing time-point averages of these epochs, temporally aligned with respect to stimulus onset. The voltage changes that emerge in the averaged waveform are then typically measured in amplitude and latency.

The neural generators of most components of the sensory evoked potentials have been located (Chiappa, 1997). The generators giving rise to the P300 and a few other ERP components have also been mapped to specific loci (e.g., Naatanen and Picton, 1987; Naatanen, 1995). However, relative to the generators of the sensory EPs, the generators of the ERP are more diffusely distributed. ERP generators can also vary in their detectability and topography as a function of the difficulty and nature of the task that is used to elicit the ERP.

An evoked potential can be elicited and studied in all 5 sensory modalities. In addition, pain can be studied as separate modality via selective electrical stimulation of tooth pulp afferents or via other means (Bromm and Treede, 1991; Thurauf et al., 1994). However, to date, the vast majority of studies of drug use and abuse have focused on potentials elicited by visual, auditory, or mild somatosensory stimulation. Only one study (Bauer and Mott, 1996) has examined olfactory evoked potentials in drug abusers. To our knowledge, gustatory evoked potentials have not been studied in this context.

Alcohol

Extensive reviews of the acute effects of alcohol on EPs and ERPs have been published (Porjesz and Begleiter, 1993; Porjesz and Begleiter, 1996). The massive literature regarding alcohol's effects will therefore be reviewed briefly.

There are virtually no published peer-reviewed articles describing the acute effects of ethanol on the human auditory brainstem response (ABR). In fact, only one such study could be located. In a 1982 publication, Church and Williams described the effects of varying ethanol doses and time since dosing on components of the ABR in nine healthy young men. Wave II was the first ABR component to show an increase in latency following the ingestion of both 0.5 and 1.0 g/kg alcohol. This latency delay emerged within 30 min after ingestion and therefore coincided with the ascending limb of the BAL curve. All of the subsequent components of the ABR, viz. Waves III–VII, were also delayed by alcohol over this interval in a dose-sensitive manner. Because ABR Wave II arises from a change in resistance as action potentials traveling along the auditory nerve (C.N. VIII) enter the brain stem (Martin et al., 1995), the delayed wave II latency detected in that study could only have resulted from an impairment in neural conduction along the auditory nerve. Yet, one should not infer that the impairment is therefore locally mediated. The changes in auditory nerve conduction time observed in this acute administration study, and in similar studies of chronic alcohol abusers, have been attributed to an indirect effect mediated by alcohol's ability to alter brain temperature and thereby change axonal conduction time (Jones et al., 1980; Lee et al., 1990).

Studies of flash or pattern-reversal visual evoked potentials (PRVEP) (Lewis et al., 1970; Colrain et al., 1993) and short latency somatosensory evoked potentials (SEP) (Salamy and Williams, 1973) have revealed minimal changes in component latencies or amplitudes following low to moderate doses of alcohol, 0.3–0.7 g/kg. Significant reductions in evoked potential amplitudes have been reported following doses that exceed 0.9 g/kg (Lewis et al., 1969). The PRVEP and SEP amplitude reductions at these higher doses are highly correlated with individual differences in blood alcohol level (BAL) and therefore may reflect individual differences in alcohol absorption or metabolism.

A small literature documents the inconsistent effects of alcohol on the P300 component of the ERP. Moderate to high doses of alcohol were found to significantly reduce P300 amplitude in some studies (Elmasian et al., 1982; Teo and Ferguson, 1986; Campbell and Lowick, 1987; Rohrbaugh et al., 1988; Colrain et al., 1993; Wall and

Ehlers, 1995), but not in others (Erwin et al., 1986; Sommer et al., 1993). The reports of delays in P300 latency following alcohol consumption (Lee et al., 1990; Colrain et al., 1993; Fowler and Adams, 1993) have also not been consistently replicated.

The effects of alcohol on other aspects of the ERP have rarely been examined. However, in two similar reports published in 1995, Naatanen and colleagues (Jaaskelainen et al., 1995a,b) detected a significant reduction in the amplitude of the mismatch negativity following administration of a 0.5 g/kg dose of ethanol. The amplitudes of P300 and the processing negativity were not affected.

As is the case for the spontaneous EEG, these inconsistent results from studies of the acute effects of alcohol on the ERP can arise from the varying doses administered across studies, the duration of the recording period, and genetic or other individual difference variables. From studies of alcohol's effects on response accuracy and reaction time (Tharp et al., 1974; Maylor et al., 1992; Ryan et al., 1996) one should also consider the possibility that the nature and/or difficulty of the information processing task is important. Indeed, there is good evidence to suggest that tasks which involve a manipulation of stimulus-response compatibility, stimulus-response mapping, or response complexity are more sensitive to the acute effects of alcohol than tasks which manipulate stimulus discriminability or probability. By inference, one would expect that ERP components which measure response selection or output, e.g., the readiness potential and premotor positivity, would be more sensitive to alcohol than ERP components that measure stimulus evaluation, e.g., P300. These components have rarely been studied (Rohrbaugh et al., 1988; Sommer et al., 1993).

Another source of the inconsistencies in ERP findings may arise from the failure to consider the role of a subject's ethnicity and family history in augmenting or reducing the effects of alcohol. In a 1995 study, Wall and Ehlers examined P300 latency and amplitude in 29 young men of Asian heritage. All of the subjects were genotyped. Fourteen subjects were heterozygous for the inactive ALDH2 allele (ALDH2*1/2*2). The remaining 15 subjects were homozygous for the active ALDH2 allele (ALDH2*1/2*1). Interestingly, Asian men with the active ALDH2*1/2*1 genotype, which is associated with low rate of facial flushing, tachycardia, and other untoward reactions to alcohol, exhibited no change in P300 after ingesting a 0.75 mL/kg dose of alcohol. In contrast, the group of Asian men with the ALDH2*1/2*2 genotype, which is associated with a "disulfiram-like" reaction to alcohol, exhibited a significant decrease in P300 amplitude and an increase in P300 latency after alcohol ingestion. Genetic factors therefore appear to play a significant role in determining the presence or absence of an effect of alcohol on the ERP.

Benzodiazepines

To date, one study of the auditory brainstem response has documented a statistically significant but modest increase in the Wave V–Wave I interpeak interval following the administration of a low dose (12.5–16 mg) of diazepam (Adams et al., 1985). A later study (Loughnan et al., 1987) failed to replicate this finding in 13 healthy volunteers receiving a higher 20 mg dose.

A larger number of studies have documented significant and reproducible effects of diazepam and other benzodiazepines on visual and somatosensory evoked potentials. Both flash-evoked and pattern-reversal visual evoked potentials are decreased in amplitude following the administration of small subhypnotic doses of diazepam (8–10 mg; Broughton et al., 1966; Ebe et al., 1969; Boker and Heinze, 1984) or midazolam (10 mg/kg; Bauer et al., 1997). Three of these investigations of VEPs (Broughton et al., 1966; Ebe et al., 1969; Boker and Heinze, 1984) also demonstrated a statistically significant increase in the latencies of the N75 or P100 components.

The cortical components (e.g., N19, P22) of the median nerve somatosensory evoked potential are decreased in amplitude following midazolam administration, but are not reliably delayed in latency by either midazolam or diazepam (Coulthard and Rood, 1993; Lauer et al., 1994). Interestingly, one published report described a reduction in cortical SEP amplitude following intravenous administration of 10 mg diazepam which was reversed by a 3-mg i.v. dose of flumazenil. The sensitivity of the somatosensory EP to benzodiazepines and benzodiazepine antagonists is consistent with the large number of benzodiazepine receptors residing in primary somatosensory cortex (Oka et al., 1986).

As is the case for sensory evoked potentials, the benzodiazepines have been shown to reduce the amplitude or increase the latency of the ERP (Saletu, 1974; Herrmann et al., 1981; Laurian et al., 1984; Milligan et al., 1989; Noldy et al., 1990; Rockstroh et al., 1991; Bond et al., 1992; van Leeuwen et al., 1992; Plourde et al., 1993; Semlitsch et al., 1995; Curran et al., 1998). The deficit in P300 amplitude following benzodiazepine administration can be reversed by flumazenil (Engelhardt et al., 1992).

Marijuana/THC

Despite the existence of a large literature demonstrating inhibitory effects of THC on evoked potentials in animals, only one published study has examined its acute effects in humans. The findings were negative (Kopell et al., 1978). In that study, 12 male college students orally ingested a marijuana extract containing 0.7 mg/kg delta-9-THC. Over a 4.5 h period following THC administration, no significant changes in auditory evoked potential amplitudes were detected relative to the placebo condition.

There have been several published reports of a significant effect of acute marijuana/THC on event related potentials. In the same subject sample described above, in which no significant changes in EPs were noted, Roth and colleagues (1977) detected a significant reduction in P300 amplitude and a delay in the 50% recovery time of the contingent negative variation. These changes were detected while subjects performed a fixed-set version of Sternberg's memory retrieval task for visually-presented digits. In the context of simpler auditory signal detection task, Herning et al. (1979) also found a reduction in P300 amplitude following THC administration.

A recent ERP study (Leweke et al., 1998) demonstrated a curious result which disagrees with those reported above. The authors of the study reported that P300 amplitude was enhanced by THC when the ERP-eliciting stimuli were words with a positive emotional connotation. The authors interpreted the P300 enhancement in terms of a congruity between the positive drug-induced mood state and the positive emotional valence of the material to be encoded. However, their P300 finding was not hypothesized a priori and should therefore be viewed cautiously. In addition, the failure to demonstrate an improvement in recognition accuracy that correlated with the P300 enhancement on positive word trials, and the failure to show a reduction in both P300 amplitude and recognition accuracy when words with a negative emotional connotation were presented, are problematic for their interpretation. A replication of the Leweke et al. finding is clearly needed before their counterintuitive results are assigned any theoretical value.

Opioids

In general, the family of auditory, visual, and somatosensory evoked potentials is unaffected by the introduction of opioids, even at the higher doses that are conventional in anesthesia practice. For example, the latencies of Wave II through the mid-latency components of the auditory brainstem response are not changed by the administration of intravenous doses of 10–100 μg/kg fentanyl (Thurner et al., 1987; Inoue et al., 1992; Schwender et al., 1993b), 100–500 μg/kg alfentanil (Schwender et al., 1993b), 1–3 mg/kg morphine (Schwender et al., 1993b), or 2–3 μg/kg sufentanil (Schwender et al., 1995). The cortical components of the median nerve somatosensory evoked potential (McPherson et al., 1986; Thurner et al., 1987) and the N75 and P100 components of the pattern reversal visual evoked potential (Thurner et al., 1987) are likewise unchanged in their latencies following the administration of opioid agonists. One exception to this pattern of opioid insensitivity are somatosensory potentials evoked by nociceptive stimuli. These so-called pain evoked potentials are significantly reduced in amplitude by alfentanil and other opioid agonists (Petersen-Felix et al., 1996). Pain EPs are also reduced in amplitude by some sedative drugs, e.g., propofol, that are not members of the opiate class (Petersen-Felix et al., 1996).

Three reports could be located in which the acute effects of an opioid agonist on P300 were examined. Kouri et al. (1996) elicited P300 event-related potentials via an auditory oddball paradigm in opiate and cocaine dependent patients undergoing a treatment trial of either buprenorphine or placebo. Compared to a group of seven non-drug dependent, untreated volunteers, the seven opiate-dependent patients receiving the placebo exhibited smaller P300 amplitudes throughout the duration of the trial. The 14 remaining patients ($n = 7$ per group) receiving either 6 or 12 mg buprenorphine exhibited a normalization in P300 over time. These findings suggest that opioid agonists acutely enhance P300 amplitude.

Two studies have examined P300 auditory ERPs as a reciprocal measure of the amount of attention directed toward a painful distracting stimulus. In one of these studies, using chronic pain patients, Lorenz and colleagues (1997) showed that the reduction in P300 amplitude occasioned by the introduction of experimentally induced pain was antagonized by morphine. Unfortunately, neither the Lorenz et al. nor the Kouri et al. studies included healthy volunteers as research subjects. It therefore remains uncertain whether opioids will enhance P300 amplitude in a normal, nonopiate dependent nervous system, or will only do so in a nervous system that has developed tolerance and other physiological abnormalities.

Cocaine

To our knowledge, no one has examined the acute effects of cocaine on auditory, visual, or somatosensory EPs in human subjects. Only two studies have examined its effects on P300 and the results have been contradictory. In a 1985 publication, Herning and colleagues (1985b) examined the effects of three i.v. and three oral doses of cocaine on P300 in recreational users of the drug. A significant reduction in P300

Table 2
Summary of Acute EP and ERP Effects of Alcohol, Benzodiazepines, Marijuana/THC, Opioids, Cocaine, and Several Other Drugs of Abuse

	Auditory EPs	Visual EPs	Somatosensory EPs	ERPs
Alcohol	–	–	–	?–?
Benzodiazepines		–	–	–
Marijuana/THC				–
Opioids			– (pain EPs only)	+
Cocaine				?+?
Hallucinogens (1–4)	+		+	
Barbiturates (5–8)	–	–		–
Amphetamine (9)				?+?
Inhalants (10–14)	–	–	–	–

("–" = inhibition of amplitude or latency, "+" = facilitation of amplitude or latency).
1. Hou et al., 1993; 2. Schwender et al., 1994; 3. Langeron et al., 1997; 4. Plourde et al., 1997; 5. Frowein et al., 1981; 6. Schwender et al., 1993a; 7. Brinciotti, 1994; 8. Fowler and Mitchell, 1997; 9. Halliday et al., 1987; 10. Hazemann et al., 1987; 11. Morrow et al., 1992; 12. Indulski et al., 1996; 13. Lindgren et al., 1997; 14. Vrca et al., 1997.

amplitude was detected regardless of the route of administration. However, in a 1994 study of subjects with extensive histories of cocaine abuse or dependence, the same investigators found that a 60–80 mg i.v. dose enhanced both P300 and slow wave amplitudes (Herning et al., 1994a).

The 1985 report of a reduction in P300 amplitude by cocaine is curious, but is not unprecedented. Studies of the acute P300 effects of amphetamine and methlyphenidate have also yielded contradictory results. One explanation for the finding of Herning et al. (1985b) may reside in the intense cardiovascular effects of cocaine, particularly among intolerant recreational users. In these subjects, the enhancement of cardiac rate and output, and the associated increase in anxiety, may have served as potent distractors which diverted attention away from the P300-eliciting stimuli and accordingly reduced P300 amplitude (Table 2).

Electroencephalographic Studies of Chronic Substance Abusers

Before the evidence for EEG, EP, or ERP anomalies in patients with histories of alcohol or drug dependence is reviewed, it would be valuable to highlight some of the methodological and interpretive problems that are inherent in studying patients with drug use histories as well as several problems that are created by researchers themselves. These problems are not specific to EEG/EP/ERP research. Rather, they generalize across all of the neuroimaging modalities.

1. It is a logical fallacy to unquestionably attribute an EEG/EP/ERP difference between one group of substance dependent patients and a group of healthy, non-drug-abusing volunteers to an effect of substance abuse. Collectively, substance-dependent patients are known to exhibit higher-than-normal rates of comorbid psychopathology, polydrug abuse, medical disorders (e.g., cirrhosis,

hepatitis, cardiovascular disorders, diabetes, HIV/AIDS, malnutrition), licit and illicit medication use, head injuries, seizures, and epilepsy (Lowinson et al., 1992). In addition, substance dependent patients exhibit low levels of compliance/motivation, below average IQ scores, and higher-than-normal rates of childhood psychopathology. Other complicating factors include dysfunctional environmental or genetic histories, and educational, social, or cultural factors (e.g., reading disability or illiteracy, language barriers, a below-average level of educational achievement that is overestimated by educational attainment)—all of which predate their substance abuse careers. The simple demonstration of a difference in EEG/EP/ERP (or other neuroimaging) indices between a group of patients and a group of healthy volunteers is therefore insufficient for inferring causation, unless the researchers have either matched the groups on all of these potential confounds, excluded all patients with these confounds, included additional control groups, or explicitly examined the role of these confounds in planned or *post hoc* analyses. It is unfortunate that many neuroimaging researchers have failed to take these complexities into account.

2. It can be misleading to report findings and derive hypotheses from studies of small numbers of patients, because of the high risk of both type II (from inadequate statistical power) and type I (from outliers, biased sampling, unrecognized confounds) errors. Many errors of inference may also derive from a failure to consider the impact of a small *N* on the assumptions and validity of the most commonly employed parametric and nonparametric inferential statistics. Furthermore, studies of small numbers of patients preclude the researcher from conducting the types of subgroup analyses which are best suited to revealing the effects of mediating and moderating variables.
3. One cannot assert that a study is examining the effects of acute withdrawal based upon the point in time at which data were collected. That is, a study examining patients several hours after their last use of a drug is not necessarily a study of withdrawal. The differences can just as reasonably be attributed to premorbid factors, a persistent chronic effect, or a protracted withdrawal phenomenon associated with the patient's prior abuse of another substance.
4. It is problematic when neuroimaging studies fail to adopt appropriate and state-of-the-art methods for psychiatric assessment and relapse monitoring. In any standard clinical trial, a failure to distinguish between abuse and dependence diagnoses, or to fully assess psychiatric and medical comorbidity in a structured interview, would be considered naïve and "fatally flawed". Similarly, failing to conduct frequent urine toxicology screens or to work with collateral informants to verify the patient's self-reported duration of abstinence would also be considered unacceptable. Yet, a number of neuroimaging studies do not meet these minimal standards.

Alcohol

A number of early, i.e., 1960–1980, studies (reviewed in Porjesz and Begleiter, 1985) indicated that the abrupt cessation of chronic alcohol dependence is accompanied by marked changes in sensory evoked potentials. These changes include an enhancement of the P100 component of the flash-evoked visual potential, and an enhancement of the amplitudes and reduction of the latencies of both auditory brainstem responses and median nerve somatosensory evoked responses. Similar changes have also been reported in the amplitudes of later evoked potential components, such as P300. These EP and ERP findings suggest that the early phase of withdrawal is marked by enhanced central nervous system arousal and excitability. The severity and duration of the acute hyperexcitability phase is determined by a number of factors, including drinking (Begleiter and Porjesz, 1979) and seizure (Brown et al., 1988; Noldy and Carlen, 1990) histories.

Consistent with the results of EP and ERP studies, the vast majority of studies of the spontaneous EEG find evidence for CNS hyperexcitability via the demonstration of enhanced power in the high frequency beta band (Coger et al., 1978; Kaplan et al., 1985; Spehr and Stemmler, 1985; Frank et al., 1986; Krauss and Niedermeyer, 1991; Bauer, 1994a; Costa and Bauer, 1997; Winterer et al., 1998) and decreased power in the slower alpha band (Zilm et al., 1980; Kaplan et al., 1985; Spehr and Stemmler, 1985). There are also scattered reports of enhanced delta or theta activity and qualitative EEG abnormalities (e.g., spiking, epileptiformlike discharges; Holmes and Korteling, 1993). The latter findings appear to be limited to the subset of alcoholic patients with histories of cerebellar or liver disease, withdrawal seizures, severe vitamin deficiency, or head injuries. Qualitative EEG abnormalities are rare in alcoholic patients without these medical complications (Begleiter and Platz, 1972).

As central nervous system hyperexcitability subsides, after approx 1–2 wk, it is replaced by a more protracted period, characterized by attenuated or delayed evoked potentials (Chan et al., 1986; Cadaveira et al., 1991, 1992), but a persistent elevation in EEG beta power (Bauer, 1994a; Costa and Bauer, 1997; Winterer et al., 1998). The attenuated sensory EPs typically normalize (Chan et al., 1986; Bauer and Easton, 1996) unless the patient is complicated by other disorders (e.g., liver disease, vitamin deficiency, Wernicke-Korsakoff's syndrome, head injury). The later, endogenous ERP components (e.g., P300) can remain attenuated, however, after as long as 1 yr of abstinence. The elevation in EEG beta power, and the attenuation of P300 amplitude, persisting beyond the initial months of abstinence appear to reflect a premorbid deficit (Elmasian et al., 1982; Pfefferbaum et al., 1991; Bauer and Hesselbrock, 1993, 1999a,b; Hesselbrock et al., 1993a,b, Bauer, 1994a; Bauer et al., 1994a,b; O'Connor et al., 1994; Polich et al., 1994) and not a persistent effect of alcohol.

Benzodiazepines

To our knowledge, only one study has examined EEG activity in benzodiazepine dependent patients without the complication of a seizure history (Hallstrom and Lader, 1981). Under controlled conditions, 10 patients, who reported an inability to discontinue benzodiazepine abuse, were prescribed either 20 or 135 mg diazepam per day. During a subsequent period in which these doses were tapered downward, patients reported heightened levels of anxiety and perceptual disturbances. Changes in EEG beta power, that were opposite to those associated with the initiation of diazepam treatment, also were found.

Marijuana/THC

It has been difficult for researchers to identify EEG, EP, or ERP differences associated with chronic marijuana/THC use. In part, the difficulty arises from the substantial variability in the intensity and frequency of use even among subjects who uniformly meet diagnostic criteria for cannabis dependence (Wert and Raulin, 1986). In addition, subjects who meet criteria for cannabis dependence often meet criteria for dependence upon other substances or possess premorbid or comorbid psychopathology. Many of the initial neuropsychological and neurophysiological findings in chronic marijuana/THC users have not been replicated for these and other reasons.

Struve and colleagues have discussed these problems and noted that many of the extant EEG studies are deficient for various reasons (Struve et al., 1989, 1994, 1998). They note, for example, that early reports of a high prevalence of qualitative EEG abnormalities among chronic marijuana users were misleading because the prevalence is in fact no greater than the base rate in the normal population. Other qualitative EEG studies reporting a high prevalence of abnormalities have been criticized for imprecise or biased definitions of abnormality, or other problems.

A recent quantitative analysis of the EEG in chronic marijuana/THC users is noteworthy for its many strengths. Struve and colleagues (1998) examined 15 subjects who reported using THC on a daily basis for 15–24 consecutive years. None of the subjects reported significant levels of use of other psychoactive drugs and all were free of serious psychopathology. A group of moderate duration (3–6 yr), daily THC abusers was recruited as a comparison group, as was a larger group of normal, non-drug-abusing volunteers. The results of the study revealed a THC duration-related increase in EEG theta power at all scalp locations. Because the design of this study included subjects with a regular and daily pattern of THC use, the power for detecting an EEG difference between users and nonusers was enhanced. By comparing long and moderate duration THC abusers, and by excluding subjects with psychiatric complications, these investigators were also able to discount alternative explanations for their results.

Studies of short latency evoked potentials have not revealed evidence for a deficit in peripheral or central processing of visual, auditory, or somatosensory stimuli (Patrick and Struve, 1994; Patrick et al., 1997) among chronic THC users. Studies of the P300 ERP have also revealed inconsistent results (Solowij et al., 1991, 1995; Patrick et al., 1995).

Opioids

An early study examined EEG activity in 63 heroin-dependent patients (Volavka et al., 1970). EEG irregularities, identified by clinical raters, were present in approx 50% of the patients. Unfortunately, no consideration was given in this study to the complicating effects of other drug use, head injury, or psychopathology.

In a 1997 study which excluded individuals with these complications (Fig. 1), we found no evidence of quantitative EEG abnormalities in a group of 19 heroin dependent patients, abstinent for 1–5 mo, compared to healthy controls (Costa and Bauer, 1997). Importantly, the patients in our study failed to exhibit the same enhancement of EEG beta power demonstrated in cocaine or alcohol dependent patients via the same

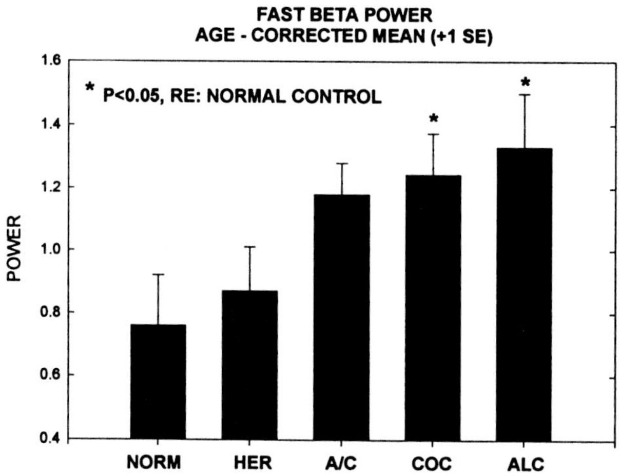

Fig. 1. Average EEG fast beta power (+1 SE) in normal control (NORM), heroin-dependent (HER), alcohol- and cocaine-dependent (A/C), cocaine-dependent (COC), and alcohol-dependent (ALC) groups. (From Costa and Bauer, 1997, with permission.)

analysis. This normal EEG pattern was problematic for our interpretation of enhanced beta power as existing premorbidly in the cocaine and alcohol-dependent groups. Indeed, why should a group of heroin dependent patients, which possessed the highest prevalence of conduct disorder, antisocial personality disorder, and other risk factors, not exhibit the largest amount of beta activity in their EEGs, if the beta enhancement was truly premorbid?

In response to this question, we have recently reanalyzed the EEG data from our 1997 publication. We limited the analysis to the 19 patients with histories of heroin dependence and the 14 non-drug-dependent controls. We hypothesized that heroin dependent patients indeed possess the enhanced EEG beta activity of premorbid origin found in the other patient groups and that the enhancement is antagonized by the cumulative effects of persistent heroin use.

Accordingly, we subdivided the heroin dependent group into two groups based upon the median number of years of heroin use. A one-way analysis of variance, with age as a covariate, was used to compare the patient groups and the normal control group. The ANCOVA revealed a significant difference in the hypothesized direction: patients with fewer years of heroin use exhibited the same enhancement in EEG beta activity found in our previous analysis of alcohol dependent or cocaine dependent patients. In contrast, patients with more years of heroin use exhibited a diminished amount of EEG beta activity (Fig. 2, left panel) and an enhanced amount of alpha activity (Fig. 2, right panel).

Thus, our 1997 demonstration of no EEG abnormalities in heroin-dependent patients now requires a caveat. Heroin-dependent patients only appeared to exhibit a normal EEG pattern because the EEG was in a transitional phase. During the early phase of opiate abuse, the EEG is characterized by an abnormal enhancement of high-frequency (beta) activity. At a later time, a slowing of the EEG occurs such that the EEG is indistinguishable from the normal pattern. However, with additional years of

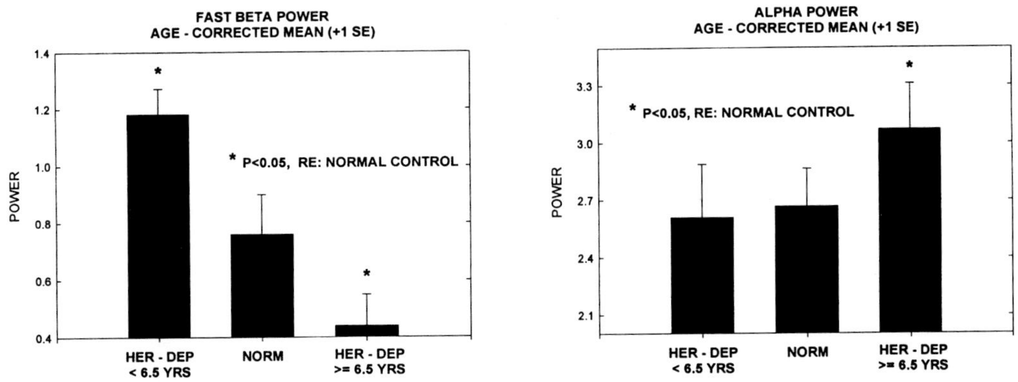

Fig. 2. Left Average EEG fast beta power in healthy, non-drug-abusing volunteers (NORM) and in heroin-dependent patients ranking below (HER-DEP < 6.5 yrs) or above (HER-DEP >= 6.5 yr) the median number of years of heroin abuse for all patients. Note that the two patient groups exhibit an opposite EEG abnormality, which when summed, yields the "normal" result shown in Fig. 1. **Right** Average EEG alpha power in healthy, non-drug-abusing volunteers (NORM) and in heroin-dependent patients ranking below (HER-DEP < 6.5 yr) or above (HER-DEP >= 6.5 yr) the median number of years of heroin abuse for all patients. Note the emergence of a slowed EEG pattern with continued years of exposure.

heroin abuse, an abnormal enhancement of lower frequency (alpha) activity emerges. Shufman and colleagues (1996) have published data indicating that active abusers of heroin and other opiates exhibit the same alpha enhancement as we now demonstrate in abstinent patients with many years of exposure.

To date, only one study has examined evoked potentials in patients abstinent from heroin and other opiates. In 1998, we examined pattern shift visual evoked potentials in 59 patients assigned to one of three groups defined by: a past history (2–4 mo abstinent) of DSM-IIIR opioid dependence (i.e., in partial remission); a recent history (7 d abstinent) of opioid dependence with ongoing methadone maintenance; and a recent history of opioid dependence, ongoing methadone maintenance, and asymptomatic HIV-1 infection (Bauer, 1998). A group of 21 healthy, non-drug-dependent volunteers was also evaluated. The analyses revealed no PSVEP differences between patients with a past history of opioid dependence and healthy volunteers. There were also no PSVEP differences between methadone-maintained patients with or without HIV-1 infection. Collectively, however, the two methadone maintenance groups exhibited significant delays in the N75 and P100 components of the PSVEP relative to the other two groups. After the data were corrected for the variance in the age of the subjects, a strong and significant correlation emerged between N75 latency and self-reported years of heroin abuse. N75 latency did not correlate with years of cocaine, alcohol, or other drug abuse; methadone blood levels; CD4+ count; or duration of abstinence. The delay in N75 latency in the two methadone maintenance groups was entirely related to their more severe and protracted level of heroin abuse and was independent of their methadone treatment and HIV-1 serostatus (Fig. 3).

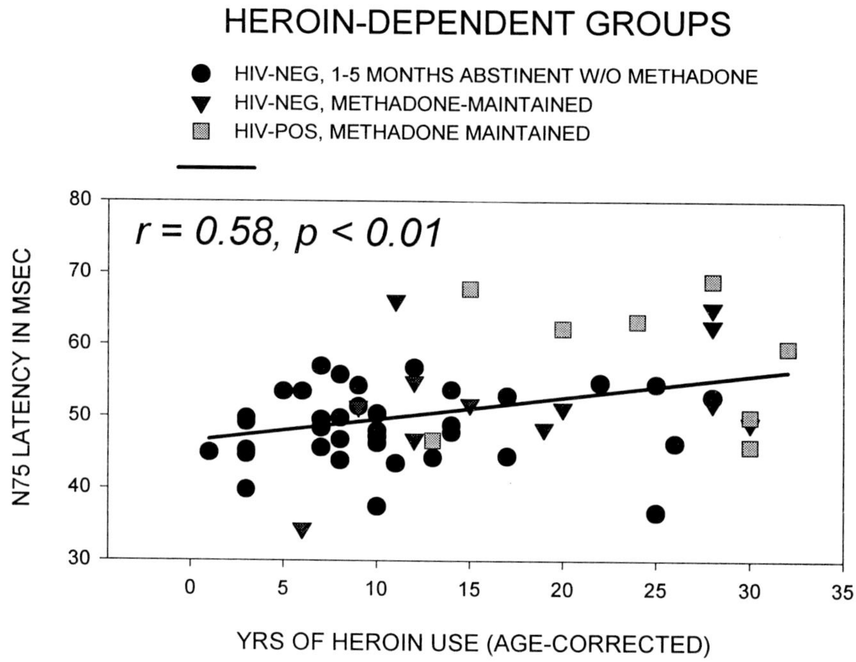

Fig. 3. Scatterplot relating years of heroin use to the latency of the N75 component of the pattern shift visual evoked potential. (From Bauer, 1998, with permission.)

Only one study (Kouri et al., 1996) has examined P300 in patients with a history of opiate dependence. The patients also met diagnostic criteria for cocaine dependence. The results showed no significant P300 amplitude differences between patients and healthy, non-drug-dependent volunteers when patients presented for detoxification. After detoxification, P300 amplitude in the seven patients assigned to the placebo arm of a treatment trial was significantly smaller than P300 amplitude in the control group.

Cocaine

The variety of EEG findings among patients with histories of cocaine dependence includes increased alpha power (Alper et al., 1990; Prichep et al., 1996; Alper et al., 1998), increased beta power (Pascual-Leone et al., 1991; Noldy et al., 1994; Costa and Bauer, 1997; Herning et al., 1997), decreased delta power (Roemer et al., 1995; Prichep et al., 1996; Alper et al., 1998), and no difference at all (Bauer, 1993, 1994b, 1996; Bauer and Kranzler, 1994; Hersh et al., 1995). This mixture of findings most likely reflects a failure to recognize many of the confounds noted above.

For example, it has long been recognized that subclinical and clinical levels of depression are associated with enhanced alpha activity in the EEG (Pollock and Schneider, 1990). The studies which have reported enhanced alpha activity in cocaine dependent patients may have been compromised by inclusion of a disproportionately large number of patients with high levels of depressive comorbidity. Indeed, one of these manuscripts (Alper et al., 1990) explicitly stated that four of the seven patients reported a history of suicide attempts. The average Beck Depression score for the entire patient group was also high (18.9/21), indicating significant depressive comorbidity. The failure to include another group of patients with high levels of depression but no cocaine abuse history, or to exclude patients with depressive symptomatology that was not drug-abuse-related, precluded these researchers from being confident in attributing the group differences to an effect of cocaine abuse.

Two laboratories have reported a decrease in delta power in the EEGs of cocaine dependent patients (Roemer et al., 1995; Prichep et al., 1996; Alper et al., 1998). One manuscript reported that the delta deficit persisted over 6 mo of continued abstinence (Alper et al., 1998). These reports are curious, because all other types of brain pathology, e.g., dementia, head injury, stroke, etc., are associated with an increase in delta power, not a decrease. Before one accepts the counterintuitive claim of a delta deficit in abstinent cocaine abusers, several sources of artifact should be considered. For example, it is noteworthy that the recording period for studies finding the delta deficit was 20–30 min in duration, whereas the duration of the recording period for studies which did not find the deficit was much shorter, i.e., typically 5 min. Although it can be argued that longer recording periods allow more data to be included in the averaged frequency spectrum, and can thereby improve the stability of the average, longer recording periods also permit drowsiness and sleep to contaminate the recording. If patients were more alert (e.g., paranoid) during the 30-minute recording period than the normal control group, they may have had difficulty relaxing and would not enter the initial stages of sleep as readily as the normal control group. In other words, the delta deficit might be the result of an interaction between the extended duration of the recording period and group differences in the inclination to sleep.

Four laboratories (Pascual-Leone et al., 1991; Noldy et al., 1994; Costa and Bauer, 1997; Herning et al., 1997) have independently detected enhanced beta power in the awake, resting EEGs of cocaine dependent patients. A noteworthy feature of the Costa and Bauer (1997) study was the inclusion of multiple patient groups with histories of either alcohol, cocaine, cocaine and alcohol, or polydrug/heroin dependence. In addition, normative data were obtained from a group of nondependent healthy volunteers who were tested over the same time frame as the patients. By contrast, some of the EEG studies described above utilized historical norms for their EEG analysis. The aforementioned studies are therefore vulnerable to the numerous problems which relate to the use of archived data (e.g., unrecognized drift in methodology, recording, or analysis methods; historical changes in subject ascertainment; incomplete knowledge of demographic, medical, and psychiatric characteristics of the normative sample).

By virtue of examining patients with various types of drug dependence, it was possible in our 1997 study to compare the effects of different drug use histories while premorbid factors, comorbid depression, and educational, social, and cultural factors were held constant. From our analysis, a significant elevation in EEG beta power was detected in cocaine dependent patients after 1–5 mo of verified abstinence. There were no differences among the groups in delta, theta, or alpha power. Interestingly, a similar elevation in EEG beta power was detected in alcohol dependent patients and to a lesser (and marginally nonsignificant) degree in patients with histories of dual alcohol and cocaine dependence (*see* Fig. 1). Thus, increased EEG beta power might not be a specific result of prior cocaine use. Rather, it is most probably related to a factor common to both cocaine and alcohol dependence. One likely possibility is the combination of a family history of alcoholism and a diagnosis of Antisocial Personality Disorder. These premorbid factors have been found to elevate EEG beta power in young men who have not yet developed alcohol or cocaine dependence (Bauer and Hesselbrock, 1993) and are prevalent in patients with psychoactive substance dependence.

Studies of EP and ERP differences among cocaine dependent patients suggest that a subtle disruption of central nervous system function is present during the first 3 mo of abstinence. These subtle anomalies include a dampened EEG frequency-following response to square wave photic stimulation (Bauer, 1993, 1996), dampened auditory P50 amplitude and gating (Fein et al., 1996), a delay in the latency of the P100 component of the pattern reversal visual evoked potential (Bauer and Easton, 1996), and a reduction in the amplitude (Herning et al., 1990; Herning and King, 1996; Bauer, 1997) or a delay in the latency (Noldy and Carlen, 1997) of the P300 response to stimuli which are both novel and demanding of attention, i.e., task relevant. The dampened P300 response to novel target stimuli normalizes over time with continued abstinence from cocaine (Herning et al., 1990; Bauer, 1997).

Two studies have shown an abnormality in a subcomponent of the P300 (Bauer, 1997; Biggins et al., 1997) that does not normalize with continued cocaine abstinence (Bauer, 1997). This subcomponent, known as P3*a*, is elicited by novel stimuli which do not otherwise command attention from the subject—that is, no button press or counting response is required. Studies of neurologic patients with identified frontal brain damage, as well as more recent fMRI studies, have suggested that the P3*a* response to novel nontarget stimuli is generated frontally, whereas the larger P3*b* response to novel target stimuli is generated by neural activity at multiple locations in both frontal and nonfrontal regions.

A study by Biggins et al. (1997) examined the P3*a* response in 10 cocaine-dependent patients, 10 cocaine- and alcohol-dependent patients, and 20 healthy, non-drug-dependent controls. The patients were studied after 2–6 wk of abstinence. Their analyses revealed no P3*a* differences between the two patient groups. P3*a* amplitude and latency were significantly inhibited in patients relative to normal controls. Curiously, the authors attributed the group difference to an effect of chronic cocaine abuse despite the fact that the correlation between severity of cocaine use and P3*a* amplitude was not significant. Furthermore, the same group of authors had previously demonstrated the same P3*a* deficit in alcohol dependent patients and attributed that deficit to alcohol dependence (Biggins et al., 1995). It is, of course, conceivable that cocaine dependence and alcohol dependence could both effect the same neurophysiological change. However, a more parsimonious explanation for the common change in frontal P3*a* might involve a common premorbid factor, such as Conduct Disorder or Antisocial Personality Disorder.

A more elaborate study by Bauer examined visual P3*a* in 49 patients with histories of either cocaine dependence or cocaine and alcohol dependence, and 20 healthy, non-drug-dependent volunteers (Bauer, 1997). The patients were objectively verified to have been abstinent for 1–5 mo. Analyses of the data revealed reduced P3*a* amplitudes at frontal electrode sites only among cocaine dependent patients meeting diagnostic criteria for childhood Conduct Disorder and Antisocial Personality Disorder (Fig. 4). In

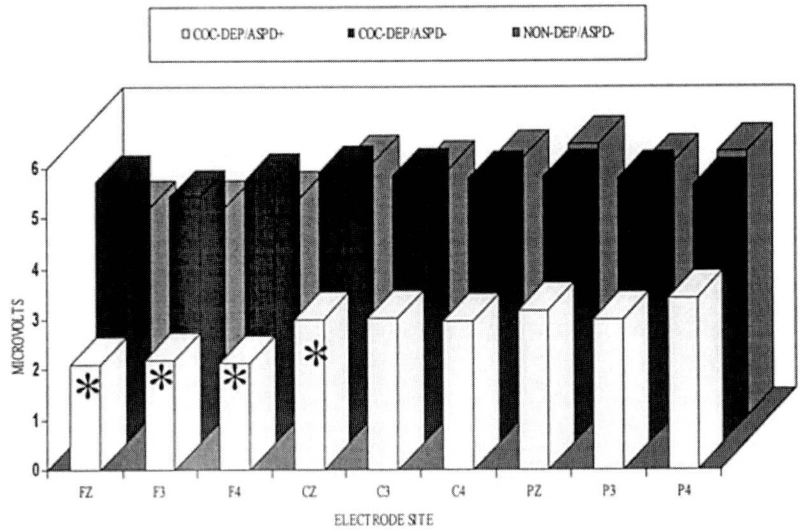

Fig. 4. Average P3*a* amplitude plotted as a function of group (ASPD+ cocaine-dependent, ASPD- cocaine-dependent, ASPD—nondrug-abusing control) and electrode site. Asterisks designate statistically significant differences between the ASPD+ Cocaine Dependent group and the two other groups. (From Bauer, 1997, with permission.)

these patients, the frontal P3*a* decrement also correlated significantly with the number of diagnostic criteria met for childhood Conduct Disorder. The results of Bauer's careful analysis therefore revealed that the ERP decrement in cocaine dependent patients was strongly related to the patients' premorbid status and independent of their drug use (Bauer, 1997).

A remarkable additional feature of Bauer's study was the demonstration that P3*a* amplitude recorded during the initial months of abstinence was significantly related to outcome. In fact, P3*a* was more strongly related to outcome than any of the traditional clinical predictors, viz., years of alcohol or cocaine abuse, family history of alcoholism, and Michigan Alcoholism Screening Test (MAST) score. A discriminant function analysis revealed that P3*a* amplitude alone accurately identified 70.6% of the patients who would later relapse and 53.3% of the patients who would remain abstinent.

Discussion

Neuroimaging Research In Context

The application of functional magnetic resonance imaging (fMRI) and positron and single photon emission tomography (PET and SPECT) to studies of the effects of psychoactive drug use has generated tremendous enthusiasm in the scientific and lay communities. High resolution structural magnetic resonance images are now frequently featured as the "backdrop" for overlaid renderings of regional variation in either glucose or oxygen utilization, or ligand binding. When such images are displayed from patients exposed to psychoactive drugs in comparison to healthy non-intoxicated or non-dependent volunteers, the results appear compelling. However, it must be recognized that these renderings are based upon assumptions which are not always recognized as important or made explicit. Nadeau and Crosson (1995) have presented an excellent and highly readable overview of the assumptions of the newer functional neuroimaging technologies.

In the present context of the enthusiasm for fMRI, PET, and SPECT, electroencephalography has sometimes been discounted. Among the criticisms is the fact that the technology is rather old and has several known limitations. In fairness, however, we must recognize that the younger neuroimaging modalities have limitations which we are only now beginning to discover and elucidate. It will be interesting to see what the future holds with regard to the relative value of these various technologies as they mature.

A second criticism of EEG research is the perception that it has entered a stagnant period in which the same questions are repeatedly being asked and answered. For example, one could reasonably ask whether the scientific literature would significantly benefit from yet another demonstration of a P300 deficit in either schizophrenic or Alzheimer's-Diseased patients. In addition, the use of the electroencephalogram in clinical practice, and the associated requirement of standardization (e.g., of the number of recording channels, electrode density and placement, and EEG scoring methods), has implicitly discouraged commercial vendors of EEG hardware and software, as well as some clinical researchers, from pursuing advancements in the technology and its application to new and interesting questions.

Fortunately, the situation with regard to EEG research and its technological development is changing. The traditional approach in EEG/ERP studies, in which data were collected from a mere 19 electrodes arranged in the standard 10/20 montage, is being replaced by high density electrode arrays, containing as many as 256 channels. With higher density electrode arrays, the spatial resolution of EEG recordings improves markedly and the ability to localize generators of normal or abnormal activity approaches that of PET or SPECT.

However, increasing the density of the electrode array is not enough. The accurate localization of a regional change in brain electrical activity also requires the solution of two problems—namely, (1) the biasing effect of the reference electrode and (2) the blurring of the scalp voltage distribution arising from volume conduction. Because EEG recordings make use of differential amplifiers, the voltage difference between the reference electrode and the "active" electrode will be related to the physical proximity of the electrodes as well as their alignment relative to the source of the voltage fluctuation (Jayakar et al., 1991). Topographic maps of EEG or evoked potential voltages cannot be accurately interpreted unless this bias is removed. In fact, a partial solution can be implemented by mathematically removing the reference and calculating a current source density (CSD) map. The calculation of this Laplacian derivative of the voltage distribution also removes much of the spatial blurring in the topographic map that arises from diffusion or volume conduction of the signal through the dura, cranium, and scalp.

Despite some remaining problems, there is much to recommend EEG technology in studies of the acute and chronic effects of psychoactive drugs. For example, the cost of a new multichannel EEG amplification system has dropped substantially in recent years. In the 1999 marketplace, a 64-channel EEG amplifier system can be purchased for <$19,000. The recurring costs for infrastructure (e.g., technicians, space), maintenance, and supplies are also minimal. When contrasted to the high initial and recurring costs of PET, SPECT, or fMRI studies, EEG studies are a remarkable value.

Related to the lower cost of EEG technology is an increase in the number of subjects or conditions that can be tested within a fixed budget. It would, for example, be difficult for any PET, SPECT, or fMRI researcher to conduct a study in which the design requires the testing of three or more groups with more than 20–30 members, and/or an interaction among two or more grouping factors. The costs of such a study would be prohibitive. By contrast, because of its lower cost, EEG techniques provide the clinical researcher with an opportunity to examine the effects of numerous mediating and moderating variables within complex multi-group experimental designs.

Because EEG recordings offer a level of temporal resolution which exceeds that of the other neuroimaging modalities, EEG technology provides a unique opportunity to study the flow of information processing in real time (cf. Gevins, 1998). With EEG data, it is a relatively simple matter to plot the distribution of CSD changes over the scalp over time and follow the activation from sensory cortex into different association areas. Because blood flow, oxygen, and glucose utilization changes lag behind the EEG, and are also slow to recover, PET, SPECT, and fMRI are less able to determine which cortical activations occurred first or how the activations relate to one another in sequence.

A final strength of EEG technology is its portability and ease of use. For example, manufacturers have recently produced multichannel EEG amplification systems that are small, lightweight, and battery-operated. EEG acquisition software has also been programmed for lightweight, portable notebook computers. Thus, the opportunity exists for assembling a portable EEG/ERP lab which could be mobilized to study patients in small clinics, rural settings, or in homes or other residences (such as prisons). This portability and ease of use can lead to a rapid translation between laboratory findings and their clinical implementation, e.g., in relapse prediction (Bauer, 1994a, 1997; Winterer et al., 1998), medication monitoring (Hersh et al., 1995), or the assessment of central nervous system recovery (Bauer, 1996).

To date, most investigations of EEG changes associated with psychoactive drug use or abuse have not included the aforementioned refinements in spatial localization. However, the absence of such refinements need not be viewed as a significant weakness or a barrier to progress. As we have seen from our review of the literature, a high level of spatial resolution is unnecessary if an investigator is interested in asking questions about dose-effect relationships, rate of recovery of brain function, medication effects, or correlations with clinical variables. The implementation of high spatial resolution techniques is only necessary for testing specific hypotheses about localization of functional differences. Of course, if the hypotheses are not location specific and are not formulated a priori, then the enormous number of data points (whether these data points be voxels, pixels, or electrode sites) associated with high spatial resolution imaging will create a massive data set that will invite "fishing expeditions" and unreproducible results.

Future Directions

One avenue by which electroencephalography and the other neuroimaging modalities could reach their common destination of elucidating the effects of drug use and abuse is by following parallel and independent tracks, i.e., the status quo. Up to the present time, it has not been necessary for EEG, fMRI, PET, or SPECT researchers to read and cite literature from other neuroimaging domains. Indeed, each of the neuroimaging technologies has a knowledge base which is somewhat specific to that technology and is undergoing rapid growth. However, it would be unfortunate if fMRI, PET, or SPECT researchers failed to examine the rich EEG/EP/ERP literature for ideas about the subject variables, activation paradigms, and analytical models which have already been shown to be useful for revealing differences associated with drug use and abuse. More specifically, fMRI, PET, and SPECT researchers might want to more closely consider the complex main effects or interactions described above involving genetics (Wall and Ehlers, 1995; Ehlers et al., 1998), childhood conduct disorder/adult antisocial personality disorder (Hesselbrock et al., 1993a,b; Bauer et al., 1994a,b; O'Connor et al., 1994; Bauer and Hesselbrock, 1999a,b), severity of dependence (Bauer, 1998; Struve et al., 1998), duration of abstinence (Bauer, 1997), and other factors, e.g., rising versus falling blood levels, alcohol's indirect effects on brain temperature, comorbid depression.

A second avenue for future research and collaboration might involve the performance of an EEG, EP, or ERP study as a preface to a subsequent study using one of the other neuroimaging modalities. That is, fMRI, PET, or SPECT researchers might consider EEG, EP, or ERP measures as a means for testing the ability of their stimuli, or their new cognitive activation paradigms, to evoke a detectable change in brain activity. Given the lower cost of EEG technology and the relative ease with which EEG assessments can be scheduled, stimulus or paradigm development might be more efficiently performed in an EEG laboratory than in a PET, SPECT, or MR facility.

A third avenue for future research and collaboration might involve the implementation of a large scale EEG/EP/ERP study using high spatial resolution EEG methods. If the EEG/EP/ERP study reveals a localizable difference in brain activity associated with a particular subject group or experimental condition, then the superior spatial resolution of fMRI, PET, or SPECT could be applied in a smaller, follow-up study using a subset of the original subject sample. This approach would reduce the high cost of neuroimaging research and would situate the more expensive technologies in a confirmatory rather than exploratory role.

A fourth possible direction for collaborative research might involve the acquisition of EEG/EP/ERP data along with either fMRI, SPECT, or PET data from all subjects under all conditions. Although expensive and somewhat impractical, this approach would allow one to complement the superior spatial resolution of fMRI, PET, and SPECT with the superior temporal resolution of the EEG. In doing so, one might develop a better understanding of neural processing in real time and how it is disrupted by drug use or abuse.

Acknowledgments

This research was supported in part by Public Health Service grants R01DA05826, R01DA08598, and P50AA03510.

REFERENCES

Adams, D. A., McClelland, R. J., Houston, H. G. and Gamble, W. G., The effects of diazepam on the auditory brain stem responses. Br. J. Audiol. 19:277–280, 1985.

Alper, K. R., Chabot, R. J., Kim, A. H., Prichep, L. S. and John, E. R., Quantitative EEG correlates of crack cocaine dependence. Psychiatry Res. 35:95–105, 1990.

Alper, K. R., Prichep, L. S., Kowalik, S., Rosenthal, M. S. and John, E. R., Persistent QEEG abnormality in crack cocaine users at 6 months of drug abstinence. Neuropsychopharmacology 19:1–9, 1998.

Ames, F., A clinical and metabolic study of acute intoxication with cannabis sativa and its role in the psychosis model. J. Ment. Sci. 104:972–999, 1958.

Bauer, L. O., Photic driving of EEG alpha activity in recovering substance abusers. Am. J. Addict. 3:49–57, 1993.

Bauer, L. O., Electroencephalographic and autonomic predictors of relapse in alcohol-dependent patients. Alcohol. Clin. Exp. Res. 18:755–760, 1994a.

Bauer, L. O., Vigilance in recovering cocaine-dependent and alcohol-dependent patients: a prospective study. Addict. Behav. 19:599–607, 1994b.

Bauer, L. O., Psychomotor and electroencephalographic sequelae of cocaine dependence. In: Majewska, M. D. (ed.) Neurotoxicity and Neuropathology Associated with Cocaine Abuse. NIDA Res. Mono. Vol.163, Rockville, MD, pp. 66–93, 1996.

Bauer, L. O., Frontal P300 decrements, childhood conduct disorder, family history and the prediction of relapse among abstinent cocaine abusers. Drug Alcohol Depend. 44:1–10, 1997.

Bauer, L. O., Effects of chronic opioid dependence and HIV-1 infection on pattern shift visual evoked potentials. Drug Alcohol Depend. 50:147–155, 1998.

Bauer, L. O. and Easton, C., Pattern shift visual evoked potentials in abstinent cocaine-dependent, alcohol-dependent and cross-dependent patients. Drug Alcohol Depend. 40:203–209, 1996.

Bauer, L. O. and Hesselbrock, V. M., EEG, autonomic and subjective correlates of the risk for alcoholism. J. Stud. Alcohol. 54:577–589, 1993.

Bauer, L. O. and Hesselbrock, V. M., P300 decrements in teenagers with conduct problems: implications for substance abuse risk and brain development. Biol. Psychiatry 46:263–272, 1999a.

Bauer, L. O. and Hesselbrock, V. M., Subtypes of family history and conduct disorder: effects on P300 during the Stroop Test. Neuropsychopharmacology 21:51–62, 1999b.

Bauer, L. O. and Kranzler, H. R., Electroencephalographic activity and mood in cocaine-dependent outpatients: effects of cocaine cue exposure. Biol. Psychiatry 36:189–197, 1994.

Bauer, L. O. and Mott, A. E., Differential effects of cocaine, alcohol and nicotine dependence on olfactory evoked potentials. Drug Alcohol Depend. 42:21–26, 1996.

Bauer, L. O., O'Connor, S. and Hesselbrock, V. M., Frontal P300 decrements in antisocial personality disorder. Alcohol. Clin. Exp. Res. 18:1300–1305, 1994a.

Bauer, L., Hesselbrock, V. M., O'Connor, S. and Roberts, L., P300 differences between non-alcoholic young men at average and above-average risk for alcoholism: effects of distraction and task modality. Prog. Neuropsychopharmacol. Biol. Psychiatry 18:263–277, 1994b.

Bauer, L. O., Gross, J. B., Meyer, R. E. and Greenblatt, D. J., Chronic alcohol abuse and the acute sedative and neurophysiologic effects of midazolam. Psychopharmacology (Berl.) 133:293–299, 1997.

Begleiter, H. and Platz, A., The effects of alcohol on the central nervous system in humans. In: Kissin, B. and Begleiter, H. (eds.) The Biology of Alcoholism, Vol. 2: Physiology and Behavior. New York, Plenum, pp. 293–344, 1972.

Begleiter, H. and Porjesz, B. Persistence of a "subacute withdrawal syndrome" following chronic ethanol intake. Drug Alcohol Depend. 4:353–357, 1979.

Berger, H., Arch. Psychiatr. Nervenkr. 94, 16–30, translated in (1969) Hans Berger on the electroencephalogram of man. In: Electroencephalogr. Clin. Neurophysiol. Suppl. 28: 95–132, 1931.

Berger, H., Arch. Psychiatr. Nervenkr. 106, 577–584, translated in (1969) Hans Berger on the electroencephalogram of man. In: Electroencephalogr. Clin. Neurophysiol. Suppl. 28:291–297, 1937.

Biggins, C. A., Fein, G., Raz, J. and Amir, A., Artifactually high coherences result from using spherical spline computation of scalp current density. Electroencephalogr. Clin. Neurophysiol. 79:413–419, 1991.

Biggins, C. A., MacKay, S., Poole, N. and Fein, G., Delayed P3A in abstinent elderly male chronic alcoholics. Alcohol. Clin. Exp. Res. 19:1032–1042, 1995.

Biggins, C. A., MacKay, S., Clark, W. and Fein, G., Event-related potential evidence for frontal cortex effects of chronic cocaine dependence. Biol. Psychiatry 42:472–485, 1997.

Biscaldi, G. P., Mingardi, M., Pollini, G., Moglia, A. and Bossi, M. C., Acute toluene poisoning: electroneurophysiological and vestibular investigations. Toxicol. Eur. Res. 3:271–273, 1981.

Boker, T. and Heinze, H. J., Influence of diazepam on visual pattern-evoked potentials with due regard to nonstationary effects: methodological problems. Neuropsychobiology 11:207–212, 1984.

Bond, A., Lader, M. and Shrotriya, R., Comparative effects of a repeated dose regime of diazepam and buspirone on subjective ratings, psychological tests and the EEG. Eur. J. Clin. Pharmacol. 24:463–467, 1983.

Bond, A.J., Silveira, J. C. and Lader, M. H., The effects of alprazolam alone and combined with alcohol on central integrative activity. Eur. J. Clin. Pharmacol. 42:495–498, 1992.

Breimer, L. T., Hennis, P. J., Burm, A. G., Danhof, M., Bovill, J. G., Spierdijk, J. and Vletter, A. A., Quantification of the EEG effect of midazolam by aperiodic analysis in volunteers. Pharmacokinetic/pharmacodynamic modelling. Clin. Pharmacokinet. 18:245–253, 1990.

Breimer, L. T., Burm, A. G., Danhof, M., Hennis, P. J., Vletter, A. A., de Voogt, J. W., Spierdijk, J. and Bovill, J. G., Pharmacokinetic-pharmacodynamic modelling of the interaction between flumazenil and midazolam in volunteers by aperiodic EEG analysis. Clin. Pharmacokinet. 20:497–508, 1991.

Brinciotti, M., Effects of chronic high serum levels of phenobarbital on evoked potentials in epileptic children. Electroencephalogr. Clin. Neurophysiol. 92:11–16, 1994.

Bromm, B. and Treede, R. D., Laser-evoked cerebral potentials in the assessment of cutaneous pain sensitivity in normal subjects and patients. Rev. Neurol. 147:625–643, 1991.

Broughton, R., Meier-Ewer, K. H. and Ebe, M., Visual and somatosensory evoked potentials of photosensitive epileptic subjects during wakefulness, sleep, and following i.v. diazepam. Electroencephalogr. Clin. Neurophysiol. 21:622–626, 1966.

Brown, C. R., Sarnquist, F. H., Canup, C. A. and Pedley, T. A., Clinical, electroencephalographic, and pharmacokinetic studies of a water-soluble benzodiazepine, midazolam maleate. Anesthesiology 50:467–470, 1979.

Brown, M. E., Anton, R. F., Malcolm, R. and Ballenger, J. C., Alcohol detoxification and withdrawal seizures: clinical support for a kindling hypothesis. Biol. Psychiatry 23:507–514, 1988.

Buhrer, M., Maitre, P. O., Hung, O. and Stanski, D. R., Electroencephalographic effects of benzodiazepines. I. Choosing an electroencephalographic parameter to measure the effect of midazolam on the central nervous system. Clin. Pharmacol. Ther. 48:544–554, 1990.

Cadaveira, F., Grau, C., Roso, M. and Sanchez-Turet, M., Multimodality exploration of event-related potentials in chronic alcoholics. Alcohol. Clin. Exp. Res. 15:607–611, 1991.

Cadaveira, F., Roso, M., Grau, C. and Sanchez-Turet, M., Effects of age on event-related potentials in chronic alcoholics: a multimodal study. Neuropsychobiology 25:166–171, 1992.

Caldwell, J. A., Caldwell, J. L., Crowley, J. S. and Jones, H. D., Sustaining helicopter pilot performance with Dexedrine during periods of sleep deprivation. Aviat. Space Environ. Med. 66:930–937, 1995.

Campbell, K. B. and Lowick, B. M., Ethanol and event-related potentials: the influence of distractor stimuli. Alcohol 4:257–263, 1987.

Chan, Y. W., McLeod, J. G., Tuck, R. R., Walsh, J. C. and Feary, P. A., Visual evoked responses in chronic alcoholics. J. Neurol. Neurosurg. Psychiatry 49:945–950, 1986.

Chiappa, K., Evoked Potentials in Clinical Medicine. Philadelphia, PA: Lippincott-Raven, 1997.

Church, M. W. and Williams, H. L., Dose- and time-dependent effects of ethanol on brain stem auditory evoked responses in young adult males. Electroencephalogr. Clin. Neurophysiol. 54:161–174, 1982.

Coger, R. W., Dymond, A. M., Serafetinides, E. A., Lowenstam, I. and Pearson, D., EEG signs of brain impairment in alcoholism. Biol. Psychiatry 13:729–739, 1978.

Cohen, H. L., Porjesz, B. and Begleiter, H., Ethanol-induced alterations in electroencephalographic activity in adult males. Neuropsychopharmacology 8:365–370, 1993a.

Cohen, H. L., Porjesz, B. and Begleiter, H., The effects of ethanol on EEG activity in males at risk for alcoholism. Electroencephalogr. Clin. Neurophysiol. 86:368–376, 1993b.

Colrain, I. M., Taylor, J., McLean, S., Buttery, R., Wise, G. and Montgomery, I., Dose dependent effects of alcohol on visual evoked potentials. Psychopharmacology (Berl.) 112:383–388, 1993.

Costa, L. and Bauer, L., Quantitative electroencephalographic differences associated with alcohol, cocaine, heroin and dual-substance dependence. Drug Alcohol Depend. 46:87–93, 1997.

Coulthard, P. and Rood, J. P., Midazolam and somatosensory evoked potentials. Br. J. Oral Maxillofac. Surg. 31:28–31, 1993.

Curran, H. V., Pooviboonsuk, P., Dalton, J. A. and Lader, M. H., Differentiating the effects of centrally acting drugs on arousal and memory: an event-related potential study of scopolamine, lorazepam and diphenhydramine. Psychopharmacology (Berl.) 135:27–36, 1998.

Davis, P. A., Gibbs, F. A., Davis, H., Jetter, W. W. and Trowbridge, L. S., The effects of alcohol upon the electroencephalogram. Q. J. Stud. Alcohol 1:626–631, 1941.

Docter, R. F., Naitoh, P. and Smith, J. C., Electroencephalographic changes and vigilance behavior during experimentally induced intoxication with alcoholic subjects. Psychosom. Med. 28:605–611, 1966.

Dornbush, R. L., Fink, M. and Freedman, A. M., Marijuana, memory, and perception. Am. J. Psychiatry 128:194–197, 1971.

Ebe, M., Meier-Ewert, K. H. and Broughton, R., Effects of intravenous diazepam (valium) upon evoked potentials of photosensitive epileptic and normal subjects. Electroencephalogr. Clin. Neurophysiol. 27:429–435, 1969.

Ehlers, C. L., Wall, T. L. and Schuckit, M. A., EEG spectral characteristics following ethanol administration in young men. Electroencephalogr. Clin. Neurophysiol. 73:179–187, 1989.

Ehlers, C. L., Garcia-Andrade, C., Wall, T. L., Sobel, D. F. and Phillips, E., Determinants of P3 amplitude and response to alcohol in Native American Mission Indians. Neuropsychopharmacology 18:282–292, 1998.

Ekman, G., Frankenhouser, M., Goldberg, L., Hagdahl, R. and Myrsten, A. L., Subjective and objective effects of alcohol as functions of dosage and time. Psychopharmacologia 6:399–410, 1964.

Elmasian, R., Neville, H., Woods, D., Schuckit, M. and Bloom, F., Event-related brain potentials are different in individuals at high and low risk for developing alcoholism. Proc. Natl. Acad. Sci. USA 79:7900–7903, 1982.

Engel, G. L. and Rosenbaum, M., Studies of the electroencephalogram in acute alcoholic intoxication. Proc. Cent. Soc. Clin. Res. 17:62–67, 1944.

Engelhardt, W., Friess, K., Hartung, E., Sold, M. and Dierks, T., EEG and auditory evoked potential P300 compared with psychometric tests in assessing vigilance after benzodiazepine sedation and antagonism. Br. J. Anaesth. 69:75–80, 1992.
Engelhardt, W., Stahl, K., Marouche, A., Hartung, E. and Dierks, T., Ketamine racemate versus S-(+)-ketamine with or without antagonism with physostigmine: a quantitative EEG study on volunteers. [German]. Anaesthesist 43 Suppl. 2:S76–82, 1994.
Erwin, C. W., Linnoila, M., Hartwell, J., Erwin, A. and Guthrie, S., Effects of buspirone and diazepam, alone and in combination with alcohol, on skilled performance and evoked potentials. J. Clin. Psychopharmacol. 6:199–209, 1986.
Fein, G., Biggins, C. and MacKay, S., Cocaine abusers have reduced auditory P50 amplitude and suppression compared to both normal controls and alcoholics. Biol. Psychiatry 39:955–965, 1996.
Feshchenko, V. A., Veselis, R. A. and Reinsel, R. A., Comparison of the EEG effects of midazolam, thiopental, and propofol: the role of underlying oscillatory systems. Neuropsychobiology 35:211–220, 1997.
Fink, M., Volavka, J., Panayiotopoulos, C. P. and Stefanis, C., Quantitative EEG studies of marijuana, delta-9-tetrahydrocannabinol and hashish in man. In: Braude, M. C. and Szara, S. (eds.) The Pharmacology of Marijuana. New York: Raven Press, pp. 383–391, 1976.
Fiset, P., Lemmens, H. L., Egan, T. E., Shafer, S. L. and Stanski, D. R., Pharmacodynamic modeling of the electroencephalographic effects of flumazenil in healthy volunteers sedated with midazolam. Clin. Pharmacol. Ther. 58:567–582, 1995.
Fowler, B. and Adams, J., Dissociation of the effects of alcohol and amphetamine on inert gas narcosis using reaction time and P300 latency. Aviat. Space Environ. Med. 64:493–499, 1993.
Fowler, B. and Mitchell, I., Biological determinants of P300: the effects of a barbiturate on latency and amplitude. Biol. Psychol. 46:113–124, 1997.
Frank, H., Heber, G. and Fritsch, M., Analysis of the EEG of alcoholic patients in the initial phase of abstinence. [German]. Nervenarzt 57:730–735, 1986.
Frowein, H. W., Gaillard, A. W. and Varey, C. A., EP components, visual processing stages, and the effect of a barbiturate. Biol. Psychol. 13:239–249, 1981.
Gevins, A., The future of electroencephalography in assessing neurocognitive functioning. Electroencephalogr. Clin. Neurophysiol. 106:165–172, 1998.
Grasso, P., Sharratt, M., Davies, D. M. and Irvine, D., Neurophysiological and psychological disorders and occupational exposure to organic solvents. Food Chem. Toxicol. 22:819–852, 1984.
Greenblatt, D. J., Ehrenberg, B. L., Gunderman, J., Locniskar, A., Scavone, J. M., Harmatz, J. S. and Shader, R. I., Pharmacokinetic and electroencephalographic study of intravenous diazepam, midazolam, and placebo. Clin. Pharmacol. Ther. 45:356–365, 1989.
Greenblatt, D. J., Harmatz, J. S., Gouthro, T. A., Locke, J. and Shader, R. I., Distinguishing a benzodiazepine agonist (triazolam) from a nonagonist anxiolytic (buspirone) by electroencephalography: kinetic-dynamic studies. Clin. Pharmacol. Ther. 56:100–111, 1994.
Halliday, R., Naylor, H., Callaway, E., Yano, L. and Walton, P., What's done can't always be undone: the effects of stimulant drugs and dopamine blockers on information processing. Electroencephalogr. Clin. Neurophysiol. Suppl. 40:532–537, 1987.
Hallstrom, C. and Lader, M., Benzodiazepine withdrawal phenomena. Int. Pharmacopsychiatry 16:235–244, 1981.
Hamilton, M. J., Smith, P. R. and Peck, A. W., Effects of bupropion, nomifensine and dexamphetamine on performance, subjective feelings, autonomic variables and electroencephalogram in healthy volunteers. Br. J. Clin. Pharmacol. 15:367–374, 1983.
Hazemann, P., Jeftic, M. and Lille, F., Somatosensory evoked potentials in alcoholics and patients occupationally exposed to solvents and lead. Electromyogr. Clin. Neurophysiol. 27:183–187, 1987.

Herning, R. I. and King, D. E., EEG and evoked potentials alterations in cocaine-dependent individuals. NIDA Res. Monogr. 163:203–223, 1996.

Herning, R. I., Jones, R. T. and Peltzman, D. J., Changes in human event related potentials with prolonged delta-9- tetrahydrocannabinol (THC) use. Electroencephalogr. Clin. Neurophysiol. 47:556–570, 1979.

Herning, R. I., Jones, R. T., Hooker, W. D., Mendelson, J. and Blackwell, L., Cocaine increases EEG beta: a replication and extension of Hans Berger's historic experiments. Electroencephalogr. Clin. Neurophysiol. 60:470–477, 1985a.

Herning, R. I., Jones, R. T., Hooker, W. D. and Tulunay, F. C., Information processing components of the auditory event related potential are reduced by cocaine. Psychopharmacology (Berl.) 87:178–185, 1985b.

Herning, R. I., Glover, B. J., Koeppl, B., Weddington, W. and Jaffe, J. H., Cognitive deficits in abstaining cocaine abusers. NIDA Res. Monogr. 101:167–178, 1990.

Herning, R. I., Glover, B. J., Koeppl, B., Phillips, R. L. and London, E. D., Cocaine-induced increases in EEG alpha and beta activity: evidence for reduced cortical processing. Neuropsychopharmacology 11:1–9, 1994a.

Herning, R. I., Glover, B. J. and Guo, X., Effects of cocaine on P3B in cocaine abusers. Neuropsychobiology 30:132–142, 1994b.

Herning, R. I., Guo, X., Better, W. E., Weinhold, L. L., Lange, W. R., Cadet, J. L. and Gorelick, D. A., Neurophysiological signs of cocaine dependence: increased electroencephalogram beta during withdrawal. Biol. Psychiatry 41:1087–1094, 1997.

Herrmann, W. M., Hofmann, W. and Kubicki, S., Psychotropic drug induced changes in auditory averaged evoked potentials: results of a double-blind trial using an objective fully automated AEP analysis method. Int. J. Clin. Pharmacol. Ther. Toxicol. 19:56–62, 1981.

Hersh, D., Bauer, L. O. and Kranzler, H. R., Carbamazepine and cocaine-cue reactivity. Drug Alcohol Depend. 39:213–221, 1995.

Hesselbrock, V., Bauer, L. O., O'Connor, S. and Gillen, R., Reduced P300 amplitude in relation to a family history of alcoholism and antisocial personality disorder among young men at risk for alcoholism. In: Taberner, P. V and Badawy, A. A. (eds.) Advances in Biomedical Alcohol Research: Proceedings of the 6th ISBRA Congress, June 21–26, 1992. Bristol, U.K, pp. 95–100, 1993a.

Hesselbrock, V., Bauer, L., O'Connor, S. and Gillen, R., Reduced P300 amplitude in relation to family history of alcoholism and antisocial personality disorder among young men at risk for alcoholism. Alcohol Alcohol. Suppl. 2:95–100, 1993b.

Hollister, L. E., Sherwood, S. L. and Cavasino, A., Marihuana and the human electroencephalogram. Pharmacol. Res. Commun. 2:305–308, 1970.

Holmes, G. L. and Korteling, F., Drug effects on the human EEG. Am. J. EEG Technol. 33: 1–26, 1993.

Hou, W. Y., Lee, W. Y., Lin, S. M., Liu, C. C., Susceto, L., Sun, W. Z. and Lin, S. Y., The effects of ketamine, propofol and nitrous oxide on visual evoked potential during fentanyl anesthesia. Ma Tsui Hsueh Tsa Chi 31:97–102, 1993.

Indulski, J. A., Sinczuk-Walczak, H., Szymczak, M. and Wesolowski, W., Neurological and neurophysiological examinations of workers occupationally exposed to organic solvent mixtures used in the paint and varnish production. Int. J. Occup. Med. Environ. Health 9:235–244, 1996.

Inoue, T., Kawasaki, H., Shiraishi, S. and Takasaki, M., Effects of high-dose fentanyl anesthesia on auditory brain stem responses. [Japanese]. Masui—Jpn. J. Anesthesiol. 41:1414–1418, 1992.

Jaaskelainen, I. P., Lehtokoski, A., Alho, K., Kujala, T., Pekkonen, E., Sinclair, J. D., Naatanen, R. and Sillanaukee, P., Low dose of ethanol suppresses mismatch negativity of auditory event-related potentials. Alcohol. Clin. Exp. Res. 19:607–610, 1995a.

Jaaskelainen, I. P., Pekkonen, E., Alho, K., Sinclair, J. D., Sillanaukee, P. and Naatanen, R., Dose-related effect of alcohol on mismatch negativity and reaction time performance. Alcohol 12:491–495, 1995b.

Jayakar, P., Duchowny, M., Resnick, T. J. and Alvarez, L. A., Localization of seizure foci: pitfalls and caveats. J. Clin. Neurophysiol. 8:414–431, 1991.

Jones, R. T. and Stone, G. C., Psychological studies of marijuana and alcohol in man. Psychopharmacologia 18:108–117, 1970.

Jones, T. A., Stockard, J. J. and Weidner, W. J., The effects of temperature and acute alcohol intoxication on brain stem auditory evoked potentials in the cat. Electroencephalogr. Clin. Neurophysiol. 49:23–30, 1980.

Kaplan, R. F., Glueck, B. C., Hesselbrock, M. N. and Reed, H. B., Jr., Power and coherence analysis of the EEG in hospitalized alcoholics and nonalcoholic controls. J. Stud. Alcohol 46:122–127, 1985.

Kaplan, R. F., Hesselbrock, V. M., O'Connor, S. and DePalma, N., Behavioral and EEG responses to alcohol in nonalcoholic men with a family history of alcoholism. Prog. Neuropsychopharmacol. Biol. Psychiatry 12:873–885, 1988.

Kinoshita, T., Michel, C. M., Yagyu, T., Lehmann, D. and Saito, M., Diazepam and sulpiride effects on frequency domain EEG source locations. Neuropsychobiology 30:126–131, 1994.

Kochs, E. and Bischoff, P., Ketamine and evoked potentials. [German]. Anaesthesist 43 Suppl. 2:S8–14, 1994.

Kopell, B. S., Roth, W. T. and Tinklenberg, J. R., Time course effects of marijuana and ethanol on event-related potentials. Psychopharmacology (Berl.) 56:15–20, 1978.

Kopun, M. and Propping, P., The kinetics of ethanol absorption and elimination in twins and supplementary repetitive experiments in singleton subjects. Eur. J. Clin. Pharmacol. 11:337–344, 1977.

Koukkou, M. and Lehmann, D., Correlations between cannabis-induced psychopathology and EEG before and after drug ingestion. Pharmakopsychiatr. Neuropsychopharmakol. 11:220–227, 1978.

Kouri, E. M., Lukas, S. E. and Mendelson, J. H., P300 assessment of opiate and cocaine users: effects of detoxification and buprenorphine treatment. Biol. Psychiatry 40:617–628, 1996.

Krauss, G. L. and Niedermeyer, E., Electroencephalogram and seizures in chronic alcoholism. Electroencephalogr. Clin. Neurophysiol. 78:97–104, 1991.

Langeron, O., Lille, F., Zerhouni, O., Orliaguet, G., Saillant, G., Riou, B. and Coriat, P., Comparison of the effects of ketamine-midazolam with those of fentanyl-midazolam on cortical somatosensory evoked potentials during major spine surgery. Br. J. Anaesth. 78:701–706, 1997.

Lauer, K., Munshi, C. and Larson, S., The effect of midazolam on median nerve somatosensory evoked potentials. J. Clin. Monit. 10:181–184, 1994.

Laurian, S., Gaillard, J. M., Le, P. K. and Schopf, J., Effects of a benzodiazepine antagonist on the diazepam-induced electrical brain activity modifications. Neuropsychobiology 11:55–58, 1984.

Laurijssens, B. E. and Greenblatt, D. J., Pharmacokinetic-pharmacodynamic relationships for benzodiazepines. Clin. Pharmacokinet. 30:52–76, 1996.

Lee, J. A., Schoener, E. P., Nielsen, D. W., Kelly, A. R., Lin, W. N. and Berman, R. F., Alcohol and the auditory brain-stem response, brain temperature, and blood alcohol curves: explanation of a paradox. Electroencephalogr. Clin. Neurophysiol. 77:362–375, 1990.

Lemmens, H. J., Dyck, J. B., Shafer, S. L. and Stanski, D. R., Pharmacokinetic-pharmacodynamic modeling in drug development: application to the investigational opioid trefentanil. Clin. Pharmacol. Ther. 56:261–271, 1994.

Lemmens, H. J., Egan, T. D., Fiset, P. and Stanski, D. R., Pharmacokinetic/dynamic assessment in drug development: application to the investigational opioid mirfentanil. Anesth. Analg. 80:1206–1211, 1995.

Leweke, M., Kampmann, C., Radwan, M., Dietrich, D. E., Johannes, S., Emrich, H. M. and Munte, T. F., The effects of tetrahydrocannabinol on the recognition of emotionally charged words: an analysis using event-related brain potentials. Neuropsychobiology 37:104–111, 1998.

Lewis, E. G., Dustman, R. E. and Beck, E. C., The effect of alcohol on sensory phenomena and cognitive motor tasks. Q. J. Stud. Alcohol 30:618–633, 1969.

Lewis, E. G., Dustman, R. E. and Beck, E. C., The effects of alcohol on visual and somatosensory evoked responses. Electroencephalogr. Clin. Neurophysiol. 28:202–205, 1970.

Lindgren, M., Osterberg, K., Orbaek, P. and Rosen, I., Solvent-induced toxic encephalopathy: electrophysiological data in relation to neuropsychological findings. J. Clin. Exp. Neuropsychol. 19:772–783, 1997.

Lorenz, J., Beck, H. and Bromm, B., Cognitive performance, mood and experimental pain before and during morphine-induced analgesia in patients with chronic non-malignant pain. Pain 73:369–375, 1997.

Loughnan, B. L., Sebel, P. S., Thomas, D., Rutherfoord, C. F. and Rogers, H., Evoked potentials following diazepam or fentanyl. Anaesthesia 42:195–198, 1987.

Lowinson, J. H., Ruiz, P. and Millman, R. B., Substance Abuse: A Comprehensive Textbook., 2nd edition. Baltimore, MD, Williams & Wilkins, 1992.

Lukas, S. E., Mendelson, J. H., Woods, B. T., Mello, N. K. and Teoh, S. K., Topographic distribution of EEG alpha activity during ethanol-induced intoxication in women. J. Stud. Alcohol 50:176–185, 1989a.

Lukas, S. E., Mendelson, J. H., Amass, L. and Benedikt, R., Behavioral and EEG studies of acute cocaine administration: comparisons with morphine, amphetamine, pentobarbital, nicotine, ethanol and marijuana. NIDA Res. Monogr. 95:146–151, 1989b.

Lukas, S. E., Mendelson, J. H., Kouri, E., Bolduc, M. and Amass, L., Ethanol-induced alterations in EEG alpha activity and apparent source of the auditory P300 evoked response potential. Alcohol 7:471–477, 1990.

Lukas, S. E., Mendelson, J. H. and Benedikt, R., Electroencephalographic correlates of marihuana-induced euphoria. Drug Alcohol Depend. 37:131–140, 1995.

Lykken, D. T., Tellegen, A. and Iacono, W. G., EEG spectra in twins: evidence for a neglected mechanism of genetic determination. Physiol. Psychol. 10:60–65, 1982.

Mandema, J. W., Sansom, L. N., Dios-Vieitez, M. C., Hollander-Jansen, M. and Danhof, M., Pharmacokinetic-pharmacodynamic modeling of the electroencephalographic effects of benzodiazepines: correlation with receptor binding and anticonvulsant activity. J. Pharmacol. Exp. Ther. 257:472–478, 1991.

Manmaru, S. and Matsuura, M., Two kinds of spatiotemporal EEG changes after discontinuation of benzodiazepine, medazepam. Jpn. J. Psychiatry Neurol. 44:85–90, 1990.

Martin, W. H., Pratt, H. and Schwegler, J. W., The origin of the human auditory brain-stem response wave II. Electroencephalogr. Clin. Neurophysiol. 96:357–370, 1995.

Maylor, E. A., Rabbitt, P. M., James, G. H. and Kerr, S. A., Effects of alcohol, practice, and task complexity on reaction time distributions. Q. J. Exp. Psychol. [A] 44:119–139, 1992.

McPherson, R. W., Sell, B. and Traystman, R. J., Effects of thiopental, fentanyl, and etomidate on upper extremity somatosensory evoked potentials in humans. Anesthesiology 65:584–589, 1986.

Merlo, F. and Lion, P., Study of the rapid EEG activity induced by midazolam. Curr. Ther. Res. Clin. Exp. 38:798–807, 1985.

Milligan, K. R., Lumsden, J., Howard, R. C., Howe, J. P. and Dundee, J. W., Use of auditory evoked responses as a measure of recovery from benzodiazepine sedation. J. R. Soc. Med. 82:595–597, 1989.

Montagu, J. D., Effects of diazepam on the EEG in man. Eur. J. Pharmacol. 17:167–170, 1972.

Morrow, L. A., Steinhauer, S. R. and Hodgson, M. J., Delay in P300 latency in patients with organic solvent exposure. Arch. Neurol. 49:315–320, 1992.

Naatanen, R., Generators of electrical and magnetic mismatch responses in humans. Brain Topogr. 7:315–320, 1995.

Naatanen, R. and Picton, T., The N1 wave of the human electric and magnetic response to sound: a review and an analysis of the component structure. Psychophysiology 24:375–425, 1987.

Nadeau, S. E. and Crosson, B., A guide to the functional imaging of cognitive processes. Neuropsychiatry Neuropsychol. Behav. Neurol. 8:143–162, 1995.

Newlin, D. B. and Thomson, J. B., Alcohol challenge with sons of alcoholics: a critical review and analysis. Psychol. Bull. 108:383–402, 1990.

Noldy, N. E. and Carlen, P. L., Acute, withdrawal, and chronic alcohol effects in man: event-related potential and quantitative EEG techniques. Ann. Med. 22:333–339, 1990.

Noldy, N. E. and Carlen, P. L., Event-related potential changes in cocaine withdrawal: evidence for long-term cognitive effects. Neuropsychobiology 36:53–56, 1997.

Noldy, N. E., Neiman, J., el-Nesr, B. and Carlen, P. L., Late auditory evoked potentials: a method for monitoring drug effects on the central nervous system. Neuropsychobiology 23:48–52, 1990.

Noldy, N. E., Santos, C. V., Politzer, N., Blair, R. D. and Carlen, P. L., Quantitative EEG changes in cocaine withdrawal: evidence for long-term CNS effects. Neuropsychobiology 30:189–196, 1994.

Nunez, P. L., Srinivasan, R., Westdorp, A. F., Wijesinghe, R. S., Tucker, D. M., Silberstein, R. B. and Cadusch, P. J., EEG coherency. I: Statistics, reference electrode, volume conduction, Laplacians, cortical imaging, and interpretation at multiple scales. Electroencephalogr. Clin. Neurophysiol. 103:499–515, 1997.

O'Connor, S., Bauer, L., Tasman, A. and Hesselbrock, V., Reduced P3 amplitudes are associated with both a family history of alcoholism and antisocial personality disorder. Prog. Neuropsychopharmacol. Biol. Psychiatry 18:1307–1321, 1994.

Oka, J. I., Jang, E. K. and Hicks, T. P., Benzodiazepine receptor involvement in the control of receptive field size and responsiveness in primary somatosensory cortex. Brain Res. 376:194–198, 1986.

Pascual-Leone, A., Dhuna, A. and Anderson, D. C., Long-term neurological complications of chronic, habitual cocaine abuse. Neurotoxicology 12:393–400, 1991.

Patrick, G. and Struve, F. A., Brainstem auditory response (BAER) in polydrug abuse. Clin. Electroencephalogr. 25:1–7, 1994.

Patrick, G., Straumanis, J. J., Struve, F. A., Nixon, F., Fitz-Gerald, M. J., Manno, J. E. and Soucair, M., Auditory and visual P300 event related potentials are not altered in medically and psychiatrically normal chronic marihuana users. Life Sci. 56:2135–2140, 1995.

Patrick, G., Straumanis, J. J., Struve, F. A., Fitz-Gerald, M. J. and Manno, J. E., Early and middle latency evoked potentials in medically and psychiatrically normal daily marihuana users: a paucity of significant findings. Clin. Electroencephalogr. 28:26–31, 1997.

Petersen-Felix, S., Arendt-Nielsen, L., Bak, P., Fischer, M. and Zbinden, A. M., Psychophysical and electrophysiological responses to experimental pain may be influenced by sedation: comparison of the effects of a hypnotic (propofol) and an analgesic (alfentanil). Br. J. Anaesth. 77:165–171, 1996.

Pfefferbaum, A., Ford, J. M., White, P. M. and Mathalon, D., Event-related potentials in alcoholic men: P3 amplitude reflects family history but not alcohol consumption. Alcohol. Clin. Exp. Res. 15:839–850, 1991.

Phillips, R. L., Herning, R. and London, E. D., Morphine effects on the spontaneous electroencephalogram in polydrug abusers: correlations with subjective self-reports. Neuropsychopharmacology 10:171–181, 1994.

Plourde, G., Joffe, D., Villemure, C. and Trahan, M., The P3a wave of the auditory event-related potential reveals registration of pitch change during sufentanil anesthesia for cardiac surgery. Anesthesiology 78:498–509, 1993.

Plourde, G., Baribeau, J. and Bonhomme, V., Ketamine increases the amplitude of the 40-Hz auditory steady-state response in humans. Br. J. Anaesth. 78:524–529, 1997.
Polich, J., Pollock, V. E. and Bloom, F. E., Meta-analysis of P300 amplitude from males at risk for alcoholism. Psychol. Bull. 115:55–73, 1994.
Pollak, L., Schiffer, J., Klein, C., Giladi, R. and Rabey, J. M., Quantified EEG in patients with vertigo of central or peripheral origin. Int. J. Neurosci. 93:35–41, 1998.
Pollock, V. E., Volavka, J., Goodwin, D. W., Mednick, S. A., Gabrielli, W. F., Knop, J. and Schulsinger, F., The EEG after alcohol administration in men at risk for alcoholism. Arch. Gen. Psychiatry 40:857–861, 1983.
Pollock, V. E., Teasdale, T. W., Gabrielli, W. F. and Knop, J., Subjective and objective measures of response to alcohol among young men at risk for alcoholism. J. Stud. Alcohol 47:297–304, 1986.
Pollock, V. E. and Schneider, L. S., Quantitative, waking EEG research on depression. Biol. Psychiatry 27:757–780, 1990.
Porjesz, B. and Begleiter, H., Evoked brain potentials and alcoholism. In: Tarter, R. and Van Thiel, D. (eds.) Neuropsychology of alcoholism: Implications for Diagnosis and Treatment. New York, Guilford, pp. 139–185, 1985.
Porjesz, B. and Begleiter, H., Neurophysiological factors associated with alcoholism. In: Hunt, W. A. and Nixon, S. J. (eds.) Alcohol induced brain damage. NIAAA Res. Mono. Vol. 22, Rockville, MD, pp. 89–120, 1993.
Porjesz, B. and Begleiter, H., Effects of alcohol on electrophysiological activity of the brain. In: Begleiter, H. and Kissin, B. (eds.) Pharmacology of Alcohol and Alcohol Dependence. New York: Oxford University Press, pp. 207–247, 1996.
Prichep, L. S., Alper, K. R., Kowalik, S., Merkin, H., Tom, M., John, E. R. and Rosenthal, M. S., Quantitative electroencephalographic characteristics of crack cocaine dependence. Biol. Psychiatry 40:986–993, 1996.
Propping, P., Genetic control of ethanol action on the central nervous system. An EEG study in twins. Hum. Genet. 35:309–334, 1977.
Propping, P., Kruger, J. and Janah, A., Effect of alcohol on genetically determined variants of the normal electroencephalogram. Psychiatry Res. 2:85–98, 1980.
Rockstroh, B., Elbert, T., Lutzenberger, W. and Altenmuller, E., Effects of the anticonvulsant benzodiazepine clonazepam on event-related brain potentials in humans. Electroencephalogr. Clin. Neurophysiol. 78:142–149, 1991.
Roemer, R. A., Cornwell, A., Dewart, D., Jackson, P. and Ercegovac, D. V., Quantitative electroencephalographic analyses in cocaine-preferring polysubstance abusers during abstinence. Psychiatry Res. 58:247–257, 1995.
Rohrbaugh, J. W., Stapleton, J. M., Frowein, H. W., Adinoff, B., Varner, J. L., Lane, E. A., Eckardt, M. J. and Linnoila, M., Acute effects of ethanol on motor performance and movement-related brain potentials. Adv. Alcohol Subst. Abuse 7:53–57, 1988.
Roth, W. T., Tinklenberg, J. R. and Kopell, B. S., Ethanol and marihuana effects on event-related potentials in a memory retrieval paradigm. Electroencephalogr. Clin. Neurophysiol. 42:381–388, 1977.
Ryan, C., Russo, K. and Greeley, J., Testing the global-slowing hypothesis: are alcohol's effects on human performance process-specific or task-general? Acta. Psychol. (Amst.) 92:59–78, 1996.
Salamy, A. and Williams, H. L., The effects of alcohol on sensory evoked and spontaneous cerebral potentials in man. Electroencephalogr. Clin. Neurophysiol. 35:3–11, 1973.
Saletu, B., Classification of psychotropic drugs based on human evoked potentials. In: Itil, T. M. (ed.) Psychotropic drugs and the human EEG. Modern problems of pharmacopsychiatry. New York: Karger, pp. 258–285, 1974.
Saletu, B., Barbanoj, M. J., Anderer, P., Sieghart, W. and Grunberger, J., Clinical-pharmacological study with the two isomers (d-, l-) of fenfluramine and its comparison with

chlorpromazine and d-amphetamine: blood levels, EEG mapping and safety evaluation. Methods Find Exp. Clin. Pharmacol. 15:291–312, 1993.

Schwender, D., Klasing, S., Madler, C., Poppel, E. and Peter, K., Effects of benzodiazepines on midlatency auditory evoked potentials. Can. J. Anaesth. 40:1148–1154, 1993a.

Schwender, D., Rimkus, T., Haessler, R., Klasing, S., Poppel, E. and Peter, K., Effects of increasing doses of alfentanil, fentanyl and morphine on mid-latency auditory evoked potentials. Br. J. Anaesth. 71:622–628, 1993b.

Schwender, D., Faber-Zullig, E., Fett, W., Klasing, S., Finsterer, U., Poppel, E. and Peter, K., Mid-latency auditory evoked potentials in humans during anesthesia with S (+) ketamine—a double-blind, randomized comparison with racemic ketamine. Anesth. Analg. 78:267–274, 1994.

Schwender, D., Weninger, E., Schnatmann, N., Mulzer, S., Klasing, S. and Peter, K., Acoustic evoked potentials mid-latency following anesthesia with sufentanil. [German]. Anaesthesist 44:478–482, 1995.

Scott, J. C., Cooke, J. E. and Stanski, D. R., Electroencephalographic quantitation of opioid effect: comparative pharmacodynamics of fentanyl and sufentanil. Anesthesiology 74:34–42, 1991.

Semlitsch, H. V., Anderer, P. and Saletu, B., Acute effects of the anxiolytics suriclone and alprazolam on cognitive information processing utilizing topographic mapping of event-related brain potentials (P300) in healthy subjects. Eur. J. Clin. Pharmacol. 49:183–191, 1995.

Shufman, E., Perl, E., Cohen, M., Dickman, M., Gandaku, D., Adler, D., Veler, A., Bar-Hamburger, R. and Ginath, Y., Electro-encephalography spectral analysis of heroin addicts compared with abstainers and normal controls. Isr. J. Psychiatry Relat. Sci. 33:196–206, 1996.

Slattum, P. W., Venitz, J. and Barr, W. H., Comparison of methods for the assessment of central nervous system stimulant response after dextroamphetamine administration to healthy male volunteers. J. Clin. Pharmacol. 36:1039–1050, 1996.

Solowij, N., Michie, P. T. and Fox, A. M., Effects of long-term cannabis use on selective attention: an event-related potential study. Pharmacol. Biochem. Behav. 40:683–688, 1991.

Solowij, N., Michie, P. T. and Fox, A. M., Differential impairments of selective attention due to frequency and duration of cannabis use. Biol. Psychiatry 37:731–739, 1995.

Sommer, W., Leuthold, H. and Hermanutz, M., Covert effects of alcohol revealed by event-related potentials. Percept. Psychophys. 54:127–135, 1993.

Sorbel, J., Morzorati, S., O'Connor, S., Li, T. K. and Christian, J. C., Alcohol effects on the heritability of EEG spectral power. Alcohol. Clin. Exp. Res. 20:1523–1527, 1996.

Spehr, W. and Stemmler, G., Postalcoholic diseases: diagnostic relevance of computerized EEG. Electroencephalogr. Clin. Neurophysiol. 60:106–114, 1985.

Srinivasan, R., Nunez, P. L. and Silberstein, R. B., Spatial filtering and neocortical dynamics: estimates of EEG coherence. IEEE Trans. Biomed. Eng. 45:814–826, 1998.

Stassen, H. H., Bomben, G. and Propping, P., Genetic aspects of the EEG: an investigation into the within-pair similarity of monozygotic and dizygotic twins with a new method of analysis. Electroencephalogr. Clin. Neurophysiol. 66:489–501, 1987.

Stenberg, G., Sano, M., Rosen, I. and Ingvar, D. H., EEG topography of acute ethanol effects in resting and activated normals. J. Stud. Alcohol 55:645–656, 1994.

Struve, F. A., Straumanis, J. J., Patrick, G. and Price, L., Topographic mapping of quantitative EEG variables in chronic heavy marihuana users: empirical findings with psychiatric patients. Clin. Electroencephalogr. 20:6–23, 1989.

Struve, F. A., Straumanis, J. J. and Patrick, G., Persistent topographic quantitative EEG sequelae of chronic marihuana use: a replication study and initial discriminant function analysis. Clin. Electroencephalogr. 25:63–75, 1994.

Struve, F. A., Patrick, G., Straumanis, J. J., Fitz-Gerald, M. J. and Manno, J., Possible EEG sequelae of very long duration marihuana use: pilot findings from topographic quantitative EEG analyses of subjects with 15 to 24 years of cumulative daily exposure to THC. Clin. Electroencephalogr. 29:31–36, 1998.

Tassinari, C. A., Ambrosetto, H. G., Peraita-Adrodos, M. R. and Gastaut, H., Neurophysiological effects of high doses of marihuana in man. Electroencephalogr. Clin. Neurophysiol. 35:404–405, 1973.

Tassinari, C. A., Ambrosetto, H. G., Peraita-Adrodos, M. R. and Gastaut, H., Effects of marihuana and delta-9-THC at high doses in man. A polygraphic study. Electroencephalogr. Clin. Neurphysiol. 36:94, 1974.

Teo, R. K. and Ferguson, D. A., The acute effects of ethanol on auditory event-related potentials. Psychopharmacology (Berl.) 90:179–184, 1986.

Tharp, V. K., Jr., Rundell, O. H., Jr., Lester, B. K. and Williams, H. L., Alcohol and information processing. Psychopharmacologia 40:33–52, 1974.

Thurauf, N., Ditterich, W. and Kobal, G., Different sensitivity of pain-related chemosensory potentials evoked by stimulation with CO2, tooth pulp event-related potentials, and acoustic event-related potentials to the tranquilizer diazepam. Br. J. Clin. Pharmacol. 38:545–555, 1994.

Thurner, F., Schramm, J. and Pasch, T., Effect of fentanyl and enflurane on sensory evoked potentials in the human in basic flunitrazepam/N2O anesthesia. [German]. Anaesthesist 36: 548–554, 1987.

Van Leeuwen, T. H., Verbaten, M. N., Koelega, H. S., Kenemans, J. L. and Slangen, J. L., Effects of bromazepam on single-trial event-related potentials in a visual vigilance task. Psychopharmacology (Berl.) 106:555–564, 1992.

Van Steveninck, A. L., Mandema, J. W., Tuk, B., Van Dijk, J. G., Schoemaker, H. C., Danhof, M. and Cohen, A. F., A comparison of the concentration-effect relationships of midazolam for EEG-derived parameters and saccadic peak velocity. Br. J. Clin. Pharmacol. 36:109–115, 1993.

Volavka, J., Zaks, A., Roubicek, J. and Fink, M., Electrographic effects of diacetylmorphine (heroin) and naloxone in man. Neuropharmacology 9:587–593, 1970.

Volavka, J., Dornbush, R., Feldstein, S., Clare, G., Zaks, A., Fink, M. and Freedman, A. M., Marihuana, EEG, and behavior. Ann. NY Acad. Sci. 191:206–215, 1971.

Volavka, J., Levine, R., Feldstein, S. and Fink, M., Short-term effects of heroin in man. Is EEG related to behavior? Arch. Gen. Psychiatry 30:677–681, 1974.

Volavka, J., Czobor, P., Goodwin, D. W., Gabrielli, W. F., Jr., Penick, E. C., Mednick, S. A., Jensen, P. and Knop, J., The electroencephalogram after alcohol administration in high-risk men and the development of alcohol use disorders 10 years later. Arch. Gen. Psychiatry 53:258–263, 1996.

Vrca, A., Bozicevic, D., Bozikov, V., Fuchs, R. and Malinar, M., Brain stem evoked potentials and visual evoked potentials in relation to the length of occupational exposure to low levels of toluene. Acta Med. Croatica 51:215–219, 1997.

Wall, T. L. and Ehlers, C. L., Acute effects of alcohol on P300 in Asians with different ALDH2 genotypes. Alcohol. Clin. Exp. Res. 19:617–622, 1995.

Weber, M., Laxenaire, M. C., Fays, J., Hottier, M. C. and Cozette, P., Electro-clinical features of short-term anaesthesia. [(author's transl)]. Rev. Electroencephalogr. Neurophysiol. Clin. 7:38–44, 1977.

Wert, R. C. and Raulin, M. L., The chronic cerebral effects of cannabis use. I. Methodological issues and neurological findings. Int. J. Addict. 21:605–628, 1986.

White, P. F., Schuttler, J., Shafer, A., Stanski, D. R., Horai, Y. and Trevor, A. J., Comparative pharmacology of the ketamine isomers: studies in volunteers. Br. J. Anaesth. 57:197–203, 1985.

Williams, E. G., Himmelsbach, C. K., Wikler, A. and Rubie, D. C., Studies on marihuana and pyrahexyl compound. Public Health Report 61:1059–1085, 1946.

Winterer, G., Kloppel, B., Heinz, A., Ziller, M., Dufeu, P., Schmidt, L. G. and Herrmann, W. M., Quantitative EEG (QEEG) predicts relapse in patients with chronic alcoholism and points to a frontally pronounced cerebral disturbance. Psychiatry Res. 78:101–113, 1998.
Zilm, D. H., Huszar, L., Carlen, P. L., Kaplan, H. L. and Wilkinson, D. A., EEG correlates of the alcohol-induced organic brain syndrome in man. Clin. Toxicol. 16:345–358, 1980.

Chapter 5

Emission Tomographic Studies in Substance Abuse

Jonathan M. Levin, MD, MPH

Introduction

Since the work of Roy and Sherrington at the end of the nineteenth century, the coupling of neural activity and cerebral blood flow (CBF) has been recognized as a fundamental principle of brain functional activity (Roy and Sherrington, 1890). For several decades, the radiotracer techniques have been mainstays in the effort to noninvasively image brain function. In the last two decades, computer-based advances in computational and data processing capacity have led to the development of tomographic techniques such as positron emission tomography (PET) and single photon emission computed tomography (SPECT). These advances have led to the ability to non-invasively measure regional CBF and cerebral blood volume (CBV), the regional metabolism of glucose (CMRglc) and oxygen ($CMRO_2$), and the regional binding of radiolabeled compounds such as neurotransmitters and their analogs.

While many of the neurochemical effects of drugs of abuse are well understood, less is known about their actual effects on brain function. Yet, drugs profoundly alter brain function, through both their immediate behavioral effects and their long-term sequellae. Thus, studying the effects of drugs on cerebral hemodynamics and metabolism has been one avenue in an attempt to understand their effects on brain function. Studying receptor binding, blockade, and dysfunction has proven to be another important and fruitful avenue. It is hoped that a more complete understanding

From: *Brain Imaging in Substance Abuse: Research, Clinical, and Forensic Applications*
M. J. Kaufman, ed. © Humana Press Inc., Totowa, New Jersey

of these effects will serve to elucidate the nature of the addictive properties of certain substances and the propensity for substance dependence in certain individuals, while suggesting and aiding in the evaluation of drug addiction therapies. To this end, important findings have been made studying functional alterations due to both acute and chronic use of various substances, and for an overview of these topics, the reader is referred to several sources (Mathew and Wilson, 1991; London, 1993; Levin and Kaufman, 1995; Volkow et al., 1996a; Gatley and Volkow, 1998).

This chapter will review the findings of emission tomographic imaging studies in man, using a variety of methodologies to study a number of different abused drugs. The chapter is organized by substance and question addressed, and to a lesser degree by technique. Every attempt has been made to focus on the most salient points made in each study and to emphasize the important message. The technical foundations for emission tomographic imaging of the brain are discussed in Chapter 2.

Alcohol and Alcoholism

Acute Alcohol Administration

Cerebral Blood Flow

The acute and chronic effects of alcohol on cerebral blood flow and metabolism in man have been studied for over half a century, for longer and to a greater extent than any other drug, sometimes with conflicting and confusing results. This may be explained not only by the evolving precision of the techniques available for performing measurements, but also by the fact that a number of early experiments controlled for fewer variables than is the trend in more recent studies. Prior to the advent of modern emission tomographic techniques, the Kety-Schmidt technique for measuring CBF was used by Hine et al. (1952) who noted reduced CBF and metabolism following ingestion of 0.5 mL/kg alcohol. In contrast, the following year, using similar techniques, Battey et al. published the results of a variety of experiments involving alcohol intoxication. They found a marked increase in CBF and reduction in cerebral oxygen metabolism in subjects administered intravenous alcohol as well as in patients admitted to the hospital with acute intoxication. In the admitted patients, these changes partially resolved with sobriety (Battey et al., 1953).

Emission tomographic techniques have generally been in agreement with regard to the acute effect of alcohol on CBF in normal subjects. Using the ^{133}Xe inhalation method, Newlin et al. (1982) studied normal social drinkers one hour following consumption of 0.75 g/kg alcohol, a time near peak blood alcohol level (BAL). They found increased CBF in all gray matter regions of interest (ROIs) with the exception of the left anterior region. Subsequent studies with this technique have also reported globally increased CBF following acute alcohol administration (Mathew and Wilson, 1986; Sano et al., 1993). However, Sano et al. also found the regional increase in CBF to vary according to alcohol dose, with flow to temporal regions continuing to increase with higher alcohol doses (0.7 vs 1.5 g/kg), while flow to prefrontal regions began to decrease at higher doses (Sano et al., 1993). Berglund et al. (1989) found markedly increased mean global CBF levels in an individual during "alcohol blackout" with a BAL of 0.38%.

PET has also been used to study the acute effects of alcohol. Volkow et al. (1988b) used the ^{15}O-labeled water ([^{15}O]H_2O) method to study the acute effect of 0.5 and 1.0 g/kg alcohol on rCBF and found reduced cerebellar CBF, as well as increased right temporal and prefrontal CBF at the higher alcohol dose. Recent PET studies have confirmed decreased cerebellar blood flow following alcohol ingestion, suggesting a possible mechanism for its effect on suppressing essential tremor (Boecker et al., 1996).

Other issues have been examined in conjunction with measurements of CBF in acute alcohol administration. Tiihonen et al. (1994) used SPECT to show that pretreatment with naloxone blocked right prefrontal cortical increase in cerebral perfusion seen with alcohol administration, implicating this area and possibly the endogenous opioid system in the mediation of euphoria. In an interesting study, Wendt et al. (1994) showed that the normal coupling of increased rCBF in response to neuronal activation remained intact following alcohol administration, although the typical right hemispheric predominance for visual activation disappeared with intoxication.

Cerebral Metabolism

The metabolic effects of acute alcohol intoxication have been studied with PET, although less work has been performed in this area than in that of perfusion. De Wit et al. (1990) examined glucose metabolism with [^{18}F]fluoro-2-deoxyglucose ([^{18}F]FDG) PET in control subjects ingesting 0.5–0.8 g/kg alcohol. While they found a global reduction in the cerebral metabolic rate for glucose metabolism (CMRglc), they detected no clear regional differences or correlation with subjective effects of intoxication (de Wit et al., 1990). Volkow et al. (1990b) also used [^{18}F]FDG PET in both controls and alcohol-dependent subjects receiving an acute alcohol (1.0 g/kg) challenge and reported reduced cortical and cerebellar glucose metabolism, particularly in the alcohol-dependent subjects, which they attributed to decreased glucose phosphorylation. Such a finding raises the intriguing possibility of a disassociation between CBF and glucose metabolism with alcohol, particularly in cortical regions.

Chronic Alcohol Effects and Alcoholism

Cerebral Blood Flow

Although observational in nature, early studies generally indicated reduced rCBF in association with alcoholic liver dysfunction (Johannesson et al., 1982; Valmier et al., 1986). Melgaard et al. (1990) used the ^{133}Xe inhalation method with SPECT to measure CBF in 20 chronic alcoholic men abstinent for at least 2 wk, finding reduced mean cerebral and cerebellar blood flow, as well as focal areas of reduced perfusion. These focal perfusion deficits (especially in the anteromesial frontal lobes) were found to correlate with severity of alcoholism, cerebral atrophy, and cognitive impairment. In an uncontrolled study, meaning that an appropriate control population was not studied as a comparison group, Erbas et al. found abnormal perfusion in 86% of chronic alcoholics studied with ^{99m}Tc-HMPAO SPECT, with the majority showing impairment of left hemispheric and frontal perfusion (Erbas et al., 1992). A subsequent and carefully controlled study was in concordance with those findings and noted that perfusion impairments were both independent of brain atrophy and reversible with abstinence (Nicolas et al., 1993). Mampunza et al. (1995) also found abnormal perfusion in recently detoxified alcoholics, more frequently in patients with a positive family history of alcoholism. Others have confirmed abnormal perfusion in chronic, detoxified alcoholics (Gunther et al., 1997).

The vascular effects of chronic, moderate alcohol consumption remain subject to debate. While alcohol consumption is generally considered to be vasoprotective, other evidence suggests a dose-related increase in vascular disease. Along these lines, Rogers et al. measured rCBF in 222 subjects with the ^{133}Xe inhalation method and found a significant inverse linear relationship between blood flow and alcohol consumption, independent of other risk factors for vascular disease (Rogers et al., 1983).

Cerebral Metabolism

The first controlled [^{18}F]FDG PET study of the effects of chronic alcoholism was performed by Sampson et al. in 1986, although the duration of abstinence was not specified. While they noted only a trend toward reduced absolute cortical CMRglc in alcoholics, and no abnormality in cerebellar glucose metabolism, they were able to establish reduced normalized metabolic index in the mesiofrontal cortices (Samson et al., 1986). In a similarly controlled study of detoxified alcoholics, using [^{18}F]FDG PET, Martin et al. (1992) also found few differences in absolute CMRglc but clear differences in normalized regional CMRglc, including decreased right hemispheric and increased left cerebellar and right parietal CMRglc. Volkow et al. (1992b) also used [^{18}F]FDG PET to study neurologically healthy alcoholics detoxified for 6–32 d, as well as controls. They found reduced whole brain CMRglc in alcoholics, correlating with time since abstinence, and reductions in left parietal and right frontal normalized regional CMRglc. Subsequent work from this group showed that metabolic deficits correlated with impaired neuropsychological performance but not with structural brain changes (Wang et al., 1993). Gilman et al. demonstrated reduced rCMRglc in the bilateral medial frontal cortex correlating with the degree of cerebral atrophy (Gilman et al., 1990). This group subsequently demonstrated that, while medial frontal hypometabolism correlated with cognitive deficits in frontal lobe function as determined by the Wisconsin Card Sorting Test and the Halstead Category Test, the metabolic abnormalities were not likely a result of cortical atrophy (Adams et al., 1993). Additional studies have also indicated that these metabolic abnormalities are not dependent on a family history of alcoholism (Adams et al., 1998). Dao-Castellana et al. (1998) demonstrated that reduced rCMRglc in the mediofrontal and left dorsolateral prefrontal cortex correlated with neuropsychological measures of frontal dysfunction.

Other methods have also been used to study cerebral glucose metabolism in chronic alcoholics. In a controlled study using [^{11}C]2-deoxyglucose PET, Sachs et al. found reduced global and regional CMRglc, as well as fewer interregional correlations and reduced metabolic response to focal right hemispheric activation, in alcoholic subjects detoxified for 8–45 d (Sachs et al., 1987). Wik et al. (1988) used [^{11}C]glucose PET in controls and in alcoholics abstinent for at least a month, also demonstrating reduced cortical and subcortical glucose metabolism.

Finally, while most studies have focused on men, Wang et al. (1998b) used [^{18}F]FDG PET to study recently detoxified female alcoholics as well as age- and sex-matched controls. They found no difference between the two groups. As studies in alcoholic men have generally demonstrated reduced glucose metabolism, these results suggest a possible sex specificity with regard to alcohol's effects on brain metabolism (Wang et al., 1998b).

Receptor Studies

The effects of chronic alcohol abuse on receptor systems have been described in several studies. Gilman et al. used [^{11}C]dihydrotetrabenazine to evaluate striatal vesicular monoamine transporter (VMAT2) binding and found reduced binding in chronic alcoholic patients, indicating reduced striatal monoaminergic terminals in this population (Gilman et al., 1998). Abi-Dargham et al. (1998b) evaluated benzodiazepine receptor binding in detoxified alcoholics with [^{123}I]iomazenil SPECT and noted reduced anterior cingulate, left occipital, and cerebellar receptor binding in alcoholics as compared to control subjects. Heinz et al. (1998) used [^{123}I]β–CIT and SPECT to evaluate serotonin and dopamine transporter availability in chronic alcoholics as compared to control subjects. They found significantly reduced (30%) brainstem [^{123}I]β–CIT binding, indicating reduced transporter availability in this group of alcoholics, consistent with an hypothesis of monoamine dysfunction (Heinz et al., 1998).

Effects of Withdrawal and Abstinence

While many studies of the effects of chronic alcohol exposure and alcoholism focus on detoxified alcoholics, the effects of withdrawal and longer-term abstinence are also of great interest. Using the ^{133}Xe inhalation CBF method during withdrawal in male alcoholics, Berglund and Risberg (1981) found global CBF to be reduced, particularly during the first 2 d of the withdrawal syndrome. A pattern of relatively high temporal and low parietal flow was also noted in cases with severe withdrawal symptoms (Berglund and Risberg, 1981). Others have demonstrated increased CBF during severe alcohol withdrawal (impending and full-blown delirium tremens), correlating with visual hallucinations and agitation (Hemmingsen et al., 1988). Caspari et al. used ^{99m}Tc-HMPAO SPECT to study alcoholics in the midst of withdrawal and then three weeks later, following resolution of withdrawal symptoms (Caspari et al., 1993). During withdrawal, they observed increased perfusion in the inferior temporal lobes and reduced perfusion in the superior temporal lobes. Using similar methodology, Tutus et al. (1998) observed reduced frontal and right hemispheric perfusion during withdrawal, which later resolved. Volkow at al. (1994) used [^{18}F]FDG PET to show increased (improved) rCMRglc 2–4 wk following detoxification, particularly in the frontal regions, but noted a persistent metabolic reduction in basal ganglia and parietal cortex. A subsequent study by this group demonstrated widespread reduction in rCMRglc during early withdrawal (2–3 wk), but more focal reductions in rCMRglc (cingulate and orbitofrontal cortex) during late withdrawal (6–8 wk) (Volkow et al., 1997d).

Interestingly, abstinence may improve not only gray matter perfusion but brain volume as well (Ishikawa et al., 1986). Berglund et al. also found improved mean rCBF (+9%) when they compared findings from abstinent alcoholics evaluated during their

1st and 7th weeks of abstinence, with the most significant increase occurring in the right hemisphere (Berglund et al., 1987). Dupont et al. (1996) compared perfusion as well as performance on Raven's Progressive Matrices (a measure of prefrontal function) in long-term (mean 7.7 yr) abstinent alcoholics, in recently detoxified subjects, and normal controls. Using [^{123}I]iodoamphetamine (IMP) SPECT, they found reduced perfusion with both short- and long-term abstinence, despite nearly normal neuropsychological testing in the latter group (Dupont et al., 1996). In a longitudinal [^{18}F]FDG PET study, Johnson-Greene et al. (1997) evaluated the effect of abstinence and relapse on cerebral glucose metabolism and neuropsychological testing of cognitive and executive function on two separate occasions separated by 10–32 mo. Although the study was limited in size, the four abstinent subjects showed improvement in rCMRglc and in neuropsychological test results, while the two relapsing subjects exhibited further decline on both measures (Johnson-Greene et al., 1997).

Modell and Mountz examined the functional correlates of alcohol in a ^{99m}Tc-HMPAO SPECT study of alcohol-dependent subjects. They found increased right caudate perfusion during the craving condition as compared to baseline, implicating this and related structures in mediating potentially abnormal craving and consumption of alcohol (Modell and Mountz, 1995).

Neurological Disorders Associated with Alcoholism

Wernicke-Korsakoff Syndrome

Functional neuroimaging is useful in assessing not only the acute and chronic effects of alcohol, but also aspects of neurological disease associated with alcoholism. One of the more common and devastating group of disorders is the Wernicke-Korsakoff syndrome, which results from nutritional (particularly thiamine) deficiency commonly associated with alcoholism. Pathological examination and structural imaging indicate damage in the periaqueductal gray matter, mamillary bodies, and medial dorsal diencephalon. While the clinical and pathological correlates of these disorders are highly variable, a clear distinction can be made between acute Wernicke's encephalopathy and Korsakoff's amnestic syndrome. Generally speaking, however, the disorders are often lumped for study purposes. An early functional imaging study demonstrated reduced temporal and parietal CBF in acute Wernicke-Korsakoff syndrome, which improved at 3 mo following treatment (Meyer et al., 1985). Others have found normal cerebral perfusion in the Korsakoff syndrome (Sharp et al., 1986). Subsequently, using ^{99m}Tc-HMPAO SPECT, Hunter et al. (1989) compared cerebral perfusion in Korsakoff's syndrome and Alzheimer's disease. In contrast to the reduced perfusion in temporoparietal cortex seen in Alzheimer's disease, patients with Korsakoff's syndrome had impaired frontal perfusion, correlating with cognitive impairment (Hunter et al., 1989). More recently, [^{15}O]H_2O PET rCBF and regional cerebral metabolic rate of oxygen (rCMRO$_2$) were found to be reduced bilaterally in the fronto-temporal regions and left thalamus in a single patient with Korsakoff's syndrome (Matsuda et al., 1997). Benson et al. (1996) conducted an elegant study of a single patient with Korsakoff's syndrome, evaluating perfusion with ^{133}Xe-calibrated ^{99m}Tc-HMPAO SPECT during the ictus of the disorder and four months later. During the acute amnestic-confabulatory phase, they found impaired perfusion in the orbital and medial frontal regions and in the medial diencephalon. At follow-up, there was improved frontal but not diencephalic perfusion, correlating with reduced confabulation and improved performance on frontal lobe neuropsychological instruments (Benson et al., 1996). Finally, Moffoot et al. (1994) have suggested improved perfusion in anterior cingulate, left dorsolateral frontal cortex, posterior cingulate, and thalamus following clonidine infusion in patients with Korsakoff's syndrome.

Cerebral metabolic studies using [^{18}F]FDG PET have also been performed in Korsakoff's syndrome. Joyce et al. (1994) found reduced cingulate and precuneate rCMRglc, findings thought to be related to the diencephalic lesions seen in Korsakoff's syndrome. Martin et al. found increased left cerebellar and parietal, and reduced right posterior and anterior temporal, rCMRglc in patients with "organic mental disorders," including Korsakoff's syndrome (Martin et al., 1992).

Marchiafava-Bignami Syndrome

Marchiafava-Bignami syndrome is a relatively rare disorder of unknown etiology, although it is almost exclusively associated with alcoholism. Although the pathology of this disorder is specific, involving regional demyelination of the corpus callosum, the symptoms and clinical course are variable, occasionally rapid and often devastating. In a case report of a patient with Marchiafava-Bignami disease studied with [^{18}F]FDG PET, Pappata et al. demonstrated reduced CMRglc in the frontal and temporo-parieto-occipital association cortices even though MRI showed structural abnormalities limited to the corpus callosum (Pappata et al., 1994). Widespread abnormalities in perfusion were noted in another case evaluated by SPECT (Humbert et al., 1992).

Cerebellar Degeneration

Clinically and pathologically, the cerebellum is particularly susceptible to the deleterious effects of alcohol. In order to understand this propensity for regionally selective damage, several functional studies have focused on the cerebellum, including cases of overt cerebellar degeneration. Gilman et al. (1990) evaluated glucose metabolism with [^{18}F]FDG PET in alcoholic patients with and without clinical signs of cerebellar degeneration. As compared to control subjects and patients without cerebellar signs, patients with clinical cerebellar abnormalities had decreased rCMRglc in the superior cerebellar vermis, although this did not correlate with atrophy. Both alcoholic groups showed decreased metabolism bilaterally in the medial frontal cortex correlating with cerebral atrophy (Gilman et al., 1990). A follow-up study confirming these observations showed additionally that benzodiazepine receptor binding was altered in the superior cerebellar vermis in patients with alcoholic cerebellar degeneration (Gilman et al., 1996b).

Hepatic Encephalopathy

Lockwood et al. (1993) evaluated the effect of what they termed "minimal hepatic encephalopathy" (alcoholic patients with compensated cirrhosis and mild hyperammonemia) on cerebral metabolism with [^{18}F]FDG PET. They found reduced CMRglc in the cingulate and increased CMRglc in visual associative areas, possibly the result of a compensatory response (Lockwood et al., 1993).

Drug Challenge and Receptor Level Studies

Effects of Treatment for Alcohol Abuse

Although most studies of the chronic effects of alcohol include detoxified and medicated patients, there is a paucity of data addressing the direct effect of those medications on brain function. The direct influence of disulfiram (Antabuse) on cerebral glucose metabolism and on benzodiazepine binding in chronic alcoholics has been examined with ^{18}F-FDG and [^{11}C]flumazenil PET, respectively. Studies by Gilman et al. (1996a) indicate reduced global CMRglc and reduced flumazenil influx and distribution volume in patients receiving disulfiram. However, because an appropriate control group was not included, the possibility remains that the patients receiving disulfiram differed in a clinically meaningful way from the comparison group, limiting the ability to generalize these findings.

Benzodiazepine Studies

Farde et al. (1994) evaluated benzodiazepine receptor binding in normal subjects and in alcoholic men using [^{11}C]flumazenil PET. Binding was unaffected in the neocortex and cerebellum following acute alcohol ingestion in normal subjects. Furthermore, no significant abnormality of benzodiazepine receptor binding was noted in the alcoholic subjects studied at rest (Farde et al., 1994). Gilman et al. also performed [^{11}C]flumazenil PET in chronic alcoholics, demonstrating reduced flumazenil influx (K_1) and volume of distribution (DV) in the medial frontal lobes, including the superior frontal gyrus and anterior cingulate (Gilman et al., 1996b). Volkow et al. (1993b) measured CMRglc before and after intravenous lorazepam in recently detoxified alcoholics and normal control subjects. Lorazepam reduced whole brain and cerebellar glucose metabolism in both groups, although the response was blunted in the alcoholic group in the thalamus, basal ganglia, and orbitofrontal cortex (Volkow et al., 1993b). In a subsequent study, this group measured CMRglc before and after intravenous lorazepam administration in alcoholics in early and late withdrawal. They found little difference in metabolic response to the benzodiazepine between alcoholics and controls, and little effect of withdrawal state (Volkow et al., 1997d).

Dopamine Studies

Hietala et al. (1994) studied postsynaptic striatal dopamine D_2 receptor binding in abstinent alcoholics and controls using the selective D_2 receptor ligand [^{11}C]raclopride and PET. Although they noted only a trend toward reduced receptor density (Bmax) and affinity (Kd) in alcoholics, there was a significant reduction in Bmax/Kd (receptor availability) (Hietala et al., 1994). Volkow et al. (1996d) measured both postsynaptic D_2 receptor binding and presynaptic dopamine transporter function with [^{11}C]raclopride and [^{11}C]d-threomethylphenidate PET, respectively. They found dopamine receptor availability to be lower in alcoholics, but found no difference in dopamine transporter availability (Volkow et al., 1996d). Tiihonen et al. (1994) also evaluated presynaptic striatal dopamine reuptake in violent and nonviolent alcoholics using the dopamine transporter analog [^{123}I]β–CIT and SPECT. Nonviolent alcoholics were found to have lower dopamine transporter density, while violent alcoholics were not significantly different from controls (Tiihonen et al., 1994). In a subsequent study, this group used

[^{18}F]DOPA PET to evaluate presynaptic striatal dopamine function, finding generally higher striatal DOPA uptake in alcoholics, although 2 of 10 subjects demonstrated lower uptake in the left caudate (Tiihonen et al., 1998). The authors speculate that higher presynaptic dopamine function in alcoholics may represent a compensatory mechanism for low postsynaptic dopamine function.

Serotonin Studies

Following infusion of the mixed serotonin agonist/antagonist *m*-chlorophenylpiperazine (mCPP), Hommer et al. examined resultant changes in glucose metabolism in alcoholics and controls using [^{18}F]FDG PET. Alcoholics had a blunted metabolic response to this serotonergic challenge in the thalamus, caudate, and orbital and middle frontal cortices, suggesting altered functional activity in limbic circuits in alcoholics (Hommer et al., 1997).

Summary

The effects of alcohol have been studied for several decades and remain the subject of conflicting assessments. Generally, however, studies in humans suggest that chronic use of ethanol is associated with reduced regional CBF and glucose metabolism, while acute ethanol ingestion, perhaps due to its vasodilatory effects, results in increased CBF and CBV. Despite the normal close coupling between blood flow and metabolism, acute alcohol ingestion also seems to be associated with reduced regional and global glucose metabolism in certain regions, possibly reflecting an alteration in neurovascular coupling.

Marijuana

Acute Intoxication

Mathew et al. (1989) used the ^{133}Xe inhalation technique to measure the effect of marijuana on CBF in both experienced and inexperienced marijuana smokers. They found increased CBF in the experienced users and reduced CBF in the inexperienced users following both marijuana and placebo inhalation. The increased CBF in the experienced users correlated with their reports of relaxation, whereas decreased CBF in the inexperienced group correlated with their reports of associated anxiety and depression (Mathew et al., 1989). Using [^{18}F]FDG PET, Volkow et al. found that although the global glucose metabolic response was variable following intravenous administration of tetrahydrocannabinol (THC), cerebellar rCMRglc increased and was correlated with plasma THC concentration and subjective report of intoxication 0.5 h after administration (Volkow et al., 1991b). The cerebellar findings are consistent with the known high density of cannabinoid type 1 (CB1) receptors in this region. Volkow et al. (1996b) confirmed increased relative cerebellar metabolism with THC, but found that only chronic abusers of marijuana also showed increased rCMRglc in orbitofrontal cortex, prefrontal cortex, and basal ganglia. With [^{15}O]H_2O PET, Mathew et al. (1997) demonstrated increased frontal, insular, and cingulate CBF 30–60 min following intravenous THC infusion, which was most prominent in the right hemisphere. Augmented right frontal CBF correlated closely with self-reported intoxication (Mathew et al., 1997). Recently, Mathew and colleagues found increased cortical and cerebellar blood flow in most subjects, most prominently in anterior cingulate, insula, and cerebellum, although those subjects reporting an impaired sense of time showed decreased cerebral and cerebellar flow (Mathew et al., 1998).

Chronic Use and Abuse

In early work, Mathew et al. (1986) found a trend toward lower baseline CBF in marijuana smokers than in controls, and an apparent worsening with increased marijuana use (Mathew et al., 1989; Mathew and Wilson, 1991). In a longitudinal ^{133}Xe inhalation CBF study, hospitalized, chronic heavy marijuana smokers exhibited reduced baseline global cortical CBF, but improved CBF following 1–8 wk of abstinence (Tunving et al., 1986). Volkow et al. (1996b) demonstrated lower baseline cerebellar rCMRglc in chronic marijuana abusers, who also showed widespread increases in rCMRglc following acute THC administration *(see above)*.

Hallucinogens

Ketamine

An antagonist of the *N*-methyl-D-aspartate (NMDA) receptor, ketamine reliably produces psychosis in healthy individuals when administered in subanesthetic doses. A PET study using [^{11}C]ketamine as a radioligand reported localization in brain regions rich in NMDA receptors, while subjective effects of the drug appeared to be dependent on plasma and brain concentrations reaching critical levels (Hartvig et al., 1995). Breier et al. used [^{18}F]FDG PET to evaluate regional cerebral metabolic activity associated with ketamine-induced psychosis in healthy subjects, noting focally increased rCMRglc in prefrontal cortex (Breier et al., 1997a). Vollenweider et al. (1997b) used similar methods to demonstrate increased frontomedial and anterior cingulate cortex rCMRglc following ketamine administration that correlated with drug-related psychotic symptomatology. These investigators also studied the effect of ketamine enantiomers on metabolic activity with [^{18}F]FDG PET. They found that (*S*)-ketamine, in a dose adequate to produce psychosis, increased rCMRglc in frontal and parietal cortex, anterior cingulate, and thalamus, while equimolar (*R*)-ketamine, producing relaxation and no psychosis, reduced rCMRglc widely, particularly in temporomedial cortex and left insula (Vollenweider et al., 1997a). This interesting investigation elegantly suggests that differential subjective effects of similar medications may correlate with markedly different cerebral metabolic effects. Breier et al. (1998) evaluated the interaction between the NMDA and dopaminergic systems, using [^{11}C]raclopride (dopamine D_2 receptor ligand) and PET to measure changes in synaptic dopamine levels in response to ketamine administration. They noted increased striatal dopamine production with displacement of [^{11}C]raclopride following ketamine as compared to saline, which is similar to changes found with amphetamine (which directly increases synaptic dopamine). Others have reported similar findings (Smith et al., 1998).

MDMA ("Ecstasy")

Using PET with [^{11}C]McN-5652 (a serotonin transporter ligand), McCann et al. (1998a) evaluated the effects of MDMA ("Ecstasy") on serotonergic neurons in currently abstinent former users. MDMA users showed reduced global and regional serotonin transporter binding as compared to controls, correlating with the extent of previous MDMA exposure but not with length of abstinence, although the permanence of these changes is uncertain (McCann et al., 1998a).

Psilocybin and Mescaline

The effect of psilocybin on cerebral glucose metabolic activity was evaluated by Vollenweider et al. (1997c) in healthy volunteers using [^{18}F]FDG PET. In doses sufficient to produce psychosis, psilocybin increased global and regional CMRglc, particularly in prefrontal and temporal cortex, anterior cingulate, and basal ganglia, correlating with psychotic symptoms (Vollenweider et al., 1997c).

Hermle et al. (1992) used SPECT perfusion imaging to evaluate the effect of a psychotomimetic dose of mescaline in normal volunteers. Psychotic symptoms were associated with right hemispheric dysfunction as assessed by neuropsychological testing, while SPECT revealed increased frontal perfusion, most markedly in the right hemisphere (Hermle et al., 1992).

Summary

Taken as a whole, the literature regarding hallucinogens is very consistent regarding the increase in frontal CBF and metabolism seen with acute drug administration at doses sufficient to produce psychosis or hallucinogenic effect.

Benzodiazepines

Effects of Acute Administration

Cerebral Blood Flow

Several studies have used the ^{133}Xe inhalation technique to measure the effects of benzodiazepine agonists and antagonists on CBF. Under normocarbic conditions, 0.15 mg/kg midazolam decreased global CBF by approximately 30%, while under hypercarbic conditions (raising CBF), midazolam decreased CBF ~6% (Forster et al., 1983). Mathew and colleagues also used the ^{133}Xe inhalation technique with a small, non-sedating dose of intravenous diazepam (0.1 mg/kg) given to normal subjects. They found a marked reduction in right hemispheric CBF, particularly in the frontal regions (Mathew et al., 1985). On the other hand, a clinically active dose (1 mg) of the benzodiazepine antagonist flumazenil did not alter global or regional CBF in healthy volunteers as measured by ^{133}Xe inhalation SPECT (Wolf et al., 1990). Roy-Byrne et al. (1993) evaluated the effect of both acute and chronic alprazolam administration on CBF as measured by [^{15}O]H_2O PET. They showed that alprazolam, given intravenously to healthy volunteers in a dose (0.014 mg/kg) producing sedation and memory disturbance, reduces whole brain CBF by 25–30% with no clear regional preference. However, one week of "chronic" oral alprazolam administration resulted in tolerance to both the behavioral and physiological effects (including CBF) of a subsequent intravenous dose of the drug, although there was a trend toward reduced baseline CBF after "chronic" use (Roy-Byrne et al., 1993). Matthew et al. (1995) used [^{15}O]H_2O PET to study the effects of lorazepam and flumazenil on CBF in healthy volunteers. Following intravenous lorazepam administration, they found time- and dose-dependent reductions in rCBF in multiple brain regions, which were reversed by flumazenil, indicating that the observed CBF effects are likely receptor-mediated (Matthew et al., 1995). Veselis et al. (1997) used [^{15}O]H_2O PET to evaluate the effects of midazolam infusion in normal volunteers, noting dose-dependent global and regional reductions in CBF, including prefrontal, insular, cingulate, and association cortices and thalamus, along with increased rCBF in occipital cortex.

Cerebral Metabolism

Several investigators have used [^{18}F]FDG PET to evaluate cerebral glucose metabolism following acute benzodiazepine challenge. Oral diazepam (0.07–0.14 mg/kg) administration in healthy volunteers was associated with reduced global CMRglc, although no regional differences or clear correlation between metabolism and subjective effects was noted (de Wit et al., 1991). Volkow et al. (1995b) found that intravenous lorazepam (30 μg/kg) administration decreased whole brain as well as thalamic and occipital regional glucose metabolism, with thalamic metabolic changes correlating most closely with sedation. Flumazenil partially reversed both rCMRglc changes and the sedative effects of lorazepam (Volkow et al., 1995b). Wang et al. reported no significant gender differences in behavioral effects or absolute metabolic changes in response to lorazepam infusion, although trends toward minor differences in gyrus rectus and cerebellar metabolism were noted (Wang et al., 1998a).

Effects of Chronic Administration

Much less is known about the effects of chronic benzodiazepine administration, abuse and dependence. In fact, the two studies of "chronic" use describe fairly short-term drug use patterns. Buchsbaum and colleagues (1987) used [^{18}F]FDG PET to evaluate patients with generalized anxiety disorder before and following 3 wk of double-blinded clorazepate treatment. They found rCMRglc to be reduced in frontal and occipital cortex, particularly in the right hemisphere, and increased in thalamus and basal ganglia. Furthermore, they found that the areas of greatest reduction in rCMRglc were also areas of greatest benzodiazepine receptor density as previously determined (Buchsbaum et al., 1987). As mentioned above, Roy-Byrne noted that one week of "chronic" alprazolam use resulted in a trend toward reduced baseline CBF, although it blunted the subjective and CBF response to an i.v. alprazolam challenge (Roy-Byrne et al., 1993). Other case reports are inconclusive.

Heroin and Opiates

Acute Administration

Cerebral Blood Flow and Receptor Studies

Firestone et al. (1996) used [^{15}O]H_2O PET to evaluate possible changes in CBF in response to intravenous administration of the potent synthetic opioid fentanyl. They found increased rCBF in cingulate, orbitofrontal and medial prefrontal cortices, as well as the caudate nuclei, while reduced rCBF was noted in frontal, temporal, and cerebellar regions (Firestone et al., 1996). In a follow-up study employing painful stimuli, they found that fentanyl augmented pain-related increases in rCBF in medial and prefrontal cortices, but did not appear to affect pain-related rCBF changes in other regions including the thalamus and cingulate (Adler et al., 1997). This result was somewhat surprising in that, as they suggested, one might expect that an analgesic would attenuate pain-related effects on cerebral function. In a study designed to differentiate between κ and μ opioid agonists, which are associated with euphoria and dysphoria, respectively, Schlaepfer et al. (1998) measured cerebral perfusion with ^{99m}Tc-HMPAO SPECT in opioid abusers. Hydromorphone (a μ agonist) increased perfusion in the anterior cingulate, amygdala, and thalamus, whereas butorphanol (a mixed agonist/antagonist) administration resulted in less distinct perfusion increases in the temporal lobes (Schlaepfer et al., 1998). A rodent study and findings in a single human subject suggest that acute fentanyl administration also increases striatal dopamine concentration as reflected by decreased SPECT [^{123}I]β–CIT binding (Bergstrom et al., 1998).

Cerebral Metabolism

London et al. (1990a) used [^{18}F]FDG PET to evaluate the effect of intramuscular (IM) injection of morphine sulfate (30 mg) in polydrug abusers in a placebo-controlled crossover study. They found reduced whole brain CMRglc (~10%), as well as reduced rCMRglc in several cortical and cerebellar regions (*see* Fig. 1), although these effects were not found to be related to euphoria (London et al., 1990a). In another placebo-controlled crossover study, Walsh and colleagues used [^{18}F]FDG PET to evaluate the effect of IM buprenorphine, a mixed opioid μ agonist / κ antagonist, in a group of drug abusers. They found that buprenorphine, in addition to producing sedation and euphoria, reduced rCMRglc in almost all brain regions studied (Walsh et al., 1994).

Chronic Administration

In studies performed in our laboratory using ^{99m}Tc-HMPAO SPECT in a group of cocaine and polydrug dependent subjects, we noted, in both women and men, that concurrent heroin and cocaine abuse resulted in far more perfusion abnormalities than did cocaine abuse alone (Levin et al., 1994). In a separate, randomized placebo-controlled study evaluating the effect of buprenorphine treatment in a group of detoxified polydrug dependent men, we evaluated cerebral perfusion with ^{99m}Tc-HMPAO SPECT at baseline, at maximal buprenorphine dose, and following its discontinuation (*see* Fig. 2). We found that buprenorphine, but not placebo, resulted in improvement in baseline cerebral perfusion abnormalities in a dose-related fashion (Levin et al., 1995b).

Krystal et al. evaluated the effects of naloxone (0.8 mg, sc) on cerebral perfusion in methadone-maintained opioid addicts and in controls, using ^{99m}Tc-HMPAO SPECT. They found baseline perfusion reductions in the opioid-dependent patients in frontal and parietal cortices, and increased perfusion in the thalamus. Following naloxone administration, patients but not controls experienced symptoms of drug withdrawal, along with generally reduced perfusion (Krystal et al., 1995). Wang et al. (1997b) measured dopamine D_2 receptor availability following naloxone-precipitated withdrawal in opiate-dependent subjects with [^{11}C]raclopride PET. They found reduced baseline D_2 receptors in the opiate-dependent subjects as compared to controls. However, while naloxone precipitated intense withdrawal symptoms, it was not associated with further changes in D_2 receptor availability (Wang et al., 1997b).

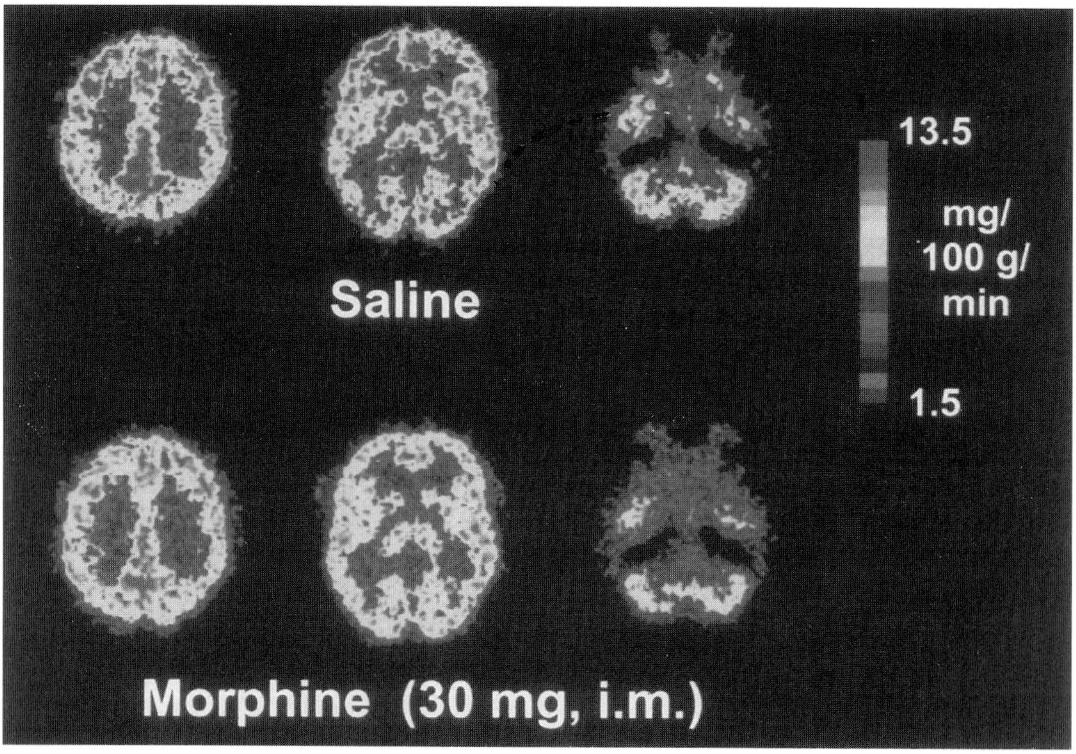

Fig. 1. Positron emission tomography (PET) scans showing reduction of cerebral glucose metabolism (an index of brain function) by 30 mg intramuscular morphine injection. Human volunteers with histories of drug abuse were subjected to PET scanning with [^{18}F]fluorodeoxyglucose as a tracer for cerebral glucose metabolism. Each volunteer was studied twice, with placebo and morphine given in pseudo-random order. Rates of cerebral glucose metabolism are indicated on the color bars. At the dose given, morphine produces euphoria while reducing activity in the cerebral cortex (seen as a shift from light to dark, or, in the color version of this figure, from red to yellow). For more details, see London et al. (1990a). (Courtesy of Dr. E.D. London, National Institute on Drug Abuse, Baltimore, MD.) (*See* color plate 5 appearing after p. 134.)

Withdrawal and Abstinence

Several studies in addition to those mentioned above have taken advantage of antagonist medications to induce and evaluate the effects of drug withdrawal. Using ^{99m}Tc-HMPAO SPECT, van Dyck and colleagues evaluated the effects of naltrexone-induced withdrawal from buprenorphine on cerebral perfusion. In this study of opiate-dependent patients maintained on buprenorphine for 1 wk, naltrexone induced symptoms of opiate withdrawal, but naltrexone was not associated with regional perfusion changes, the severity of the withdrawal it precipitated inversely correlated with perfusion in the anterior cingulate (van Dyck et al., 1994). Results in methadone-maintained addicts with a similar protocol revealed a more widespread reduction in perfusion following naloxone-induced withdrawal (Krystal et al., 1995).

The effects of withdrawal and abstinence from heroin were studied by Rose et al. (1996) using ^{99m}Tc-HMPAO SPECT to evaluate associated cerebral perfusion changes

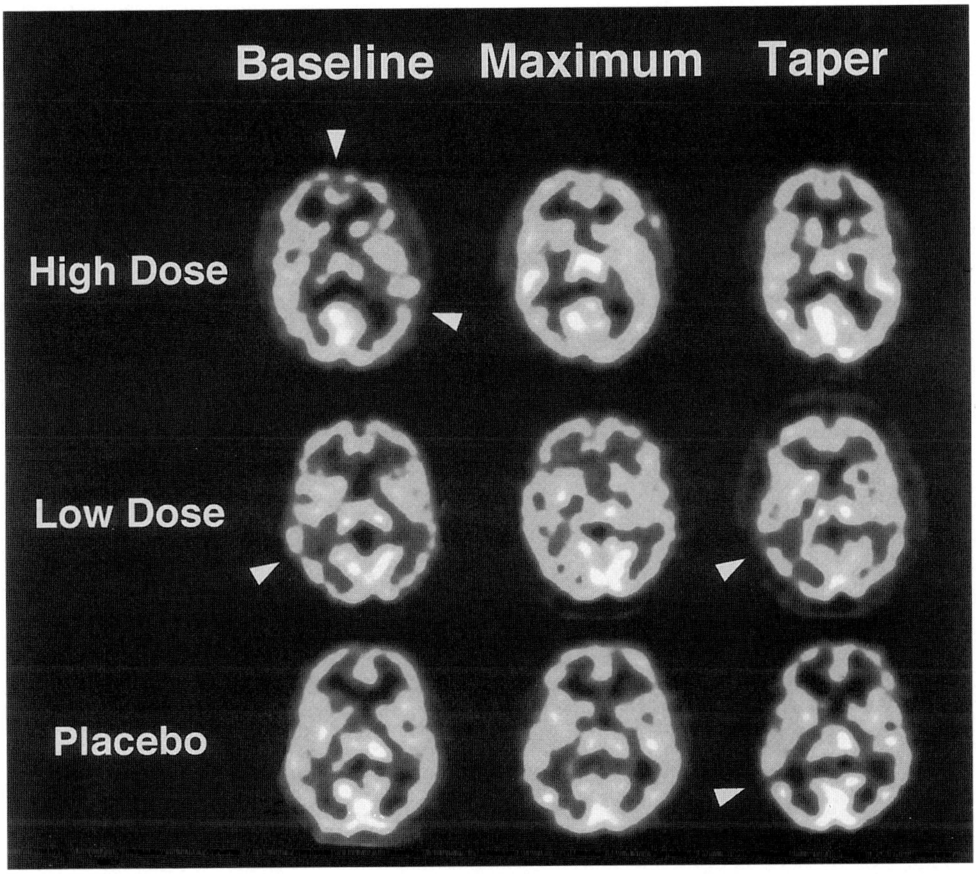

Fig. 2. Comparison of representative brain SPECT images of heroin- and cocaine-abusing men enrolled in a placebo-controlled trial of the partial opiate agonist buprenorphine for the treatment of polydrug dependence. Images are from three subjects, receiving high or low dose buprenorphine (12 or 6 mg, respectively) or placebo, and studied at three separate time points (at baseline, at maximum dose during buprenorphine treatment, and following a taper off treatment). A comparable midcortical slice includes the basal ganglia, thalamus, and frontal, temporal, parietal, and occipital cortex. Arrows indicate perfusion defects. The subject receiving high dose buprenorphine shows marked improvement in perfusion, seen as dark (purple) areas becoming light (orange or yellow), whereas the patient receiving the low dose shows more mild improvement. The patient receiving placebo shows no improvement in perfusion. Following drug taper, buprenorphine treatment groups show reduced perfusion. These data illustrate a dose-related effect of buprenorphine on improving cerebral perfusion abnormalities seen in chronic cocaine dependence, and demonstrate the potential for functional neuroimaging methods to aid in the assessment of drug abuse treatment strategies. (From Levin et al., 1995b, with permission.) (*See* color plate 7 appearing after p. 134.)

in opiate-dependent men on an inpatient drug rehabilitation unit. At 1 wk following opiate discontinuation, when symptoms of withdrawal had subsided, multiple discrete cortical perfusion defects were noted. Improvement was seen 2 wk later in all nine subjects with abnormal scans (Rose et al., 1996). However, it is unclear whether the perfusion defects noted on the initial scan (1 wk following opiate discontinuation) resulted from chronic heroin exposure or from withdrawal.

Danos et al. (1998) used ^{99m}Tc-HMPAO SPECT to measure perfusion changes associated with withdrawal in a group of heroin-dependent patients, most of whom were also receiving methadone. Regional hypoperfusion, most notably in the temporal lobes, was seen in a majority of the patients, although such hypoperfusion lacked clear clinical correlation (Danos et al., 1998). In addition, ^{99m}Tc-HMPAO SPECT was used by Gerra and colleagues to evaluate cerebral perfusion in a group of detoxified opiate-dependent subjects. Compared with normal subjects, the detoxified addicts were found to have a trend toward reduced whole brain perfusion, with significant regional hypoperfusion correlating most significantly with mood and behavioral traits (Gerra et al., 1998).

COCAINE

Cocaine is one of the most addictive and dangerous drugs of abuse, and in addition to having profound behavioral effects, it has been associated with a variety of medical and neurological sequellae. Of all the drugs of abuse, cocaine's effects on cerebral blood flow and metabolism are perhaps the most fully understood. In addition, emission tomographic studies have contributed greatly to our understanding of the neurochemical and neurotransmitter basis for cocaine's euphoric, reinforcing and addictive effects.

Acute Cocaine Administration

Cerebral Blood Flow

Cocaine is a powerful sympathomimetic compound with effects on central and peripheral vasculature. The first study of the effect of acute cocaine administration on cerebral perfusion was reported by Pearlson et al. in 1993. In a double-blind crossover study, they administered 48 mg of intravenous (iv) cocaine hydrochloride or placebo to abstinent cocaine users and compared high-resolution ^{99m}Tc-HMPAO SPECT perfusion scans at baseline and 1–5 min following cocaine administration. They found that cocaine was associated with reduced relative perfusion in frontal and inferior cingulate cortex and left basal ganglia, correlating with behavioral changes (Pearlson et al., 1993). Other frontal areas showed trends toward reduced relative perfusion, and no areas showed meaningfully increased perfusion. Wallace et al. (1996) used a quantitative ^{99m}Tc-HMPAO ASPECT imaging procedure to measure changes in absolute CBF in response to a 40 mg iv dose of cocaine hydrochloride administered to briefly abstinent cocaine-dependent men. At the time of peak "high," they found reduced rCBF in all regions studied (basal ganglia, thalamus, anterior cingulate, prefrontal cortex, occipital cortex, cerebellum), and a 30% mean reduction in whole brain CBF (Wallace et al., 1996). The reduction in cerebellar CBF would indicate that studies measuring cerebral perfusion relative to that of the cerebellum (a common practice) might not be sensitive to cocaine-associated changes in hemodynamics. Johnson et al. employed a ^{99m}Tc-ECD SPECT method for quantifying rCBF to assess changes brought about by acute iv administration of cocaine hydrochloride (0.325–0.65 mg/kg) or placebo to recently abstinent cocaine-dependent subjects. This study demonstrated dose-dependent reduction in global CBF, as well as reduction in rCBF in prefrontal, frontal, and temporal cortical regions, 5–10 min following cocaine injection, the time of peak behavioral effects (Johnson et al., 1998b).

In a preliminary study, Gottschalk et al. (1997) evaluated the time course of the rCBF response to 0.45 mg/kg iv cocaine hydrochloride or placebo in cocaine abusing subjects with quantitative ^{133}Xe-SPECT. They found the hemodynamic effect of cocaine to depend upon time following injection, with a trend toward increased rCBF noted at 4–8 min, but decreased rCBF 18–22 min postinjection, although the results were not statistically significantly different in the placebo group (Gottschalk et al., 1997). Finally, Mathew and colleagues used the ^{133}Xe inhalation technique to measure the CBF response to 0.3 mg/kg iv cocaine hydrochloride in cocaine abusing men. On separate occasions, each subject received both cocaine and placebo. This cocaine dose, adequate to produce euphoria as well as increased heart rate and blood pressure, resulted in increased CBF both immediately after and 30 min following injection, in regions located in frontal, central and parietal cortex (Mathew et al., 1996). A similar reduction in CBF was noted with placebo, at both time points. Aside from possible differences in technique and cocaine dose, it is nevertheless difficult to reconcile these findings with other evidence in the literature pointing to the vasoconstrictive effects of acute cocaine administration. The authors speculate that the initial increase in CBF they saw might represent acute neuronal activation resulting from cocaine, which overwhelms the vasoconstrictive effects, even after correcting for the vasoconstrictive effects of reduced arterial pCO_2, a finding that persists. Clearly, it will be necessary to sort out more fully the complex, and possibly competing, central vascular and functional effects of cocaine, as well as its possible influence on cerebral autoregulation.

Cerebral Metabolism

Interestingly, there has only been a single report of metabolic changes in association with cocaine administration in humans. In a carefully controlled and executed study, London and colleagues administered 40 mg cocaine hydrochloride intravenously to polydrug abusers in a double-blind, placebo-controlled crossover study employing [^{18}F]FDG PET, EEG, and behavioral assessment (*see* Fig. 3). Associated with euphoria was a 14% reduction in global glucose utilization, as well as a reduction in rCMRglc in nearly all of 29 brain regions studied, including all cortical regions, striatum, amygdala, and thalamus (London et al., 1990b). No changes were noted in the pons or cerebellum.

Similarly, ex vivo autoradiographic studies in nonhuman primates have demonstrated reduced regional metabolism following acute cocaine administration in a group of interconnected subcortical and cortical limbic structures. Such areas include the ventral striatum, especially in the nucleus accumbens, as well as the anterior thalamus, locus ceruleus, the raphe nuclei, medial temporal regions, and the ventral prefrontal cortex, with little or no neocortical involvement (Lyons et al., 1996). These findings reinforce the importance of the mesolimbic system postulated to underlie the reinforcing effects of cocaine.

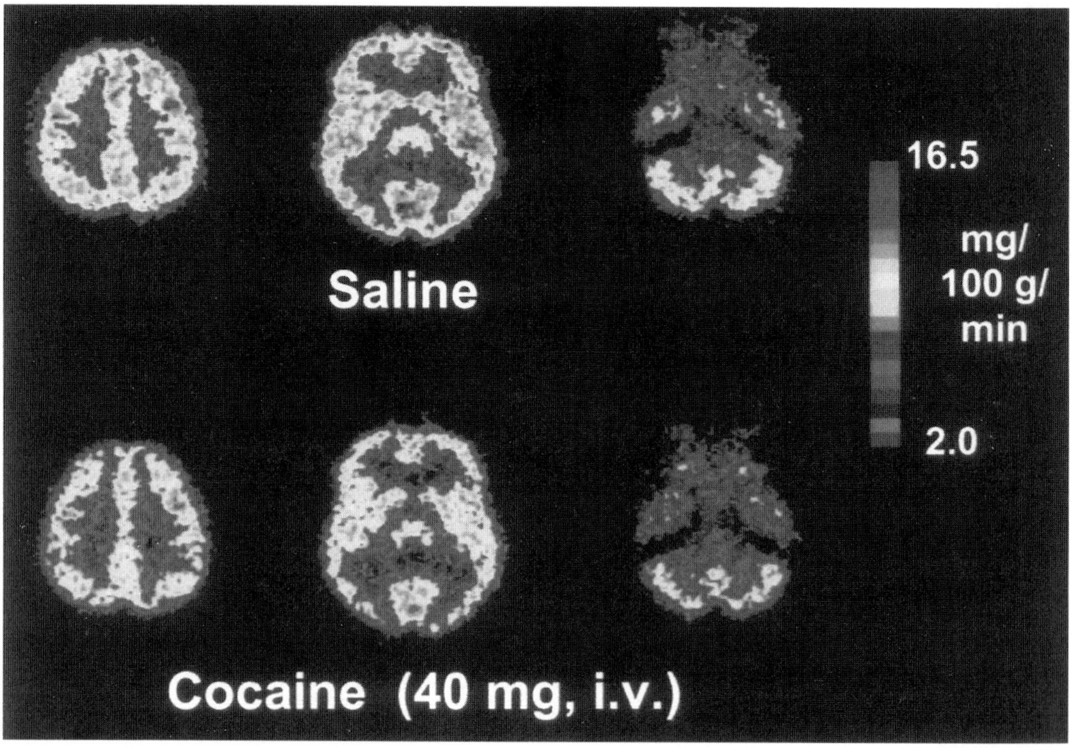

Fig. 3. Positron emission tomography (PET) scans showing reduction of cerebral glucose metabolism (an index of brain function) by 40 mg intravenous cocaine hydrochloride injection. Human volunteers with histories of drug abuse were subjected to PET scanning with [^{18}F]fluorodeoxyglucose as a tracer for cerebral glucose metabolism. Each volunteer was studied twice, with placebo and cocaine given in pseudorandom order. Rates of cerebral glucose metabolism are indicated on the color bars. At the dose given, cocaine produces euphoria while reducing activity in the cerebral cortex (seen as a shift from light to dark, or, in the color version of this figure, from red to yellow). For more details, see London et al. (1990b). (Courtesy of Dr. E.D. London, National Institute on Drug Abuse, Baltimore, MD.) (*See* color plate 6 appearing after p. 134.)

Cocaine Binding and Receptor Studies

Much work has focused on characterizing the in vivo distribution and pharmacological properties of central cocaine binding sites. Fowler et al. (1989) used a subpharmacological, or tracer, dose of [^{11}C]cocaine to map cocaine binding sites in the human brain with PET. They found peak binding of [^{11}C]cocaine in the striatum at 4–10 min after iv injection, with clearance to half-peak binding at 25 min, paralleling the documented time course of cocaine's euphoric effects. Concurrent baboon studies employing pretreatment with nomifensine (a dopamine reuptake inhibitor) noted reduced striatal uptake of [^{11}C]cocaine, demonstrating the selectivity of striatal cocaine binding to the presynaptic dopamine transporter (DAT) (Fowler et al., 1989). Malison et al. used SPECT with the radiolabeled cocaine congener [^{123}I]β–CIT, which has high DAT binding potency, and SPECT to provide evidence that euphorigenic doses of cocaine bind in a fairly selective fashion to DAT sites (Malison et al., 1995). Logan and colleagues subsequently measured the concentration, and effective occupancy by cocaine, of striatal DAT sites in cocaine abusers with [^{11}C]cocaine and PET, but found the estimates of DAT concentration to be fairly unstable (Logan et al., 1997). Schlaepfer et al. (1997) used PET with [^{11}C]raclopride, a selective postsynaptic dopamine D_2 receptor ligand, to assess the effect of cocaine on D_2 binding. Following a dose of 48 mg cocaine hydrochloride, which produced euphoric effects in the iv drug users studied, striatal [^{11}C]raclopride binding was reduced (displaced), supporting the contention that cocaine administration increases synaptic dopamine concentration (Schlaepfer et al., 1997). Volkow and colleagues further demonstrated the importance of DAT blockade in producing the euphoric effects of cocaine. Using euphorigenic (0.3–0.6 mg/kg) doses of [^{11}C]cocaine as a DAT ligand in cocaine-dependent subjects, they estimated that at least half the DAT sites must be occupied to produce behavioral effects (Volkow et al., 1997a).

The interaction between cocaine and alcohol has received increasing attention. It has been suggested that increased behavioral and toxic effects associated with coabuse of cocaine and alcohol may result from the formation of cocaethylene (Hearn et al., 1991; McCance et al., 1995). Fowler et al. used PET with [^{11}C]cocaine to evaluate the uptake, clearance, and distribution volume of cocaine before and during alcohol ingestion. They found no significant differences with alcohol, and no detectable radiolabeled cocaethylene, suggesting that the enhanced response to the combination is not directly due to altered cocaine metabolism (Fowler et al., 1992).

Chronic Cocaine Abuse and Dependence

Cerebral Blood Flow

The chronic effects of cocaine on cerebral hemodynamics have been studied in great detail in a number of controlled studies. The first report of abnormal baseline cerebral perfusion in chronic cocaine users was published by Volkow et al. in 1988. Using [^{15}O]H_2O PET in 20 chronic cocaine-abusing men, they demonstrated multifocal, patchy regions of reduced perfusion (perfusion defects) as well as decreased rCBF in prefrontal cortex (Volkow et al., 1988a). These defects were present during detoxification and again 10 days later when patients showed no signs of withdrawal. Tumeh et al. (1990) used SPECT with [^{123}I]IMP in a group of neurologically normal, polydrug abusing, HIV-negative men. They also found multifocal cortical perfusion defects, which were more common in the frontal and temporal lobes (Tumeh et al., 1990). Follow-up studies with high-resolution ^{99m}Tc-HMPAO annular SPECT (ASPECT) in HIV-negative, cocaine- and polydrug-dependent men, many of whom tested positive for cocaine metabolites at the time of the examination, confirmed multifocal perfusion defects (*see* Fig. 4), generally in inferoparietal, temporal and anterofrontal cortex and basal ganglia (Holman et al., 1991). Subsequent work comparing cocaine-dependent subjects and patients with the AIDS dementia complex (ADC) demonstrated the non-specificity and similarity of perfusion defects in the two groups (Holman et al., 1992). Weber et al., using [^{123}I]IMP SPECT, found similar focal perfusion defects and "patchy" tracer uptake in a large percentage of crack abusers with no history of intravenous drug use or dependence on any other drugs (Weber et al., 1993). Similar perfusion abnormalities have been noted by others (Miller et al., 1992; Strickland et al., 1993).

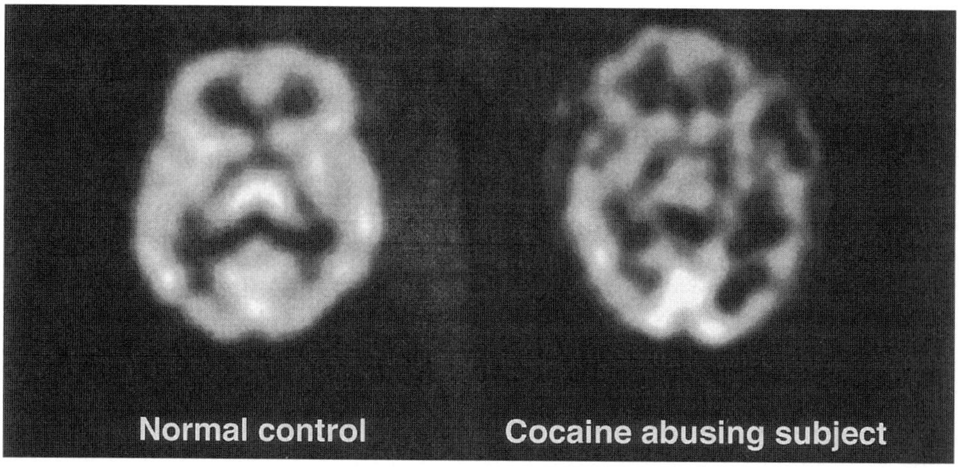

Fig. 4. Single photon emission computed tomography (SPECT) perfusion scans of a chronic cocaine-dependent subject on the right and an age-matched normal volunteer the left. Both subjects were men. Each was injected with the radiotracer ^{99m}Tc-HMPAO and imaged several minutes later in the resting state with eyes open. In the normal subject, cerebral perfusion is uniform and robust, as represented by hues of white and orange. By contrast, in the cocaine-dependent subject, in addition to an overall picture of less robust cerebral perfusion, there are focal reductions in numerous brain regions, as seen by replacement of white and orange hues with blue and black. (*See* color plate 8 appearing after p. 134.)

The abovementioned studies focused mainly on cocaine-dependent men. However, we subsequently demonstrated that cocaine-dependent women have far fewer perfusion abnormalities than do men with similar cocaine use histories (Levin et al., 1994). Furthermore, although cocaine-dependent women were difficult to distinguish from normal control subjects, and cocaine-dependent men had multiple abnormalities, polydrug-dependent subjects of both sexes displayed more abnormalities than did cocaine-dependent subjects. Therefore, both male gender and polydrug abuse appear to be among the greatest risk factors for the development of cerebral perfusion abnormalities in chronic cocaine dependence.

Fortunately, cocaine-associated cerebral perfusion defects appear to be limited to adults. Konkol et al. found normal cerebral perfusion in high-resolution ^{99m}Tc-HMPAO SPECT measurements of 21 neonates with a history of in utero cocaine exposure (Konkol et al., 1994). This was in contrast to their findings of behavioral or electroencephalographic abnormalities in all but four newborns, as well as microcephaly in five. Although neonates do not appear to escape significant toxic effects of in utero cocaine exposure, this study indicates that they may escape some of the cerebrovascular effects.

Cerebral Metabolism

The metabolic effects of chronic cocaine use are less clear than the hemodynamic effects. Much of this work overlaps with studies in various phases of cocaine withdrawal and will be discussed in that context below.

In studies employing [^{18}F]FDG PET, Volkow et al. (1993a) demonstrated reduced orbitofrontal and anterior cingulate rCMRglc in abstinent cocaine-dependent men. Subsequently, in order to assess the effect of cocaine abuse on GABA-ergic systems, this group evaluated the effect of chronic cocaine abuse on the metabolic response to the benzodiazepine lorazepam. Compared to controls, cocaine abusers responded to lorazepam with greater reduction in global and regional glucose metabolism, particularly in the striatum, thalamus, and parietal cortex. These group effects were noted despite lower lorazepam plasma levels in the cocaine abusers (Volkow et al., 1998b).

Withdrawal

Using [^{18}F]FDG PET, Baxter et al. (1988) found no abnormality in left lateral prefrontal cortical glucose metabolism in a cohort of cocaine-dependent subjects early in withdrawal, but these data are incomplete and inconclusive. Volkow and colleagues also used [^{18}F]FDG PET in cocaine-dependent men both during and following withdrawal, and compared them to normal subjects. They found increased global CMRglc and increased rCMRglc in orbitofrontal cortex and basal ganglia, with normalization following withdrawal (Volkow et al., 1991a).

Kosten et al. (1998) evaluated cerebral perfusion with ^{99m}Tc-HMPAO SPECT in cocaine-dependent subjects in acute (1–3 d) and midterm (21 d) abstinence, with no signs of withdrawal. Frontal and parietal perfusion abnormalities were not found to change over the course of abstinence, although they seemed to be limited to subjects with a history of concomitant alcohol abuse (Kosten et al., 1998). This finding of greater perfusion abnormalities in polydrug abusing patients than in those abusing cocaine alone is consistent with previous work in our laboratory (Levin et al., 1994).

Cocaine Craving

In order to determine the functional correlates of craving, Grant et al. (1996) exposed cocaine-abusing subjects to cocaine-related cues while undergoing [^{18}F]FDG PET (*see* Fig. 5). They demonstrated increases in rCMRglc in the dorsolateral prefrontal cortex, amygdala, and cerebellum that correlated with the subjects' reports of cocaine craving (Grant et al., 1996). Liu et al. (1998) evaluated both glucose metabolism and EEG in cocaine abusers and controls presented with cocaine-related cues. Cocaine abusers, but not controls, demonstrated reduced alpha power on EEG, correlating with increased glucose metabolism. However, these measures did not correlate with the time course or magnitude of cocaine craving, suggesting that cue-elicited craving is not directly related to these electrophysiological and metabolic measures (Liu et al., 1998).

Most recently, using [^{15}O]H_2O PET, Childress and colleagues measured brain activation (relative increase in rCBF) in response to cue-induced cocaine craving in limbic and control regions in detoxified cocaine users. Despite having lower baseline rCBF in limbic regions, cocaine users, but not controls, showed increased limbic activation in response to cocaine-related cues, particularly in the left amygdala and anterior cingulate cortex. The two groups did not differ in terms of activation in control regions (dorsolateral prefrontal cortex, cerebellum, thalamus, and visual cortex),

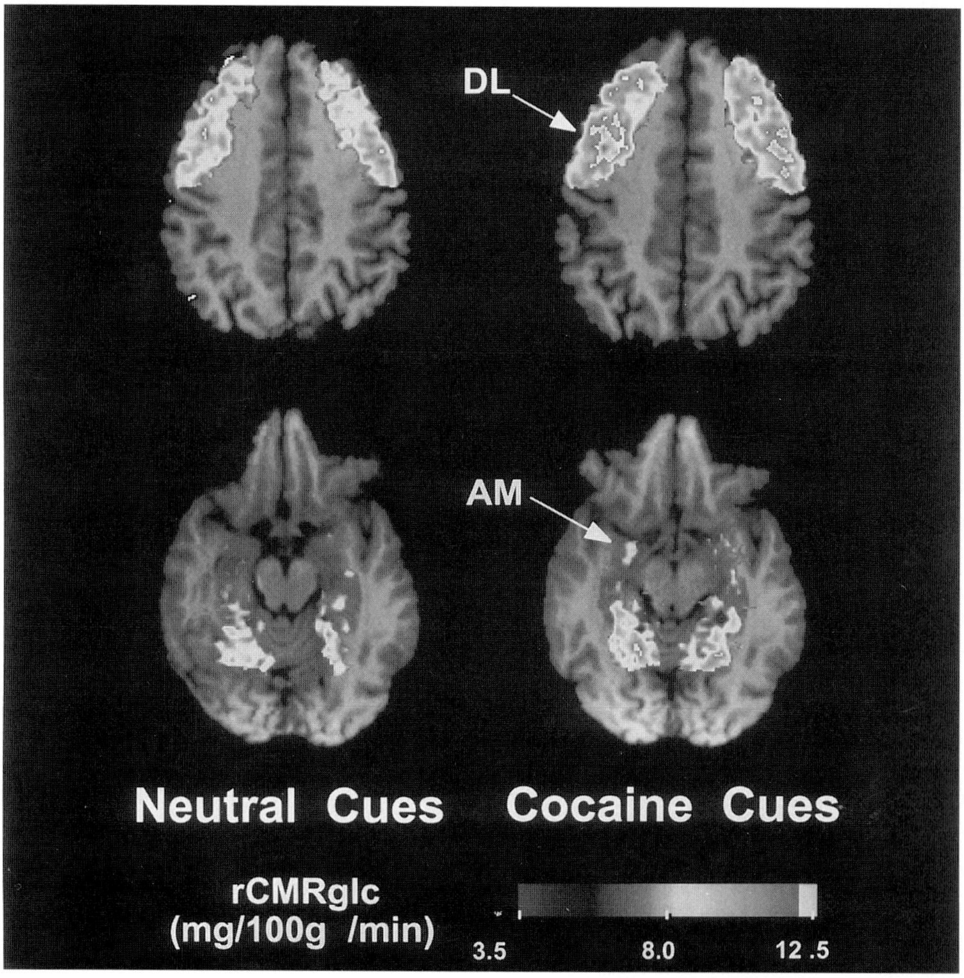

Fig. 5. Positron emission tomography (PET) scanning with [^{18}F]fluorodeoxyglucose as a tracer for cerebral glucose metabolism, showing increased activity in brain regions implicated in several forms of memory, when human volunteers who abused cocaine were exposed to drug-related stimuli. Cocaine abusers were studied under a neutral condition (left) and also in a test session in which they were presented with drug-related stimuli, such as a videotape of cocaine self-administration. They reported varying degrees of craving. A subject who reported high cocaine craving when viewing the cocaine cues (right) showed brain activation in the dorsolateral prefrontal cortex (DL) (*upper scans*), a brain region that is important in short-term memory, and the amygdala (AM) (*lower scans*), a brain region that is important in emotional aspects of memory. The findings, which have implications for treatment of cocaine addiction, suggest that a distributed network, which integrates emotional and other aspects of memory, links environmental cues with cocaine craving. For more details, see Grant et al. (1996). (Courtesy of Dr. E.D. London, National Institute on Drug Abuse, Baltimore, MD.) (*See* color plate 9 appearing after p. 134.)

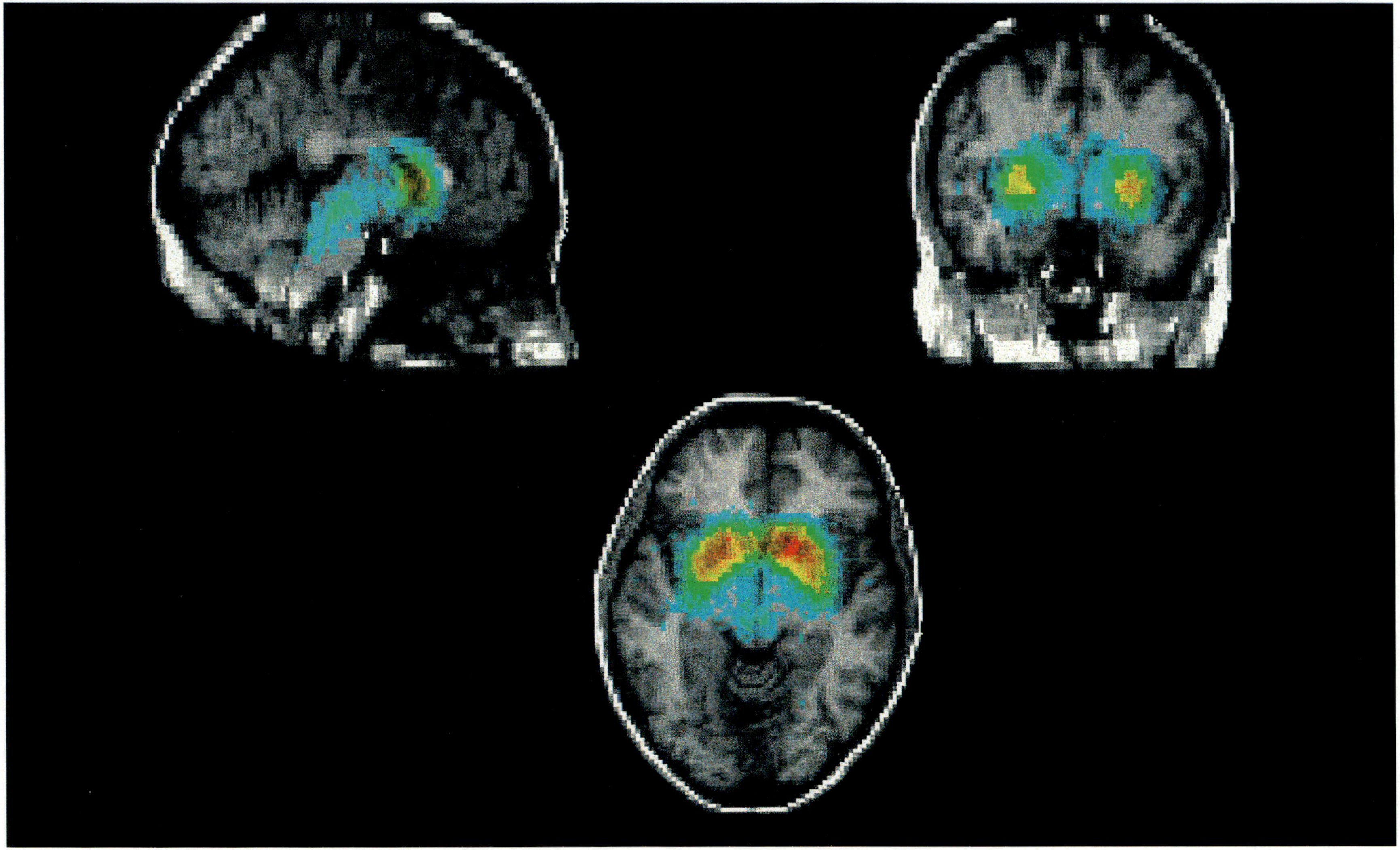

Plate 3. Sagittal (top left), coronal (top right), and transaxial (bottom) views of the in vivo distribution of the cocaine analog $[^{123}I]\beta$-CIT as imaged by SPECT and coregistered with MRI. *See Chapter 2, Fig. 4, p. 34.*

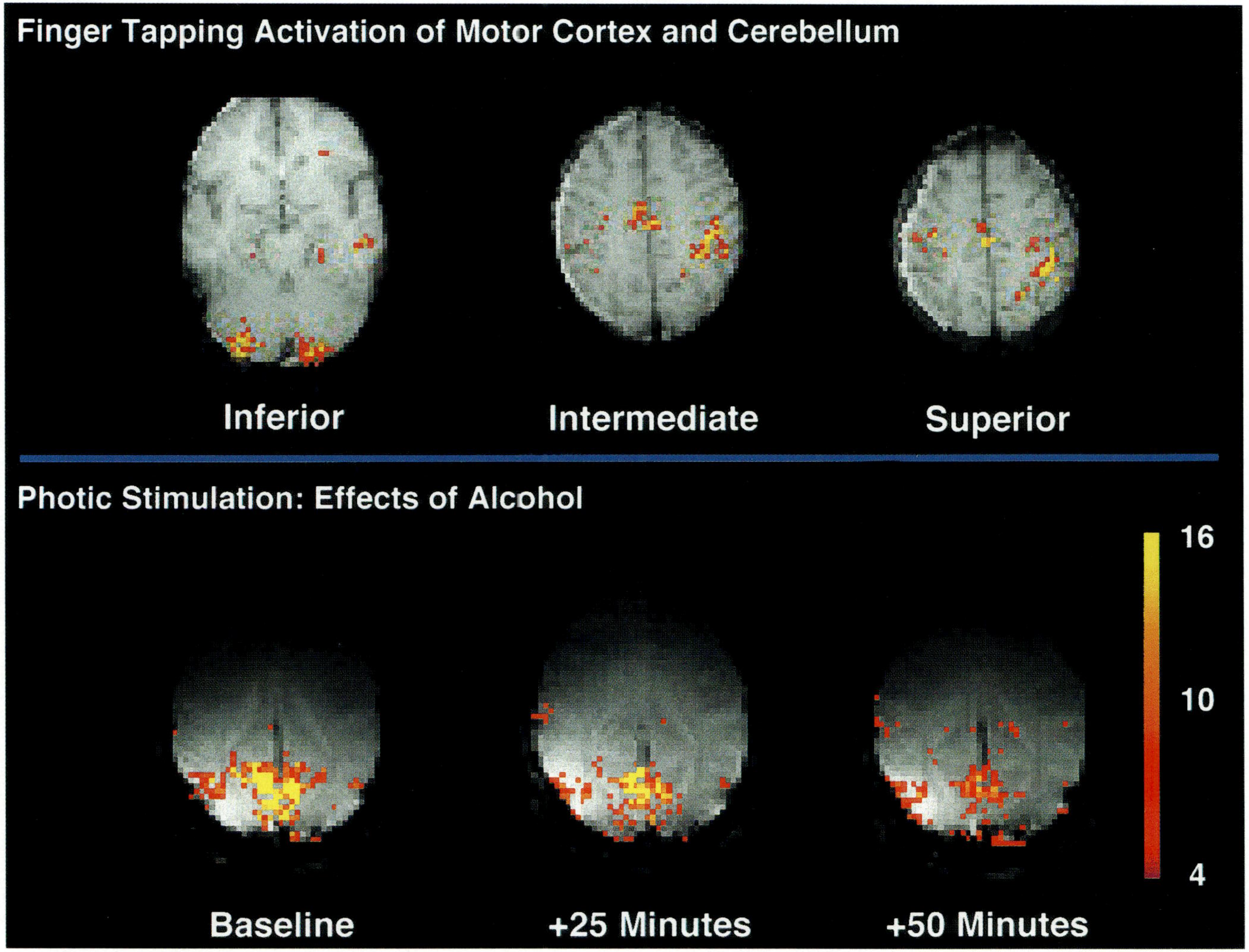

Plate 4. BOLD fMRI srudies of brain activation during finger tapping (top) and during photic stimulation at baseline and during alcohol intoxication (bottom). Cortical activation (colored pixels) are mapped onto axial MRI images. *For details (top panel), see Chapter 3, Fig. 14, p. 63 and for (bottom panel), Chapter 6, Fig. 4, p. 160.*

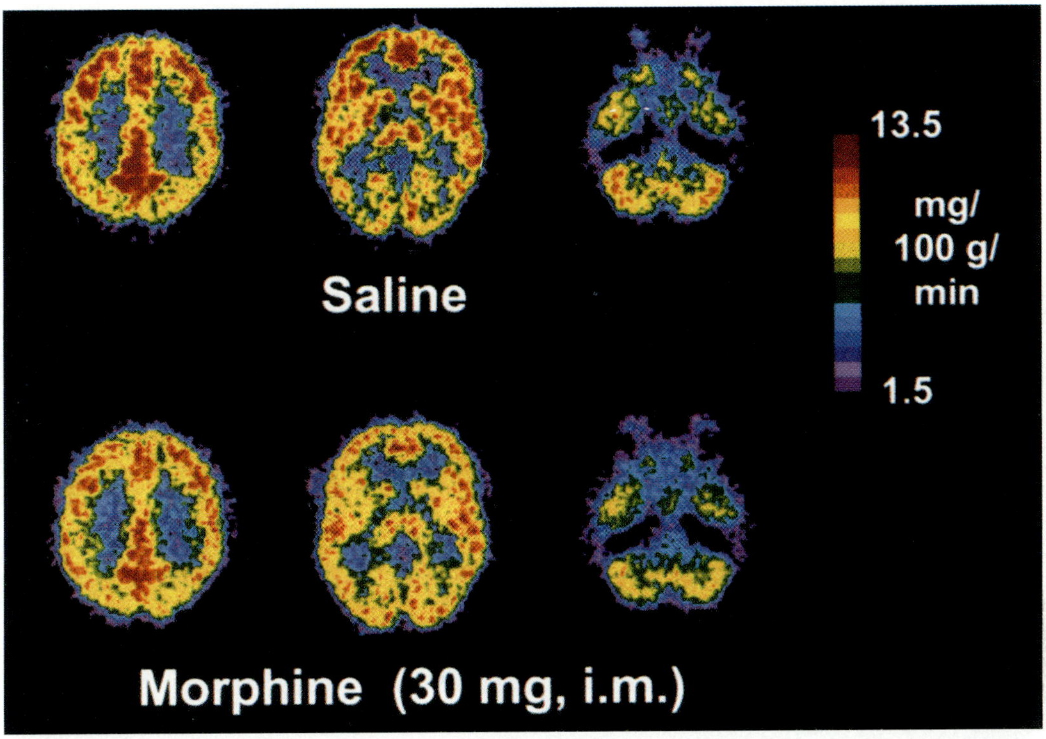

Plate 5. Positron emission tomography (PET) scan showing reduction of cerebral glucose metabolism following intramuscular morphine injection (Courtesy, Dr. E. D. London). *See Chapter 5, Fig. 1, p. 126.*

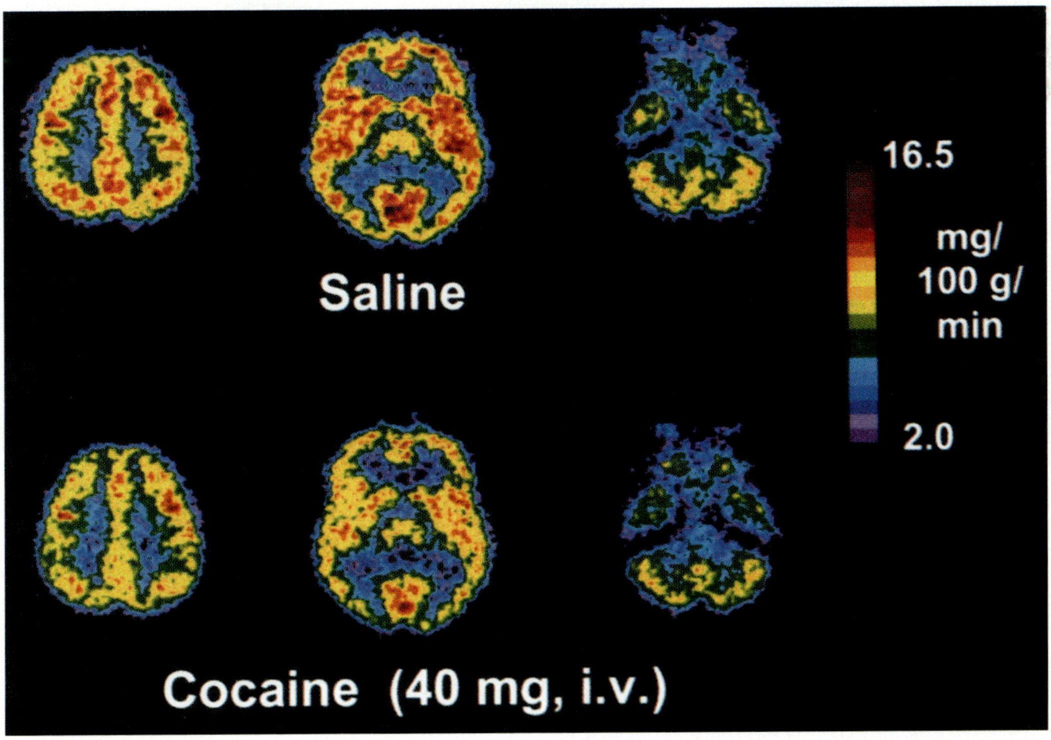

Plate 6. Positron emission tomography (PET) scan showing reduction of cerebral glucose metabolism following intravenous cocaine injection (Courtesy, Dr. E. D. London). *See Chapter 5, Fig. 3, p. 130.*

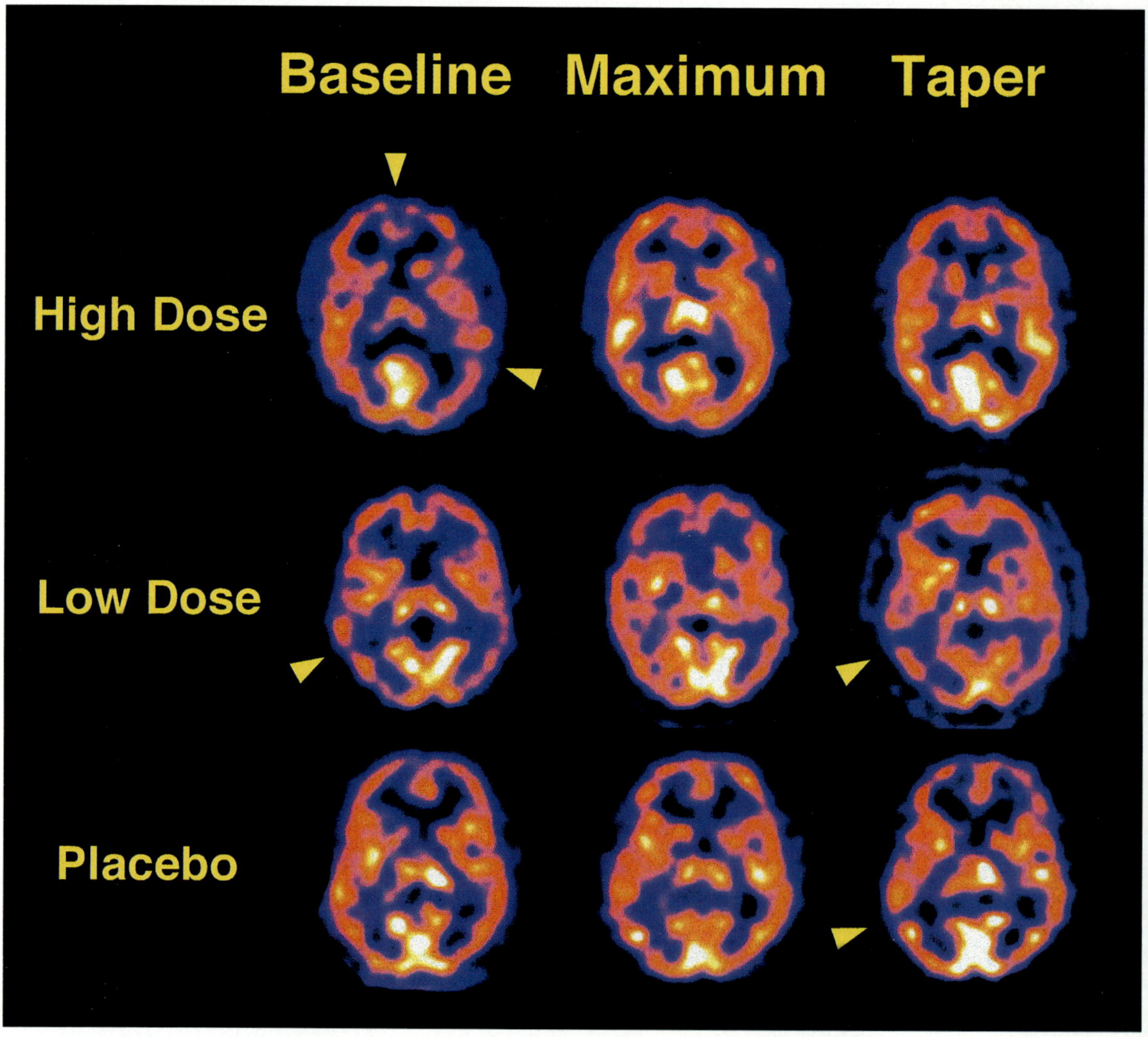

Plate 7. Single photon emission computed tomography (SPECT) perfusion scans of heroin- and cocaine-dependent polydrug abusers treated with buprenorphine or placebo. Arrows indicate perfusion defects (From Levin et al., 1995b, with permission). *See Chapter 5, Fig. 2, p. 127.*

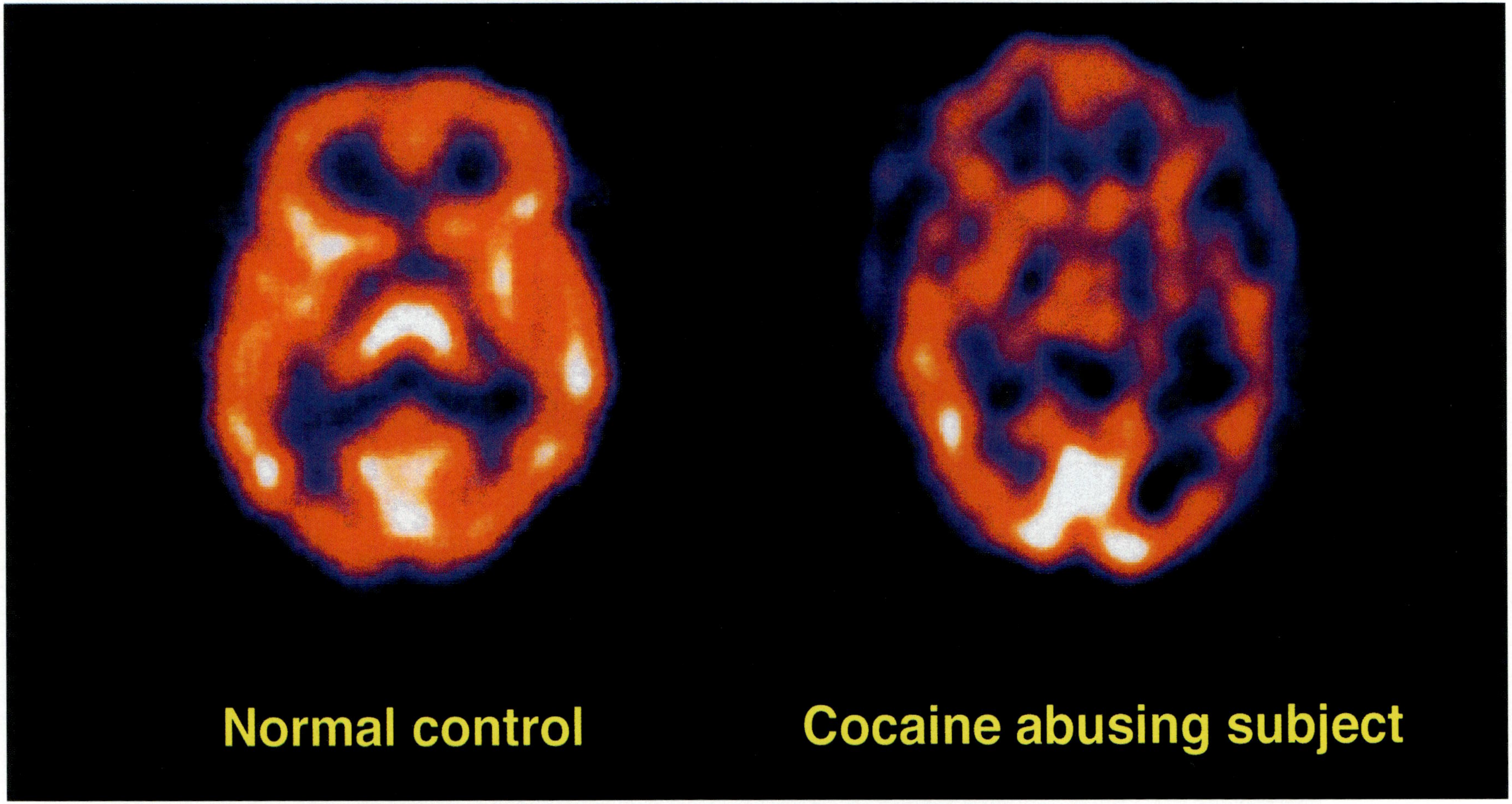

Plate 8. Single photon emission computed tomography (SPECT) perfusion scans of a control and a cocaine-dependent subject. *See Chapter 5, Fig. 4, p. 132.*

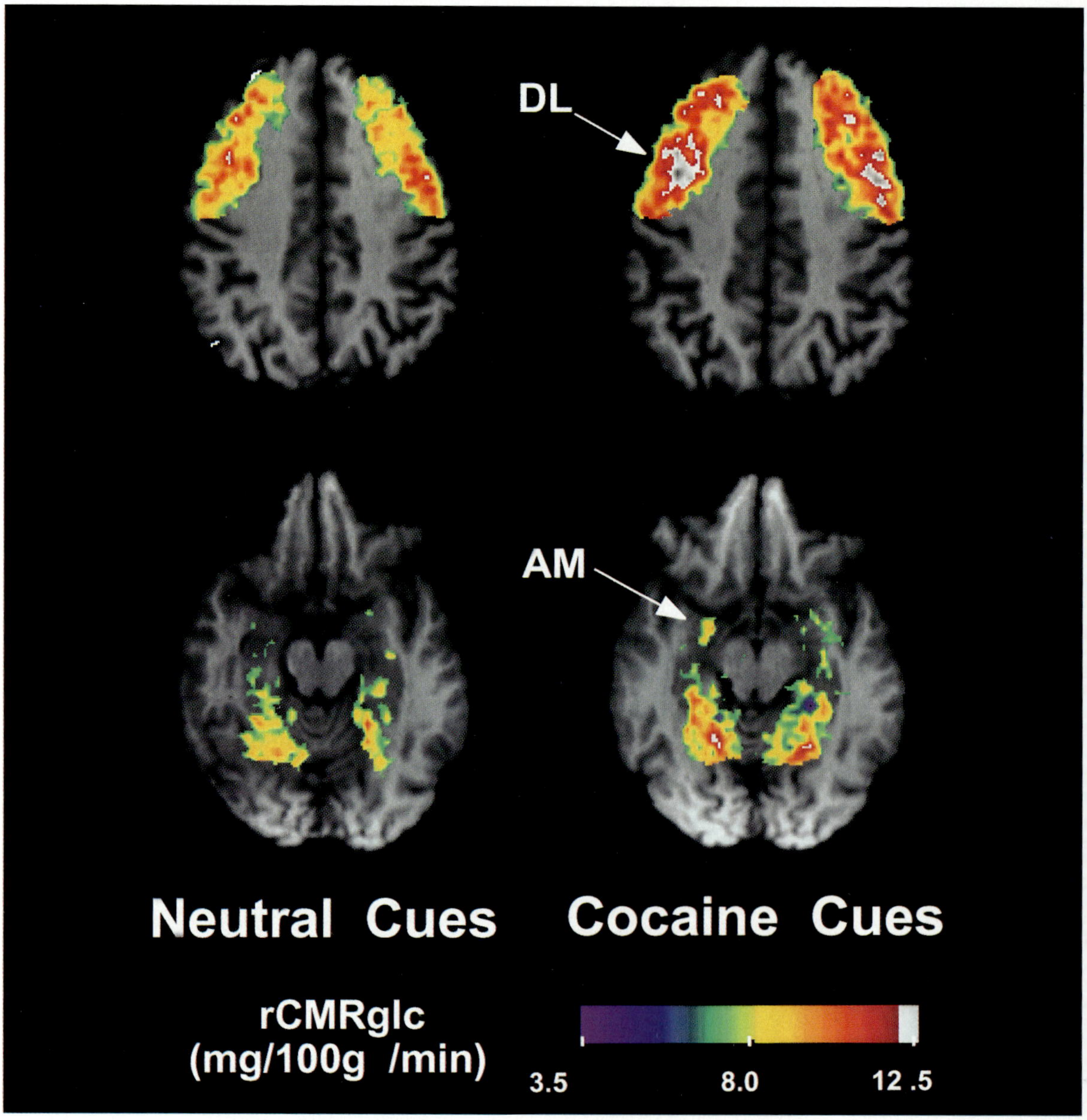

Plate 9. Positron emission tomography (PET) scan showing increased brain metabolism in a cocaine abuser in response to cocaine-related stimuli. Arrows highlight dorsolateral prefrontal cortex (DL) and amygdala (AM), which are activated during cocaine craving (Courtesy, Dr. E. D. London). *See Chapter 5, Fig. 5, p. 134.*

although the cocaine users did respond to cues with reduced rCBF in the basal ganglia (Childress et al., 1999). Thus, the authors confirmed their initial hypothesis regarding selective limbic activation with craving, and thereby demonstrate the potential for functional imaging to address complex questions regarding the neurobiology of addiction on a systems level.

Abstinence

Although several studies of the chronic effects of cocaine abuse include both current and abstinent users, the effect of abstinence has been directly addressed. Using [^{18}F]FDG PET, Volkow et al. demonstrated reduced frontal (particularly left hemispheric) glucose metabolism in chronic cocaine-abusing men during late withdrawal that persisted for 3–4 mo following detoxification (Volkow et al., 1992a). Strickland et al. measured cerebral perfusion with both ^{133}Xe and ^{99m}Tc-HMPAO SPECT in crack-abusing HIV-negative subjects who were drug free for at least 6 mo prior to examination. They found multifocal cerebral perfusion defects, as well as numerous neuropsychological abnormalities, such as deficits in attention, concentration, learning, memory and language (Strickland et al., 1993).

Receptor/Transporter Effects

The role of dopamine and the dopamine transporter (DAT) in subserving the behavioral and reinforcing effects of cocaine has received increasing attention. As a result, numerous emission tomographic studies have focused on this issue and have contributed to our understanding of the neurobiology of addiction. Volkow et al. (1990a) first evaluated binding to striatal postsynaptic dopamine D_2 receptors using [^{18}F]*N*-methylspiroperidol and PET in a group of detoxified cocaine abusers. Subjects in early abstinence (1 wk or less) showed reduced D_2 receptor binding, whereas normal binding was seen in those in midterm abstinence (1 mo), demonstrating impaired postsynaptic dopamine receptor availability associated with cocaine abuse, and its possible recovery with abstinence (Volkow et al., 1990a). However, subsequent work indicated persistently reduced dopamine D_2 receptor binding at up to 3–4 mo of abstinence (Volkow et al., 1993a). This work combining [^{18}F]*N*-methylspiroperidol and [^{18}F]FDG PET also indicated correlations between D_2 receptor binding and CMRglc in prefrontal, orbitofrontal, motor, inferior temporal, and cingulate cortex. Reduced dopamine D_2 receptor binding could reflect either reduced numbers of D_2 receptors with chronic cocaine abuse, or the presence of increased levels of synaptic dopamine that could competitively block receptors, although the former is the more likely possibility. In order to determine whether increased dopamine could reverse the abnormally low glucose metabolism seen in chronic cocaine dependence, this group evaluated the effect of methylphenidate administration in a group of chronic cocaine-dependent men in early abstinence. While response to methylphenidate was variable, they found that subjects with reduced D_2 receptor density at baseline (as measured by [^{11}C]raclopride binding) had reduced metabolism, while those with increased D_2 receptor density had the opposite response. Furthermore, while methylphenidate was associated with increased metabolism in superior cingulate, right thalamus, and cerebellum, only increased metabolism in right orbitofrontal cortex and right striatum correlated with craving, and only increased metabolism in prefrontal cortex correlated with enhanced mood (Volkow et al., 1999a, 1999b).

Other studies of the dopaminergic system have also been performed. Wu et al. (1997) measured striatal 6-[^{18}F]fluorodopa uptake (an index of presynaptic dopaminergic activity) in abstinent cocaine addicts. They found that in early abstinence (1–10 d), striatal dopamine nerve terminal function in addicts was similar to that in controls, although in later abstinence (11–30 d) it was significantly reduced (Wu et al., 1997). This would imply that dopaminergic dysfunction develops with prolonged abstinence. Volkow et al. assessed the capacity for abstinent cocaine-dependent subjects to increase synaptic dopamine by using PET to assess binding of a competitive postsynaptic dopamine D_2 receptor ligand, [^{11}C]raclopride, in association with iv injection of methylphenidate. Striatal dopamine release and methylphenidate "high" were impaired in the addicts relative to controls. However, thalamic dopamine release was slightly augmented in the addicts. These findings raise the issue of the relative importance of striatal and thalamic dopamine pathway involvement in addiction (Volkow et al., 1997c).

Cocaine binding to the dopamine transporter is believed to be an important component of the drug's reinforcing effects, and studies of the DAT in cocaine use and abuse are of extreme interest. Volkow et al. measured cocaine uptake, DAT availability, and D_2 receptor availability in the brains of abstinent cocaine abusers by using PET with [^{11}C]cocaine and [^{18}F]*N*-methylspiroperidol. Cocaine abusers showed reduced cocaine binding as compared to controls in the basal ganglia, cortex, thalamus, and cerebellum, as well as reduced D_2 receptor availability, although DAT availability appeared to be normal. The authors speculate that chronic DAT blockade by cocaine may protect against normal age-related loss of the DAT (Volkow et al., 1996e; Wang et al., 1997a). Malison et al. used [^{123}I]β–CIT SPECT and found elevated levels of striatal DAT during acute abstinence (NB:1–4 d, not described as in withdrawal) in a group of cocaine abusers (Malison et al., 1998a).

Other neurotransmitter systems are also of interest in cocaine abuse. Upregulation of opioid μ receptors in recently abstinent cocaine-dependent men was demonstrated with [^{11}C]carfentanil and PET, and persisted for at least four weeks of verified abstinence (Zubieta et al., 1996). These results support the contention that the endogenous opioid system may be involved in cocaine dependence and craving. On the other hand, Wang et al. were unable to demonstrate changes in serotonin 5-HT_2 receptor availability in chronic cocaine abusers as compared to controls using [^{18}F]*N*-methylspiperone PET (Wang et al., 1995).

Treatment for Cocaine Abuse and Dependence

Preliminary studies using ^{99m}Tc-HMPAO SPECT indicated improvement in abnormal cerebral perfusion in cocaine-dependent men undergoing treatment with the partial opioid agonist buprenorphine, although the effect of abstinence from cocaine exposure alone could not be excluded (Holman et al., 1993). Our subsequent placebo-controlled study demonstrated a dose-dependent improvement in perfusion in patients receiving buprenorphine, and a worsening in perfusion in patients receiving placebo (*see* Fig. 2), demonstrating that drug treatment, and not abstinence alone, accounted for this improvement (Levin et al., 1995b). The effect of the L-type calcium channel antagonist isradipine on cerebral perfusion abnormalities resulting from acute cocaine infusion (0.325 mg/kg) was assessed with quantitative Tc-ECD SPECT. Cocaine alone resulted in reduced CBF in numerous regions, while isradipine pre-treatment appeared to block this effect and even increase blood flow in several areas, including prefrontal cortex and caudate (Johnson et al., 1998a).

Non-euphorigenic DAT blockade has been suggested as a possible avenue for treatment of cocaine dependence. Using SPECT, Malison et al. (1998b) studied the potency of mazindol binding to striatal dopamine transporter sites in cocaine-dependent subjects by evaluating subsequent binding of [^{123}I]β–CIT, a cocaine congener of high binding potency at the dopamine transporter. They found the potency of mazindol to be low, providing a possible explanation for the lack of clinical efficacy reported with its use to treat cocaine dependence (Malison et al., 1998b).

Summary

Cocaine's effects on cerebral hemodynamics, metabolism, and receptor systems are complex, but numerous studies have resulted in an increasingly clear understanding of the neurobiology of cocaine reinforcement and addiction, thus providing an avenue into understanding how this drug affects brain function. Volkow and colleagues (1988a) first demonstrated patchy regions of relatively diminished CBF in chronic cocaine-abusing men throughout the cerebral cortex. Subsequent perfusion studies with PET and SPECT have confirmed these focal perfusion defects in cocaine- and polydrug-dependent men (Tumeh et al., 1990; Holman et al., 1991; Miller et al., 1992; Weber et al., 1993), although not in women (Levin et al., 1994). Further work has demonstrated improvement in perfusion abnormalities coincident with drug abuse treatment (Holman et al., 1993; Levin et al., 1995b), and increased metabolism during withdrawal (Volkow et al., 1991a). In addition, studies of acute intravenous administration of cocaine have demonstrated global and regional reduction in glucose metabolism associated with euphoria (London et al., 1990b), as well as decreased frontal regional CBF (Pearlson et al., 1993). Finally, numerous imaging studies have confirmed the association between the behavioral and reinforcing effects of cocaine and measures of striatal DAT occupancy.

Amphetamine and Methamphetamine

Amphetamine

Cerebral Blood Flow

Studies of the acute effects of amphetamines on CBF with the ^{133}Xe inhalation method have been inconsistent. When Berglund and Risberg first studied a single male addict, they found increased CBF following amphetamine administration, particularly in frontal regions and in the left hemisphere (Berglund and Risberg, 1980). However, Mathew and Wilson reported reduced global CBF, with no regional differences, following intravenous *d*-amphetamine administration in both schizophrenic patients and control subjects (Mathew and Wilson, 1985; Mathew and Wilson, 1989). Kahn et al. (1989) noted a trend toward reduced CBF in normal volunteers following amphetamine infusion. More recently, Mattay et al. (1996) measured [^{15}O]H_2O PET rCBF responses to several cognitive tasks both before and following *d*-amphetamine administration in healthy volunteers. Baseline global CBF was unchanged following amphetamine. However, rCBF responses to the cognitive tasks were affected in a complex pattern by the *d*-amphetamine infusion, with both increased and decreased task-related activation depending upon task and location (Mattay et al., 1996).

Cerebral Metabolism

Early [^{18}F]FDG PET studies indicated that oral administration of *d*-amphetamine resulted in reduced frontal, temporal, and striatal rCMRglc in both schizophrenic patients and control subjects, and that these metabolic effects correlated with plasma drug levels (Wolkin et al., 1994). Ernst et al. found that intravenous *d*-amphetamine administration in healthy volunteers resulted in increased subcortical, limbic, frontal, and cerebellar rCMRglc, but reduced temporal rCMRglc (Ernst et al., 1997). More recently, Vollenweider and colleagues evaluated the effect of high dose *d*-amphetamine (1 mg/kg p.o.), which was sufficient to produce mania in healthy volunteers. They found a resultant widespread increase in absolute rCMRglc in anterior cingulate, striatum, and thalamus, with certain rCMRglc changes correlating with the mania, while others correlated with plasma drug levels (Vollenweider et al., 1998).

Receptor Studies

Laruelle et al. (1995) used the dopamine D_2 receptor radioligand [^{123}I]IBZM and SPECT to evaluate striatal dopamine release following intravenous (0.3 mg/kg) *d*-amphetamine administration to healthy subjects. They found that striatal dopamine D_2 receptor availability decreased by ~15%, reflecting increased synaptic dopamine and correlating with the behavioral effects of the drug (Laruelle et al., 1995). Subsequent work by this group suggested that D_2 receptor availability decreased more in drug-free schizophrenic patients (~20%) than in control subjects (~8%) despite similar baseline D_2 receptor density. This finding is consistent with the hypothesis of augmented responsiveness of dopaminergic neurons in schizophrenia, although the discrepancy with the previous report of 15% reduction in D_2 receptor availability in control subjects is not explained (Laruelle et al., 1996). A recent study confirmed the differential effects of amphetamine in schizophrenics and controls, although the effect size was somewhat smaller (Abi-Dargham et al., 1998a). Breier et al. (1997b) reached similar conclusions using [^{11}C]raclopride (another D_2 radioligand) and PET, again indicating greater striatal dopamine release following intravenous amphetamine (0.3 mg/kg) in schizophrenics than in controls, despite similar plasma drug levels. Detection of dopamine release depends upon the relative selectivity and affinity of the radioligand. This was demonstrated by the studies of Tibbo and colleagues using SPECT and [^{123}I]epidepride, a D_2 radioligand with high D_2 specific binding and affinity. In this study, no effect of amphetamine was seen, most likely because epidepride occupancy of D_2 receptors was unaffected by augmented endogenous dopamine release (Tibbo et al., 1997).

Chronic Effects

The first case report of a patient with a history of amphetamine and thinner use revealed multifocal perfusion defects with ^{123}IMP SPECT (Ohta et al., 1992). Kao et al. (1994) performed a more systematic study of amphetamine abusers, whose drug use ranged from 1 mo to several years. This ^{99m}Tc-HMPAO SPECT study documented small multifocal perfusion defects in 95% of subjects, although the degree of abnormality did not correlate with amount or duration of drug abuse or with the severity of neuropsychological abnormalities (Kao et al., 1994).

Methamphetamine

Methamphetamine abuse has increased dramatically in recent years and is nearly epidemic in certain regions of the United States, yet few human functional imaging studies involving this drug have been performed. Iyo et al. used [^{11}C]methylspiperone and PET to determine that an imbalance between striatal dopamine receptors and frontal serotonin receptors may underlie methamphetamine-induced psychosis (Iyo et al., 1993). McCann et al. (1998b) used PET and the selective cocaine congener [^{11}C]WIN-35,428 (also known as [^{11}C]CFT) to determine striatal DAT density in long-term abstinent (average 3 yr) methamphetamine abusers. Compared to younger controls, these former abusers had striatal DAT density reductions of ~25%. Although this reduction was less than that seen in older patients with Parkinson's disease (50–70% reduction), the validity of these comparisons is questionable since the groups were not age-matched (McCann et al., 1998b). Similar studies performed in baboons suggest that such DAT loss may occur after a limited exposure to methamphetamine in doses typical of a recreational human user, and that the effects may be dose-related (Villemagne et al., 1998). Finally, using ^{99m}Tc-HMPAO SPECT, Iyo et al. (1997) found multifocal perfusion defects in 66% of methamphetamine abusers, detected even after relatively long periods of abstinence.

Methylphenidate

Cerebral Blood Flow and Metabolism

Wang et al. used [^{15}O]H_2O PET to study the effect of intravenous methylphenidate (0.5 mg/kg) on CBF in healthy men. They found a 20–25% reduction in whole brain CBF at 5–30 min following administration, with little regional variation, which they attributed to a direct vascular effect of the drug (Wang et al., 1994). Volkow et al. (1997b) used [^{18}F]FDG and [^{11}C]raclopride PET to evaluate both metabolic response and dopamine release (by measuring D_2 receptor availability) following methylphenidate administration in healthy subjects. They found increased absolute and relative rCMRglc in cerebellum and decreased relative rCMRglc in the basal ganglia following methylphenidate, with a variable response in other brain regions. Moreover, they found that frontal, temporal, and cerebellar metabolic changes correlated with D_2 receptor availability (Volkow et al., 1997b). Further investigation has established that the metabolic response to methylphenidate is dependent upon whether single or multiple doses are administered (Volkow et al., 1998c).

Receptor Studies

Volkow and colleagues (1995a) also compared striatal methylphenidate and cocaine binding sites in healthy men using [^{11}C]methylphenidate PET. They found [^{11}C]methylphenidate binding sites to be similar to those of cocaine, maximal in the striatum, and competitive. However, there was marked difference with regard to pharmacokinetics: methylphenidate clearance (90 min) was significantly slower than cocaine (20 min). Furthermore, while the high of both drugs paralleled their rapid uptake in the striatum, the rapid decline in high with both drugs paralleled cocaine's clearance from brain but not methylphenidate's (Volkow et al., 1995a). While rapid clearance may be a factor in the abuse liability of cocaine and may promote frequent self-administration, slow clearance with methylphenidate may underlie its relatively safe profile. A subsequent study by this group found selective [^{11}C]methylphenidate uptake in the basal ganglia and that physiological changes as well as a feeling of "restlessness" closely paralleled methylphenidate's brain pharmacokinetics, while "high" and "anxiety" followed a shorter time course (Volkow et al., 1996f).

The dopaminergic system is of considerable interest when considering methylphenidate. Booij et al. (1997) used the dopamine D_2 receptor radioligand [^{123}I]IBZM and SPECT to demonstrate methylphenidate-induced dopamine release in the striatum. Volkow and colleagues at the Brookhaven National Laboratory have performed the balance of the work in this area. Initially, they examined the relationship between DAT occupancy or blockade and euphoria in studies using [^{11}C]methylphenidate and PET in studies with normal subjects given sequential intravenous doses of methylphenidate. They found 80% residual DAT occupancy 60 min after initial methylphenidate administration, despite significant attenuation in "high." Furthermore, despite continued DAT occupancy, a second methylphenidate dose could produce a "high" similar to that produced by the initial dose, thus indicating that DAT blockade is not in and of itself sufficient for euphoria (Volkow et al., 1996c). Subsequently, this group used tracer doses of [^{11}C]cocaine and PET to evaluate DAT binding following various doses of oral methylphenidate administration in control subjects. They found a dose-related response, with a dose of 0.25 mg/kg (17.5 mg in a 70 kg person) producing blockade of 50% (ED_{50}) of DAT 2 h after administration (Volkow et al., 1998a). They also evaluated uptake of oral [^{11}C]methylphenidate in baboon brain with PET, finding peak brain concentration 60 min following administration (Volkow et al., 1998a). Similar studies have not been performed in humans. Yet, while methylphenidate clearly blocks striatal DAT sites, the relationship of this blockade to drug-induced euphoria is less clear. More recently, Volkow et al. (1999a) performed [^{11}C]cocaine PET studies of DAT binding following intravenous methylphenidate administration in control subjects and found the ED_{50} to be 0.075 mg/kg. They also found that while DAT binding was significantly correlated with self reports of "high," half of the subjects did not report a "high" despite significant DAT blockade (Volkow et al., 1999a). Therefore they concluded that DAT blockade might be necessary but not sufficient to produce the behavioral effects associated with methylphenidate.

Solvents ("Thinners") and Toluene

Functional studies in solvent and toluene exposure are somewhat confounded by the fact that these subjects often exhibit considerable structural brain abnormalities, such as atrophy, white matter and thalamic lesions (Rosenberg et al., 1988; Hirai and Ikeuchi, 1993). Ohta et al. (1992) reported multifocal perfusion defects seen with [^{123}I]IMP SPECT in a patient with a history of thinner exposure, although the case is confounded by the subject's abuse of amphetamine. Another case report details diffuse reduction in absolute CBF and oxygen metabolism, particularly in the hippocampi, in a man with a history of toluene abuse (Terashi et al., 1997). Ryu et al. report a case of toluene abuse in which no structural abnormalities were noted on MRI, but with multifocal perfusion abnormalities noted on a ^{99m}Tc-ECD SPECT study (Ryu et al., 1998).

In a controlled study, Arlien-Soborg and colleagues used the ^{133}Xe inhalation method to evaluate CBF in house painters exposed to organic solvents for an average of 22 yr. They found CBF reduced by ~20%, as well as mild to moderate intellectual impairment, in house painters as compared to controls (Arlien-Soborg et al., 1982). However, it is unclear whether the intellectual differences predated the solvent exposure. Maximilian et al. also used the ^{133}Xe inhalation method to evaluate CBF in industrial workers with a mean exposure to organic solvents of 24.5 yr, with no control group. Although baseline CBF was reduced ~17% from the expected value in controls, when controlled for age, no clear effect of exposure was seen. However, matched for age, more heavily exposed workers had reduced frontal activation in response to a cognitive task (Maximilian et al., 1982).

Risberg and Hagstadius (1983) used the ^{133}Xe inhalation method in paint-factory workers with long-term exposure to organic solvents, with age-matched sugar-refinery workers serving as controls. Minor, dose-related reductions in CBF were seen at baseline, but the exposed group had a somewhat augmented CBF response to a cognitive task (Risberg and Hagstadius, 1983). Hagstadius et al. (1989) used the ^{133}Xe inhalation method to compare resting CBF in patients with chronic solvent exposure with and without encephalopathy, and in normal controls. They found mildly reduced CBF in encephalopathic as compared to nonencephalopathic exposed patients, and as compared to controls, most significantly in the frontotemporal areas. At 2–7 yr follow-up, most CBF differences had resolved (Hagstadius et al., 1989).

More recently, Edling and coworkers have used [^{11}C]*l*-DOPA and [^{11}C]nomifensine with PET to evaluate in vivo dopamine synthesis activity and to estimate the number of presynaptic terminals, respectively, following short-term toluene exposure in healthy volunteers. They found that 15 min of 100 ppm toluene exposure had no effect on these measures (Edling et al., 1997b). This group also performed a similar study looking at the long-term effects of organic solvent exposure in a group of patients with chronic exposure and concurrent neuropsychiatric deficits. After controlling for age, they found minimally increased dopamine synthesis in subjects with long-term organic solvent exposure as compared to controls, and no significant differences in presynaptic terminals or postsynaptic dopamine receptors (Edling et al., 1997a).

Conclusions

The above is a summary of the major emission tomographic studies involving abused substances in man. An attempt has been made to present both the strengths and the weaknesses of these methods, but several general comments merit consideration.

First of all, emission tomographic studies are often subject to design and analysis considerations, and subtle technical differences can lead to dramatically different results. As these techniques continue to evolve, it is not always possible to compare findings across or even among specific methods. It is beyond the scope of this review to discuss the merits and pitfalls of each study and each procedure. As such, these studies are best considered on their own, while only broad conclusions can be drawn from the literature as a whole.

A number of additional limitations pertain to human studies of substance abuse, including dependence upon self-reported drug use histories, the reliability of which vary considerably. Furthermore, many studies purporting to address the effects of a single substance are likely confounded by polysubstance abuse, which is the rule rather than the exception. In addition, substance abuse is often associated with comorbid psychiatric disease. As we learn more about the neurobiology of psychiatric disorders, the relative influence of these conditions on functional neuroimaging findings is becoming increasingly clear.

Finally, as is often true in clinical research, the respective roles of cause and effect are not easily discriminated in the area of substance abuse. Whether differences in CBF, metabolism, or receptor activity and function are a result of substance abuse, or represent its cause, remains at the scientific heart of these investigations. As study design becomes more inventive, and as study control and execution become more rigorous, it will be easier to address such questions. Such work represents the future and the promise of investigation in this challenging field.

Acknowledgment

This work was supported, in part, by a grant from the National Institute on Drug Abuse (DA00297). The author gratefully acknowledges the editorial assistance of Jonathan F. Fox.

References

Abi-Dargham, A., Gil, R., Krystal, J., Baldwin, R. M., Seibyl, J. P., Bowers, M., van Dyck, C. H., Charney, D. S., Innis, R. B. and Laruelle, M., Increased striatal dopamine transmission in schizophrenia: confirmation in a second cohort. Am. J. Psychiatry 155:761–767, 1998a.

Abi-Dargham, A., Krystal, J., Anjilvel, S., Scanley, B. E., Zoghbi, S., Baldwin, R. M., Rajeevan, N., Ellis, S., Petrakis, I. L., Seibyl, J. P., Charney, D. S., Laruelle, M. and Innis, R. B., Alterations of benzodiazepine receptors in type II alcoholic subjects measured with SPECT and [^{123}I]iomazenil. Am. J. Psychiatry 155:1550–1555, 1998b.

Adams, K. M., Gilman, S., Koeppe, R. A., Kluin, K. J., Brunberg, J. A., Dede, D., Berent, S. and Kroll, P. D., Neuropsychological deficits are correlated with frontal hypometabolism in positron emission tomography studies of older alcoholic patients. Alcohol. Clin. Exp. Res. 17:205–210, 1993.

Adams, K. M., Gilman, S., Johnson-Greene, D., Koeppe, R. A., Junck, L., Kluin, K. J., Martorello, S., Johnson, M. J., Heumann, M. and Hill, E., The significance of family history status in relation to neuropsychological test performance and cerebral glucose metabolism studied with positron emission tomography in older alcoholic patients. Alcohol. Clin. Exp. Res. 22:105–110, 1998.

Adler, L. J., Gyulai, F. E., Diehl, D. J., Mintun, M. A., Winter, P. M. and Firestone, L. L., Regional brain activity changes associated with fentanyl analgesia elucidated by positron emission tomography. Anesth. Analg. 84:120–126, 1997.

Arlien-Soborg, P., Henriksen, L., Gade, A., Gyldensted, C. and Paulson, O. B., Cerebral blood flow in chronic toxic encephalopathy in house painters exposed to organic solvents. Acta Neurol. Scand. 66:34–41, 1982.

Battey, L. L., Heyman, A. and Patterson, J. L., Effects of ethyl alcohol on cerebral blood flow and metabolism. JAMA 152:6–10, 1953.
Baxter, L. R., Jr., Schwartz, J. M., Phelps, M. E., Mazziotta, J. C., Barrio, J., Rawson, R. A., Engel, J., Guze, B. H., Selin, C. and Sumida, R., Localization of neurochemical effects of cocaine and other stimulants in the human brain. J. Clin. Psychiatry 49:23–26, 1988.
Benson, D. F., Djenderedjian, A., Miller, B. L., Pachana, N. A., Chang, L., Itti, L. and Mena, I., Neural basis of confabulation. Neurology 46:1239–1243, 1996.
Berglund, M. and Risberg, J., Regional cerebral blood flow in a case of amphetamine intoxication. Psychopharmacology (Berl.) 70:219–221, 1980.
Berglund, M. and Risberg, J., Regional cerebral blood flow during alcohol withdrawal. Arch. Gen. Psychiatry 38:351–355, 1981.
Berglund, M., Hagstadius, S., Risberg, J., Johanson, T. M., Bliding, A. and Mubrin, Z., Normalization of regional cerebral blood flow in alcoholics during the first 7 weeks of abstinence. Acta Psychiatr. Scand. 75:202–208, 1987.
Berglund, M., Prohovnik, I. and Risberg, J., Regional cerebral blood flow during alcoholic blackout. Psychiatry Res. 27:49–54, 1989.
Bergstrom, K. A., Jolkkonen, J., Kuikka, J. T., Akerman, K. K., Viinamaki, H., Airaksinen, O., Lansimies, E. and Tiihonen, J., Fentanyl decreases β-CIT binding to the dopamine transporter. Synapse 29:413–415, 1998.
Boecker, H., Wills, A. J., Ceballos-Baumann, A., Samuel, M., Thompson, P. D., Findley, L. J. and Brooks, D. J., The effect of ethanol on alcohol-responsive essential tremor: a positron emission tomography study. Ann. Neurol. 39:650–658, 1996.
Booij, J., Korn, P., Linszen, D. H. and van Royen, E. A., Assessment of endogenous dopamine release by methylphenidate challenge using iodine-123 iodobenzamide single-photon emission tomography. Eur. J. Nucl. Med. 24:674–677, 1997.
Breier, A., Malhotra, A. K., Pinals, D. A., Weisenfeld, N. I. and Pickar, D., Association of ketamine-induced psychosis with focal activation of the prefrontal cortex in healthy volunteers. Am. J. Psychiatry 154:805–811, 1997a.
Breier, A., Su, T. P., Saunders, R., Carson, R. E., Kolachana, B. S., de Bartolomeis, A., Weinberger, D. R., Weisenfeld, N., Malhotra, A. K., Eckelman, W. C. and Pickar, D., Schizophrenia is associated with elevated amphetamine-induced synaptic dopamine concentrations: evidence from a novel positron emission tomography method. Proc. Natl. Acad. Sci. USA 94:2569–2574, 1997b.
Breier, A., Adler, C. M., Weisenfeld, N., Su, T. P., Elman, I., Picken, L., Malhotra, A. K. and Pickar, D., Effects of NMDA antagonism on striatal dopamine release in healthy subjects: application of a novel PET approach. Synapse 29:142–147, 1998.
Buchsbaum, M. S., Wu, J., Haier, R., Hazlett, E., Ball, R., Katz, M., Sokolski, K., Lagunas-Solar, M. and Langer, D., Positron emission tomography assessment of effects of benzodiazepines on regional glucose metabolic rate in patients with anxiety disorder. Life Sci. 40:2393–2400, 1987.
Caspari, D., Trabert, W., Heinz, G., Lion, N., Henkes, H. and Huber, G., The pattern of regional cerebral blood flow during alcohol withdrawal: a single photon emission tomography study with ^{99m}Tc-HMPAO. Acta Psychiatr. Scand. 87:414–417, 1993.
Childress, A. R., Mozley, P. D., McElgin, W., Fitzgerald, J., Reivich, M. and O'Brien, C. P., Limbic activation during cue-induced cocaine craving. Am. J. Psychiatry 156:11–18, 1999.
Danos, P., Kasper, S., Grunwald, F., Klemm, E., Krappel, C., Broich, K., Hoflich, G., Overbeck, B., Biersack, H. J. and Moller, H. J., Pathological regional cerebral blood flow in opiate-dependent patients during withdrawal: a HMPAO-SPECT study. Neuropsychobiology 37:194–199, 1998.
Dao-Castellana, M. H., Samson, Y., Legault, F., Martinot, J. L., Aubin, H. J., Crouzel, C., Feldman, L., Barrucand, D., Rancurel, G., Feline, A. and Syrota, A., Frontal dysfunction

in neurologically normal chronic alcoholic subjects: metabolic and neuropsychological findings. Psychol. Med. 28:1039–1048, 1998.

de Wit, H., Metz, J., Wagner, N. and Cooper, M., Behavioral and subjective effects of ethanol: relationship to cerebral metabolism using PET. Alcohol. Clin. Exp. Res. 14:482–489, 1990.

de Wit, H., Metz, J., Wagner, N. and Cooper, M., Effects of diazepam on cerebral metabolism and mood in normal volunteers. Neuropsychopharmacology 5:33–41, 1991.

Dupont, R. M., Rourke, S. B., Grant, I., Lehr, P. P., Reed, R. J., Challakere, K., Lamoureux, G. and Halpern, S., Single photon emission computed tomography with iodoamphetamine-123 and neuropsychological studies in long-term abstinent alcoholics. Psychiatry Res. 67:99–111, 1996.

Edling, C., Hellman, B., Arvidson, B., Andersson, J., Hartvig, P., Lilja, A., Valind, S. and Langstrom, B., Do organic solvents induce changes in the dopaminergic system? Positron emission tomography studies of occupationally exposed subjects. Int. Arch. Occup. Environ. Health 70:180–186, 1997a.

Edling, C., Hellman, B., Arvidson, B., Johansson, G., Andersson, J., Hartvig, P., Valind, S. and Langstrom, B., Positron emission tomography studies of healthy volunteers: no effects on the dopamine terminals and synthesis after short-term exposure to toluene. Hum. Exp. Toxicol. 16:171–176, 1997b.

Erbas, B., Bekdik, C., Erbengi, G., Enunlu, T., Aytac, S., Kumbasar, H. and Dogan, Y., Regional cerebral blood flow changes in chronic alcoholism using Tc-99m HMPAO SPECT: comparison with CT parameters. Clin. Nucl. Med. 17:123–127, 1992.

Ernst, M., Zametkin, A. J., Matochik, J., Schmidt, M., Jons, P. H., Liebenauer, L. L., Hardy, K. K. and Cohen, R. M., Intravenous dextroamphetamine and brain glucose metabolism. Neuropsychopharmacology 17:391–401, 1997.

Farde, L., Pauli, S., Litton, J. E., Halldin, C., Neiman, J. and Sedvall, G., PET-determination of benzodiazepine receptor binding in studies on alcoholism. EXS 71:143–153, 1994.

Firestone, L. L., Gyulai, F., Mintun, M., Adler, L. J., Urso, K. and Winter, P. M., Human brain activity response to fentanyl imaged by positron emission tomography. Anesth. Analg. 82:1247–1251, 1996.

Forster, A., Juge, O. and Morel, D., Effects of midazolam on cerebral hemodynamics and cerebral vasomotor responsiveness to carbon dioxide. J. Cereb. Blood Flow Metab. 3:246–249, 1983.

Fowler, J. S., Volkow, N. D., Wolf, A. P., Dewey, S. L., Schlyer, D. J., Macgregor, R. R., Hitzemann, R., Logan, J., Bendriem, B., Gatley, S. J. and Christman, D., Mapping cocaine binding sites in human and baboon brain in vivo. Synapse 4:371–377, 1989.

Fowler, J. S., Volkow, N. D., Logan, J., MacGregor, R. R., Wang, G. J. and Wolf, A. P., Alcohol intoxication does not change [^{11}C]cocaine pharmacokinetics in human brain and heart. Synapse 12:228–235, 1992.

Gatley, S. J. and Volkow, N. D., Addiction and imaging of the living human brain. Drug Alcohol Depend. 51:97–108, 1998.

Gerra, G., Calbiani, B., Zaimovic, A., Sartori, R., Ugolotti, G., Ippolito, L., Delsignore, R., Rustichelli, P. and Fontanesi, B., Regional cerebral blood flow and comorbid diagnosis in abstinent opioid addicts. Psychiatry Res. 83:117–126, 1998.

Gilman, S., Adams, K., Koeppe, R. A., Berent, S., Kluin, K. J., Modell, J. G., Kroll, P. and Brunberg, J. A., Cerebellar and frontal hypometabolism in alcoholic cerebellar degeneration studied with positron emission tomography. Ann. Neurol. 28:775–785, 1990.

Gilman, S., Adams, K. M., Johnson-Greene, D., Koeppe, R. A., Junck, L., Kluin, K. J., Martorello, S., Heumann, M. and Hill, E., Effects of disulfiram on positron emission tomography and neuropsychological studies in severe chronic alcoholism. Alcohol. Clin. Exp. Res. 20:1456–1461, 1996a.

Gilman, S., Koeppe, R. A., Adams, K., Johnson-Greene, D., Junck, L., Kluin, K. J., Brunberg, J., Martorello, S. and Lohman, M., Positron emission tomographic studies of cerebral benzodiazepine-receptor binding in chronic alcoholics. Ann. Neurol. 40:163–171, 1996b.

Gilman, S., Koeppe, R. A., Adams, K. M., Junck, L., Kluin, K. J., Johnson-Greene, D., Martorello, S., Heumann, M. and Bandekar, R., Decreased striatal monoaminergic terminals in severe chronic alcoholism demonstrated with (+)[^{11}C]dihydrotetrabenazine and positron emission tomography. Ann. Neurol. 44:326–333, 1998.

Gottschalk, P. C. H., Van Heertum, R. L., Perera, G. M., Pozniakoff, T. A., Moeller, J. R., Young, W. L., Volkow, N. D., Foltin, R. W. and Fischman, M. W., Cerebral blood flow response to IV cocaine in humans: quantitative xenon-133-SPECT studies [abstract]. Coll. Probl. Drug Depend. 174:117, 1997.

Grant, S., London, E. D., Newlin, D. B., Villemagne, V. L., Liu, X., Contoreggi, C., Phillips, R. L., Kimes, A. S. and Margolin, A., Activation of memory circuits during cue-elicited cocaine craving. Proc. Natl. Acad. Sci. USA 93:12040–12045, 1996.

Gunther, W., Muller, N., Knesewitsch, P., Haag, C., Trapp, W., Banquet, J. P., Stieg, C. and Alper, K. R., Functional EEG mapping and SPECT in detoxified male alcoholics. Eur. Arch. Psychiatry Clin. Neurosci. 247:128–136, 1997.

Hagstadius, S., Orbaek, P., Risberg, J. and Lindgren, M., Regional cerebral blood flow at the time of diagnosis of chronic toxic encephalopathy induced by organic-solvent exposure and after the cessation of exposure. Scand. J. Work Environ. Health 15:130–135, 1989.

Hartvig, P., Valtysson, J., Lindner, K. J., Kristensen, J., Karlsten, R., Gustafsson, L. L., Persson, J., Svensson, J. O., Oye, I., Antoni, G., Westerberg, G. and Långstrom, B., Central nervous system effects of subdissociative doses of (S)-ketamine are related to plasma and brain concentrations measured with positron emission tomography in healthy volunteers. Clin. Pharmacol. Ther. 58:165–173, 1995.

Hearn, W. L., Flynn, D. D., Hime, G. W., Rose, S., Cofino, J. C., Mantero-Atienze, E., Wetli, C. V. and Mash, D. C., Cocaethylene: a unique cocaine metabolite displays high affinity for the dopamine transporter. J. Neurochem. 56:698–701, 1991.

Heinz, A., Ragan, P., Jones, D. W., Hommer, D., Williams, W., Knable, M. B., Gorey, J. G., Doty, L., Geyer, C., Lee, K. S., Coppola, R., Weinberger, D. R. and Linnoila, M., Reduced central serotonin transporters in alcoholism. Am. J. Psychiatry 155:1544–1549, 1998.

Hemmingsen, R., Vorstrup, S., Clemmesen, L., Holm, S., Tfelt-Hansen, P., Sorensen, A. S., Hansen, C., Sommer, W. and Bolwig, T. G., Cerebral blood flow during delirium tremens and related clinical states studied with xenon-133 inhalation tomography. Am. J. Psychiatry 145:1384–1390, 1988.

Hermle, L., Funfgeld, M., Oepen, G., Botsch, H., Borchardt, D., Gouzoulis, E., Fehrenbach, R. A. and Spitzer, M., Mescaline-induced psychopathological, neuropsychological, and neurometabolic effects in normal subjects: experimental psychosis as a tool for psychiatric research. Biol. Psychiatry 32:976–991, 1992.

Hietala, J., West, C., Syvalahti, E., Nagren, K., Lehikoinen, P., Sonninen, P. and Ruotsalainen, U., Striatal D_2 dopamine receptor binding characteristics in vivo in patients with alcohol dependence. Psychopharmacology (Berl.) 116:285–290, 1994.

Hine, C. H., Shick, A. F., Margolis, L., Burbridge, T. N. and Simon, A., Effects of alcohol in small doses and tetraethylthiuramdisulphide (Antabuse) on cerebral blood flow and cerebral metabolism. J. Pharmacol. Exp. Ther. 106:253–260, 1952.

Hirai, H. and Ikeuchi, Y. MRI of chronic toluene intoxication. Rinsho Shinkeigaku 33:552–555, 1993.

Holman, B. L., Carvalho, P. A., Mendelson, J., Teoh, S. K., Nardin, R., Hallgring, E., Hebben, N. and Johnson, K. A., Brain perfusion is abnormal in cocaine-dependent polydrug users: a study using technetium-99m-HMPAO and ASPECT. J. Nucl. Med. 32:1206–1210, 1991.

Holman, B. L., Garada, B., Johnson, K. A., Mendelson, J. H., Hallgring, E., Teoh, S. K., Worth, J. and Navia, B., A comparison of brain perfusion SPECT in cocaine abuse and AIDS dementia complex. J. Nucl. Med. 33:1312–1315, 1992.

Holman, B. L., Mendelson, J., Garada, B., Teoh, S. K., Hallgring, E., Johnson, K. A. and Mello, N. K., Regional cerebral blood flow improves with treatment in chronic cocaine polydrug users. J. Nucl. Med. 34:723–727, 1993.

Hommer, D., Andreasen, P., Rio, D., Williams, W., Ruttimann, U., Momenan, R., Zametkin, A., Rawlings, R. and Linnoila, M., Effects of m-chlorophenylpiperazine on regional brain glucose utilization: a positron emission tomographic comparison of alcoholic and control subjects. J. Neurosci. 17:2796–2806, 1997.

Humbert, T., De Guilhermier, P., Maktouf, C., Grasset, G., Lopez, F. M. and Chabrand, P., Marchiafava-Bignami disease. A case studied by structural and functional brain imaging. Eur. Arch. Psychiatry Clin. Neurosci. 242:69–71, 1992.

Hunter, R., McLuskie, R., Wyper, D., Patterson, J., Christie, J. E., Brooks, D. N., McCulloch, J., Fink, G. and Goodwin, G. M., The pattern of function-related regional cerebral blood flow investigated by single photon emission tomography with ^{99m}Tc-HMPAO in patients with presenile Alzheimer's disease and Korsakoff's psychosis. Psychol. Med. 19:847–855, 1989.

Ishikawa, Y., Meyer, J. S., Tanahashi, N., Hata, T., Velez, M., Fann, W. E., Kandula, P., Motel, K. F. and Rogers, R. L., Abstinence improves cerebral perfusion and brain volume in alcoholic neurotoxicity without Wernicke-Korsakoff syndrome. J. Cereb. Blood Flow Metab. 6:86–94, 1986.

Iyo, M., Nishio, M., Itoh, T., Fukuda, H., Suzuki, K., Yamasaki, T., Fukui, S. and Tateno, Y., Dopamine D_2 and serotonin S_2 receptors in susceptibility to methamphetamine psychosis detected by positron emission tomography. Psychiatry Res. 50:217–231, 1993.

Iyo, M., Namba, H., Yanagisawa, M., Hirai, S., Yui, N. and Fukui, S., Abnormal cerebral perfusion in chronic methamphetamine abusers: a study using 99MTc-HMPAO and SPECT. Prog. Neuropsychopharmacol. Biol. Psychiatry 21:789–796, 1997.

Johannesson, G., Berglund, M. and Ingvar, D. H., Reduction of blood flow in cerebral white matter in alcoholics related to hepatic function. Acta Neurol. Scand. 65:190–202, 1982.

Johnson, B., Barron, B., Fang, B., Lamki, L., Wagner, L., Wells, L., Kenny, P., Overton, D., Dhother, S., Abramson, D., Chen, R. and Kramer, L., Isradipine prevents global and regional cocaine-induced changes in brain blood flow: a preliminary study. Psychopharmacology (Berl.) 136:335–341, 1998a.

Johnson, B., Lamki, L., Fang, B., Barron, B., Wagner, L., Wells, L., Kenny, P., Overton, D., Dhother, S., Abramson, D., Chen, R. and Kramer, L., Demonstration of dose-dependent global and regional cocaine-induced reductions in brain blood flow using a novel approach to quantitative single photon emission computerized tomography. Neuropsychopharmacology 18:377–384, 1998b.

Johnson-Greene, D., Adams, K. M., Gilman, S., Koeppe, R. A., Junck, L., Kluin, K. J., Martorello, S. and Heumann, M., Effects of abstinence and relapse upon neuropsychological function and cerebral glucose metabolism in severe chronic alcoholism. J. Clin. Exp. Neuropsychol. 19:378–385, 1997.

Joyce, E. M., Rio, D. E., Ruttimann, U. E., Rohrbaugh, J. W., Martin, P. R., Rawlings, R. R. and Eckardt, M. J., Decreased cingulate and precuneate glucose utilization in alcoholic Korsakoff's syndrome. Psychiatry Res. 54:225–239, 1994.

Kahn, D. A., Prohovnik, I., Lucas, L. R. and Sackeim, H. A., Dissociated effects of amphetamine on arousal and cortical blood flow in humans. Biol. Psychiatry 25:755–767, 1989.

Kao, C. H., Wang, S. J. and Yeh, S. H., Presentation of regional cerebral blood flow in amphetamine abusers by 99Tcm-HMPAO brain SPECT. Nucl. Med. Commun. 15:94–98, 1994.

Konkol, R. J., Tikofsky, R. S., Wells, R., Hellman, R. S., Nemeth, P., Walsh, D. J., Heimler, R. and Sty, J. R., Normal high-resolution cerebral ^{99m}Tc-HMPAO SPECT scans in symptomatic neonates exposed to cocaine. J. Child Neurol. 9:278–283, 1994.

Kosten, T. R., Cheeves, C., Palumbo, J., Seibyl, J. P., Price, L. H. and Woods, S. W., Regional cerebral blood flow during acute and chronic abstinence from combined cocaine-alcohol abuse. Drug Alcohol Depend. 50:187–195, 1998.

Krystal, J. H., Woods, S. W., Kosten, T. R., Rosen, M. I., Seibyl, J. P., van Dyck, C. C., Price, L. H., Zubal, I. G., Hoffer, P. B. and Charney, D. S., Opiate dependence and withdrawal: preliminary assessment using single photon emission computerized tomography (SPECT). Am. J. Drug Alcohol Abuse 21:47–63, 1995.

Laruelle, M., Abi-Dargham, A., van Dyck, C. H., Rosenblatt, W., Zea-Ponce, Y., Zoghbi, S. S., Baldwin, R. M., Charney, D. S., Hoffer, P. B., Kung, H. F. and Innis, R. B., SPECT imaging of striatal dopamine release after amphetamine challenge. J. Nucl. Med. 36:1182–1190, 1995.

Laruelle, M., Abi-Dargham, A., van Dyck, C. H., Gil, R., D'Souza, C. D., Erdos, J., McCance, E., Rosenblatt, W., Fingado, C., Zoghbi, S. S., Baldwin, R. M., Seibyl, J. P., Krystal, J. H., Charney, D. S. and Innis, R. B., Single photon emission computerized tomography imaging of amphetamine-induced dopamine release in drug-free schizophrenic subjects. Proc. Natl. Acad. Sci. USA 93:9235–9240, 1996.

Levin, J. M., Holman, B. L., Mendelson, J. H., Teoh, S. K., Garada, B., Johnson, K. A. and Springer, S., Gender differences in cerebral perfusion in cocaine abuse: ^{99m}Tc-HMPAO SPECT study of drug abusing women. J. Nucl. Med. 35:1902–1909, 1994.

Levin, J. M. and Kaufman, M. J., Functional studies in substance abuse: imaging and beyond. J. Nucl. Med. 36:1298–1300, 1995a.

Levin, J. M., Mendelson, J. H., Holman, B. L., Teoh, S. K., Garada, B., Schwartz, R. B. and Mello, N. K., Improved regional cerebral blood flow in chronic cocaine polydrug users treated with buprenorphine. J. Nucl. Med. 36:1211–1215, 1995b.

Liu, X., Vaupel, D. B., Gran, S. and London, E. D., Effect of cocaine-related environmental stimuli on the spontaneous electroencephalogram in polydrug abusers. Neuropsychopharmacology 19:10–17, 1998.

Lockwood, A. H., Murphy, B. W., Donnelly, K. Z., Mahl, T. C. and Perini, S., Positron-emission tomographic localization of abnormalities of brain metabolism in patients with minimal hepatic encephalopathy. Hepatology 18:1061–1068, 1993.

Logan, J., Volkow, N. D., Fowler, J. S., Wang, G. J., Fischman, M. W., Foltin, R. W., Abumrad, N. N., Vitkun, S., Gatley, S. J., Pappas, N., Hitzemann, R. and Shea, C. E., Concentration and occupancy of dopamine transporters in cocaine abusers with [^{11}C]cocaine and PET. Synapse 27:347–356, 1997.

London, E. D., Imaging Drug Action in the Brain. Boca Raton, FL: CRC Press, 1993.

London, E. D., Broussolle, E. P., Links, J. M., Wong, D. F., Cascella, N. G., Dannals, R. F., Sano, M., Herning, R., Snyder, F. R., Rippetoe, L. R., Toung, T. J. K., Jaffe, J. H. and Wagner, H. N. Jr., Morphine-induced metabolic changes in human brain; studies with positron emission tomography and [fluorine 18]fluorodeoxyglucose. Arch. Gen. Psychiatry 47:73–81, 1990a.

London, E. D., Cascella, N. G., Wong, D. F., Phillips, R. L., Dannals, R. F., Links, J. M., Herning, R., Grayson, R., Jaffe, J. H. and Wagner, H. N. Jr., Cocaine-induced reduction of glucose utilization in human brain: a study using positron emission tomography and [fluorine 18]-fluorodeoxyglucose. Arch. Gen. Psychiatry 47:567–574, 1990b.

Lyons, D., Friedman, D. P., Nader, M. A. and Porrino, L. J., Cocaine alters cerebral metabolism within the ventral striatum and limbic cortex of monkeys. J. Neurosci. 16:1230–1238, 1996.

Malison, R. T., Best, S. E., Wallace, E. A., McCance, E., Laruelle, M., Zoghbi, S. S., Baldwin, R. M., Seibyl, J. S., Hoffer, P. B., Price, L. H., Kosten, T. R. and Innis, R. B., Euphorigenic doses of cocaine reduce [^{123}I]β-CIT SPECT measures of dopamine transporter availability in human cocaine addicts. Psychopharmacology (Berl.) 122:358–362, 1995.

Malison, R. T., Best, S. E., van Dyck, C. H., McCance, E. F., Wallace, E. A., Laruelle, M., Baldwin, R. M., Seibyl, J. P., Price, L. H., Kosten, T. R. and Innis, R. B., Elevated striatal dopamine transporters during acute cocaine abstinence as measured by [^{123}I]β-CIT SPECT. Am. J. Psychiatry 155:832-834, 1998a.

Malison, R. T., McCance, E., Carpenter, L. L., Baldwin, R. M., Seibyl, J. P., Price, L. H., Kosten, T. R. and Innis, R. B., [^{123}I]β-CIT SPECT imaging of dopamine transporter availability after mazindol administration in human cocaine addicts. Psychopharmacology (Berl.) 137:321–325, 1998b.

Mampunza, S., Verbanck, P., Verhas, M., Martin, P., Paternot, J., LeBon, O., Kornreich, C., Den Bulk, A. and Pelc, I., Cerebral blood flow in just detoxified alcohol dependent patients: a 99m Tc-HMPAO-SPECT study. Acta Neurol. Belg. 95:164–169, 1995.

Martin, P. R., Rio, D., Adinoff, B., Johnson, J. L., Bisserbe, J. C., Rawlings, R. R., Rohrbaugh, J. W., Stapleton, J. M. and Eckardt, M. J., Regional cerebral glucose utilization in chronic organic mental disorders associated with alcoholism. J. Neuropsychiatry Clin. Neurosci. 4:159–167, 1992.

Mathew, R. J. and Wilson, W. H., Dextroamphetamine-induced changes in regional cerebral blood flow. Psychopharmacology (Berl.) 87:298–302, 1985.

Mathew, R. J. and Wilson, W. H., Regional cerebral blood flow changes associated with ethanol intoxication. Stroke 17:1156–1159, 1986.

Mathew, R. J. and Wilson, W. H., Changes in cerebral blood flow and mental state after amphetamine challenge in schizophrenic patients. Neuropsychobiology 21:117–123, 1989.

Mathew, R. J. and Wilson, W. H., Substance abuse and cerebral blood flow. Am. J. Psychiatry 148:292–305, 1991.

Mathew, R. J., Wilson, W. H. and Daniel, D. G., The effect of nonsedating doses of diazepam on regional cerebral blood flow. Biol. Psychiatry 20:1109–1116, 1985.

Mathew, R. J., Tant, S. and Burger, C., Regional cerebral blood flow in marijuana smokers. Br. J. Addict. 81:567–571, 1986.

Mathew, R. J., Wilson, W. H. and Tant, S. R., Acute changes in cerebral blood flow associated with marijuana smoking. Acta Psychiatr. Scand. 79:118–128, 1989.

Mathew, R. J., Wilson, W. H., Lowe, J. V. and Humphries, D., Acute changes in cranial blood flow after cocaine hydrochloride. Biol. Psychiatry 40:609–616, 1996.

Mathew, R. J., Wilson, W. H., Coleman, R. E., Turkington, T. G. and DeGrado, T. R., Marijuana intoxication and brain activation in marijuana smokers. Life Sci. 60:2075–2089, 1997.

Mathew, R. J., Wilson, W. H., Turkington, T. G. and Coleman, R. E., Cerebellar activity and disturbed time sense after THC. Brain Res. 797:183–189, 1998.

Matsuda, K., Yamaji, S., Ishii, K., Sasaki, M., Sakamoto, S., Kitagaki, H., Imamura, T. and Mori, E., Regional cerebral blood flow and oxygen metabolism in a patient with Korsakoff syndrome. Ann. Nucl. Med. 11:33–35, 1997.

Mattay, V. S., Berman, K. F., Ostrem, J. L., Esposito, G., Van Horn, J. D., Bigelow, L. B. and Weinberger, D. R., Dextroamphetamine enhances "neural network-specific" physiological signals: a positron-emission tomography rCBF study. J. Neurosci. 16:4816–4822, 1996.

Matthew, E., Andreason, P., Pettigrew, K., Carson, R. E., Herscovitch, P., Cohen, R., King, C., Johanson, C. E., Greenblatt, D. J. and Paul, S. M., Benzodiazepine receptors mediate regional blood flow changes in the living human brain. Proc. Natl. Acad. Sci. USA 92:2775–2779, 1995.

Maximilian, V. A., Risberg, J., Prohovnik, I., Rehnstrom, S. and Haeger-Aronsen, B., Regional cerebral blood flow and verbal memory after chronic exposure to organic solvents. Brain Cogn. 1:196–205, 1982.

McCance, E. F., Price, L. H., Kosten, T. R. and Jatlow, P. I., Cocaethylene: Pharmacology, physiology, and behavioral effects in humans. J. Pharmacol. Exp. Ther. 274:215–223, 1995.
McCann, U. D., Szabo, Z., Scheffel, U., Dannals, R. F. and Ricaurte, G. A., Positron emission tomographic evidence of toxic effect of MDMA ("Ecstasy") on brain serotonin neurons in human beings. Lancet 352:1433–1437, 1998a.
McCann, U. D., Wong, D. F., Yokoi, F., Villemagne, V., Dannals, R. F. and Ricaurte, G. A., Reduced striatal dopamine transporter density in abstinent methamphetamine and methcathinone users: evidence from positron emission tomography studies with [^{11}C]WIN-35,428. J. Neurosci. 18:8417–8422, 1998b.
Melgaard, B., Henrikson, L., Ahlgren, P., Danielsen, U. T., Sorensen, H. and Paulson, O. B., Regional cerebral blood flow in chronic alcoholics measured by single photon emission computerized tomography. Acta Neurol. Scand. 82:87–93, 1990.
Meyer, J. S., Tanahashi, N., Ishikawa, Y., Hata, T., Velez, M., Fann, W. E., Kandula, P., Mortel, K. F. and Rogers, R. L., Cerebral atrophy and hypoperfusion improve during treatment of Wernicke-Korsakoff syndrome. J. Cereb. Blood Flow Metab. 5:376–385, 1985.
Miller, B. L., Mena, I., Giombetti, R., Villanueva-Meyer, J. and Djenderedjian, A. H., Neuropsychiatric effects of cocaine: SPECT measurements. J. Addict. Dis. 11:47–58, 1992.
Modell, J. G. and Mountz, J. M., Focal cerebral blood flow change during craving for alcohol measured by SPECT. J. Neuropsychiatry Clin. Neurosci. 7:15–22, 1995.
Moffoot, A., O'Carroll, R. E., Murray, C., Dougall, N., Ebmeier, K. and Goodwin, G. M., Clonidine infusion increases uptake of ^{99m}Tc-exametazime in anterior cingulate cortex in Korsakoff's psychosis. Psychol. Med. 24:53–61, 1994.
Newlin, D. B., Golden, C. J., Quaife, M. and Graber, B., Effect of alcohol ingestion on regional cerebral blood flow. Int. J. Neurosci. 17:145–150, 1982.
Nicolas, J. M., Catafau, A. M., Estruch, R., Lomena, F. J., Salamero, M., Herranz, R., Monforte, R., Cardenal, C. and Urbano-Marquez, A., Regional cerebral blood flow-SPECT in chronic alcoholism: relation to neuropsychological testing. J. Nucl. Med. 34:1452–1459, 1993.
Ohta, H., Komibuchi, T., Nishino, I., Enomoto, Y. and Miyata, M., Brain perfusion abnormalities in a thinner and amphetamine abuser detected by I-123 IMP scintigraphy. Ann. Nucl. Med. 6:273–275, 1992.
Pappata, S., Chabriat, H., Levasseur, M., Legault-Demare, F. and Baron, J. C., Marchiafava-Bignami disease with dementia: severe cerebral metabolic depression revealed by PET. J. Neural. Transm. Park. Dis. Dement. Sect. 8:131–137, 1994.
Pearlson, G. D., Jeffery, P. J., Harris, G. J., Ross, C. A., Fischman, M. W. and Camargo, E. E., Correlation of acute cocaine-induced changes in local cerebral blood flow with subjective effects. Am. J. Psychiatry 150:495–497, 1993.
Risberg, J. and Hagstadius, S., Effects on the regional cerebral blood flow of long-term exposure to organic solvents. Acta Psychiatr. Scand. Suppl. 303:92–99, 1983.
Rogers, R. L., Meyer, J. S., Shaw, T. G. and Mortel, K. F., Reductions in regional cerebral blood flow associated with chronic consumption of alcohol. J. Am. Geriatr. Soc. 31:540–543, 1983.
Rose, J. S., Branchey, M., Buydens-Branchey, L., Stapleton, J. M., Chasten, K., Werrell, A. and Maayan, M. L., Cerebral perfusion in early and late opiate withdrawal: a technetium-99m-HMPAO SPECT study. Psychiatry Res. 67:39–47, 1996.
Rosenberg, N. L., Kleinschmidt-DeMasters, B. K., Davis, K. A., Dreisbach, J. N., Hormes, J. T. and Filley, C. M., Toluene abuse causes diffuse central nervous system white matter changes. Ann. Neurol. 23:611–614, 1988.
Roy, C. S. and Sherrington, C. S., On the regulation of the blood supply of the brain. J. Physiol. 11:85–108, 1890.
Roy-Byrne, P., Fleishaker, J., Arnett, C., Dubach, M., Stewart, J., Radant, A., Veith, R. and Graham, M., Effects of acute and chronic alprazolam treatment on cerebral blood flow, memory, sedation, and plasma catecholamines. Neuropsychopharmacology 8:161–169, 1993.

Ryu, Y. H., Lee, J. D., Yoon, P. H., Jeon, P., Kim, D. I. and Shin, D. W., Cerebral perfusion impairment in a patient with toluene abuse. J. Nucl. Med. 39:632–633, 1998.

Sachs, H., Russell, J. A., Christman, D. R. and Cook, B., Alteration of regional cerebral glucose metabolic rate in non-Korsakoff chronic alcoholism. Arch. Neurol. 44:1242–1251, 1987.

Samson, Y., Baron, J.-C., Feline, A., Bories, J. and Crouzel, C., Local cerebral glucose utilisation in chronic alcoholics: a positron tomographic study. J. Neurol. Neurosurg. Psychiatry 49:1165–1170, 1986.

Sano, M., Wendt, P. E., Wirsen, A., Stenberg, G., Risberg, J. and Ingvar, D. H., Acute effects of alcohol on regional cerebral blood flow in man. J. Stud. Alcohol 54:369–375, 1993.

Schlaepfer, T. E., Pearlson, G. D., Wong, D. F., Marenco, S. and Dannals, R. F., PET study of competition between intravenous cocaine and [^{11}C]raclopride at dopamine receptors in human subjects. Am. J. Psychiatry 154:1209–1213, 1997.

Schlaepfer, T. E., Strain, E. C., Greenberg, B. D., Preston, K. L., Lancaster, E., Bigelow, G. E., Barta, P. E. and Pearlson, G. D., Site of opioid action in the human brain: mu and kappa agonists' subjective and cerebral blood flow effects. Am. J. Psychiatry 155:470–473, 1998.

Sharp, P., Gemmell, H., Cherryman, G., Besson, J., Crawford, J. and Smith, F., Application of iodine-123-labeled isopropylamphetamine imaging to the study of dementia. J. Nucl. Med. 27:761–768, 1986.

Smith, G. S., Schloesser, R., Brodie, J. D., Dewey, S. L., Logan, J., Vitkun, S. A., Simkowitz, P., Hurley, A., Cooper, T., Volkow, N. D. and Cancro, R., Glutamate modulation of dopamine measured in vivo with positron emission tomography (PET) and ^{11}C-raclopride in normal human subjects. Neuropsychopharmacology 18:18–25, 1998.

Strickland, T. L., Mena, I., Villanueva-Meyer, J., Miller, B. L., Cummings, J., Mehringer, C. M., Satz, P. and Myers, H., Cerebral perfusion and neuropsychological consequences of chronic cocaine use. J. Neuropsychiatry Clin. Neurosci. 5:419–427, 1993.

Terashi, H., Nagata, K., Satoh, Y., Hirata, Y. and Hatazawa, J., Hippocampal hypoperfusion underlying dementia due to chronic toluene intoxication. Rinsho Shinkeigaku 37:1010–1013, 1997.

Tibbo, P., Silverstone, P. H., McEwan, A. J., Scott, J., Joshua, A. and Golberg, K., A single photon emission computed tomography scan study of striatal dopamine D_2 receptor binding with ^{123}I-epidepride in patients with schizophrenia and controls. J. Psychiatry Neurosci. 22:39–45, 1997.

Tiihonen, J., Kuikka, J., Hakola, P., Paanila, J., Airaksinen, J., Eronen, M. and Hallikainen, T., Acute ethanol-induced changes in cerebral blood flow. Am. J. Psychiatry 151:1505–1508, 1994.

Tiihonen, J., Vilkman, H., Rasanen, P., Ryynanen, O. P., Hakko, H., Bergman, J., Hamalainen, T., Laakso, A., Haaparanta-Solin, M., Solin, O., Kuoppamaki, M., Syvalahti, E. and Hietala, J., Striatal presynaptic dopamine function in type 1 alcoholics measured with positron emission tomography. Mol. Psychiatry 3:156–161, 1998.

Tumeh, S. S., Nagel, J. S., English, R. J., Moore, M. and Holman, B. L., Cerebral abnormalities in cocaine abusers: demonstration by SPECT perfusion brain scintigraphy. Work in progress. Radiology 176:821–824, 1990.

Tunving, K., Thulin, S. O., Risberg, J. and Warkentin, S., Regional cerebral blood flow in long-term heavy cannabis use. Psychiatry Res. 17:15–21, 1986.

Tutus, A., Kugu, N., Sofuoglu, S., Nardali, M., Simsek, A., Karaaslan, F. and Gonul, A. S., Transient frontal hypoperfusion in Tc-99m hexamethylpropyleneamineoxime single photon emission computed tomography imaging during alcohol withdrawal. Biol. Psychiatry. 43:923–928, 1998.

Valmier, J., Touchon, J., Zanca, M., Fauchere, V., Bories, P. and Baldy-Moulinier, M., Correlations between cerebral grey matter flow and hepatic histology in alcoholism. Eur. Neurol. 25:428–435, 1986.

van Dyck, C. H., Rosen, M. I., Thomas, H. M., McMahon, T. J., Wallace, E. A., O'Connor, P. G., Sullivan, M., Krystal, J. H., Hoffer, P. B., Woods, S. W. and Kosten, T. R., SPECT regional cerebral blood flow alterations in naltrexone-precipitated withdrawal from buprenorphine. Psychiatry Res. 55:181–191, 1994.

Veselis, R. A., Reinsel, R. A., Beattie, B. J., Mawlawi, O. R., Feshchenko, V. A., DiResta, G. R., Larson, S. M. and Blasberg, R. G., Midazolam changes cerebral blood flow in discrete brain regions: an $H2(^{15})O$ positron emission tomography study. Anesthesiology 87:1106–1117, 1997.

Villemagne, V., Yuan, J., Wong, D. F., Dannals, R. F., Hatzidimitriou, G., Mathews, W. B., Ravert, H. T., Musachio, J., McCann, U. D. and Ricaurte, G. A., Brain dopamine neurotoxicity in baboons treated with doses of methamphetamine comparable to those recreationally abused by humans: evidence from $[^{11}C]$WIN-35,428 positron emission tomography studies and direct in vitro determinations. J. Neurosci. 18:419–427, 1998.

Volkow, N. D., Mullani, N., Gould, K. L., Adler, S. and Krajewski, K., Cerebral blood flow in chronic cocaine users: a study with positron emission tomography. Br. J. Psychiatry 152:641–648, 1988a.

Volkow, N. D., Mullani, N., Gould, L., Adler, S. S., Guynn, R. W., Overall, J. E. and Dewey, S., Effects of acute alcohol intoxication on cerebral blood flow measured with PET. Psychiatry Res. 24:201–209, 1988b.

Volkow, N. D., Fowler, J. S., Wolf, A. P., Schlyer, D., Shiue, C. Y., Alpert, R., Dewey, S. L., Logan, J., Bendriem, B., Christman, D., Hitzemann, R. and Henn, F., Effects of chronic cocaine abuse on postsynaptic dopamine receptors. Am. J. Psychiatry 147:719–724, 1990a.

Volkow, N. D., Hitzemann, R., Wolf, A. P., Logan, J., Fowler, J. S., Christman, D., Dewey, S. L., Schlyer, D., Burr, G., Vitkun, S. and Hirschowitz, J., Acute effects of ethanol on regional brain glucose metabolism and transport. Psychiatry Res. 35:39–48, 1990b.

Volkow, N., Fowler, J., Wolf, A., Hitzemann, R., Dewey, S., Bendriem, B., Alpert, R. and Hoff, A., Changes in brain glucose metabolism in cocaine dependence and withdrawal. Am. J. Psychiatry 148:621–626, 1991a.

Volkow, N. D., Gillespie, H., Mullani, N., Tancredi, L., Grant, C., Ivanovic, M. and Hollister, L., Cerebellar metabolic activation by delta-9-tetrahydro-cannabinol in human brain: a study with positron emission tomography and ^{18}F-2-fluoro-2-deoxyglucose. Psychiatry Res. 40:69–78, 1991b.

Volkow, N., Hitzemann, R., Wang, G., Fowler, J., Wolf, A., Dewey, S. and Handlesman, L., Long-term frontal brain metabolic changes in cocaine abusers. Synapse 11:184–190, 1992a.

Volkow, N. D., Hitzemann, R., Wang, G. J., Fowler, J. S., Burr, G., Pascani, K., Dewey, S. L. and Wolf, A. P., Decreased brain metabolism in neurologically intact healthy alcoholics. Am. J. Psychiatry 149:1016–1022, 1992b.

Volkow, N. D., Fowler, J. S., Wang, G. J., Hitzemann, R., Logan, J., Schlyer, D. J., Dewey, S. L. and Wolf, A. P., Decreased dopamine D_2 receptor availability is associated with reduced frontal metabolism in cocaine abusers. Synapse 14:169–177, 1993a.

Volkow, N. D., Wang, G. J., Hitzemann, R., Fowler, J. S., Wolf, A. P., Pappas, N., Biegon, A. and Dewey, S. L., Decreased cerebral response to inhibitory neurotransmission in alcoholics. Am. J. Psychiatry 150:417–422, 1993b.

Volkow, N. D., Wang, G. J., Hitzemann, R., Fowler, J. S., Overall, J. E., Burr, G. and Wolf, A. P., Recovery of brain glucose metabolism in detoxified alcoholics. Am. J. Psychiatry 151:178–183, 1994.

Volkow, N. D., Ding, Y.-S., Fowler, J. S., Wang, G.-J., Logan, J., Gatley, J. S., Dewey, S., Ashby, C., Liebermann, J., Hitzemann, R. and Wolf, A. P., Is methylphenidate like cocaine? Studies on their pharmacokinetics and distribution in the human brain. Arch. Gen. Psychiatry 52:456–463, 1995a.

Volkow, N. D., Wang, G. J., Hitzemann, R., Fowler, J. S., Pappas, N., Lowrimore, P., Burr, G., Pascani, K., Overall, J. and Wolf, A. P., Depression of thalamic metabolism by lorazepam is associated with sleepiness. Neuropsychopharmacology 12:123–132, 1995b.
Volkow, N. D., Ding, Y. S., Fowler, J. S. and Wang, G. J., Cocaine addiction: hypothesis derived from imaging studies with PET. J. Addict. Dis. 15:55–71, 1996a.
Volkow, N. D., Gillespie, H., Mullani, N., Tancredi, L., Grant, C., Valentine, A. and Hollister, L., Brain glucose metabolism in chronic marijuana users at baseline and during marijuana intoxication. Psychiatry Res. 67:29–38, 1996b.
Volkow, N. D., Wang, G. J., Fowler, J. S., Gatley, S. J., Ding, Y. S., Logan, J., Dewey, S. L., Hitzemann, R. and Lieberman, J., Relationship between psychostimulant-induced "high" and dopamine transporter occupancy. Proc. Natl. Acad. Sci. USA 93:10388–10392, 1996c.
Volkow, N. D., Wang, G. J., Fowler, J. S., Logan, J., Hitzemann, R., Ding, Y. S., Pappas, N., Shea, C. and Piscani, K., Decreases in dopamine receptors but not in dopamine transporters in alcoholics. Alcohol. Clin. Exp. Res. 20:1594–1598, 1996d.
Volkow, N. D., Wang, G. J., Fowler, J. S., Logan, J., Hitzemannn, R., Gatley, S. J., MacGregor, R. R. and Wolf, A. P., Cocaine uptake is decreased in the brain of detoxified cocaine abusers. Neuropsychopharmacology 14:159–168, 1996e.
Volkow, N. D., Wang, G. J., Gatley, S. J., Fowler, J. S., Ding, Y. S., Logan, J., Hitzemann, R., Angrist, B. and Lieberman, J., Temporal relationships between the pharmacokinetics of methylphenidate in the human brain and its behavioral and cardiovascular effects. Psychopharmacology (Berl.) 123:26–33, 1996f.
Volkow, N. D., Wang, G. J., Fischman, M. W., Foltin, R. W., Fowler, J. S., Abumrad, N. N., Vitkun, S., Logan, J., Gatley, S. J., Pappas, N., Hitzemann, R. and Shea, C. E., Relationship between subjective effects of cocaine and dopamine transporter occupancy. Nature 386:827–830, 1997a.
Volkow, N. D., Wang, G. J., Fowler, J. S., Logan, J., Angrist, B., Hitzemann, R., Lieberman, J. and Pappas, N., Effects of methylphenidate on regional brain glucose metabolism in humans: relationship to dopamine D_2 receptors. Am. J. Psychiatry 154:50–55, 1997b.
Volkow, N. D., Wang, G. J., Fowler, J. S., Logan, J., Gatley, S. J., Hitzemann, R., Chen, A. D., Dewey, S. L. and Pappas, N., Decreased striatal dopaminergic responsiveness in detoxified cocaine-dependent subjects. Nature 386:830–833, 1997c.
Volkow, N. D., Wang, G. J., Overall, J. E., Hitzemann, R., Fowler, J. S., Pappas, N., Frecska, E. and Piscani, K., Regional brain metabolic response to lorazepam in alcoholics during early and late alcohol detoxification. Alcohol. Clin. Exp. Res. 21:1278–1284, 1997d.
Volkow, N. D., Wang, G. J., Fowler, J. S., Gatley, S. J., Logan, J., Ding, Y. S., Hitzemann, R. and Pappas, N., Dopamine transporter occupancies in the human brain induced by therapeutic doses of oral methylphenidate. Am. J. Psychiatry 155:1325–1331, 1998a.
Volkow, N. D., Wang, G. J., Fowler, J. S., Hitzemann, R., Gatley, S. J., Dewey, S. S. and Pappas, N., Enhanced sensitivity to benzodiazepines in active cocaine-abusing subjects: a PET study. Am. J. Psychiatry 155:200–206, 1998b.
Volkow, N. D., Wang, G. J., Fowler, J. S., Hitzemann, R. J., Gatley, J., Ding, Y. S., Wong, C. and Pappas, N. R., Differences in regional brain metabolic responses between single and repeated doses of methylphenidate. Psychiatry Res. 83:29–36, 1998c.
Volkow, N. D., Wang, G. J., Fowler, J. S., Gatley, S. J., Logan, J., Ding, Y. S., Dewey, S. L., Hitzemann, R., Gifford, A. N. and Pappas, N. R., Blockade of striatal dopamine transporters by intravenous methylphenidate is not sufficient to induce self-reports of high. J. Pharmacol. Exp. Ther. 288:14–20, 1999a.
Volkow, N. D., Wang, G. J., Fowler, J. S., Hitzemann, R., Angrist, B., Gatley, S. J., Logan, J., Ding, Y. S. and Pappas, N., Association of methylphenidate-induced craving with changes in right striato-orbitofrontal metabolism in cocaine abusers: implications in addiction. Am J Psychiatry 156:19–26, 1999b.

Vollenweider, F. X., Leenders, K. L., Oye, I., Hell, D. and Angst, J., Differential psychopathology and patterns of cerebral glucose utilisation produced by (S)- and (R)-ketamine in healthy volunteers using positron emission tomography (PET). Eur. Neuropsychopharmacol. 7:25–38, 1997a.

Vollenweider, F. X., Leenders, K. L., Scharfetter, C., Antonini, A., Maguire, P., Missimer, J. and Angst, J., Metabolic hyperfrontality and psychopathology in the ketamine model of psychosis using positron emission tomography (PET) and [^{18}F]fluorodeoxyglucose (FDG). Eur. Neuropsychopharmacol. 7:9–24, 1997b.

Vollenweider, F. X., Leenders, K. L., Scharfetter, C., Maguire, P., Stadelmann, O. and Angst, J., Positron emission tomography and fluorodeoxyglucose studies of metabolic hyperfrontality and psychopathology in the psilocybin model of psychosis. Neuropsychopharmacology 16:357–372, 1997c.

Vollenweider, F. X., Maguire, R. P., Leenders, K. L., Mathys, K. and Angst, J., Effects of high amphetamine dose on mood and cerebral glucose metabolism in normal volunteers using positron emission tomography. Psychiatry Res 83:149–162, 1998.

Wallace, E. A., Wisniewski, G., Zubal, G., vanDyck, C. H., Pfau, S. E., Smith, E. O., Rosen, M. I., Sullivan, M. C., Woods, S. W. and Kosten, T. R., Acute cocaine effects on absolute cerebral blood flow. Psychopharmacology (Berl.) 128:17–20, 1996.

Walsh, S. L., Gibson, S. F., Jasinski, D. R., Stapleton, J. M., Phillips, R. L., Dannals, R. F., Schmidt, J., Preston, K. L., Grayson, R., Bigelow, G. E., Sullivan, J. T., Contoreggi, C. and London, E. D., Buprenorphine reduces cerebral glucose metabolism in poly drug users. Neuropsychopharmacology 10:157–170, 1994.

Wang, G. J., Volkow, N. D., Roque, C. T., Cestaro, V. L., Hitzemann, R. J., Cantos, E. L., Levy, A. V. and Dhawan, A. P., Functional importance of ventricular enlargement and cortical atrophy in healthy subjects and alcoholics as assessed with PET, MR imaging, and neuropsychologic testing. Radiology 186:59–65, 1993.

Wang, G. J., Volkow, N. D., Fowler, J. S., Ferrieri, R., Schlyer, D. J., Alexoff, D., Pappas, N., Lieberman, J., King, P., Warner, D., Wong, C., Hitzemann, R. J. and Wolf, A. P., Methylphenidate decreases regional cerebral blood flow in normal human subjects. Life Sci. 54:PL143–PL146, 1994.

Wang, G. J., Volkow, N. D., Logan, J., Fowler, J. S., Schlyer, D., MacGregor, R. R., Hitzemann, R. J., Gjedde, A. and Wolf, A. P., Serotonin 5-HT_2 receptor availability in chronic cocaine abusers. Life Sci. 56:PL299–PL303, 1995.

Wang, G. J., Volkow, N. D., Fowler, J. S., Fischman, M., Foltin, R., Abumrad, N. N., Logan, J. and Pappas, N. R., Cocaine abusers do not show loss of dopamine transporters with age. Life Sci. 61:1059–1065, 1997a.

Wang, G. J., Volkow, N. D., Fowler, J. S., Logan, J., Abumrad, N. N., Hitzemann, R. J., Pappas, N. S. and Pascani, K., Dopamine D_2 receptor availability in opiate-dependent subjects before and after naloxone-precipitated withdrawal. Neuropsychopharmacology 16:174–182, 1997b.

Wang, G. J., Volkow, N. D., Fowler, J. S., Hitzemann, R. J., Pappas, N. R. and Netusil, N., Evaluation of gender difference in regional brain metabolic responses to lorazepam. Psychiatry Res. 82:37–46, 1998a.

Wang, G. J., Volkow, N. D., Fowler, J. S., Pappas, N. R., Wong, C. T., Pascani, K., Felder, C. A. and Hitzemann, R. J., Regional cerebral metabolism in female alcoholics of moderate severity does not differ from that of controls. Alcohol. Clin. Exp. Res. 22:1850–1854, 1998b.

Weber, D. A., Franceschi, D., Ivanovic, M., Atkins, H. L., Cabahug, C., Wong, C. T. C. and Susskind, H., SPECT and planar brain imaging in crack abuse: iodine-123-iodoamphetamine uptake and localization. J. Nucl. Med. 34:899–907, 1993.

Wendt, P. E., Risberg, J., Stenberg, G., Rosen, I. and Ingvar, D. H., Ethanol reduces asymmetry of visual rCBF responses. J. Cereb. Blood Flow Metab. 14:963–973, 1994.

Wik, G., Borg, S., Sjogren, I., Wiesel, F. A., Blomqvist, G., Borg, J., Greitz, T., Nyback, H., Sedvall, G., Stone-Elander, S. and Widen, L., PET determination of regional cerebral glucose metabolism in alcohol-dependent men and healthy controls using ^{11}C-glucose. Acta Psychiatr. Scand. 78:234–241, 1988.

Wolf, J., Friberg, L., Jensen, J., Hansen, P. B., Andersen, A. R. and Lassen, N. A., The effect of the benzodiazepine antagonist flumazenil on regional cerebral blood flow in human volunteers. Acta Anaesthesiol. Scand. 34:628–631, 1990.

Wolkin, A., Sanfilipo, M., Angrist, B., Duncan, E., Wieland, S., Wolf, A. P., Brodie, J. D., Cooper, T. B., Laska, E. and Rotrosen, J. P., Acute d-amphetamine challenge in schizophrenia: effects on cerebral glucose utilization and clinical symptomatology. Biol. Psychiatry 36:317–325, 1994.

Wu, J. C., Bell, K., Najafi, A., Widmark, C., Keator, D., Tang, C., Klein, E., Bunney, B. G., Fallon, J. and Bunney, W. E., Decreasing striatal 6-FDOPA uptake with increasing duration of cocaine withdrawal. Neuropsychopharmacology 17:402–409, 1997.

Zubieta, J.-K., Gorelick, D. A., Stauffer, R., Ravert, H. T., Dannals, R. F. and Frost, J. J., Increased mu opioid receptor binding detected by PET in cocaine-dependent men is associated with cocaine craving. Nat. Med. 2:1225–1229, 1996.

Chapter 6

Magnetic Resonance Findings in Substance Abuse

Marc J. Kaufman, PhD, and Jonathan M. Levin, MD, MPH

INTRODUCTION

To date, magnetic resonance (MR) technologies have been used primarily for clinical evaluation of patients with substance abuse-related neurologic complications. The MR literature contains several types of reports. The largest segment consists of MR imaging findings regarding the effects of chronic alcohol abuse on gross brain structure. A smaller segment includes case report descriptions of relatively infrequent cerebrovascular abnormalities found in neurologically impaired illicit drug users. The smallest but most rapidly growing segment consists of experimental studies using MR to monitor the effects of drugs and alcohol on brain physiology and neurochemistry. The MR modalities used in those investigations include functional MRI (fMRI), which is capable of detecting brain activation and blood flow changes, MR spectroscopy (MRS), which can monitor both brain metabolism and neurochemistry, and MR angiography (MRA), which can assess cerebrovascular abnormalities.

MR imaging modalities have several advantages over other clinical brain imaging techniques. They do not use ionizing radiation, are not invasive, and in general offer superior spatial and temporal resolution. Consequently, they are well-suited for human studies. Additionally, their high safety margin makes them particularly advantageous for use in longitudinal studies evaluating treatments designed to diminish drug use, protect individuals from continued drug abuse, and improve brain function in chronic

From: *Brain Imaging in Substance Abuse: Research, Clinical, and Forensic Applications*
M. J. Kaufman, ed. © Humana Press Inc., Totowa, New Jersey

substance abusers. The following overview will describe the existing MR literature in substance abuse. For each substance of abuse, findings related to acute effects of will be discussed initially, followed by findings from studies of chronic exposure to those substances. The primary focus will be on peer-reviewed reports of studies conducted in humans, although results from preliminary studies published in abstract form or from studies using animal models will be included, when peer-reviewed human data are not available. While space limitations do not permit inclusion of all published work, citations for studies not covered in this review can be found in the bibliography section at the end of this book. An overview of the technical foundations for these techniques can be found in Chapter 3.

Alcohol and Alcoholism

Acute Effects

MR Imaging

Although alcohol is not an illicit drug, alcohol abuse and alcoholism are perhaps the greatest substance abuse problems facing society, causing an estimated 148 billion dollar yearly expenditure in the United States alone (Harwood et al., 1999). In spite of the fact that MR imaging has been extremely useful for detecting structural brain changes associated with chronic alcohol abuse (see below), there are no MR imaging studies documenting brain structural changes induced by acute alcohol exposure. However, alcohol is a diuretic, and several MR imaging studies have focused on determining whether alcohol alters brain hydration state, which can be assessed with MR imaging by measuring T1 and T2 relaxation times (relaxometry). Frontal T1 relaxation times were found to be reduced in two intoxicated alcoholics studied at the time of hospital admission (Besson et al., 1981), but whole-brain T1 was decreased in control subjects after an acute alcohol challenge producing blood alcohol levels (BALs) of 140–200 mg/dL (Mander et al., 1985). By contrast, a subsequent study failed to demonstrate alcohol-induced T1 or T2 changes (peak BALs of 50–100 mg/dL (Logsdail et al., 1987). Those contradictory findings could imply that brain tissue relaxation changes occur only at higher blood alcohol levels.

MR Spectroscopy

Several studies have exploited the fact that ethyl alcohol can be detected with proton MR spectroscopy (^{1}H MRS) (Fig. 1), and at intoxicating BALs (approx. 100 mg/dL or 20 mmol/L) can be monitored in brain with ^{1}H MRS. Brain alcohol detection had been reported during intoxication in humans (Hetherington et al., 1989; Hanstock et al., 1990; Mendelson et al., 1990) and subjective reports of intoxication have been shown to parallel ^{1}H MRS measures of brain alcohol levels (Mendelson et al., 1990; Lukas et al., 1993). However, using T2-weighted spectroscopy methods, ^{1}H MRS is nonquantitative because it detects less than 60% of the alcohol known to be in brain based on a concurrent blood or breath alcohol determination (Mendelson et al., 1990; Kaufman et al., 1994). This may be explained by the fact that just as water is present in tissue environments with different T1 and T2 relaxation properties (the basis for

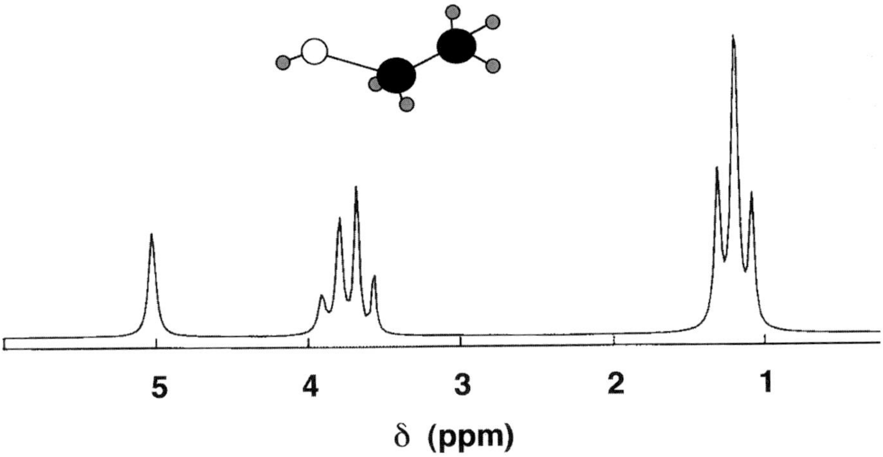

Fig. 1. Proton (^{1}H) MRS spectrum acquired from a bottle of white Bordeaux wine (12% alcohol by volume). The gray, black, and white spheres in the ethyl alcohol molecule cartoon represent hydrogen (proton), carbon, and oxygen nuclei, respectively. The spectrum contains information regarding the concentration and local chemical environment of proton nuclei. The methyl proton triplet ($\delta = 1.2$ ppm) is typically measured in in vivo MRS studies.

certain types of tissue contrast in MR imaging), alcohol also appears to partition into multiple molecular environments with fast and slow T2-relaxation properties that are differentially detectable with T2-weighted spectroscopy methods. Alcohol molecules in pools with constrained mobility (e.g., those hydrogen-bonded to lipids or membrane proteins) relax quickly (short T2) and produce small MRS signals in T2-weighted spectroscopy acquisitions. In contrast, molecules with larger molecular mobilities (e.g. alcohol in the cerebrospinal fluid not associated with tissue lipids or proteins) which relax more slowly and have longer T2 produce larger MRS signals. Proton MR spectroscopic imaging (^{1}H MRSI), which can simultaneously acquire spectra from gray matter, white matter, and cerebrospinal fluid, has been used to demonstrate differential brain alcohol concentration and visibility in these tissue types (Spielman et al., 1993). Figure 2 is an example showing ^{1}H MRSI brain alcohol spectra.

While partial brain alcohol detectability may be an artifact of T2-weighted acquisitions, the phenomenon may have clinical utility for detecting alcohol tolerance. In this regard, our group published two studies suggesting relationships between brain alcohol detectability and alcohol tolerance. In the first study, acute alcohol challenges induced larger ^{1}H MRS brain alcohol signals in alcohol-tolerant subjects than in controls, even though spectrum acquisitions were conducted in both groups at statistically equivalent BALs (Chiu et al., 1994). In the second study, in which controls were sequentially administered two alcoholic drinks and brain alcohol was measured at statistically equivalent BALs after each drink, brain alcohol detectability was greater following the second drink (Fig. 3) after the development of acute alcohol tolerance (Kaufman et al., 1996). We postulated that alcohol-tolerant individuals had altered membrane partitioning of brain alcohol, resulting in increased molecular mobility and

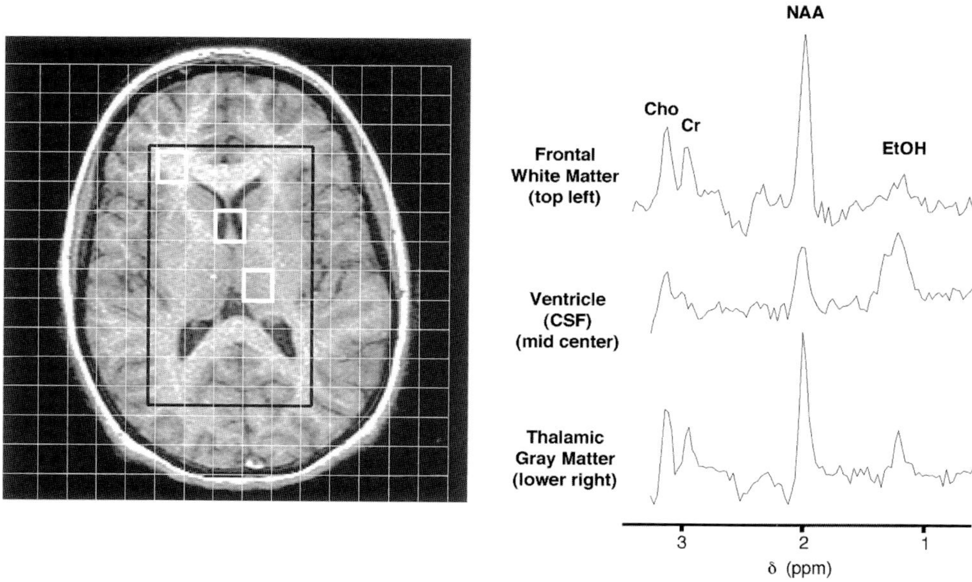

Fig. 2. [1]H magnetic resonance spectroscopic imaging (^{1}H MRSI) of brain alcohol. An axial brain slice localizer image (left) is superimposed with a 16 × 16 spectroscopic imaging voxel grid. The grid contains three voxels with thick white borders from which sample spectra (right) were extracted. The data were acquired from a 23-yr-old woman 30 min after consuming alcohol (0.6 g/kg), at which time her breath alcohol level was 60 mg/dL. Acquisition parameters: PRESS sequence; TR/TE = 2000/272 ms. Note the small alcohol signal ($\delta = 1.2$ ppm) in white matter (right top), intermediate signal in gray matter (right middle) and large signal in the ventricle (right bottom). Cho, choline-containing compounds; Cr, creatine containing compounds; NAA, *N*-acetylaspartate-containing compounds; EtOH, ethyl alcohol.

increased MRS visibility. Meyerhoff and colleagues subsequently used magnetization transfer to document that alcohol exists in different pools (with different relaxation properties) in both rodent and human brain, supporting the possibility of differential pool occupation after the development of alcohol tolerance (Meyerhoff et al., 1996; Meyerhoff, 1998).

Functional MRI

We have also utilized the blood oxygen level dependent (BOLD) fMRI method to evaluate the effects of an acute alcohol challenge on visual cortex activation, subsequent to photic stimulation. In normal subjects, the fMRI response to photic stimulation was reduced in a dose-dependent manner following alcohol administration, while placebo was without effect (Fig. 4). The complex nature of the BOLD fMRI response precluded a determination as to whether the inhibitory effect of alcohol was due to hemodynamic factors or to alterations in neuronal function (Levin et al., 1998). However, alcohol's inhibitory effects were greater in the right hemisphere, consistent with the known lateralization of the functional effects of alcohol (Levin et al., 1998).

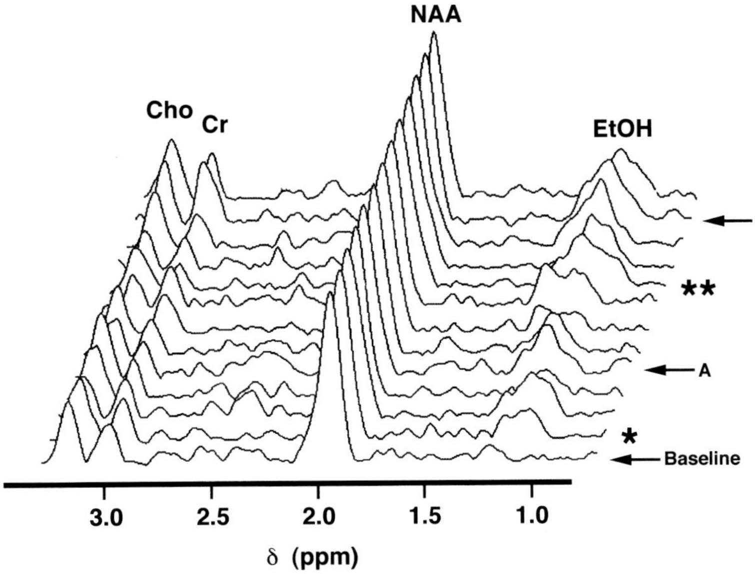

Fig. 3. Stacked plot of ^1H MR spectra acquired from the left basal ganglia following the sequential administration of two alcoholic drinks (0.6 g/kg). Results are shown for a single male subject. Seven spectra acquired continuously after drink 1 was administered (*) are shown. A second drink (**) was administered 6 h into the study followed by spectrum acquisitions. Spectrum A was acquired 80 min after drink 1 was administered, at a blood alcohol level (BAL) of 65.5 mg/dL. The brain alcohol resonance (δ = 1.2 ppm) was calculated to be 5 mg/dL. Spectrum B was acquired 86 min after drink 2 was administered, at a BAL of 65.7 mg/dL. The corresponding brain alcohol resonance was 11.3 mg/dL, or more than twice that observed at the same BAL after drink 1. Details of this study are described in Kaufman et al. (1996). The following resonances are shown: Cho, choline containing compounds; Cr, creatine + phosphocreatine; NAA, *N*-acetylaspartate; EtOH, ethyl alcohol methyl triplet.

Chronic Effects

MR Imaging

Tissue Relaxation Abnormalities

As alluded to previously, chronic alcohol abuse has been associated with structural brain changes that can be visualized with MR imaging. However, the earliest MR imaging studies of alcoholics used relaxometry to determine whether tissue dehydration had occurred. Besson (1981) first reported frontal gray and white matter T1 increases in alcoholics during abstinence, implying increased tissue hydration during the post-alcohol period (Besson et al., 1981). A number of subsequent reports also documented elevated brain T1 in abstinent alcoholics (Smith et al., 1985, 1998; Mander et al., 1988, 1989b; Chick et al., 1989). Correlations between cognitive impairment and whole brain T1 (Chick et al., 1989) and between cerebral atrophy and whole brain T1 (Mander et al., 1989b) were described. In contrast, one study reported decreased T1 during early

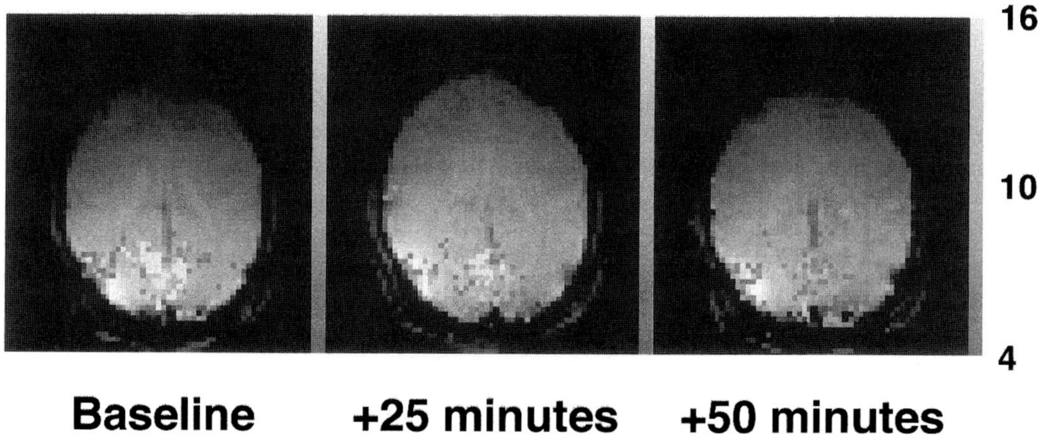

Fig. 4. Acute alcohol inhibits occipital cortex photic activation. Shown are fMRI images superimposed with photic stimulation activation profiles (bright pixels). **(Left)** Baseline study of occipital cortex activation at a blood alcohol level (BAL) of 0 mg/dL. **(Center)** Study at 25 minutes following alcohol administration (BAL = 63 mg/dl). **(Right)** Study at 50 min following alcohol administration (BAL = 85 mg/dL). Note the alcohol concentration-dependent decrease of photic activation, seen as a change from bright to darker pixels, or in the color version of this figure from yellow to red pixels. (*See* color plate 4 appearing after p. 134.)

abstinence (Mander et al., 1989a) and several studies failed to find either T1 (Agartz et al., 1991) or T2 (Schroth et al., 1988; Mann et al., 1989; Agartz et al., 1991) differences in alcoholics after the initiation of abstinence. These conflicting findings appear to be inconsistent with a rehydration hypothesis. However, since these reports studied patients in different stages of alcoholism (e.g. continued drinking, withdrawal, early abstinence, prolonged abstinence) the discrepancies could have resulted from T1 and T2 variations as a function of those clinical stages.

Ventricular Enlargement

Chronic alcohol-induced brain atrophy and ventricular enlargement had been well-established and described in autopsy and X-ray computed tomography (CT) studies prior to the advent of MR imaging. However, MR imaging affords distinct advantages over CT imaging by offering greatly increased spatial resolution, different tissue contrast options (e.g., T1-weighted, T2-weighted, or proton density images) and the ability to acquire images in sagittal, coronal, and oblique planes, making it possible to visualize structures not easily detected in axial images (the image plane available in CT studies). Accordingly, numerous additional MR investigations of alcohol-induced brain atrophy and ventricular and sulcal enlargement have been conducted and published (e.g., Mann et al., 1989; Zipursky et al., 1989) (Table 1). One study failed to detect ventricular enlargement in a group of alcoholic women (Kroft et al., 1991). However, the women in that study were young, leading the authors to suggest that age differences may have been the basis for negative study results (Kroft et al., 1991). This interpretation is supported by reports documenting an absence of ventricular volume abnormalities in young alcoholic men (Wang et al., 1993; Pfefferbaum et al., 1997).

Cortical Atrophy

Sulcal volume increases and brain tissue volume decreases have been noted in alcoholics (Table 1). While these changes are generally believed to be related, one study noted sulcal changes in alcoholics in the absence of cortical volume reduction (Jernigan et al., 1991a), suggesting that sulcal and cortical volume changes could occur by independent processes. Several reports described correlations between these different measures of brain atrophy and brain function (Table 1); correlations were noted between sulcal or thalamic volumes and olfactory function (Ditraglia et al., 1991; Shear et al., 1992), sulcal volumes and neuropsychological performance (Jernigan et al., 1991a), frontal and cingulate cortex volumes and both cingulate metabolism and Wisconsin Card Sorting Test performance (Adams et al., 1993), and cortical volume and neuropsychological test performance (Wang et al., 1993). Importantly, neuropsychological impairments were found in long-abstinent alcoholics who did not have global atrophy, suggesting either that cognitive dysfunction and brain volume abnormalities may be induced by independent processes or that they may be reversible to different extents (Di Sclafani et al., 1995). Agartz and colleagues (1999) noted global cerebral and proportional hippocampal atrophy, and that alcoholic women had smaller left hippocampi and nonhippocampal brain volumes than alcoholic men, despite having consumed less alcohol over their lifetimes.

Corpus Callosum Atrophy

Atrophy of the corpus callosum has also been noted in association with chronic alcohol use (*see* Fig. 5). Reduced callosal cross sectional areas along with a negative association between age and callosal volume were found in alcoholic men (Pfefferbaum et al., 1996). Callosal volume reductions have also been reported in alcoholic women (Hommer et al., 1996), although that study failed to find callosal abnormalities in a comparison group of alcoholic men with similar cumulative alcohol exposures. The conflicting findings in men in the Pfefferbaum (1996) and Hommer (1996) studies may have resulted from the fact that men in the latter study had an estimated lifetime alcohol consumption averaging only one-third of the amount of the group evaluated in the former study. Indeed, a link between lifetime alcohol consumption and callosal area was substantiated by Estruch and colleagues (1997). That study also reported an association between callosal areas and neuropsychological impairment (Estruch et al., 1997). The gender discrepancy noted by Hommer (1996) was attributed to the fact that women generally achieve higher blood alcohol levels than men, effectively resulting in greater brain alcohol exposure (Hommer et al., 1996). Callosal abnormalities are present in several alcohol-related conditions including Marchiafava-Bignami Disease (MBD, *see* Marchifava-Bignami Disease) and in fetal alcohol exposure (*see* Fetal Alcohol Exposure) suggesting that the corpus callosum is an important target for the effects of alcohol.

Cerebellar Degeneration

Cerebellar atrophy is one of the most important and prominent clinical indicators of alcoholic brain damage (*see* Fig. 5), and several MR imaging reports have described alcohol-induced cerebellar structural changes. Cerebellar vermal atrophy, shrinkage, or sulcal widening have been noted in alcoholics (Okudaira et al., 1988; Blansjaar

Table 1
MR Studies of Brain Abnormalities in Alcohol Abuse and Alcoholism

Study	Year	Age[a]	Drinking[a]	Abstinence[a]	Ventricular volume	Sulcal volume	Gray matter volume	White matter volume	Functional findings
Ditraglia	1991	50	14	10		↑			Sulcal volumes correlated with UPSIT scores; lower UPSITs in relapsed subjects at retest
Jernigan	1991a	50	12	~35	↑	↑	Global ↓; caudate nucleus and diencephalon ↓	T2 hyperintensities	Sulcal volumes correlated with both Trails B and Stroop; ventricular volumes correlated with Trails A/B, DSST, RAVLT
Hayakawa	1992	31–61	13		↑	↑	Subcortical T1 hypointensities; age correlated	Periventricular T2 hyperintensities; age correlated	
Pfefferbaum	1992	45	19	33	↑, Age correlated	↑, Age correlated	Global ↓, age correlated	Global ↓	Cortical gray, white. and CSF volumes correlated with both NART IQ and Vocabulary age SS
Shear	1992	48	12	12	↑	↑	Global ↓; lateral cortex↓; caudate nucleus and lenticular nucleus ↓		Sulcal and thalamic volumes correlated with UPSIT scores
Adams	1993	51	22	25/31 patients: ≥ 28			Anterior frontal and cingulate volumes age correlated		Anterior frontal and cingulate volumes correlated with both cingulate PET metabolism and WCST scores
Pfefferbaum	1993	42	24	≥ 21	↑, Age correlated	↑, Age correlated			
Wang	1993	37	>15	6–32	Normal in young men		Global ↓		Ventricular and cortical volumes correlated with mental control; cortical volumes correlated with both SDMT and BDI

Di Sclafani	1995	60	27	280	Age correlated	Age correlated			Persistent WMS, Trails B, and HVOT impairments in the absence of global atrophy
Pfefferbaum	1995	43–49	20	Varies	↓ Lateral early abstinence;↓ 3rd ventr. late abstin.	↓ Posterior in early abstinence	↑ Anterior in early abstinence	↓ In relapsers	
Sullivan	1995	44	27	33	↑, Age correlated	↑ Temporal	↓ Temporal lobe and anterior hippocampus volumes, age correlated	Temporal, age correlated	Anterior hippocampal volumes correlated with both Trails A and B
Sullivan	1996	43–45	19–21	~28	↑; Age correlated	↑ Temporal and frontoparietal; temp. age correl.	↓ Anterior hippocampus, temporal and frontopar.; temporal age correlated	↓ Temporal and frontoparietal	Alcoholics with seizures had greater temporal lobe white matter deficits
Pfefferbaum	1997	38–53	17–20	28	↑; Larger ↑ in older subjects	↑; Larger ↑ in older subjects	↓ Cortical; larger global and frontal ↓ in older subjects	↓ Cortical and frontal only in older subjects	
Pfefferbaum	1998	45	16–23	29	Abstinent subjects had normal age-related changes	↑ Correl. with alcohol consumption	↓ Correl. with alcohol consumption		
Sullivan	1998	45	19	33	↑	↑	↓ Global	↓ Global and prefrontal and temporal	

[a]Shown are means (or ranges) for ages and years of drinking as well as mean number of days (or ranges) of abstinence for each study. Abbreviations: abstin: abstinent; ant.: anterior; CSF: cerebrospinal fluid; frontopar.: frontoparietal; temp.: temporal; UPSIT: University of Pennsylvania Smell Identification Test; DSST: Digit Symbol Subtraction Test; RAVLT: Rey Auditory Verbal Learning Test; NART IQ; National Adult Reading Test IQ; Vocabulary Age SS: Vocabulary subtest of the Wechsler Adult Intelligence Test; SDMT: Symbol Digit Modalities Test, Written; BDI: Beck Depression Inventory, psychiatric scale; PET: positron emission tomography; WCST: Wisconsin Card Sorting Task; WMS: Wechsler Memory Scale; HVOT: Hooper Visual Organization Test.

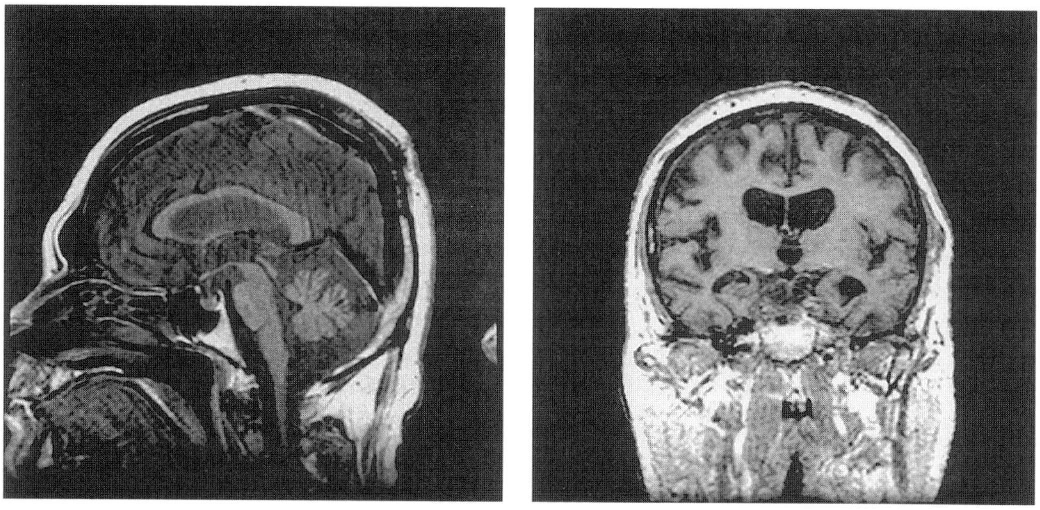

Fig. 5. MR images of a patient with Wernicke's encephalopathy. T1-weighted midline sagittal image **(Left)** and coronal 3D SPGR images through the thalamus and temporal lobes **(Right)** reveal brain volume changes typically noted in alcoholics and in patients with the Wernicke-Korsakoff syndrome. The corpus callosum is abnormally thin (left), the cerebellum vermis is atrophic (left), and the ventricles are enlarged (left and right). The mamillary bodies (normally visible on midline sagittal images, e.g., at arrow in the left panel of Fig. 6), are extremely atrophic and cannot be resolved in this case (left).

et al., 1992; Hayakawa et al., 1992; Tsuchiya et al., 1993; Davila et al., 1994; Shear et al., 1996; Seitz et al., 1999) and in polydrug abusers who had histories of prior or current alcohol abuse (Aasly et al., 1993). Prenatal alcohol exposure also has been shown to result in cerebellar developmental abnormalities (see the section Fetal Alcohol Exposure).

White Matter Lesions

Frontal, occipital and periventricular white matter hyperintensities have been found in T2-weighted scans of asymptomatic alcoholics, suggestive of demyelination (Gallucci et al., 1989). That study also reported a correlation between daily alcohol consumption and the number of large (>3 mm) white matter hyperintensities. Hayakawa and colleagues (1992) noted focal T2 hyperintensities and T1 hypointensities in over 60 and 20% of alcoholic subjects, respectively, as well as basal ganglia and pontine T2 hyperintensities. A high proportion (~50%) of young alcoholics were noted to have white matter T2 hyperintensities (Meyerhoff et al., 1995).

Effects of Aging

Pfefferbaum (1992) reported the first MR study documenting that brain gray matter, white matter and CSF volume abnormalities were correlated with age, but not with total lifetime alcohol consumption (Pfefferbaum et al., 1992). A number of subsequent reports confirmed and expanded on these findings in both whole brain and in a number of brain regions (Table 1), including age associated volume changes in frontal and cingulate cortex (Adams et al., 1993), and in the anterior hippocampus, temporal lobe, and frontoparietal cortex (Sullivan et al., 1995, 1996). Frontal gray matter volume reductions were detected in young alcoholics, implying that the frontal cortex is especially sensitive to alcoholism (Pfefferbaum et al., 1997). A longitudinal (5-yr) follow-up study of alcoholics and controls noted accelerated cortical and sulcal volume changes in alcoholics and confirmed that the prefrontal cortex was particularly sensitive to the combined effects of aging and alcohol (Pfefferbaum et al., 1998). As described above, age effects on callosal size (Pfefferbaum et al., 1996) and the severity of T2 hyperintensities (Hayakawa et al., 1992) have been noted. Together, these findings suggest that the aged brain is more susceptible to the effects of alcohol abuse. This increased sensitivity appears to result from an enhanced toxic effect of alcohol on the aged brain (Pfefferbaum et al., 1992, 1993; Sullivan et al., 1995).

Abstinence and Relapse

MR Imaging

While most studies of chronic alcoholics have been conducted during the post-alcohol period (e.g. during detoxification or abstinence), few studies have employed repeated MR measurements to document brain changes associated with prolonged abstinence or relapse. Several of these studies reported reversibilty of alcohol-induced ventricular enlargements (Schroth et al., 1988; Mann et al., 1989; Zipursky et al., 1989). The Zipursky study also demonstrated ventricular volume stability over time in controls, suggesting that ventricular volume normalization in abstinent alcoholics is associated with abstinence (Zipursky et al., 1989). A study of alcoholic women repeatedly scanned over a 6-week interval noted no ventricular volume changes; however, baseline ventricular volumes in those women were nearly normal and abstinence-associated changes may have been too small to detect (Kroft et al., 1991). Subsequent longitudinal studies of abstinent alcoholics reported improved brain white matter, ventricular, sulcal, and anterior gray matter cortical volumes (Shear et al., 1994; Pfefferbaum et al., 1995). By contrast, studies of relapsed alcoholics noted persistent white matter and ventricular abnormalities (Shear et al., 1994) and white matter volume reductions (Pfefferbaum et al., 1995). In a long-term (5-yr) longitudinal study, Pfefferbaum (1998) noted a correlation between alcohol consumption and cortical gray matter volume changes in relapsed alcoholics, and also found that abstinent alcoholics experienced ventricular volume rates of change comparable to those found in controls (Pfefferbaum et al., 1998).

MR Spectroscopy

Martin and colleagues (1995) first used ^{1}H MRS to study neurochemical changes in alcoholics during prolonged abstinence. Elevated cerebellar vermis choline/*N*-acetylaspartate (Cho/NAA) ratios were noted, along with a correlation between Cho/NAA ratios and neuropsychological test performance (Martin et al., 1995). The findings were interpreted to suggest remyelination or reversal of cholinergic deafferentation, although the authors pointed out that the Cho/NAA ratio might also have reflected NAA abnormalities (Martin et al., 1995). Elevated Cho/NAA ratios were subsequently detected in the cerebellum, frontal lobe, and thalamus in abstinent alcoholics (Jagannathan et al., 1996). That study also reported decreased NAA levels in all three brain regions, suggestive of neuronal loss (Jagannathan et al., 1996). The presence of NAA abnormalities suggests that metabolite ratios using NAA in the denominator might not provide stable measures in alcoholics. Seitz and colleagues (1999) reported both reduced cerebellar volumes and reduced NAA/Cr ratios in recently abstinent alcoholics, consistent with neuronal loss. Phosphorus (^{31}P) MRS has also been used to evaluate the neurochemical effects of chonic alcohol abuse. White matter phosphocreatine (PCr) and phosphodiester (PDE) levels were reduced in alcoholics, and correlations between white matter PDE levels and both age and ventricular volumes were found (Meyerhoff et al., 1995). PCr abnormalities implied bioenergetic dysfunction while abnormal PDE levels were interpreted to reflect either altered phospholipid concentration or phospholipid relaxation rates (Meyerhoff et al., 1995).

Special Syndromes Associated with Alcohol Abuse

Hepatic Cirrhosis and Encephalopathy

MR Imaging

Cerebral volume changes including frontal and parietal sulcal width increases were described in nonencephalopathic cirrhotic alcoholics (Moore et al., 1989). Cirrhotic alcoholics were found to have more frontal and parietal lobe morphologic abnormalities than noncirrhotic alcoholics (Barthauer et al., 1992). One study noted associations between brain atrophy and both memory and frontal-premotor function (Kulisevsky et al., 1992). In addition to cerebral volume abnormalities, symmetric globus pallidus T1 hyperintensites have been described in alcoholics with chronic hepatic encephalopathy (CHE) (Zeneroli et al., 1991). Additionally, correlations between pallidal signal intensity and plasma ammonia levels (Kulisevsky et al., 1992), severity of hepatic dysfunction (Pujol et al., 1993), and brain atrophy (Kulisevsky et al., 1993) have been identified. Reversibility of the T1 abnormality was confirmed by a study documenting the disappearance of pallidal T1 hyperintensites following liver transplantation (Pujol et al., 1993). Two reports failed to find correlations between pallidal T1 abnormalities and cognitive dysfunction, suggesting that T1 abnormalities are associated with, but not markers for, CHE (Thuluvath et al., 1995; Krieger et al., 1996). Abnormal basal ganglia, thalamic, and white matter T1 and T2 relaxation times were also noted in cirrhotic patients and were attributed to elevated manganese levels (Vymazal et al., 1996). The manganese deposition hypothesis was supported by a postmortem study (in non-alcoholic cirrhotic patients) revealing elevated manganese levels only in patients whose MRIs showed pallidal T1 hyperintensities (Maeda et al., 1997).

MR Spectroscopy

MR spectroscopy has been characterized as an "ideal modality" for evaluating CHE because it is capable of monitoring neurochemical events related to the pathogenesis of the disorder (Seery and Taylor-Robinson, 1996). Kreis and coworkers (1992) reported increased parietal cortex glutamine (Glx) levels and decreased myo-inositol (mI) and choline levels (Cho) in CHE (Kreis et al., 1992). Subsequently, reduced parietal white matter Cho/total creatine (Cr), parietal white and occipital gray matter mI/Cr, and elevated Glx/Cr ratios were noted in CHE (Ross et al., 1994). Ross and colleagues (1994) proposed that ^{1}H MRS may be helpful in detecting early brain changes in this disorder, a conclusion that was subsequently supported by a study finding ^{1}H MRS abnormalities in patients who were judged to be unimpaired on neuropsychological tests (Geissler et al., 1997). The mI/Cr ratio was not normalized in patients receiving liver tranplants, although the Cho/Cr ratio was increased in these subjects (Huda et al., 1998). Using ^{1}H MR spectroscopic imaging (MRSI), Taylor-Robinson (1994a) detected increased Glx/Cr and reduced Cho/Cr ratios in the basal ganglia and in temporal and occipital cortices. A subsequent ^{31}P MRS study by this group found reduced whole brain and basal ganglia phosphomono- (PME) and diesters (PDE), expressed as PME/nucleoside polyphosphate (β-NP) and PDE/β-NP ratios, respectively, suggestive of abberant phospholipid metabolism; this report also noted an association between phospholipid abnormality and disease severity (Taylor-Robinson et al., 1994b). A study employing both ^{1}H MRS and ^{1}H-decoupled-^{31}P MRS documented reduced mI and Cho, increased Glx, and reduced phosphocreatine (PCr) and β-NP levels in CHE (Bluml et al., 1998). That metabolite profile led the authors to conclude that CHE was associated with cerebral osmoregulatory and energetic disturbances (Bluml et al., 1998).

Wernicke and Korsakoff's Syndromes

Wernicke's encephalopathy and Korsakoff's psychosis, or the Wernicke-Korsakoff syndrome, result from nutritional deficiencies, particularly thiamine deficiencies. The syndrome can be precipitated by glucose administration to thiamine-deficient alcoholics. These syndromes are not exclusive to alcoholism, having been documented with MR imaging in nonalcoholic individuals with severe nutritional deficiencies (Doraiswamy et al., 1994) and in patients with thalamic lesions not resulting from alcoholism (Cole et al., 1992). Early studies of alcoholic Korsakoff's syndrome patients indicated increased whole brain and frontal white matter T1 values (Christie et al., 1988; Besson et al., 1989). T1 increases also have been described in several other brain regions in Korsakoff's patients including parietal white matter, caudate nucleus, and thalamus (Emsley et al., 1996).

The anatomical change most widely associated with the Wernicke-Korsakoff syndrome is mamillary body atrophy (Fig. 5). This abnormality has been suggested to be a basis for differential diagnosis of alcoholic and nonalcoholic forms of dementia (Charness and DeLaPaz, 1987; Bigler et al., 1989; Squire et al., 1990). However, mamillary body abnormalities are absent in some Korsakoff's cases (Welch et al., 1996; Matsuda et al., 1997) but are present in alcoholics who do not have the Wernicke-Korsakoff syndrome and who are not memory impaired (Davila et al., 1994).

Thalamic abnormalities as well as orbitofrontal and mesial temporal lobe gray matter volume reductions have also been reported in the Wernicke-Korsakoff syndrome (Kitaguchi et al., 1987; Donnal et al., 1990; Gallucci et al., 1990; Jernigan et al., 1991b; Kopelman et al., 1997). Lesion patterns similar to those found in Korsakoff's patients have been detected in alcoholics who are not cognitively impaired (Blansjaar et al., 1992; Davila et al., 1994; Shear et al., 1996), suggesting that at least some of the neuroanatomical changes ascribed to the Wernicke and Korsakoff's syndromes may be antecedent to the full-blown syndrome. As is the case in therapy for Marchiafava-

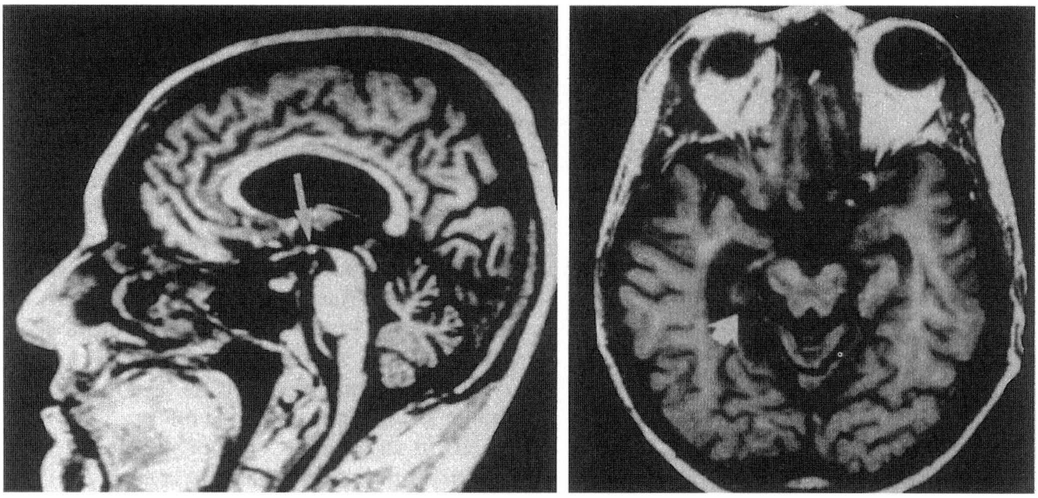

Fig. 6. MR images of a patient with alcohol-associated amnesia but absent the characteristic structural abnormalities seen in the Wernicke-Korsakoff syndrome. The sagittal T1 image **(Left)** shows a prominent mammillary body (thin arrow). The axial T1 image **(Right)** reveals a prior right temporal lobe infarct and hippocampal atrophy (thick arrow). (From Welch et al., 1996, with permission, courtesy of P. R. Martin, MD Vanderbilt University Medical Center, Nashville TN.)

Bignami Disease, nutritional intervention has been reported to reverse thalamic volume and T2 abnormalities in the Wernicke-Korsakoff syndrome (Donnal et al., 1990; Gallucci et al., 1990). One interesting case of alcohol-associated amnesia, absent the typical mamillary body and thalamic neuroanatomical abnormalities was described by Welch and colleagues (1996). This case was characterized by a right temporal lobe infarct, hippocampal atrophy (Fig. 6), and a left diencephalic metabolic asymmetry that was noted in a positron emission tomography scan. The study authors concluded that amnesia resulted from a functional asymmetry of diencephalic structures (Welch et al., 1996).

Central Pontine Myelinolysis

Central pontine myelinolysis (CPM) is a rarely occurring demyelination syndrome that is characterized by symmetric pontine lesions. It is typically though not exclusively detected in alcoholics. It has been postulated that CPM is induced by rapid correction of the electrolyte imbalance occurring in severe hyponatremia (Brunner et al., 1990). However, CPM occurs in normonatremic or partially hypernatremic patients, and it has been suggested that hypokalaemia may be significant (Bahr et al., 1990). DeWitt et al. (1984) reported the first case of CPM diagnosed with MR imaging, which was characterized by abnormal pontine signals that partially resolved during treatment. Extrapontine lesions have been found in CPM patients in the cerebellar peduncles (Steller et al., 1988), the basal ganglia (Price et al., 1987; Demaerel et al., 1992; Tien et al., 1992) and the thalamus (Rippe et al., 1987; Koci et al., 1990; Demaerel et al., 1992; Tien et al., 1992; Mascalchi et al., 1993). One report documented gadolinium-DTPA enhancement of pontine lesions, indicating local blood-brain-barrier compromise

(Mascalchi et al., 1993). T2 hypointensities were described early in the course of CPM prior to symptom emergence (Rouanet et al., 1994). This stands in contrast to the pontine T2-*hyper*intense signals typically observed after symptom onset. An abnormally low pontine magnetization transfer ratio (MTR) was noted in a case of CPM, indicative of demyelination (Silver et al., 1996).

Marchiafava-Bignami Disease

Marchiafava-Bignami disease (MBD) is a rare hemispheric disconnection syndrome typically associated with chronic alcoholism. The characteristic corpus callosum lesion appears hypodense or hyperdense on T1- or T2-weighted images, respectively, suggestive of callosal demyelination. Because MBD symptoms are quite variable, prior to the advent of noninvasive brain imaging techniques such as X-ray computerized tomography (CT) or MR imaging, antemortem diagnosis was not possible. A number of early MR descriptions of this syndrome were published (Kawamura et al., 1985; Bracard et al., 1986; Mayer et al., 1987; Baron et al., 1989; Ikeda et al., 1989). One longitudinal study of two MBD patients revealed the early phase of the disorder characterized by callosal T2 hyperintensities, indicative of callosal swelling at hospital admission (Chang et al., 1992). This was followed by reduced callosal swelling within a week, followed later by focal T2 hypointensities indicative of callosal atrophy and necrosis (Chang et al., 1992). Gadolinium enhancement of callosal lesions was noted during an early phase of the disorder, suggestive of blood brain barrier compromise (Caparros-Lefebvre et al., 1994). Transient callosal T2-weighted image hyperintensities have been reported in several acute MBD cases, reflecting reversible white matter edema (Tobita et al., 1997; Yamashita et al., 1997; Gass et al., 1998). Alcohol discontinuation and nutritional supplementation (including thiamine treatment and/or vitamin B substitution therapy) appear to contribute to recovery from this syndrome (Kawamura et al., 1985; Izquierdo et al., 1992; Pappata et al., 1994; Tobita et al., 1997; Gass et al., 1998).

Fetal Alcohol Exposure

The numbers of pregnant women who consume alcohol and who binge drink are increasing (Ebrahim et al., 1998; 1999). Accordingly, it is expected that the case report literature of brain abnormalities associated with fetal alcohol exposure will grow steadily. One of the first reports of MR follow up in a case of chronic fetal alcohol exposure noted multifocal T2 hyperintensities and poor gray-white matter differentiation (Gabrielli et al., 1990). Partial agenesis and displacement of the corpus callosum was described in an infant born to a binge-drinking mother (Schaefer et al., 1991). A hypoplastic corpus callosum, agenesis of the corpus callosum, and/or reduced caudate nucleus, thalamic, diencephalic, cranial and cerebellar vault volumes have been found in subjects exposed prenatally to alcohol (Mattson et al., 1992, 1994, 1996). Anterior cerebellar vermis volume was significantly reduced in adolescents exposed prenatally to alcohol compared to controls (Sowell et al., 1996). Two surveys comparing MR findings and craniofacial features in fetal alcohol syndrome patients revealed abnormalities consistent with midline developmental field disruptions (Johnson et al., 1996; Swayze et al., 1997). Although prenatal alcohol exposure is difficult to mimic in the laboratory, a nonhuman primate study of controlled fetal alcohol exposure documented normal brain morphology (Astley et al., 1995). However, that study also reported elevated basal ganglia ^{1}H MRS choline (Cho) over total creatine (Cr) ratios, as well as associations between Cho/Cr ratios and both duration of alcohol exposure and degree of developmental impairment (Astley et al., 1995).

Methanol

Methanol intoxication occurs when methanol-containing preparations are substituted for alcohol, in cases of accidental ingestion, or in suicide attempts. An early case report with MR follow-up described a woman with bilateral lesions of the claustrum, external capsule, putamen, and head of the caudate nucleus, who presented clinically with a Parkinson-like syndrome (Mozaz et al., 1991). Bilateral and symmetric putaminal lesions (Pelletier et al., 1992) as well as basal ganglia hemorrhages and white matter degeneration in the frontal and parietal lobes have been noted (Glazer and Dross, 1993). Methanol-induced lesions also have been reported in the pontine tegmentum, cerebellar white matter, and the optic nerves (Gaul et al., 1995), as well as in the hypothalamus (Anderson et al., 1997). The latter study reported gadolinium enhancing lesions indicating blood–brain barrier breakdown (Anderson et al., 1997). Methanol intoxication may be associated with delayed lesion development, as a case report documented MR-detectable putaminal, cingulate and white matter lesions 2 d after a normal CT examination (Rubinstein et al., 1995). Hantson et al. (1997) noted that regression of methanol-induced MR lesions at followup was associated with lower probability for developing extrapyramidal disturbances (Hantson et al., 1997).

Marijuana and Hallucinogens

In spite of the widespread use of marijuana and the increasing popularity of hallucinogens, only a handful of MR reports have been published studying the effects of these drugs. A single MR report from our group has examined the effects of marijuana use. In that study, chronic marijuana users were found to have abnormal dorsolateral prefrontal cortex BOLD fMRI activation during a working memory task (Fig. 7), when studied after both short- and long-term abstinence (24 h and 28 d, respectively). Those findings suggested that chronic marijuana use resulted in persistently abnormal brain activation patterns during a cognitive challenge (Yurgelun-Todd et al., 1998).

A case report of anabolic steroid abuse (classified as hallucinogen abuse by the National Institute on Drug Abuse) utilized MR imaging to document a right basal ganglia ischemic infarction, in a young man with a 6 wk history of steroid abuse who presented with left hemiparesis (Akhter et al., 1994). A study in anesthetized rodents using long echo time gradient echo fMRI imaging found increased cerebral blood flow (rCBF) in the hippocampus, cortex, and olfactory bulb following ketamine administration, which implied a selective receptor-mediated effect of the drug on rCBF (Burdett et al., 1995). A case report of acute inflammatory CNS disease in association with methylenedioxymethamphetamine (MDMA) abuse was described (Bitsch et al., 1996). Low baseline ^{1}H MRS choline (Cho) levels were found in a case report of a chronic MDMA abuser, and total creatine (Cr) levels were elevated in that subject 2 wk after an acute MDMA (0.5 mg/kg) challenge (Grob et al., 1996).

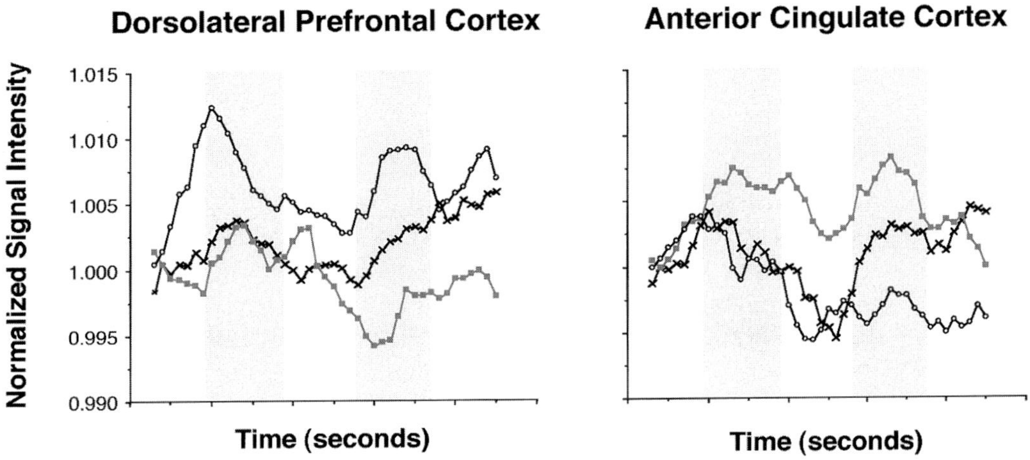

Fig. 7. Functional MRI detects abnormal dorsolateral prefrontal cortex activity in chronic heavy marijuana users. Heavy marijuana smokers ($N = 8$) tested at abstinence d 1 and 28 showed decreased dorsolateral prefrontal cortex activity during a spatial working memory task (shaded bar epochs) compared to controls. The anterior cingulate cortex was activated in marijuana smokers but not in controls. Open circles, control subjects; crosses, smokers, abstinence day 1; filled squares, smokers, abstinence d 28. (Courtesy of D. A. Yurgelun-Todd, PhD, Brain Imaging Center, McLean Hospital, Belmont, MA.)

Benzodiazepines

Two MR studies of the acute effects of benzodiazepines on brain function have been published. The first study determined that acute diazepam (10 or 20 mg) administration had no effect on ^{31}P MRS metabolites (Deicken et al., 1992). The second study used the dynamic susceptibility contrast fMRI (DSC MRI) method, in which MR constrast agents can be used to detect relative changes in cerebral blood volume (CBV), to map CBV changes following an alprazolam challenge. Alprazolam (1 mg) reduced global, left caudate nucleus, and left inferior prefrontal cortex CBV in subjects who were family history positive for alcoholism, 1 h after drug administration, and reduced right inferior prefrontal and anterior cingulate CBV in controls 2 h after drug administration (Streeter et al., 1998).

Heroin and Opiates

Acute Effects

An fMRI study by Sell and colleagues (1997) reported an acute heroin-induced reduction in the BOLD fMRI photic stimulation response in opiate-dependent subjects. The study could not determine whether fMRI signal changes were attributable to drug-induced changes in cerebral blood flow, changes in cerebrovascular reactivity, changes in cerebral activation, or some combination of those events.

Cerebrovascular Effects

While reports of major cerebrovascular complications accompanying heroin use are rare, several case reports have documented vascular effects of the drug. White matter demyelination was found in two chronic heroin abusers, and was attributed to vascular pathology (Volkow et al., 1988b). A case of anterior choroidal artery infarction was reported in a heroin abuser who "sniffed" the drug (Bartolomei et al., 1992). Heroin "snorting" has also been associated with the development of globus pallidus infarcts (Benassi et al., 1996; Zuckerman et al., 1996). Vila and Chamorro reported two cases of basal ganglia ischemic strokes associated with intravenous heroin administration (Vila and Chamorro, 1997). In both cases, patients demonstrated ballistic movements, yet the subthalamic nuclei were spared, an unusual finding in cases of vascular ballism (Vila and Chamorro, 1997). Additional cases of basal ganglia infarctions in heroin abusers have been reported along with a single case of thoracic spinal cord infarction (Niehaus et al., 1997; Niehaus and Meyer, 1998).

Leukoencephalopathy

Toxic leukoencephalopathy has been described in heroin abusers who inhale vaporized heroin using a method known as "Chinese Blowing" or "Chasing the Dragon." This syndrome is infrequently observed, is found only in patients who abuse the drug via this route, and is often found in clusters of cases. Consequently, it has been concluded that unidentified lipophilic adulterants activated by pyrolysis are the toxic agents (Tan et al., 1994). In the earliest report of this phenomenon with MRI followup, symmetric cerebellar and cerebral white matter lesions were noted in two patients (Hungerbuhler and Waespe, 1990). One of four patients studied by Tan (1994) and one patient studied by Celius (1996) had improved MRIs at follow-up along with other clinical improvements, suggesting that leukoencephalopathy may at least partially resolve. An interesting finding in the latter study was the observation that the girlfriend of the affected subject, who used greater amounts of the same batch of heroin, did not develop leukoencephalopathy or have an abnormal neurological examination, implying that sex differences might play a role in this syndrome (Celius and Andersson, 1996). This syndrome was reported in an infant whose mother was heroin-dependent; however, the child made a full recovery (Roulet Perez et al., 1992).

A more recent report of the first occurance of this phenomenon in Taiwan suggests that heroin-induced toxic leukoencephalopathy may be underdiagnosed, particularly in regions in which this method of heroin self-administration is common (Chang et al., 1997b). Kriegstein and colleagues (1997) presented two case reports of heroin-induced progressive spongiform leukoencephalopathy (Fig. 8), one of which improved clinically following coenzyme Q therapy. These authors underscored the point that inhalation of heroin vapors is gaining popularity in the United States, and that more people may be at risk for developing leukoencephalopathy (Kriegstein et al., 1997). Subsequently, this group employed ^{1}H MRS to document increased lactate and reduced *N*-acetylaspartate (NAA) levels in cortex and cerebellar white matter in three leukoencephalopathic subjects, which they interpreted as reflecting increased glycolysis and neuronal damage, respectively (Shungu et al., 1998). Metabolite normalization was

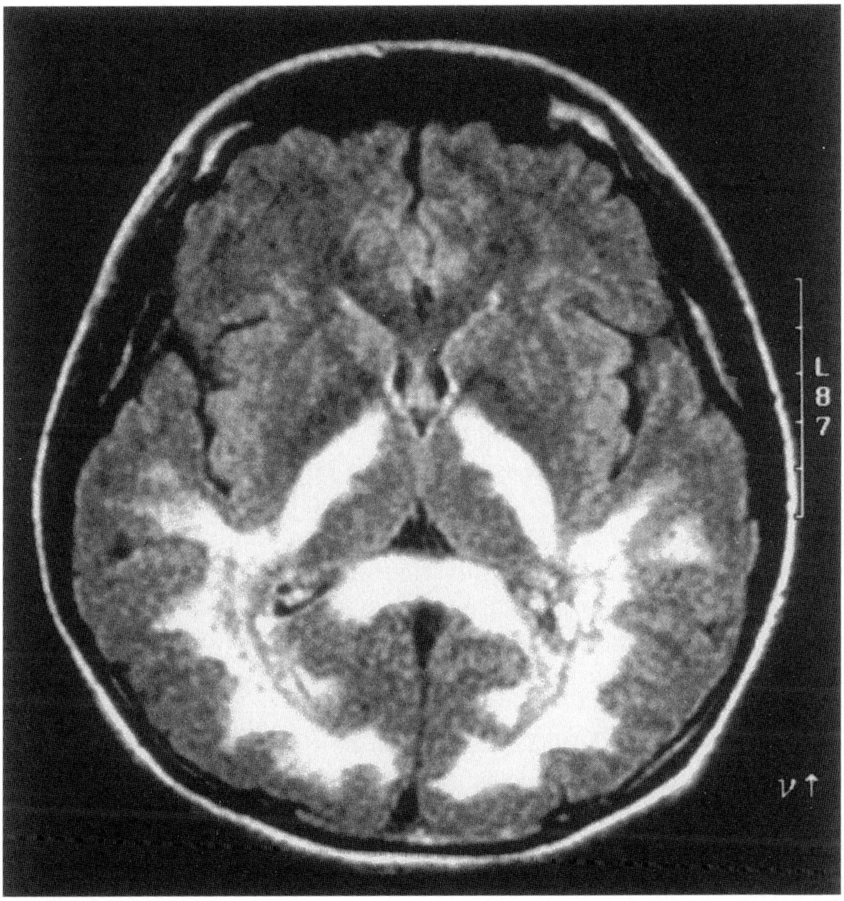

Fig. 8. Heroin pyrolysis-induced progressive spongiform encephalopathy. This axial fluid attenuated inversion recovery (FLAIR) image shows the characteristic lesion including symmetric involvement of the posterior cerebral white matter, internal capsule, and splenium of the corpus callosum. (Courtesy of A. R. Kriegstein, MD, PhD, Columbia University College of Physicians and Surgeons, New York, NY.)

not noted in follow-up scans from two of those subjects, although both had improved clinically (Shungu et al., 1998). Weber and colleagues presented a classic case of heroin leukoencephalopathy along with a comprehensive review of the epidemiology and biology of the disorder (Weber et al., 1998).

These reports illustrate an important confound in studies of substance abuse; namely, that adulterants must be considered as factors in pathology associated with illicit substance abuse, because they can have profound and deleterious effects. The potential effects of contaminants, as well as the confound introduced by polydrug abuse, underscore the importance of conducting controlled clinical studies of abused substances in which these factors are not present, in order to accurately characterize the biological effects of the substance of interest.

Chronic Effects

A number of literature reports have described MR imaging or spectroscopy findings in chronic heroin-dependent subjects (Amass et al., 1992; Teoh et al., 1993; Christensen et al., 1996; Liu et al., 1998; Kaufman et al., 1999). Because the subjects in those studies were polydrug abusers, their findings are reviewed in the Polydrug Abuse section of this chapter.

COCAINE

Acute Effects

Cocaine is profoundly vasoactive, which likely explains the increased incidence of stroke and cerebrovascular dysfunction observed in cocaine abusers (Daras, 1996). While the incidence of stroke associated with cocaine abuse is low *(see below)*, there is mounting evidence suggesting that chronic repetitive cocaine abuse may be associated with subtle (Volkow et al., 1988a; Holman et al., 1991; Levin et al., 1995) but progressive (Kaufman et al., 1998c) cerebrovascular dysfunction. Consequently, cocaine-associated stroke may result from cumulative insults to the cerebral vasculature during chronic drug use that compromise its integrity to withstand the acute effects of the drug. However, for the purposes of this review, reports of stroke will be categorized as an acute effect of the drug.

Mody and colleagues (1988) presented one of the earliest reports of cocaine-associated stroke with MR follow-up, documenting a left medullary hemorrhagic infarct in a man who experienced strokelike symptoms shortly after snorting cocaine and drinking beer. This report and others have highlighted coabuse of cocaine and alcohol, and because both drugs are vasoactive, their combination may induce additive deleterious effects. The Mody study (1988) estimated a startlingly high stroke incidence (36%) in self-reported first time cocaine users, a prevalence much higher than the overall incidence (<3%) reported in epidemiological studies of hospital admissions involving neurologic complications related to cocaine use (Jacobs et al., 1989; Peterson et al., 1991). These reports do not include cases of asymptomatic stroke, such as the ones depicted in Fig. 9, suggesting that the true incidence of cocaine-associated stroke may be higher than suggested by epidemiological studies. In this regard, Chang and colleagues (1999) described an incidence rate of asymptomatic stroke of 3% (Fig. 9) in a group of currently abstinent former cocaine users and also noted a case of asymptomatic stroke in a methamphetamine abuser (*see* Fig. 10). Another report documented a fourfold higher incidence of clinically silent cerebrovascular abnormalities, as reflected by the presence of T2 hyperintensities, in cocaine-dependent (CD) subjects as compared to controls, and that older CD subjects experienced more cerebrovascular abnormalities than younger subjects (Bartzokis et al., 1999). However, in contrast to the Chang study (1999) which excluded subjects with a history of alcohol abuse, nearly half of the CD subjects in the Bartzokis study had histories of current or prior alcohol dependence, precluding a determination as to whether cerebrovascular abnormalities were associated with cocaine, alcohol, or their combined abuse. Yet together, these findings suggest that the incidence of stimulant-associated stroke may be substantial, including a large proportion of clinically silent stroke cases.

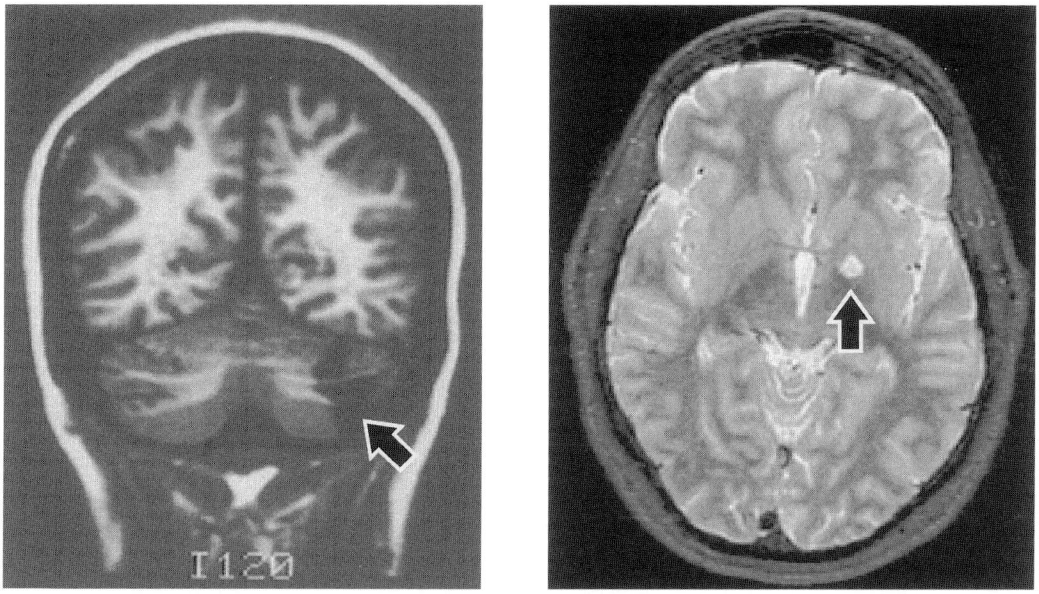

Fig. 9. Two cases of asymptomatic strokes occurring in chronic cocaine abusers. **(Left)** A coronal inversion recovery image through the cerebellum shows an old infarct as a dark spot in the left cerebellar hemisphere (arrow) in a 32-yr-old woman with a history of chronic cocaine abuse. **(Right)** An axial T2-weighted image shows a left globus pallidus infarct in a 33-yr-old man with a 2-year history of crack cocaine smoking. (Right image courtesy of L. Chang, MD and T. Ernst, PhD, Harbor UCLA Medical Center, Torrance, CA.)

Additional reports of symptomatic cocaine-associated strokes in the thalamus, cerebellum, white matter, and occipital cortex have been published (Klonoff et al., 1989; Nalls et al., 1989; Aggarwal and Byrne, 1991). The patient in the latter case had a normal conventional angiogram leading the authors to conclude that stroke symptoms were likely caused by transient vasoconstriction (Aggarwal and Byrne, 1991). Cocaine use in the form of "crack" has also been associated with stroke, as documented in a report of pontine intraparenchymal hemorrhage (Ramadan et al., 1991). While leukoencephalopathy is typically associated with certain modes of heroin abuse (*see above*), two cases of cocaine-associated leukoencephalopathy have been reported (Yamazaki et al., 1994; Nuytten et al., 1998). The latter case featured fronto-temporal white matter lesions that improved at 5-mo followup (Nuytten et al., 1998).

Research Studies

MR Spectroscopy

We have employed ^{1}H MRS to assess whether acute administration of small doses of cocaine to healthy young subjects could alter basal ganglia ^{1}H MRS metabolites. We found elevated choline (Cho) and *N*-acetylaspartate (NAA) levels, and attributed those

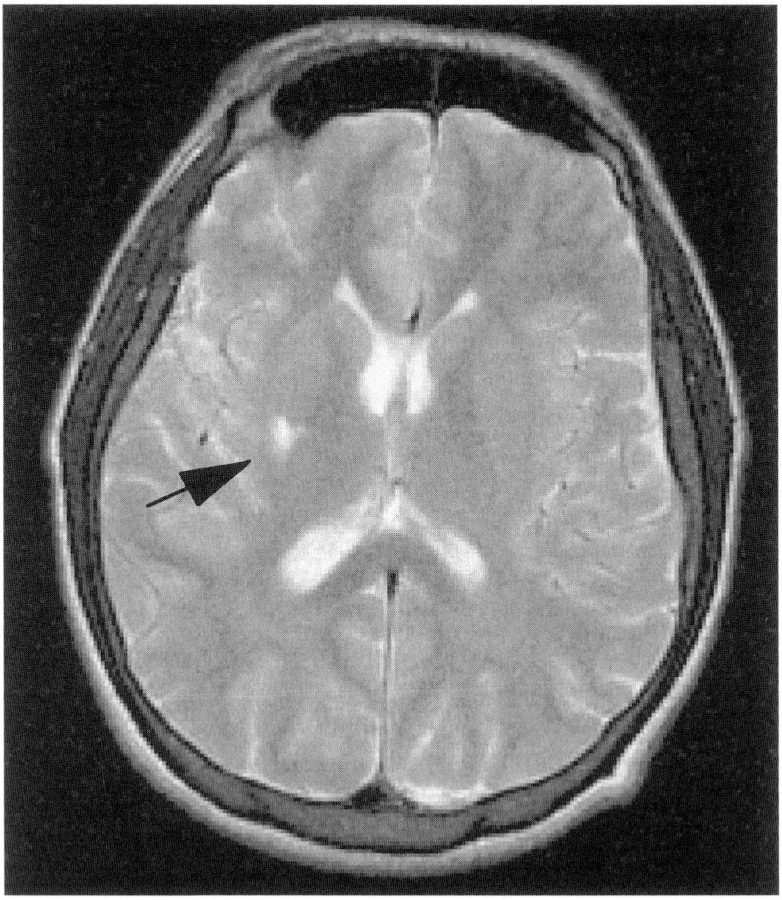

Fig. 10. Asymptomatic stroke in association with chronic methamphetamine abuse. Axial T2-weighted image from a 24-yr-old man with a 2-yr history of chronic methamphetamine abuse. A silent infact, visible as an area of increased signal intensity (arrow) is present in the right putamen. The subject had been abstinent for 1 yr at the time of scanning. (Courtesy of L. Chang, MD and T. Ernst, PhD, Harbor UCLA Medical Center, Torrance, CA.)

changes to osmotic stress and neuronal swelling (Christensen et al., 1997). Similar cocaine-induced increases in basal ganglia and thalamic NAA/total creatine ratios (NAA/Cr) have been reported in chronic cocaine users, although baseline NAA/Cr ratios in the basal ganglia, frontal lobe, and thalamus in those subjects were lower than control levels (Li et al., 1996, 1998).

Functional MRI

Breiter and colleagues published the first fMRI study of the acute effects of cocaine on human brain activation using the BOLD technique (Breiter et al., 1997). This report described rapid and transient activation of numerous brain regions, including the cingulate and lateral prefrontal cortex, basal forebrain, caudate nucleus, ventral tegmentum, and pons. In contrast, more gradual but sustained activation of the nucleus

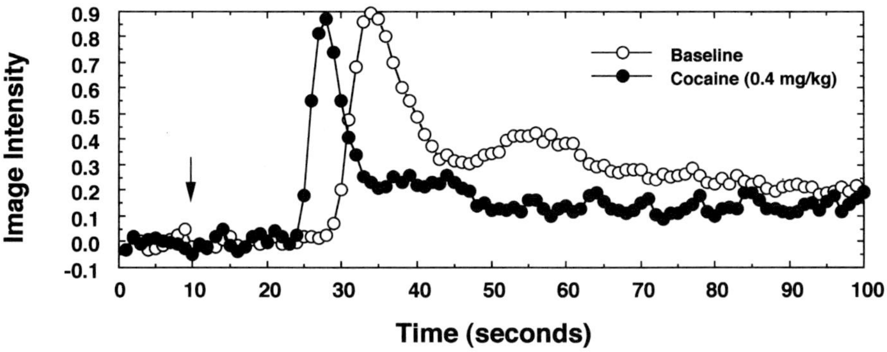

Fig. 11. Detection of cocaine-induced cerebral vasoconstriction with Dynamic Susceptibility Contrast MRI (DSC MRI). A gadolinium chelate was intravenously administered 10 s into each acquisition (arrow) and used to map cerebral blood volume (CBV). The data shown are from a 29-yr-old man at baseline *(open circles)* and 10 min after intravenous cocaine (0.4 mg/kg) administration (*filled circles*). After cocaine, the area under the curve (integrated over the first 12 s) was 30% smaller indicating cerebral vasoconstriction. Cocaine induced a heart rate increase in this subject which resulted in the contrast bolus appearing in the imaging plane earlier than at baseline.

accumbens was noted, leading the authors to conclude that they had mapped the regions participating in the early and late behavioral effects of cocaine, "rush" and "craving," respectively (Breiter et al., 1997). In a preliminary study, this group also reported cocaine activation of brainstem areas including the locus coeruleus and raphe nuclei (Breiter et al., 1998). They also reported that cocaine's vascular effects did not confound the ability to detect photic stimulation-induced occipital cortex activation, when measured 25 min after drug administration (Gollub et al., 1998). However, these data do not address whether cocaine's immediate vascular effects, which are profound, complicate measurement of occipital cortex or other brain activation responses in BOLD fMRI paradigms. In this regard, in a preliminary communication we reported that visual cortex BOLD fMRI activation is sensitive to the effects of cocaine if measurements are made at the time of peak plasma drug levels and cardiovascular effects (Levin et al., 1999).

In acute cocaine administration studies, it is important to be aware of potential confounds such as vascular dysfunction, since a number of reports have documented vasoconstrictive effects of the drug in human brain. For example, we noted a global cocaine-induced reduction of cerebral blood volume (CBV), indicative of vasoconstriction, using DSC MRI (Kaufman et al., 1998b) (Fig. 11). In that study, we found a negative correlation between the degree of global cerebral vasoconstriction and subjective ratings of cocaine-induced "high." We interpreted this finding to suggest that the cocaine "high" was associated with brain activation and increased CBV; this partially opposed cocaine's vasoconstrictive effect which is accompanied by a CBV reduction (Kaufman et al., 1998b). Subsequent preliminary DSC MRI findings from our group documented smaller vasoconstrictive effects of cocaine in women compared to men, as well as a minimal vasoconstrictive effect in women during the follicular menstrual cycle phase (Kaufman et al., 1998a). Those sex and menstrual cycle phase

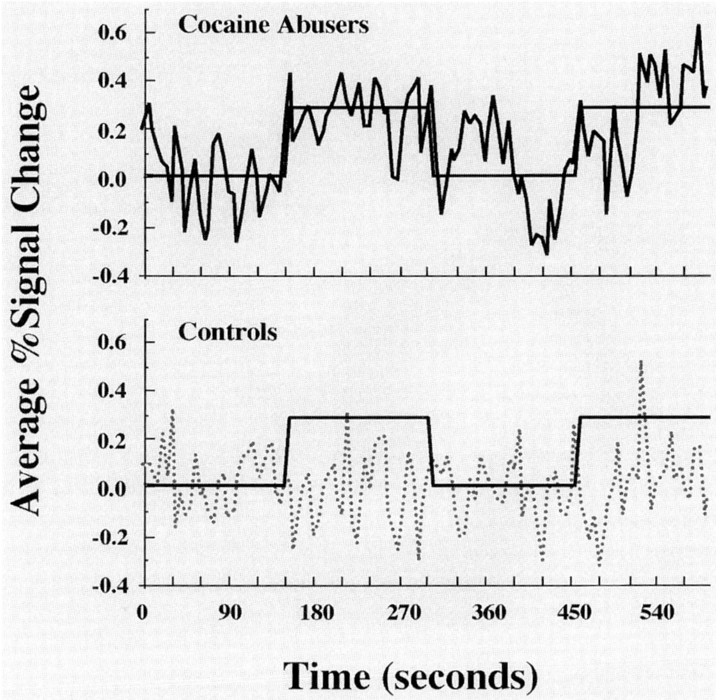

Fig. 12. Functional MRI detection of cue-induced cocaine "craving". An audiovisual program containing alternating scenes of neutral cues (epochs 1 and 3, 0–150 and 300–450 s, respectively) and cocaine-related cues (epochs 2 and 4, 150–300 and 450–600 s, respectively) was shown to subjects who were undergoing a BOLD fMRI study. Only subjects with histories of chronic cocaine abuse (top) showed consistent activation in the anterior cingulate cortex, and this activation only occurred during epochs containing cocaine related cues. Shown are composite results averaged from six subjects in each group. (Courtesy of L. C. Maas III, MD, PhD, McLean Hospital Brain Imaging Center, Belmont, MA.)

differences are consistent with prior reports of greater cerebrovascular sensitivity to cocaine in men (Levin et al., 1994) and modulation of cocaine's effects by gonadal steroids (Church and Subramanian, 1997). We suggested that gonadal steroids might modulate the effects of cocaine on cerebral hemodynamics (Kaufman et al., 1998a), which if true would suggest novel therapeutic approaches for the treatment of cocaine-induced cerebrovascular dysfunction.

Cocaine Craving

Cocaine "craving" is a behavioral phenomonon in which cocaine users, upon exposure to cues they associate with illicit cocaine use, feel strongly compelled to use more cocaine. Maas and colleagues (1998) used the BOLD fMRI technique to map brain activation during cue-induced cocaine "craving" (Maas et al., 1998). That study found increased brain activation in the cingulate and left dorsolateral prefrontal cortices (Fig. 12) during the presentation of an audiovisual program containing cocaine "cues" in cocaine abusers, but not in controls (Maas et al., 1998). The anatomical activation pattern paralleled findings from emission tomographic studies (Grant et al., 1996; Childress et al., 1999), suggesting that the fMRI technique may be useful both for measuring the craving response and for determining the efficacy of treatments designed to diminish cocaine craving. The results also suggest the presence of an additional confound in BOLD fMRI studies using cocaine-dependent subjects; namely, that craving-associated brain BOLD fMRI activation may complicate detection of drug-induced BOLD fMRI brain activation.

MR Angiography

In addition to our studies of cocaine's effects on microvasculature, we have also been interested in the drug's effects on large cerebral vessel reactivity, and have used MR Angiography (MRA), which permits detection of blood flow abnormalities in large cerebral arteries, to study such effects. The MRA signal is derived from flowing blood, and this signal is used to create an image of cerebral arterial, or, using different image acquisition parameters, venous structure. MRA has been used clinically to suggest a diagnosis of cerebral vasculitis in a cocaine abuser (Gradon and Wityk, 1995). Subsequently, we used MRA experimentally and found that low doses of cocaine could promote cerebral artery vasoconstriction in healthy, young subjects (Fig. 13). Surprisingly, we found high incidences of vessel narrowing in healthy men administered cocaine doses within the range of those typically used in illicit settings; vessel narrowing was observed in more than half of the subjects administered 0.4 mg/kg cocaine and in one third of the subjects receiving half of that dose. These data suggested a dose-effect relationship between cocaine and arterial vasoconstriction. We also determined that as few as 10 lifetime cocaine exposures increased the likelihood of experiencing cerebral artery vasoconstriction (Kaufman et al., 1998c). Those findings provide a basis to explain the increased frequency of stroke in cocaine abuse populations, and suggest that cerebrovascular function is very sensitive to cocaine's effects.

Chronic Effects

An MR imaging study documented an association between premorbid brain size, as estimated by MR measurement of the intracranial volume, and neuropsychological deficit, in abstinent, formerly cocaine-dependent subjects (Disclafani et al., 1998). The authors of this study concluded that larger premorbid brain volumes might provide a functional reserve in subjects that would at least partially protect them from cocaine-induced brain dysfunction (Disclafani et al., 1998). As noted above in Acute Effects of Cocaine, Bartzokis and colleagues (1999) reported an increased incidence of hyperintense white matter lesions on T2-weighted images in cocaine-dependent subjects. However, this study was confounded by the fact that nearly half of the subjects had a current or prior diagnosis of alcohol dependence, which itself is associated with the development of white matter hyperintensities (*see* the section White Matter Lesions).

Several studies have employed MRS to evaluate the neurochemical effects of chronic cocaine use. The first of these reports was published by MacKay and colleagues, who used phosphorus (^{31}P) MRS to document subcortical phospholipid abnormalities in chronic cocaine users (MacKay et al., 1993). Cocaine abusers abstinent for at least 3 wk had low phospholipid levels in subcortical white matter, and this was attributed

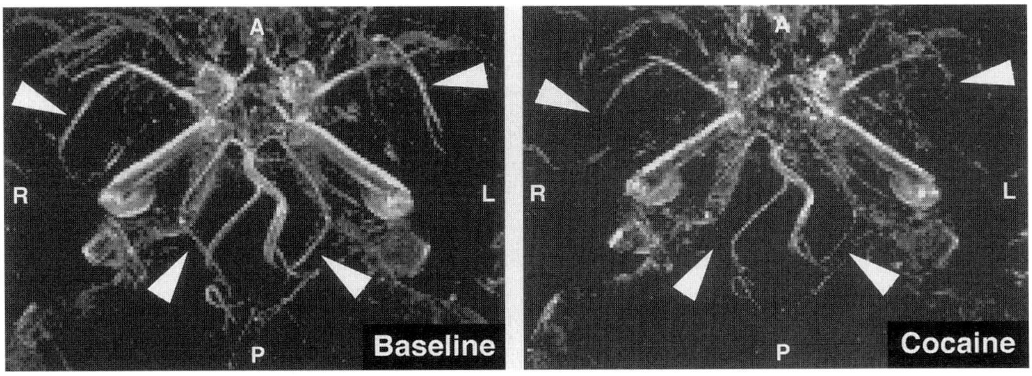

Fig. 13. Magnetic resonance angiography detection of cocaine-induced cerebral artery vasoconstriction. These axial Circle of Willis maximum intensity projection images were obtained from a healthy young man at baseline **(left)** and 20 min after intravenous cocaine (0.4 mg/kg) administration **(right)**. Cocaine induced a signal loss at distal segments of the middle cerebral arteries (upper arrowheads) and the posterior cerebral arteries (lower arrowheads), indicative of vessel narrowing. A, anterior; P, posterior; R, right; L, left. (From Kaufman et al., 1998c, with permission.)

to abnormal synthesis or breakdown of myelin phospholipids (MacKay et al., 1993). A proton spectroscopy (^{1}H MRS) study of chronic cocaine users evaluated after a median 12 mo of abstinence revealed elevated white matter total creatine (Cr) and myoinositol (Ino) levels (Chang et al., 1997a). Several correlations between ^{1}H MRS metabolites and drug use demographics were found, including negative correlations between *N*-acetylaspartate/Cr (NAA/Cr) ratios and both frequency and duration of cocaine use (Chang et al., 1997a). Another MRS study of chronic cocaine users revealed abnormally low NAA/Cr ratios in basal ganglia and frontal cortex (Li et al., 1996).

Chang and colleagues (1999) found increased gray and white matter mI levels in abstinent, asymptomatic crack users, which they interpreted to indicate neuronal loss and glial proliferation. Li et al. (1999) reported reduced thalamic NAA levels in cocaine-dependent subjects, an abnormality that was interpreted to reflect neurotoxicity. Sex differences were noted in the Chang (1999) study, including elevated Cho levels, mI/Cr ratios, and increased percentage of cerebrospinal fluid within gray matter voxels in men, consistent with prior reports of sex differences in cocaine's effects. A ^{1}H magnetic resonance spectroscopic imaging (MRSI) study of abstinent cocaine-dependent and cocaine/alcohol codependent subjects revealed low frontal cortical gray matter NAA/Cr ratios in both groups compared with controls, and reduced frontal cortical gray and white matter NAA/Cho ratios in cocaine/alcohol codependent subjects (Meyerhoff et al., 1998). That study also noted positive correlations between frontal cortical NAA/Cr ratios and abstinence duration as well as between frontal Cho levels and duration of drug use (Meyerhoff et al., 1998). The reduced frontal cortex NAA levels and increased Cho levels were interpreted to indicate neuronal loss and gliosis (Meyerhoff et al., 1998). Importantly, all of the metabolite abnormalities reported above were found in asymptomatic subjects, suggesting that MRS measures may be sensitive indicators of brain dysfunction associated with cocaine and or alcohol abuse.

As was the case with opiate abuse, a number of literature reports have documented subtle structural and neurochemical changes in cocaine-dependent subjects who were also polydrug abusers (Amass et al., 1992; Teoh et al., 1993; Christensen et al., 1996; Liu et al., 1998; Kaufman et al., 1999), and these findings are reviewed in the section Polydrug Abuse.

Prenatal Effects

Cocaine's ability to reduce placental blood flow was graphically illustrated in a nonhuman primate MRA study, which documented a drug-induced disruption of umbilical blood flow (Panigel et al., 1993). Several reports have noted developmental abnormalities in cases of prenatal cocaine exposure. A retrospective MR imaging study found higher incidences of neonatal cerebral infarction and congenital abnormalities including encephalocele, holoprosencephaly, intraspinal lipoma, and hypoplastic cerebellum, in infants whose mothers met criteria for cocaine abuse (Heier et al., 1991). Gieron-Korthals (1994) described teratogenic findings including a large interhemispheric cyst, absence of a corpus callosum, agyria, left parietal open lip schizencephaly, and partial absence of the septum pellucidum in two infants who had chronical prenatal cocaine exposure (Gieron-Korthals et al., 1994). A subsequent case report of an 11-mo-old infant exposed to cocaine throughout gestation noted diffuse severe pachygyria and corpus callosum dysgenesis (Gomez-Anson and Ramsey, 1994). Although the findings in these case reports are remarkable, the incidence of prenatal cocaine-induced teratogenic effects appears to be low, as evidenced by two studies reporting MR imaging defects in 0 of 8 (Link et al., 1991) and only 1 of 14 (Konkol et al., 1994) neonates.

Amphetamine and Other Stimulants

Amphetamine

Amphetamine, like cocaine, is a stimulant and a potent vasoconstrictor, and can produce similar effects to those reported in cocaine abuse. For example, a case report described an association between prenatal amphetamine exposure and brain developmental abnormalities, using *in utero* MR imaging to detect alobar holoprosencephaly, a monoventricle, and fused thalami (Tsai et al., 1993). Because the fetus had trisomy 13, the authors of that study cautioned that the association between prenatal amphetamine exposure and holoprosencephaly might have been concidental (Tsai et al., 1993). In adults, amphetamine-associated ischemic strokes have been described in two case reports (Lambrecht et al., 1993; Heye and Hankey, 1996). Experimental studies have also revealed amphetamine-induced cerebrovascular changes. An arterial spin labeling (ASL) perfusion imaging study in rodents, in which magnetically labelled arterial water spins served as tracers for cerebral blood flow, revealed amphetamine-induced increases in cortical, cingulate, caudate-putamen and olfactory tubercle blood flow, and decreases in hippocampal blood flow (Silva et al., 1995). A subsequent rodent fMRI study documented an amphetamine-induced increase in the BOLD fMRI signal in striatum, and in the frontal, cingulate, and parietal cortices, and those effects were abolished by dopamine nerve terminal lesions (Chen et al.,

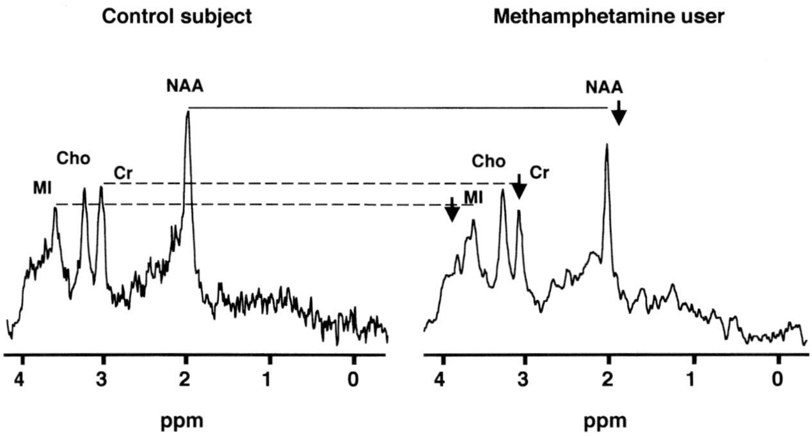

Fig. 14. Cerebral ^{1}H MRS metabolite abnormalities in a chronic methamphetamine abuser. The frontal cortex spectrum **(Right)** was obtained from a 36-year-old man with a 12-year history of heavy methamphetamine abuse (~3.5 g/d). The subject had been abstinent for 1 month prior to study. When compared with the control spectrum **(Left)**, the methamphetamine abuser had decreased *N*-acetylaspartate (NAA) levels suggesting neuronal loss and decreased myoinositol (MI) levels suggestive of glial loss. Spectrum parameters: PRESS sequence, TR/TE = 3000/30 ms. (Courtesy of L. Chang, MD and T. Ernst, PhD, Harbor UCLA Medical Center, Torrance, CA.)

1997). In humans, acute dexamphetamine administration reduced visual and auditory brain BOLD fMRI activation in control subjects (Howard et al., 1996).

Methamphetamine

Sachdeva and Woodward (1989) described a case of right thalamic T2 hyperintensity indicative of infarction, in a man who reported strokelike symptoms approx 36 h after snorting methamphetamine. Multiple cavernous angiomas were found in a chronic cocaine user who developed strokelike symptoms shortly after methamphetamine use (Ellis and Speed, 1998). Although the strokes in these two cases were symptomatic, clinically silent strokes similar to those found in cocaine abusers have been noted in association with methamphetamine abuse, such as the one shown in Fig. 10. Gadolinium-induced focal nodular enhancement of cortical sulci found in a young amphetamine abuser with AIDS was interpreted to reflect arterial ectasia and vasculitis (Lazar et al., 1992). That patient subsequently developed hemiparesis, and MR followup revealed a newly appeared right basal ganglia intracerebral hematoma (Lazar et al., 1992). ^{1}H MRS abnormalities suggestive of neuronal loss and glial dysfunction have been detected in chronic methamphetamine abusers (Fig. 14).

Methylphenidate

Methylphenidate (MPH) is the active compound in the drug Ritalin, which is prescribed widely to treat attention deficit hyperactivity disorder (ADHD). It is increasingly being used illicitly as a drug of abuse. Vaidya and colleagues (1998) used the BOLD fMRI method to evaluate the acute effects of MPH in children performing a stimulus control task. MPH decreased and increased basal ganglia activation in controls and in subjects with attention deficit hyperactivity disorder (ADHD), respectively, while it increased frontal activation in both study groups (Vaidya et al., 1998). The findings were interpreted to indicate selective modulation of the fronto-striatal connections by MPH, and dopaminergic modulation of inhibitory control in healthy children (Vaidya et al., 1998).

SOLVENT ABUSE AND OCCUPATIONAL EXPOSURE

Acute Effects

Solvent abuse is a widespread problem in adolescents, with 15–20% of high school students reporting lifetime exposure. Solvent abuse is pervasive because many easily accessible household products contain the most widely abused solvent, toluene. The acute effects of solvents have been documented with MR imaging followup in three case reports. Bilateral basal ganglia T2 hyperintensities were found in a case of 1,1,1-trichloroethane overdose induced by typewriter correction fluid inhalation (del Amo et al., 1996). Communicating hydrocephalus, cranial nerve inflammation, and gadolinium enhancement of the fifth cranial nerve were noted in a case of ethylene glycol intoxication (Lewis et al., 1997). Neurological signs were first noted in this case 10 days after hospitalization; the delayed time frame was suggested to be consistent with the time required to mount an inflammatory response to oxalate microcrystal deposition (Lewis et al., 1997). A normal follow-up MRI was acquired 3 mo later, indicating resolution of the disorder (Lewis et al., 1997). Similarly, a delay between intoxication and the detection of neuroanatomical abnormalities was noted in a subject with toluene and methyl ethyl ketone intoxication (Welch et al., 1991).

Chronic Effects

Long-term solvent abuse has been associated with loss of gray-white matter tissue differentiation, increased periventricular white matter signal intensity, and cerebral atrophy (Rosenberg et al., 1988a). These abnormalities were associated with cognitive deficits and electrophysiologic abnormalities, some of which persisted with prolonged abstinence, implying irreversible structural damage (Rosenberg et al., 1988a). Prolonged T1 and T2 relaxation times were noted in six additional subjects along with a correlation between the number of white matter abnormalities and the degree of cognitive impairment (Rosenberg et al., 1988b; Filley et al., 1990). Corpus callosum atrophy, internal capsule T2 hyperintensities, and the presence of multifocal white matter T2 hyperintensities have also been reported in chronic toluene abusers (Ikeda and Tsukagoshi, 1990; Xiong et al., 1993). Caldemeyer (1993) described a case of progressive white matter hyperintensity and extrapyramidal hypointensity and attributed the latter finding to excess brain iron deposition. The iron hypothesis was subsequently challenged by Unger et al. (1994) who suggested that toluene partitioning directly into lipid membranes caused T2 shortening. A gadolinium enhancing lesion was described in one case report along with a worsening of imaging findings in two patients who continued to abuse toluene (Caldemeyer et al., 1996).

Chronic low level occupational solvent exposure has been associated with both symptomatic (Leira et al., 1992) and asymptomatic (Thuomas et al., 1996) MR imaging abnormalities, including cerebellar atrophy, basal ganglia and thalamic T2-

hypointensities, and white matter T2-hyperintensities. A rare case of prenatal organic solvent exposure noted bilateral temporal lobe defects resembling other embryopathies, suggesting that prenatal toluene exposure may be teratogenic (Arai et al., 1997). Numerous additional reports of solvent abuse with MR follow-up have been published and can be found in the bibliography at the end of the book.

Polydrug Abuse

Polydrug abuse is probably the most typical form of illicit substance abuse, yet it is difficult if not impossible to mimic under controlled laboratory situations. The reader should note that with the exception of studies involving acute drug challenges performed in subjects with minimal drug use histories, most clinical research studies of substance abuse are likely to be portraying at least in part the results of polydrug abuse.

MR Imaging

The absence of brain T1 and T2 relaxation abnormalities was noted in opiate- and cocaine-dependent polydrug abusers, suggesting normal tissue hydration state (Amass et al., 1992). That finding stands in contrast to emission tomography reports of high incidences of multifocal cerebral perfusion impairments in comparable populations of polydrug abusers (Holman et al., 1991; Levin et al., 1995; Rose et al., 1996). This may suggest that cerebral perfusion abnormalities are not associated with T1 and T2 changes. A subsequent MR imaging study in men with concurrent heroin- and cocaine-dependence noted increased pituitary volumes, and this was attributed to pituitary hyperplasia (Teoh et al., 1993). Liu and colleagues (1998) reported reduced prefrontal and temporal cortex volumes along with reduced prefrontal gray matter volume in chronic heroin and cocaine polydrug abusers (Liu et al., 1998). Additionally, this report noted marginal negative correlations between years of heroin use and right prefrontal cortex volume, with statistically stronger negative correlations between years of cocaine use and prefrontal cortex volumes. These authors cautioned that reduced cortical volumes in polydrug abusers might have reflected a preexisting condition, as opposed to an effect of chronic substance abuse (Liu et al., 1998). An association between intracranial volume, an index of premorbid brain size, and neuropsychological impairment was detected in cocaine- and alcohol-dependent polydrug abusers (Disclafani et al., 1998). That finding supports a "functional reserve" hypothesis, which suggests that larger premorbid brain sizes confer protection against the brain damaging effects of polydrug abuse (Disclafani et al., 1998).

MR Spectroscopy

Our group has employed phosphorus (^{31}P) MRS to evaluate the effects of polydrug use on cerebral phosphorus metabolite levels. Our initial study of cocaine- and heroin-dependent polydrug abusers found increased cerebral phosphomonoesters (PME) and decreased β-NP (adenosine triphosphate, ATP) levels during the first week of medicated withdrawal. These metabolite abnormalities were attributed to membrane breakdown and bioenergetic dysfunction, respectively (Christensen et al., 1996). ^{31}P MRS studies of methadone-maintained, opiate-dependent subjects (with minimal cocaine use histories) documented increased PME and phosphodiesters (PDE) and decreased phosphocreatine (PCr) levels (Kaufman et al., 1999). These two studies used the same ^{31}P MRS technique, and we interpreted their discrepant metabolite profiles as reflective of neurochemical abnormalities associated either with different drug abuse patterns in the two study groups or with different drug use states (acute withdrawal in the first study versus prolonged methadone maintenance in the second study). An interesting and potentially important finding in the latter study was that long-term methadone-maintained subjects had nearly normal PCr and PME levels, implying that prolonged methadone treatment might be associated with cerebral metabolite improvements (Kaufman et al., 1999). However, the cross-sectional study design precluded a determination as to whether metabolite changes occurred in those patients.

Concluding Remarks

This review has illustrated the contribution MR techniques have made toward understanding brain changes associated with substance abuse. The existing MR literature is limited by many of the same shortcomings noted for other imaging modalities by other contributors to this monograph, including small sample sizes and heterogeneous subject populations. Two additional limitations of note are a consequence of the fact that MR techniques have been used in substance abuse research for a relatively short time period: there are very few instances in which experimental research findings have been replicated by more than a single laboratory, and substantial gaps exist in important areas of substance abuse. For example, a recent resurgence of opiate abuse (NIDA, 1997) as well as high levels of methamphetamine abuse in several American cities (NIDA, 1998) stand in stark contrast to the relatively few MR studies of these drugs on human brain function. With regard to the most widely abused illicit drug, marijuana, we are aware of only a single research report employing MR technology to evaluate the consequences of marijuana use on brain function (Yurgelun-Todd et al., 1998). However, as more research centers implement MR techniques in the study of substance abuse, it is likely that replication studies will be published and that the existing literature gaps will narrow.

As we look to the future, we see the approach of a period in which the baby-boom generation, perhaps the largest drug-using generation in history, will constitute a substantial proportion of the geriatric population. This convergence has important public health implications, given the findings noted in this overview documenting that alcohol and illicit substance abuse can superimpose excess brain dysfunction upon age-associated brain dysfunction. Consequently, it is likely that our health care system will experience greater numbers and possibly earlier onsets of neurological complications in the elderly. We anticipate that MR techniques, with their inherent safety, noninvasive nature, and ease of use in vulnerable populations such as the the aged, combined with their ability to detect subtle forms of brain dysfunction, will play a pivotal role in helping us to understand, diagnose, and develop treatments for drug-induced brain disorders.

Acknowledgments

We thank the National Institute on Drug Abuse for generous grant support (DA00329, MJK) and (DA00297, JML) and our colleagues at McLean Hospital who contributed substantially to the body of literature covered in this review.

REFERENCES

Aasly, J., Storsaeter, O., Nilsen, G., Smevik, O. and Rinck, P., Minor structural brain changes in young drug abusers. A magnetic resonance study. Acta Neurol. Scand. 87:210–214, 1993.

Adams, K. M., Gilman, S., Koeppe, R. A., Kluin, K. J., Brunberg, J. A., Dede, D., Berent, S. and Kroll, P. D., Neuropsychological deficits are correlated with frontal hypometabolism in positron emission tomography studies of older alcoholic patients. Alcohol. Clin. Exp. Res. 17:205–210, 1993.

Agartz, I., Saaf, J., Wahlund, L. O. and Wetterberg, L., T1 and T2 relaxation time estimates and brain measures during withdrawal in alcoholic men. Drug Alcohol Depend. 29:157–169, 1991.

Agartz, I., Momenan, R., Rawlings, R. R., Kerich, M. J. and Hommer, D. W., Hippocampal volume in patients with alcohol dependence. Arch. Gen. Psychiatry 56:356–363, 1999.

Aggarwal, S. and Byrne, B. D., Massive ischemic cerebellar infarction due to cocaine use. Neuroradiology 33:449–450, 1991.

Akhter, J., Hyder, S. and Ahmed, M., Cerebrovascular accident associated with anabolic steroid use in a young man. Neurology 44:2405–2406, 1994.

Amass, L., Nardin, R., Mendelson, J. H., Teoh, S. K. and Woods, B. T., Quantitative magnetic resonance imaging in heroin- and cocaine- dependent men: a preliminary study. Psychiatry Res. 45:15–23, 1992.

Anderson, C. A., Rubinstein, D., Filley, C. M. and Stears, J. C., MR enhancing brain lesions in methanol intoxication. J. Comput. Assist Tomogr. 21:834–836, 1997.

Arai, H., Yamada, M., Miyake, S., Yamashita, S., Iwamoto, H., Aida, N. and Hara, M., Two cases of toluene embryopathy with severe motor and intellectual disabilities syndrome. [Japanese]. No To Hattatsu 29:361–366, 1997.

Astley, S. J., Weinberger, E., Shaw, D. W., Richards, T. L. and Clarren, S. K., Magnetic resonance imaging and spectroscopy in fetal ethanol exposed Macaca nemestrina. Neurotoxicol. Teratol. 17:523–530, 1995.

Bahr, M., Sommer, N., Petersen, D., Wietholter, H. and Dichgans, J., Central pontine myelinolysis associated with low potassium levels in alcoholism. J. Neurology 237:275–276, 1990.

Baron, R., Heuser, K. and Marioth, G., Marchiafava-Bignami disease with recovery diagnosed by CT and MRI: demyelination affects several CNS structures. J. Neurology 236:364–366, 1989.

Barthauer, L., Tarter, R., Hirsch, W. and Van Thiel, D., Brain morphologic characteristics of cirrhotic alcoholics and cirrhotic nonalcoholics: an MRI study. Alcohol. Clin. Exp. Res. 16:982–985, 1992.

Bartolomei, F., Nicoli, F., Swiader, L. and Gastaut, J. L., Ischemic cerebral vascular stroke after heroin sniffing. A new case. [French]. Presse Med. 21:983–986, 1992.

Bartzokis, G., Backson, M., Hance, D. B., Lu, P. H., Foster, J. A., Mintz, J., Ling, W. and Bridge, P., Magnetic resonance imaging evidence of "silent" cerebrovascular toxicity in cocaine dependence. Biol. Psychiatry 45:1203–1211, 1999.

Benassi, G., Rinaldi, R., Azzimondi, G., Stracciari, A., D'Alessandro, R. and Pazzaglia, P., Acute generalized dystonia due to a bilateral lesion of basal ganglia mainly affecting the nuclei pallidi. Ital. J. Neurol. Sci. 17:71–73, 1996.

Besson, J. A. O., Glen, A. I. M., Foreman, E. I., MacDonald, A., Smith, F. W., Hutchison, J. M. S., Mallard, J. R. and Ashcroft, G. W., Nuclear magnetic resonance observations in alcoholic cerebral disorder and the role of vasopressin. Lancet 2:923–924, 1981.

Besson, J. A., Crawford, J. R., Parker, D. M. and Smith, F. W., Magnetic resonance imaging in Alzheimer's disease, multi-infarct dementia, alcoholic dementia and Korsakoff's psychosis. Acta Psychiatr. Scand. 80:451–458, 1989.

Bigler, E. D., Nelson, J. E. and Schmidt, R. D., Identification of mamillary body atrophy in Korsakoff's syndrome using magnetic resonance imaging. J. Neuropsychiatry Clin. Neurosci. 1:341–342, 1989.

Bitsch, A., Thiel, A., Rieckmann, P. and Prange, H., Acute inflammatory CNS disease after MDMA ('ecstasy'). [Case Report]. Eur. Neurol. 36:328–329, 1996.

Blansjaar, B. A., Vielvoye, G. J., van Dijk, J. G. and Rijnders, R. J., Similar brain lesions in alcoholics and Korsakoff patients: MRI, psychometric and clinical findings. Clin. Neurol. Neurosurg. 94:197–203, 1992.

Bluml, S., Zuckerman, E., Tan, J. and Ross, B. D., Proton-decoupled ^{31}P magnetic resonance spectroscopy reveals osmotic and metabolic disturbances in human hepatic encephalopathy. J. Neurochem. 71:1564–1576, 1998.

Bracard, S., Claude, D., Vespignani, H., Almeras, M., Carsin, M., Lambert, H. and Picard, L., Computerized tomography and MRI in Marchiafava-Bignami disease. J. Neuroradiol. 13:87–94, 1986.

Breiter, H. C., Gollub, R. L., Weisskoff, R. M., Kennedy, D. N., Makris, N., Berke, J. D., Goodman, J. M., Kantor, H. L., Gastfriend, D. R., Riorden, J. P., Mathew, R. T., Makris, N., Rosen, B. R. and Hyman, S. E., Acute effects of cocaine on human brain activity and emotion. Neuron 19:591–611, 1997.

Breiter, H., Gollub, R., Edmister, W., Talavage, T., Makris, N., Melcher, J., Kennedy, D., Kantor, H., Elman, I., Riorden, J., Gastfriend, D., Campbell, T., Foley, M., Weisskoff, R. and Rosen, B., Cocaine induced brainstem and subcortical activity observed through fMRI with cardiac gating. International Society for Magnetic Resonance in Medicine Sixth Scientific Meeting and Exhibition. Sydney, Australia, p. 499, 1998.

Brunner, J. E., Redmond, J. M., Haggar, A. M., Kruger, D. F. and Elias, S. B., Central pontine myelinolysis and pontine lesions after rapid correction of hyponatremia: a prospective magnetic resonance imaging study. Ann. Neurol. 27:61–66, 1990.

Burdett, N. G., Menon, D. K., Carpenter, T. A., Jones, J. G. and Hall, L. D., Visualisation of changes in regional cerebral blood flow (rCBF) produced by ketamine using long TE gradient-echo sequences: preliminary results. Magn. Reson. Imaging 13:549–553, 1995.

Caldemeyer, K. S., Pascuzzi, R. M., Moran, C. C. and Smith, R. R., Toluene abuse causing reduced MR signal intensity in the brain. AJR Am. J. Roentgenol. 161:1259–1261, 1993.

Caldemeyer, K. S., Armstrong, S. W., George, K. K., Moran, C. C. and Pascuzzi, R. M., The spectrum of neuroimaging abnormalities in solvent abuse and their clinical correlation. J. Neuroimaging 6:167–173, 1996.

Caparros-Lefebvre, D., Pruvo, J. P., Josien, E., Pertuzon, B., Clarisse, J. and Petit, H., Marchiafava-Bignami disease: use of contrast media in CT and MRI. Neuroradiology 36:509–511, 1994.

Celius, E. G. and Andersson, S., Leucoencephalopathy after inhalation of heroin: a case report. J. Neurol. Neurosurg. Psychiatry 60:694–695, 1996.

Chang, K. H., Cha, S. H., Han, M. H., Park, S. H., Nah, D. L. and Hong, J. H., Marchiafava-Bignami disease: serial changes in corpus callosum on MRI. Neuroradiology 34:480–482, 1992.

Chang, L., Mehringer, C. M., Ernst, T., Melchor, R., Myers, H., Forney, D. and Satz, P., Neurochemical alterations in asymptomatic abstinent cocaine users: a proton magnetic resonance spectroscopy study. Biol. Psychiatry 42:1105–1114, 1997a.

Chang, Y. J., Tsai, C. H. and Chen, C. J., Leukoencephalopathy after inhalation of heroin vapor. J. Formos. Med. Assoc. 96:758–760, 1997b.

Chang, L., Ernst, T., Strickland, T. and Mehringer, C. M., Gender effects on persistent cerebral metabolite changes in the frontal lobes of abstinent cocaine users. Am. J. Psychiatry 156:716–722, 1999.

Charness, M. E. and DeLaPaz, R. L., Mamillary body atrophy in Wernicke's encephalopathy: antemortem identification using magnetic resonance imaging. Ann. Neurol. 22:595–600, 1987.

Chen, Y. C., Galpern, W. R., Brownell, A. L., Matthews, R. T., Bogdanov, M., Isacson, O., Keltner, J. R., Beal, M. F., Rosen, B. R. and Jenkins, B. G., Detection of dopaminergic neurotransmitter activity using pharmacologic MRI: correlation with PET, microdialysis, and behavioral data. Magn. Reson. Med. 38:389–398, 1997.

Chick, J. D., Smith, M. A., Engleman, H. M., Kean, D. M., Mander, A. J., Douglas, R. H. and Best, J. J., Magnetic resonance imaging of the brain in alcoholics: cerebral atrophy, lifetime alcohol consumption, and cognitive deficits. Alcohol. Clin. Exp. Res. 13:512–518, 1989.

Childress, A. R., Mozley, P. D., McElgin, W., Fitzgerald, J., Reivich, M. and O'Brien, C. P., Limbic activation during cue-induced cocaine craving. Am. J. Psychiatry 156:11–18, 1999.

Chiu, T.-M., Mendelson, J. H., Woods, B. T., Teoh, S. K., Levisohn, L. and Mello, N. K., In vivo proton magnetic resonance spectroscopy detection of human alcohol tolerance. Magn. Reson. Med. 32:511–516, 1994.

Christensen, J. D., Kaufman, M. J., Levin, J. M., Mendelson, J. H., Holman, B. L., Cohen, B. M. and Renshaw, P. F., Abnormal cerebral metabolism in polydrug abusers during early withdrawal: a ^{31}P MR spectroscopy study. Magn. Reson. Med. 35:658–663, 1996.

Christensen, J. D., Kaufman, M. J., Rose, S. L., Mendelson, J. H., Moore, C. M., Cohen, B. M. and Renshaw, P. F., ^{1}H MRS of human basal ganglia response to acute cocaine administration. International Society for Magnetic Resonance in Medicine Fifth Scientific Meeting and Exhibition. Vancouver, B.C., p. 994, 1997.

Christie, J. E., Kean, D. M., Douglas, R. H., Engleman, H. M., St. Clair, D. and Blackburn, I. M., Magnetic resonance imaging in pre-senile dementia of the Alzheimer-type, multi-infarct dementia and Korsakoff's syndrome. Psychol. Med. 18:319–329, 1988.

Church, M. W. and Subramanian, M. G., Cocaine's lethality increases during late gestation in the rat: a study of "critical periods" of exposure. Am. J. Obstet. Gynecol. 176:901–906, 1997.

Cole, M., Winkelman, M. D., Morris, J. C., Simon, J. E. and Boyd, T. A., Thalamic amnesia: Korsakoff syndrome due to left thalamic infarction. J. Neurol. Sci. 110:62–67, 1992.

Daras, M., Neurologic complications of cocaine. In: Majewska, M.D. (ed.) Neurotoxicity and Neuropathology Associated with Cocaine Abuse. NIDA Research Monograph Vol. 163. Washington D.C., U.S. Govt. Printing Office, Dept. of Health and Human Services Pub. No. (NIH)96-4019, pp. 43–65, 1996.

Davila, M. D., Shear, P. K., Lane, B., Sullivan, E. V. and Pfefferbaum, A., Mammillary body and cerebellar shrinkage in chronic alcoholics: an MRI and neuropsychological study. Neuropsychology 8:433–444, 1994.

Deicken, R. F., Calabrese, G., Raz, J., Sappey-Marinier, D., Meyerhoff, D., Dillon, W. P., Weiner, M. W. and Fein, G., A 31phosphorous magnetic resonance spectroscopy study of diazepam does not affect brain phosphorous metabolism. Biol. Psychiatry 32:628–631, 1992.

del Amo, M., Berenguer, J., Pujol, T. and Mercader, J. M., MR in trichloroethane poisoning. AJNR Am. J. Neuroradiol. 17:1180–1182, 1996.

Demaerel, P., Wilms, G., De, B. P., Vanderwegen, L., Casteels, M., Carton, H. and Baert, A. L., Magnetic resonance imaging of extrapontine lesions in central pontine myelinolysis. J. Belge Radiol. 75:186–187, 1992.

DeWitt, L. D., Buonanno, F. S., Kistler, J. P., Zeffiro, T., DeLaPaz, R. L., Brady, T. J., Rosen, B. R. and Pykett, I. L., Central pontine myelinolysis: demonstration by nuclear magnetic resonance. Neurology 34:570–576, 1984.

Di Sclafani, V., Ezekiel, F., Meyerhoff, D. J., MacKay, S., Dillon, W. P., Weiner, M. W. and Fein, G., Brain atrophy and cognitive function in older abstinent alcoholic men. Alcohol. Clin. Exp. Res. 19:1121–1126, 1995.

Disclafani, V., Clark, H. W., Tolou-shams, M., Bloomer, C., Salas, G. A., Norman, D. and Fein, G., Premorbid brain size is a determinant of functional reserve in abstinent crack-cocaine and crack-cocaine-alcohol-dependent adults. J. Int. Neuropsychol. Soc. 4:559–565, 1998.

Ditraglia, G. M., Press, D. S., Butters, N., Jernigan, T. L., Cermak, L. S., Velin, R. A., Shear, P. K., Irwin, M. and Schuckit, M., Assessment of olfactory deficits in detoxified alcoholics. Alcohol 8:109–115, 1991.

Donnal, J. F., Heinz, E. R. and Buerger, P. C., MR of reversible thalamic lesions in Wernicke syndrome. AJNR Am. J. Neuroradiol. 11:893–894, 1990.

Doraiswamy, P. M., Massey, E. W., Enright, K., Palese, V. J., Lamonica, D. and Boyko, O., Wernicke-Korsakoff syndrome caused by psychogenic food refusal: MR findings. AJNR Am. J. Neuroradiol. 15:594–596, 1994.

Ebrahim, S. H., Luman, E. T., Floyd, R. L., Murphy, C. C., Bennett, E. M. and Boyle, C. A., Alcohol consumption by pregnant women in the United States during 1988–1995. Obstet. Gynecol. 92:187–192, 1998.

Ebrahim, S. H., Diekman, S. T., Floyd, R. L. and Decoufle, P., Comparison of binge drinking among pregnant and nonpregnant women, United States, 1991–1995. Am. J. Obstet. Gynecol. 180:1–7, 1999.

Ellis, K. L. and Speed, J., Pharmacologic management of movement disorder after midbrain haemorrhage. Brain Inj. 12:623–628, 1998.

Emsley, R., Smith, R., Roberts, M., Kapnias, S., Pieters, H. and Maritz, S., Magnetic resonance imaging in alcoholic Korsakoff's syndrome: evidence for an association with alcoholic dementia. Alcohol Alcohol. 31:479–486, 1996.

Estruch, R., Nicolas, J. M., Salamero, M., Aragon, C., Sacanella, E., Fernandez-Sola, J. and Urbano-Marquez, A., Atrophy of the corpus callosum in chronic alcoholism. J. Neurol. Sci. 146:145–151, 1997.

Filley, C. M., Heaton, R. K. and Rosenberg, N. L., White matter dementia in chronic toluene abuse. Neurology 40:532–534, 1990.

Gabrielli, O., Salvolini, U., Coppa, G. V., Catassi, C., Rossi, R., Manca, A., Lanza, R. and Giorgi, P. L., Magnetic resonance imaging in the malformative syndromes with mental retardation. Pediatr. Radiol. 21:16–19, 1990.

Gallucci, M., Amicarelli, I., Rossi, A., Stratta, P., Masciocchi, C., Zobel, B. B., Casacchia, M. and Passariello, R., MR imaging of white matter lesions in uncomplicated chronic alcoholism. J. Comput. Assist. Tomogr. 13:395–398, 1989.

Gallucci, M., Bozzao, A., Splendiani, A., Masciocchi, C. and Passariello, R., Wernicke Encephalopathy: MR findings in five patients. AJNR Am. J. Neuroradiol. 11:887–892, 1990.

Gass, A., Birtsch, G., Olster, M., Schwartz, A. and Hennerici, M. G., Marchiafava-Bignami disease: reversibility of neuroimaging abnormality. J. Comput. Assist. Tomogr. 22:503–504, 1998.

Gaul, H. P., Wallace, C. J., Auer, R. N. and Fong, T. C., MR findings in methanol intoxication. AJNR Am. J. Neuroradiol. 16:1783–1786, 1995.

Geissler, A., Lock, G., Frund, R., Held, P., Hollerbach, S., Andus, T., Scholmerich, J., Feuerbach, S. and Holstege, A., Cerebral abnormalities in patients with cirrhosis detected by proton magnetic resonance spectroscopy and magnetic resonance imaging. Hepatology 25:48–54, 1997.

Gieron-Korthals, M. A., Helal, A. and Martinez, C. R., Expanding spectrum of cocaine induced central nervous system malformations. Brain Dev. 16:253–256, 1994.

Glazer, M. and Dross, P., Necrosis of the putamen caused by methanol intoxication: MR findings. AJR Am. J. Roentgenol. 160:1105–1106, 1993.

Gollub, R. L., Breiter, H. C., Kantor, H., Kennedy, D., Gastfriend, D., Mathew, R. T., Makris, N., Guimaraes, A., Riorden, J., Campbell, T., Foley, M., Hyman, S. E., Rosen, B. and Weisskoff, R., Cocaine decreases cortical cerebral blood flow but does not obscure regional activation in functional magnetic resonance imaging in human subjects. J. Cereb. Blood Flow Metab. 18:724–734, 1998.

Gomez-Anson, B. and Ramsey, R. G., Pachygyria in a neonate with prenatal cocaine exposure: MR features. J. Comput. Assist. Tomogr. 18:637–639, 1994.

Gradon, J. D. and Wityk, R., Diagnosis of probably cocaine-induced cerebral vasculitis by magnetic resonance angiography. South. Med. J. 88:1264–1266, 1995.

Grant, S., London, E. D., Newlin, D. B., Villemagne, V. L., Liu, X., Contoreggi, C., Phillips, R. L., Kimes, A. S. and Margolin, A., Activation of memory circuits during cue-elicited cocaine craving. Proc. Natl. Acad. Sci. USA 93:12040–12045, 1996.

Grob, C. S., Poland, R. E., Chang, L. and Ernst, T., Psychobiologic effects of 3,4-methylenedioxymethamphetamine in humans: methodological considerations and preliminary observations. Behav. Brain Res. 73:103–107, 1996.

Hanstock, C. C., Rothman, D. L., Shulman, R. G., Novotny, E. J., Jr., Petroff, O. A. and Prichard, J. W., Measurement of ethanol in the human brain using NMR spectroscopy. J. Stud. Alcohol 51:104–107, 1990.

Hantson, P., Duprez, T. and Mahieu, P., Neurotoxicity to the basal ganglia shown by magnetic resonance imaging (MRI) following poisoning by methanol and other substances. J. Toxicol. Clin. Toxicol. 35:151–161, 1997.

Harwood, H., Fountain, D. and Livermore, G., Cost estimates for alcohol and drug abuse. Addiction 94:631–635, 1999.

Hayakawa, K., Kumagai, H., Suzuki, Y., Furusawa, N., Haga, T., Hoshi, T., Fujiwara, Y. and Yamaguchi, K., MR imaging of chronic alcoholism. Acta Radiol. 33:201–206, 1992.

Heier, L. A., Carpanzano, C. R., Mast, J., Brill, P. W., Winchester, P. and Deck, M. D. F., Maternal cocaine abuse: the spectrum of radiologic abnormalities in the neonatal CNS. AJNR Am. J. Neuroradiol. 12:951–956, 1991.

Hetherington, H. P., Rowley, H., Peterson, K., Boska, M., Diamond, I. and Weiner, M. W., The kinetics of alcohol uptake in human brain and blood by volume selective ^{1}H MRS. Soc. Magn. Resonance Abstr., Vol. 3, p. 370, 1989.

Heye, N. and Hankey, G. J., Amphetamine-associated stroke. Cerebrovasc. Dis. 6:149–155, 1996.

Holman, B. L., Carvalho, P. A., Mendelson, J., Teoh, S. K., Nardin, R., Hallgring, E., Hebben, N. and Johnson, K. A., Brain perfusion is abnormal in cocaine-dependent polydrug users: a study using technetium-99m-HMPAO and ASPECT. J. Nucl. Med. 32:1206–1210, 1991.

Hommer, D., Momenan, R., Rawlings, R., Ragan, P., Williams, W., Rio, D. and Eckardt, M., Decreased corpus callosum size among alcoholic women. Arch. Neurol. 53:359–363, 1996.

Howard, R. J., Ellis, C., Bullmore, E. T., Brammer, M., Mellers, J. D., Woodruff, P. W., David, A. S., Simmons, A., Williams, S. C. R. and Parkes, J. D., Functional echoplanar imaging correlates of amphetamine administration to normal subjects and subjects with the narcoleptic syndrome. Magn. Reson. Imaging 14:1013–1016, 1996.

Huda, A., Guze, B. H., Thomas, M. A., Bugbee, M., Fairbanks, L., Strouse, T. and Fawzy, F. I., Clinical correlation of neuropsychological tests with ^{1}H magnetic resonance spectroscopy in hepatic encephalopathy. Psychosom. Med. 60:550–556, 1998.

Hungerbuhler, H. and Waespe, W., Leukoencephalopathy following inhalation of heroin pyrolysate. [German]. Schweiz. Med. Wochenschr. 120:1801–1805, 1990.

Ikeda, A., Antoku, Y., Abe, T., Nishimura, H. and Iwashita, H., Marchiafava-Bignami disease: consecutive observation at acute stage by magnetic resonance imaging and computerized tomography. Jpn. J. Med. 28:740–743, 1989.

Ikeda, M. and Tsukagoshi, H., Encephalopathy due to toluene sniffing: report of a case with magnetic resonance imaging. Eur. Neurol. 30:347–349, 1990.

Izquierdo, G., Quesada, M. A., Chacon, J. and Martel, J., Neuroradiologic abnormalities in Marchiafava-Bignami disease of benign evolution. Eur. J. Radiol. 15:71–74, 1992.

Jacobs, I. G., Roszler, M. H., Kelly, J. K., Klein, M. A. and Kling, G. A., Cocaine abuse: Neurovascular complications. Radiology 170:223–227, 1989.

Jagannathan, N. R., Desai, N. G. and Raghunathan, P., Brain metabolite changes in alcoholism: an in vivo proton magnetic resonance spectroscopy (MRS) study. Magn. Reson. Imaging 14:553–557, 1996.

Jernigan, T. L., Butters, N., DiTraglia, G., Schafer, K., Smith, T., Irwin, M., Grant, I., Schuckit, M. and Cermak, L. S., Reduced cerebral grey matter observed in alcoholics using magnetic resonance imaging. Alcohol. Clin. Exp. Res. 15:418–427, 1991a.

Jernigan, T. L., Schafer, K., Butters, N. and Cermak, L. S., Magnetic resonance imaging of alcoholic Korsakoff patients. Neuropsychopharmacology 4:175–186, 1991b.

Johnson, V. P., Swayze, V. W., II., Sato, Y. and Andreasen, N. C., Fetal alcohol syndrome: craniofacial and central nervous system manifestations. Am. J. Med. Genet. 61:329–339, 1996.

Kaufman, M. J., Chiu, T. M., Mendelson, J. H., Woods, B. T., Mello, N. K., Lukas, S. E., Fivel, P. A. and Wighton, L. G., In vivo proton magnetic resonance spectroscopy of alcohol in rhesus monkey brain. Magn. Reson. Imaging 12:1245–1253, 1994.

Kaufman, M. J., Chiu, T.-M., Mendelson, J. H., Woods, B. T., Teoh, S. K., Eros-Sarnyai, M., Mercer, G. and Mello, N. K., Brain alcohol detectability increase with repeated administration in humans: a proton spectroscopy study. Magn. Reson. Med. 35:435–440, 1996.

Kaufman, M. J., Levin, J. M., Kukes, T. J., Villafuerte, R. A., Hsia, S. B., Lukas, S. E., Mendelson, J. H., Cohen, B. M. and Renshaw, P. F., Menstrual cycle phase modulates cocaine-induced cerebral blood volume reduction in women. International Society of Magnetic Resonance in Medicine Sixth Scientific Meeting and Exhibition. Sydney, Australia, p. 1581, 1998a.

Kaufman, M. J., Levin, J. M., Maas, L. C., Rose, S. L., Lukas, S. E., Mendelson, J. H., Cohen, B. M. and Renshaw, P. F., Cocaine decreases relative cerebral blood volume in humans: a dynamic susceptibility contrast magnetic resonance imaging study. Psychopharmacology (Berl.) 138:76–81, 1998b.

Kaufman, M. J., Levin, J. M., Ross, M. H., Lange, N., Rose, S. L., Kukes, T. J., Mendelson, J. H., Lukas, S. E., Cohen, B. M. and Renshaw, P. F., Cocaine-induced cerebral vasoconstriction detected in humans with magnetic resonance angiography. JAMA 279:376–380, 1998c.

Kaufman, M. J., Pollack, M. H., Villafuerte, R. A., Kukes, T. J., Rose, S. L., Mendelson, J. H., Cohen, B. M. and Renshaw, P. F., Cerebral phosphorus metabolite abnormalities in opiate-dependent polydrug abusers in methadone maintenance. Psychiatry Res. 90:143–152, 1999.

Kawamura, M., Shiota, J., Yagashita, T. and Hirayama, K., Marchiafava-Bignami disease: computed tomographic scan and magnetic resonance imaging. Ann. Neurol. 18:103–104, 1985.

Kitaguchi, T., Kobayashi, T., Tobimatsu, S., Goto, I. and Kuroiwa, Y., Computed tomography and magnetic resonance imaging in a young patient with Wernicke's encephalopathy. J. Neurology 234:449–450, 1987.

Klonoff, D., Andrews, B. and Obana, W., Stroke associated with cocaine use. Arch. Neurol. 46:989–993, 1989.

Koci, T. M., Chiang, F., Chow, P., Wang, A., Chiu, L. C., Itabashi, H. and Mehringer, C. M., Thalamic extrapontine lesions in central pontine myelinolysis. AJNR Am. J. Neuroradiol. 11:1229–1233, 1990.

Konkol, R. J., Tikofsky, R. S., Wells, R., Hellman, R. S., Nemeth, P., Walsh, D. J., Heimler, R. and Sty, J. R., Normal high-resolution cerebral 99mTc-HMPAO SPECT scans in symptomatic neonates exposed to cocaine. J. Child Neurol. 9:278–283, 1994.

Kopelman, M. D., Stanhope, N. and Kingsley, D., Temporal and spatial context memory in patients with focal frontal, temporal lobe, and diencephalic lesions. Neuropsychologia 35: 1533–1545, 1997.

Kreis, R., Ross, B. D., Farrow, N. A. and Ackerman, Z., Metabolic disorders of the brain in chronic hepatic encephalopathy detected with H-1 MR spectroscopy. Radiology 182:19–27, 1992.

Krieger, S., Jauss, M., Jansen, O., Theilmann, L., Geissler, M. and Krieger, D., Neuropsychiatric profile and hyperintense globus pallidus on T1-weighted magnetic resonance images in liver cirrhosis. Gastroenterology 111:147–155, 1996.

Kriegstein, A. R., Armitage, B. A. and Kim, P. Y., Heroin inhalation and progressive spongiform leukoencephalopathy. N. Engl. J. Med. 336:589–590, 1997.

Kroft, C. L., Gescuk, B., Woods, B. T., Mello, N. K., Weiss, R. D. and Mendelson, J. H., Brain ventricular size in female alcoholics: an MRI study. Alcohol 8:31–34, 1991.

Kulisevsky, J., Pujol, J., Balanzo, J., Junque, C., Deus, J., Capdevilla, A. and Villanueva, C., Pallidal hyperintensity on magnetic resonance imaging in cirrhotic patients: clinical correlations. Hepatology 16:1382–1388, 1992.

Kulisevsky, J., Pujol, J., Junque, C., Deus, J., Balanzo, J. and Capdevila, A., MRI pallidal hyperintensity and brain atrophy in cirrhotic patients: two different MRI patterns of clinical deterioration? Neurology 43:2570–2573, 1993.

Lambrecht, G. L., Malbrain, M. L., Chew, S. L., Baeck, E. and Verbraeken, H., Intranasal caffeine and amphetamine causing stroke. Acta Neurol. Belg. 93:146–149, 1993.

Lazar, E. B., Russell, E. J., Cohen, B. A., Brody, B. and Levy, R. M., Contrast-enhanced MR of cerebral arteritis: intravascular enhancement related to flow stasis within areas of focal arterial ectasia. AJNR Am. J. Neuroradiol. 13:271–276, 1992.

Leira, H. L., Myhr, G., Nilsen, G. and Dale, L. G., Cerebral magnetic resonance imaging and cerebral computerized tomography for patients with solvent-induced encephalopathy. Scand. J. Work Environ. Health 18:68–70, 1992.

Levin, J. M., Holman, B. L., Mendelson, J. H., Teoh, S. K., Garada, B., Johnson, K. A. and Springer, S., Gender differences in cerebral perfusion in cocaine abuse: 99mTc-HMPAO SPECT study of drug abusing women. J. Nucl. Med. 35:1902–1909, 1994.

Levin, J. M., Mendelson, J. H., Holman, B. L., Teoh, S. K., Garada, B., Schwartz, R. B. and Mello, N. K., Improved regional cerebral blood flow in chronic cocaine polydrug users treated with buprenorphine. J. Nucl. Med. 36:1211–1215, 1995.

Levin, J. M., Ross, M. H., Mendelson, J. H., Kaufman, M. J., Lange, N., Maas, L. C., Mello, N. K., Cohen, B. M. and Renshaw, P. F., Reduction in BOLD fMRI response to primary visual stimulation following alcohol ingestion. Psychiatry Res. 82:135–146, 1998.

Levin, J. M., Kaufman, M. J., Ross, M. H., Roc, A. C., Maas, L. C., Mendelson, J. H., Cohen, B. M. and Renshaw, P. F., Cocaine increases BOLD fMRI response to photic stimulation. International Society for Magnetic Resonance in Medicine, Seventh Scientific Meeting and Exhibition. Philadelphia, PA, p. 838, 1999.

Lewis, L. D., Smith, B. W. and Mamourian, A. C., Delayed sequelae after acute overdoses or poisonings: cranial neuropathy related to ethylene glycol ingestion. Clin. Pharmacol. Ther. 61:692–699, 1997.

Li, S.-J., Wang, Y., Prost, R. W., Harsch, H., Pankiewicz, J., Bloom, A. S. and Stein, E. A., Reversible neurochemical alterations in cocaine abusers assessed by ^{1}H magnetic resonance spectroscopy. International Society for Magnetic Resonance in Medicine Fourth Scientific Meeting and Exhibition. New York, NY, p. 993, 1996.

Li, S.-J., Wang, Y., Risinger, R., Rainey, C., Harsch, H., Pankiewicz, J., Sperry, L., Cho, J.-K., Bloom, A. S. and Stein, E. A., Acute cocaine administration induces NAA increase detected by ^{1}H MRS. International Society for Magnetic Resonance in Medicine Sixth Scientific Meeting and Exhibition. Sydney, Australia, p. 1714, 1998.

Li, S. J., Wang, Y., Pankiewicz, J. and Stein, E. A., Neurochemical adaptation to cocaine abuse: reduction of N-acetyl aspartate in thalamus of human cocaine abusers. Biol. Psychiatry 45:1481–1487, 1999.

Link, E. A., Weese-Mayer, D. W. and Bryd, S. E., Magnetic resonance imaging in infants exposed to cocaine prenatally: a preliminary report. Clin. Pediatr. (Phila.) 30:506–508, 1991.

Liu, X., Matochick, J. A., Cadet, J. L. and London, E. D., Smaller volume of prefrontal lobe in polysubstance abusers: a magnetic resonance imaging study. Neuropsychopharmacology 18:243–252, 1998.

Logsdail, S., Miller, D., Macmanus, D., Johnson, G., Lolin, Y. and O'Gorman, P., The effect of moderate blood alcohol levels on T1 and T2 relaxation times in the brains of normal volunteers. Magn. Reson. Med. 4:378–379, 1987.

Lukas, S. E., Dobrosielski, M., Chiu, T. M., Woods, B. T., Teoh, S. K. and Mendelson, J. H., A nonferrous instrumental joystick device for recording behavioral responses during magnetic resonance imaging and spectroscopy. Pharmacol. Biochem. Behav. 46:781–785, 1993.

Maas, L. C., Lukas, S. E., Kaufman, M. J., Weiss, R. D., Daniels, S. L., Rogers, V. W., Kukes, T. J. and Renshaw, P. F., Functional magnetic resonance imaging of human brain activation during cue-induced cocaine craving. Am. J. Psychiatry 155:124–126, 1998.

MacKay, S., Meyerhoff, D. J., Dillon, W. P., Weiner, M. W. and Fein, G., Alteration of brain phospholipid metabolites in cocaine-dependent polysubstance abusers. Biol. Psychiatry 34:261–264, 1993.

Maeda, H., Sato, M., Yoshikawa, A., Kimura, M., Sonomura, T., Terada, M. and Kishi, K., Brain MR imaging in patients with hepatic cirrhosis: relationship between high intensity signal in basal ganglia on T1-weighted images and elemental concentrations in brain. Neuroradiology 39:546–550, 1997.

Mander, A. J., Smith, M. A., Kean, D. M., Chick, J., Douglas, R. H., Rehman, A. U., Weppner, G. J. and Best, J. J., Brain water measured in volunteers after alcohol and vasopressin. Lancet 2:1075, 1985.

Mander, A. J., Weppner, G. J., Chick, J. D., Morton, J. J. and Best, J. J., An NMR study of cerebral oedema and its biological correlates during withdrawal from alcohol. Alcohol Alcohol. 23:97–102, 1988.

Mander, A. J., Young, A., Chick, J. D., Ridgway, J. and Best, J. J., NMR T1 relaxation time of the brain during alcohol withdrawal and its lack of relationship with symptom severity. Br. J. Addiction 84:669–672, 1989a.

Mander, A. J., Young, A., Chick, J. D. and Best, J. J., The relationship of cerebral atrophy and T1 in alcoholics: an MRI study. Drug Alcohol Depend. 24:57–59, 1989b.

Mann, K., Opitz, H., Petersen, D., Schroth, G. and Heimann, H., Intracranial CSF volumetry in alcoholics: studies with MRI and CT. Psychiatry Res. 29:277–279, 1989.

Martin, P. R., Gibbs, S. J., Nimmerrichter, A. A., Riddle, W. R., Welch, L. W. and Willcott, M. R., Brain proton magnetic resonance spectroscopy studies in recently abstinent alcoholics. Alcohol. Clin. Exp. Res. 19:1078–1082, 1995.

Mascalchi, M., Cincotta, M. and Piazzini, M., Case report: MRI demonstration of pontine and thalamic myelinolysis in a normonatremic alcoholic. Clin. Radiol. 47:137–138, 1993.

Matsuda, K., Yamaji, S., Ishii, K., Sasaki, M., Sakamoto, S., Kitagaki, H., Imamura, T. and Mori, E., Regional cerebral blood flow and oxygen metabolism in a patient with Korsakoff syndrome. Ann. Nucl. Med. 11:33–35, 1997.

Mattson, S. N., Riley, E. P., Jernigan, T. L., Ehlers, C. L., Delis, D. C., Jones, K. L., Stern, C., Johnson, K. A., Hesselink, J. R. and Bellugi, U., Fetal alcohol syndrome: a case report of neuropsychological, MRI and EEG assessment of two children. Alcohol. Clin. Exp. Res. 16:1001–1003, 1992.

Mattson, S. N., Riley, E. P., Jernigan, T. L., Garcia, A., Kaneko, W. M., Ehlers, C. L. and Jones, K. L., A decrease in the size of the basal ganglia following prenatal alcohol exposure: a preliminary report. Neurotoxicol. Teratol. 16:283–289, 1994.

Mattson, S. N., Riley, E. P., Sowell, E. R., Jernigan, T. L., Sobel, D. F. and Jones, K. L., A decrease in the size of the basal ganglia in children with fetal alcohol syndrome. Alcohol. Clin. Exp. Res. 20:1088–1093, 1996.

Mayer, J. M., de Liege, P., Netter, J. M., Danze, F. and Reizine, D., Computerized tomography and nuclear magnetic resonance imaging in Marchiafava-Bignami disease. J. Neuroradiol. 14:152–158, 1987.

Mena, I., Giombetti, R. J., Miller, B. L., Garrett, K., Villanueva-Meyer, J., Mody, C. and Goldberg, M. A., Cerebral blood flow changes with acute cocaine intoxication: Clinical correlations with SPECT, CT and MRI. In: Sorer, H. and Rapaka, R.S. (eds.) Imaging Techniques in Medications Development: Preclinical and Clinical Aspects, NIDA Research Monograph Vol. 138, NIH Public. No. 94-3728. Rockville, MD, U.S. Dept. of Health and Human Services, pp. 161–173, 1994.

Mendelson, J. H., Woods, B. T., Chiu, T. M., Mello, N. K., Lukas, S. E., Teoh, S. K., Sintavanarong, P., Cochin, J., Hopkins, M. A. and Dobrosielski, M., In vivo proton magnetic resonance spectroscopy of alcohol in human brain. Alcohol 7:443–447, 1990.

Meyerhoff, D. J., Ethanol in human brain: relaxation and magnetization transfer. International Society for Magnetic Resonance in Medicine, Sixth Scientific Meeting and Exhibition. Sydney, Australia, p. 193, 1998.

Meyerhoff, D. J., MacKay, S., Sappey-Marinier, D., Deicken, R., Calabrese, G., Dillon, W. P., Weiner, M. W. and Fein, G., Effects of chronic alcohol abuse and HIV infection on brain phosphorus metabolites. Alcohol. Clin. Exp. Res. 19:685–692, 1995.

Meyerhoff, D. J., Rooney, W. D., Tokumitsu, T. and Weiner, M. W., Evidence of multiple ethanol pools in the brain: an in vivo proton magnetization transfer study. Alcohol. Clin. Exp. Res. 20:1283–1288, 1996.

Meyerhoff, D. J., Bloomer, C., Salas, G., Schuff, N., Norman, D., Weiner, M. W. and Fein, G., Cortical metabolite alterations in recently abstinent cocaine and cocaine/alcohol dependent subjects. International Society for Magnetic Resonance in Medicine Sixth Scientific Meeting and Exhibition. Sydney, Australia, p. 1715, 1998.

Mody, C. K., Miller, B. L., McIntyre, H. B., Cobb, S. K. and Goldberg, M. A., Neurologic complications of cocaine abuse. Neurology 38:1189–1193, 1988.

Moore, J. W., Dunk, A. A., Crawford, J. R., Deans, H., Besson, J. A. O., De Lacey, G., Sinclair, T. S., Mowat, N. A. G. and Brunt, P. W., Neuropsychological deficits and morphological MRI brain scan abnormalities in apparently healthy non-encephalopathic patients with cirrhosis. J. Hepatology 9:319–325, 1989.

Mozaz, M. J., Wyke, M. A. and Indakoetxea, B., Parkinsonism and defects of praxis following methanol poisoning. J. Neurol. Neurosurg. Psychiatry 54:843–844, 1991.

Nalls, G., Disher, A., Daryabagi, J., Zant, Z. and Eisenman, J., Subcortical cerebral hemorrhages associated with cocaine abuse: CT and MR findings. J. Comput. Assist. Tomogr. 13:1–5, 1989.

NIDA Research Report: Heroin Abuse and Addiction., U.S. Dept. of Health and Human Services, NIH Pub. No. 97-4165, http://www.nida.nih.gov/ResearchReports/Heroin/Heroin.html, 1997.

NIDA Research Report. Methamphetamine Abuse and Addiction., National Institute on Drug Abuse, NIH Pub. No 98-4210, April, 1998.

Niehaus, L., Roricht, S., Meyer, B. U. and Sander, B., Nuclear magnetic resonance tomography detection of heroin-associated CNS lesions. [German]. Aktuelle Radiol. 7:309–311, 1997.

Niehaus, L. and Meyer, B. U., Bilateral borderzone brain infarctions in association with heroin abuse. J. Neurol. Sci. 160:180–182, 1998.

Nuytten, D., Wyffels, E., Michiels, K., Ferrante, M., Verbraeken, H., Daelemans, R., Baeck, E. and Cras, P., Drug-induced spongiform leucoencephalopathy, a case report with review of the literature. Acta Neurol. Belg. 98:32–35, 1998.

Okudaira, K., Endo, S., Saito, A., Nagano, K., Masaoka, A. and Kaneko, Y., Clinical course and MRI findings of two cases of alcoholic cerebellar degeneration. [Japanese]. Arukoru Kenkyuto Yakubutsu Ison 23:170–175, 1988.

Panigel, M., Dixon, T., Constantinidis, I., Sheppard, S., Swenson, R., McLure, H., Campbell, W. E., Huddleston, J., Polliotti, B. and Nahmias, A., Fast scan magnetic resonance imaging and Doppler ultrasonography of uteroplacental hemodynamics in the rhesus monkey (*Macaca mulatta*). J. Med. Primatol. 22:393–399, 1993.

Pappata, S., Chabriat, H., Levasseur, M., Legault-Demare, F. and Baron, J. C., Marchiafava-Bignami disease with dementia: severe cerebral metabolic depression revealed by PET. J. Neural. Transm. Park. Dis. Dement. Sect. 8:131–137, 1994.

Pelletier, J., Habib, M. H., Khalil, R., Salamon, G., Bartoli, D. and Jean, P., Putaminal necrosis after methanol intoxication. J. Neurol. Neurosurg. Psychiatry 55:234–235, 1992.

Peterson, P. L., Roszler, M., Jacobs, I. and Wilner, H. I., Neurovascular complications of cocaine abuse. J. Neuropsychiatry Clin. Neurosci. 3:143–149, 1991.

Pfefferbaum, A., Lim, K. O., Zipursky, R. B., Mathalon, D. H., Rosenbloom, M. J., Lane, B., Ha, C. N. and Sullivan, E. V., Brain gray and white matter volume loss accelerates with aging in chronic alcoholics: a quantitative MRI study. Alcohol. Clin. Exp. Res. 16:1078–1089, 1992.

Pfefferbaum, A., Sullivan, E. V., Rosenbloom, M. J., Shear, P. K., Mathalon, D. H. and Lim, K. O., Increase in brain cerebrospinal fluid volume is greater in older than in younger alcoholic patients: a replication study and CT/MRI comparison. Psychiatry Res. 50:257–274, 1993.

Pfefferbaum, A., Sullivan, E. V., Mathalon, D. H., Shear, P. K., Rosenbloom, M. J. and Lim, K. O., Longitudinal changes in magnetic resonance imaging brain volumes in abstinent and relapsed alcoholics. Alcohol. Clin. Exp. Res. 19:1177–1191, 1995.

Pfefferbaum, A., Lim, K. O., Desmond, J. E. and Sullivan, E. V., Thinning of the corpus callosum in older alcoholic men: a magnetic resonance imaging study. Alcohol. Clin. Exp. Res. 20:752–757, 1996.

Pfefferbaum, A., Sullivan, E. V., Mathalon, D. H. and Lim, K. O., Frontal lobe volume loss observed with magnetic resonance imaging in older chronic alcoholics. Alcohol. Clin. Exp. Res. 21:521–529, 1997.

Pfefferbaum, A., Sullivan, E. V., Rosenbloom, M. J., Mathalon, D. H. and Lim, K. O., A controlled study of cortical gray matter and ventricular changes in alcoholic men over a 5-year interval. Arch. Gen. Psychiatry 55:905–912, 1998.

Price, D. B., Kramer, J., Hotson, G. C. and Loh, J. P., Central pontine myelinolysis: report of a case with distinctive appearance on MR imaging. AJNR Am. J. Neuroradiol. 8:576–577, 1987.

Pujol, A., Pujol, J., Graus, F., Rimola, A., Peri, J., Mercader, J. M., Garcia-Pagan, J. C., Bosch, J., Rodes, J. and Tolosa, E., Hyperintense globus pallidus on T1-weighted MRI in cirrhotic patients is associated with severity of liver failure. Neurology 43:65–69, 1993.

Ramadan, N. M., Levine, S. R. and Welch, K. M., Pontine hemorrhage following "crack" cocaine use. Neurology 41:946–947, 1991.

Rippe, D. J., Edwards, M. K., D'Amour, P. G., Holden, R. W. and Roos, K. L., MR imaging of central pontine myelinolysis. [Case Report]. J. Comput. Assist. Tomogr. 11:724–726, 1987.

Rose, J. S., Branchey, M., Buydens-Branchey, L., Stapleton, J. M., Chasten, K., Werrell, A. and Maayan, M. L., Cerebral perfusion in early and late opiate withdrawal: a technetium-99m-HMPAO SPECT study. Psychiatry Res. 67:39–47, 1996.

Rosenberg, N. L., Spitz, M. C., Filley, C. M., Davis, K. A. and Schaumburg, H. H., Central nervous system effects of chronic toluene abuse—clinical, brainstem evoked response and magnetic resonance imaging studies. Neurotoxicol. Teratol. 10:489–495, 1988a.

Rosenberg, N. L., Kleinschmidt-DeMasters, B. K., Davis, K. A., Dreisbach, J. N., Hormes, J. T. and Filley, C. M., Toluene abuse causes diffuse central nervous system white matter changes. Ann. Neurol. 23:611–614, 1988b.

Ross, B. D., Jacobson, S., Villamil, F., Korula, J., Kreis, R., Ernst, T., Shonk, T. and Moats, R. A., Subclinical hepatic encephalopathy: proton MR spectroscopic abnormalities. Radiology 193:457–463, 1994.

Rouanet, F., Tison, F., Dousset, V., Corand, V. and Orgogozo, J. M., Early T_2 hypointense signal abnormality preceding clinical manifestations of central pontine myelinolysis. Neurology 44:979–980, 1994.

Roulet Perez, E., Maeder, P., Rivier, L. and Deonna, T., Toxic leucoencephalopathy after heroin ingestion in a 21/2-year-old child. Lancet 340(8821):729, 1992.

Rubinstein, D., Escott, E. and Kelly, J. P., Methanol intoxication with putaminal and white matter necrosis: MR and CT findings. AJNR Am. J. Neuroradiol. 16:1492–1494, 1995.

Sachdeva, K. and Woodward, K. G., Caudal thalamic infarction following intranasal methamphetamine use. Neurology 39:305–306, 1989.

Schaefer, G. B., Shuman, R. M., Wilson, D. A., Saleeb, S., Domek, D. B., Johnson, S. F. and Bodensteiner, J. B., Partial agenesis of the anterior corpus callosum: correlation between appearance, imaging, and neuropathology. [Case Report]. Pediatr. Neurol. 7:39–44, 1991.

Schroth, G., Naegele, T., Klose, U., Mann, K. and Petersen, D., Reversible brain shrinkage in abstinent alcoholics, measured by MRI. Neuroradiology 30:385–389, 1988.

Seery, J. P. and Taylor-Robinson, S. D., The application of magnetic resonance spectroscopy to the study of hepatic encephalopathy. J. Hepatology 25:988–998, 1996.

Seitz, D., Widmann, U., Seeger, U., Nagele, T., Klose, U., Mann, K. and Grodd, W., Localized proton magnetic resonance spectroscopy of the cerebellum in detoxifying alcoholics. Alcohol. Clin. Exp. Res. 23:158–163, 1999.

Sell, L. A., Simmons, A., Lemmens, G. M., Williams, S. C. R., Brammer, M. and Strang, J., Functional magnetic resonance imaging of the acute effect of intravenous heroin administration on visual activation in long-term heroin addicts: results from a feasibility study. Drug Alcohol Depend. 49:55–60, 1997.

Shear, P. K., Butters, N., Jernigan, T. L., DiTraglia, G. M., Irwin, M., Schuckit, M. A. and Cermak, L. S., Olfactory loss in alcoholics: correlations with cortical and subcortical MRI indices. Alcohol 9:247–255, 1992.

Shear, P. K., Jernigan, T. L. and Butters, N., Volumetric magnetic resonance imaging quantification of longitudinal brain changes in abstinent alcoholics. Alcohol. Clin. Exp. Res. 18:172–176, 1994.

Shear, P. K., Sullivan, E. V., Lane, B. and Pfefferbaum, A., Mammillary body and cerebellar shrinkage in chronic alcoholics with and without amnesia. Alcohol. Clin. Exp. Res. 20:1489–1495, 1996.

Shungu, D. C., Millar, W. S., Kreigstein, A. R., Lynch, T. and DeLaPaz, R. L., "Chasing the Dragon" with multislice ^{1}H MRSI of the human brain exposed to heroin vapors. International Society for Magnetic Resonance in Medicine, Sixth Scientific Meeting and Exhibition. Sydney, Australia, p. 1713, 1998.

Silva, A. C., Zhang, W., Williams, D. S. and Koretsky, A. P., Multi-slice MRI of rat brain perfusion during amphetamine stimulation using arterial spin labeling. Magn. Reson. Med. 33:209–214, 1995.

Silver, N. C., Barker, G. J., MacManus, D. G., Miller, D. H., Thorpe, J. W. and Howard, R. S., Decreased magnetisation transfer ratio due to demyelination: a case of central pontine myelinolysis. J. Neurol. Neurosurg. Psychiatry 61:208–209, 1996.

Smith, M. A., Chick, J., Kean, D. M., Douglas, R. H., Singer, A., Kendell, R. E. and Best, J. J., Brain water in chronic alcoholic patients measured by magnetic resonance imaging. Lancet 1:1273–1274, 1985.

Smith, M. A., Chick, J. D., Engleman, H. M., Kean, D. M., Mander, A. J., Douglas, R. H. and Best, J. J., Brain hydration during alcohol withdrawal in alcoholics measured by magnetic resonance imaging. Drug Alcohol Depend. 21:25–28, 1988.

Sowell, E. R., Jernigan, T. L., Mattson, S. N., Riley, E. P., Sobel, D. F. and Jones, K. L., Abnormal development of the cerebellar vermis in children prenatally exposed to alcohol: size reduction in lobules I-V. Alcohol. Clin. Exp. Res. 20:31–34, 1996.

Spielman, D. M., Glover, G. H., Macovski, A. and Pfefferbaum, A., Magnetic resonance spectroscopic imaging of ethanol in the human brain: a feasibility study. Alcohol. Clin. Exp. Res. 17:1072–1077, 1993.

Squire, L. R., Amaral, D. G. and Press, G. A., Magnetic resonance imaging of the hippocampal formation and mammillary nuclei distinguish medial temporal lobe and diencephalic amnesia. J. Neurosci. 10:3106–3117, 1990.

Steller, U., Koschorek, F. and Strenge, H., Cerebellar ataxia with recovery related to central pontine myelinolysis. J. Neurol. 235:379–381, 1988.

Streeter, C. C., Ciraulo, D. A., Harris, G. J., Kaufman, M. J., Lewis, R. F., Knapp, C. M., Ciraulo, A. M., Maas, L. C., Ungeheuer, M., Szulewski, S. and Renshaw, P. F., Functional magnetic resonance imaging of alprazolam-induced changes in humans with familial alcoholism. Psychiatry Res. 82:69–82, 1998.

Sullivan, E. V., Marsh, L., Mathalon, D. H., Lim, K. O. and Pfefferbaum, A., Anterior hippocampal volume deficits in nonamnesic, aging chronic alcoholics. Alcohol. Clin. Exp. Res. 19:110–122, 1995.

Sullivan, E. V., Marsh, L., Mathalon, D. H., Lim, K. O. and Pfefferbaum, A., Relationship between alcohol withdrawal seizures and temporal lobe white matter volume deficits. Alcohol. Clin. Exp. Res. 20:348–354, 1996.

Sullivan, E. V., Mathalon, D. H., Lim, K. O., Marsh, L. and Pfefferbaum, A., Patterns of regional cortical dysmorphology distinguishing schizophrenia and chronic alcoholism. Biol. Psychiatry 43:118–131, 1998.

Swayze, V. W., 2nd., Johnson, V. P., Hanson, J. W., Piven, J., Sato, Y., Giedd, J. N., Mosnik, D. and Andreasen, N. C., Magnetic resonance imaging of brain anomalies in fetal alcohol syndrome. Pediatrics 99:232–240, 1997.

Tan, T. P., Algra, P. R., Valk, J. and Wolters, E. C., Toxic leukoencephalopathy after inhalation of poisoned heroin: MR findings. AJNR Am. J. Neuroradiol. 15:175–178, 1994.

Taylor-Robinson, S. D., Sargentoni, J., Marcus, C. D., Morgan, M. Y. and Bryant, D. J., Regional variations in cerebral proton spectroscopy in patients with chronic hepatic encephalopathy. Metab. Brain Dis. 9:347–359, 1994a.

Taylor-Robinson, S. D., Sargentoni, J., Mallalieu, R. J., Bell, J. D., Bryant, D. J., Coutts, G. A. and Morgan, M. Y., Cerebral phosphorus-31 magnetic resonance spectroscopy in patients with chronic hepatic encephalopathy. Hepatology 20:1173–1178, 1994b.

Teoh, S. K., Mendelson, J. H., Woods, B. T., Mello, N. K., Hallgring, E., Anfinsen, P., Douglas, A. and Mercer, G., Pituitary volume in men with concurrent heroin and cocaine dependence. J. Clin. Endocrinol. Metab. 76:1529–1532, 1993.

Thuluvath, P. J., Edwin, D., Yue, N. C., DeVilliers, C., Hochman, S. and Klein, A., Increased signals seen in globus pallidus in T1-weighted magnetic resonance imaging in cirrhotics are not suggestive of chronic hepatic encephalopathy. Hepatology 21:440–442, 1995.

Thuomas, K. A., Moller, C., Odkvist, L. M., Flodin, U. and Dige, N., MR imaging in solvent-induced chronic toxic encephalopathy. Acta Radiol. 37:177–179, 1996.

Tien, R., Arieff, A. I., Kucharczyk, W., Wasik, A. and Kucharczyk, J., Hyponatremic encephalopathy: is central pontine myelinolysis a component? Am. J. Med. 92:513–522, 1992.

Tobita, M., Mochizuki, H., Takahashi, S., Onodera, H., Itoyama, Y. and Iwasaki, Y., A case of Marchiafava-Bignami disease with complete recovery: sequential imaging documenting improvement of callosal lesions. Tohoku J. Exp. Med. 182:175–179, 1997.

Tsai, E. M., Lee, J. N., Chao, M. C. and Chai, C. Y., Holoprosencephaly and trisomy 13 in a fetus with maternal early gestational amphetamine abuse: a case report. Kaohsiung J. Med. Sci. 9:703–706, 1993.

Tsuchiya, K., Watabiki, S., Shiojiri, T., Matsumoto, A. and Tsukagoshi, H., Alcoholic cerebellar degeneration with pyramidal sign—in relation to alcoholic myelopathy. [Japanese]. No To Shinkei 45:169–175, 1993.

Unger, E., Alexander, A., Fritz, T., Rosenberg, N. and Dreisbach, J., Toluene abuse: physical basis for hypointensity of the basal ganglia on T_2-weighted MR images. Radiology 193:473–476, 1994.

Vaidya, C. J., Austin, G., Kirkorian, G., Ridlehuber, H. W., Desmond, J. E., Glover, G. H. and Gabrieli, J. D., Selective effects of methylphenidate in attention deficit hyperactivity disorder: a functional magnetic resonance study. Proc. Natl. Acad. Sci. USA 95:14494–14499, 1998.

Vila, N. and Chamorro, A., Ballistic movements due to ischemic infarcts after intravenous heroin overdose: report of two cases. Clin. Neurol. Neurosurg. 99:259–262, 1997.

Volkow, N. D., Mullani, N., Gould, K. L., Adler, S. and Krajewski, K., Cerebral blood flow in chronic cocaine users: a study with positron emission tomography. Br. J. Psychiatry 152:641–648, 1988a.

Volkow, N. D., Valentine, A. and Kulkarni, M., Radiological and neurological changes in the drug abuse patient: a study with MRI. J. Neuroradiol. 15:288–293, 1988b.

Vymazal, J., Babis, M., Brooks, R. A., Filip, K., Dezortova, M., Hrncarkova, H. and Hajek, M., T1 and T2 alterations in the brains of patients with hepatic cirrhosis. AJNR Am. J. Neuroradiol. 17:333–336, 1996.

Wang, G. J., Volkow, N. D., Roque, C. T., Cestaro, V. L., Hitzemann, R. J., Cantos, E. L., Levy, A. V. and Dhawan, A. P., Functional importance of ventricular enlargement and cortical atrophy in healthy subjects and alcoholics as assessed with PET, MR imaging, and neuropsychologic testing. Radiology 186:59–65, 1993.

Weber, W., Henkes, H., Moller, P., Bade, K. and Kuhne, D., Toxic spongiform leucoencephalopathy after inhaling heroin vapour. Eur. Radiol. 8:749–755, 1998.

Welch, L., Kirshner, H., Heath, A., Gilliland, R. and Broyles, S., Chronic neuropsychological and neurological impairment following acute exposure to a solvent mixture of toluene and methyl ethyl ketone (MEK). J. Toxicol. Clin. Toxicol. 29:435–445, 1991.

Welch, L. W., Nimmerrichter, A., Kessler, R., King, D., Hoehn, R., Margolin, R. and Martin, P. R., Severe global amnesia presenting as Wernicke-Korsakoff syndrome but resulting from atypical lesions. Psychol. Med. 26:421–425, 1996.

Xiong, L., Matthes, J. D., Li, J. and Jinkins, J. R., MR imaging of "spray heads": toluene abuse via aerosol paint inhalation. AJNR Am. J. Neuroradiol. 14:1195–1199, 1993.

Yamashita, K., Kobayashi, S., Yamaguchi, S., Koide, H. and Nishi, K., Reversible corpus callosum lesions in a patient with Marchiafava-Bignami disease: serial changes on MRI. Eur. Neurol. 37:192–193, 1997.

Yamazaki, K., Katayama, S., Iwai, T. and Hirata, K., A case of malignant syndrome with leukoencephalopathy due to cocaine abuse. [Japanese]. Rinsho Shinkeigaku 34:582–586, 1994.

Yurgelun-Todd, D. A., Gruber, S. A., Hanson, R. A., Baird, A. A., Renshaw, P. F. and Pope, H. G., Jr., Residual effects of marijuana use: an fMRI study. College on Problems of Drug Dependence, 60th Annual Scientific Meeting. Scottsdale, AZ, p. 167, 1998.

Zeneroli, M. L., Cioni, G., Crisi, G., Vezzelli, C. and Ventura, E., Globus pallidus alterations and brain atrophy in liver cirrhosis patients with encephalopathy: an MR imaging study. Magn. Reson. Imaging 9:295–302, 1991.

Zipursky, R. B., Lim, K. C. and Pfefferbaum, A., MRI study of brain changes with short-term abstinence from alcohol. Alcohol. Clin. Exp. Res. 13:664–666, 1989.

Zuckerman, G. B., Ruiz, D. C., Keller, I. A. and Brooks, J., Neurologic complications following intranasal administration of heroin in an adolescent. Ann. Pharmacother. 30:778–781, 1996.

Chapter 7

Neuropsychological Correlates of Drug Abuse

Staci A. Gruber, ED M, *and Deborah A. Yurgelun-Todd,* PHD

INTRODUCTION

As technology continues to advance at an unprecedented rate, it has become increasingly possible to examine the human brain in vivo through the application of a range of neuroimaging modalities. This progress in technology is paralleled by the rapidly evolving knowledge base in cognitive neurobiology. The implementation of sophisticated neuroimaging methods provides us with the opportunity to measure brain processes with increased spatial and temporal resolution, but we are left with the challenge of relating these imaging findings to meaningful units of human behavior. In general, investigators strive to design experiments that measure levels of brain function which can be reasonably associated with their neuroimaging methods. However, the modeling of brain–behavior relationships is dependent on the definition of a number of important factors including the identification of the level of brain function to be studied. For example, should analyses of behavior be defined on the basis of tasks, symptoms or syndromes, and should these behavioral units be related to individual brain regions, to local circuits, or to network systems? One discipline which has been able to address the multiple functional levels of the brain and has contributed significantly to the interpretation of the neuroimaging data is the field of neuropsychology.

From: *Brain Imaging in Substance Abuse: Research, Clinical, and Forensic Applications*
M. J. Kaufman, ed. © Humana Press Inc., Totowa, New Jersey

Emerging from the disciplines of neurology and psychology, the field of neuropsychology has focused on the reliable objective assessment of higher cortical brain functions (Lezak, 1985). At its core, neuropsychological science relies heavily on the study of the interrelationships between behavioral function and neuroanatomy (Kolb and Whishaw, 1990). These relationships were initially based on the examination of patients who experienced acute lesions either from battle (gunshot wounds), trauma (focal accident), or from cardiovascular events (Walsh, 1978). However, behavioral and cortical changes associated with other clinical conditions including dementia and alcoholism, and psychiatric disorders including "functional" psychoses have also contributed substantially to neuropsychological models of brain function. As with other disciplines based in the neurosciences, neuropsychological theories have continued to evolve in accordance with neurobiological findings (Mesulam, 1985). Contemporary theories combine a comprehensive knowledge of neurology with cognitive and emotional processing theories in order to model function of both healthy and clinical populations.

The use of the term "neuropsychology" has increasingly broadened as the discipline has continued to evolve. In fact, a literature review using the keyword "neuropsychology" will produce a large number of studies which include a single neurocognitive test, such as reaction time, to assess cortical function. It is important to distinguish between studies that use a single assessment measure and those that apply a more traditional neuropsychological approach. The latter use multiple neuropsychological measures in order to provide converging evidence for cognitive dysfunction in one or more domains which in turn may be related to neurobiological substrates. Although many neuropsychological tests are putative markers of specific cortical regions or functional domains, it is not possible to characterize localized deficits on the basis of a single measure. The neuropsychological assessment is therefore comprised of multiple test measures that assess a range of functional domains. The pattern of responses to these measures will provide a basis for identifying the type of neuropsychological deficit and the region of cortical or subcortical impairment.

It is important to note, however, that the interpretation of neuropsychological data can be done on multiple levels, and can therefore be incorporated into a number of study designs including neuroimaging studies. One important consideration in designing and understanding functional imaging studies is the neurobiologic theory on which the study is based. In recent years, the assumption underlying the interpretation of most functional brain imaging data is that human cognition can be parsed into separate components (Wise et al., 1991). The modular approach to human cognition hypothesizes that neuropsychological processing is the result of a sequence of individual cognitive components each with its own neuroanatomic locus. Within this framework, loss of cognitive function would occur when discrete brain regions are impaired. Regional cerebral blood flow studies of visual and motor cortex (primary sensory cortex) have supported this view with demonstrations of regional cerebral activation in discrete anatomic regions in response to sensory stimulation paradigms (Fox et al., 1985).

The interpretation of functional imaging data for more complex higher cognitive functions has not been as clear. One reason is that higher order functions, such as language processing, are subserved by widely distributed networks. Furthermore, models for language processing, are complex and include elements of dynamic interactive activation and parallel processing (Wise, 1991). These factors reduce the likelihood of finding unique anatomical correlates for higher cognitive functions, and may contribute to the relatively small cortical activation observed during cognitive tasks compared with primary sensory activation (Kwong et al., 1992). Nevertheless, previous PET studies have successfully used cognitive challenge procedures to enhance localization of language processing areas in the brain (Parks et al., 1988; Petersen et al., 1988; Frith et al., 1991).

In general, new imaging studies based on clinical populations emerge from previous research findings which have identified physiologic, neurologic or neuropsychological dysfunction in patients with a specified history. Investigators are interested in developing cognitive challenge paradigms that can be used in combination with functional neuroimaging technology as a means of visualizing neural systems which underlie discrete cognitive functions. The transfer of robust, clearly delineated methods, such as those refined in off-line studies, provides a strong foundation for the extension of functional imaging studies. Brain dysfunction in subjects with substance abuse has been described for a number of functional areas including language based processes such as verbal memory, semantic priming and thought disorder. Our focus will be on neuropsychological findings that have theoretical implications for understanding the pathophysiology and etiology of substance abuse. Additional references to neuropsychological findings in substance abuse may be found in the bibliography section at the end of the book. Readers may consult Table 1 for a listing and description of commonly used neuropsychological tests, as well as the glossary for descriptions of unfamiliar neuropsychological terms.

Alcohol

Little doubt exists as to the neurotoxic effects of alcohol on the human nervous system, and multiple, though often mild, neuropsychological deficits have been documented in long-term chronic alcoholics. People generally consider the most extreme alcohol related condition, Korsakoff's disease, as reflective of all individuals who abuse alcohol. It is important to note that although this disease occurs in some individuals, the majority of individuals who use alcohol chronically do not manifest this disorder. Clinical research on alcoholic patients is sometimes difficult to interpret given the varied subject populations and the length of use or abstinence in these subjects. Factors including age, past psychiatric history, history of head trauma, length and type of abuse, and premorbid medical status may greatly affect test results. Nevertheless, several patterns of behavioral alterations and neuropsychological deficits have been associated with alcohol use and abuse.

Acute Effects

The acute neuropsychological effects of alcohol use are somewhat conflicting. At the time of acute intoxication, the alcohol abuser will generally present in a somewhat confused state with decreased attention and deficits in most cognitive areas assessed. Studies examining the relationship between the amount and frequency of alcohol consumption and neuropsychological deficits have found a slight association between

Table 1
Neuropsychology Test Descriptions

Bender Visuomotor Gestalt Test: A test designed to demonstrate the tendency to organize visual stimuli into configurational wholes; this task is also sensitive to perseverative tendencies.

Benton Visual Retention Test: A test of visuospatial memory.

Buschke's Selective Reminding Test: A test designed to measure verbal learning and memory during a multiple trial list learning task.

Category Test: One of the subtests of the Halstead-Reitan neuropsychological test battery, this test measures abstraction ability and includes a visuospatial component.

Continuous Performance Test: A test of sustained attention in which the subject is required to respond to either a specific letter or a particular pattern of letters as they continuously flash on a computer screen.

Critical Flicker Fusion Test: One of the original seven subtests comprising the Halstead-Reitan Battery, this test uses a stroboscope to measure the rate at which flashing lights appear steady or fused into a constant light.

Digit Span Forward and Backward: A subtest of the WAIS-R, this test measures the efficiency of attention through repetition of digits either in the order presented by the examiner (Digit Span Forward) or in the reverse order of presentation (Digit Span Backward).

Digit Symbol Test: A subtest of the WAIS-R, this test of psychomotor performance assesses motor persistence, sustained attention, response speed, and visuomotor coordination.

Embedded Figures Test: A test designed to examine visual search and tracing of a figure embedded in the background.

Finger Tapping Test: A test that measures the motor speed of the index finger of each hand.

Grooved Pegboard Test: A test of manual dexterity taken from the Wisconsin Neuropsychological Test Battery.

Halstead Category Test: Subtest of the Halstead-Reitan Test Battery. Measures a patient's abstraction or concept formation ability.

Mini Mental State Exam (MMSE): A brief and simple test of cognitive functions that has been standardized, this exam is useful in assessing changes in intellectual functioning for progressive dementias and psychiatric patients.

Neuropsychological Screening Battery (NSB): Consists of six tests: Word Fluency, Phrase Construction, Rey's 15 Word Memory Test, Modified Raven's Colored Progressive Matrices, Immediate Visual Memory, Copying Drawings. This battery is designed to examine major areas of cognitive functioning.

Paced Auditory Serial Addition Test: This test is a serial-addition task used to assess the rate of information processing and sustained attention.

Rey Auditory Verbal Learning Test: A test to assess verbal learning and memory during a multiple trial list learning task.

Rey-Osterrieth Complex Figure Test: A test to assess visuospatial constructional ability and visual memory. A stimulus design is presented which the subject first copies (copy condition), then must immediately recall from memory (immediate recall condition), and then is asked again to recall from memory after a delay period (delay condition).

Sternberg Task: A continuous-performance, choice-reaction-time test that relies on working memory and is thought to be mediated by attentional networks.

Symbol-Digit Modalities Test: A test of attentional functions sensitive to visual perceptual, visual scanning, oculomotor defects, or general mental or motor slowing.

Tactual Performance Test: A test that assesses tactile form recognition, memory for shapes, and spatial location, as well as psychomotor problem solving.

Trail Making Test: A test of speed for visual search, attention, mental flexibility, and motor function. It requires the connection, by making pencil lines, between 25 encircled numbers randomly arranged on a page in proper order (Trail Making A) and of 25 encircled numbers and letters in alternating order (Trail Making B).

Visual Search Test: Requires the patient to visually scan a page in order to match a specific stimulus figure.

Wechsler Adult Intelligence Scale-Revised (WAIS-R): An estimate of overall intellectual ability, consisting of six verbal scale subtests and five performance scale subtests.

WAIS-R Arithmetic Subtest: A test to measure general arithmetic knowledge. Assesses knowledge of and ability to apply arithmetic operations only.

WAIS-R Block Design Subtest: Two dimensional space constructional task; best measure of visuospatial organization.

Wisconsin Card Sorting Test: Test devised to assess the ability to form abstract concepts, and shift and maintain set.

Wechsler Memory Scale (WMS): A battery consisiting of seven subtests: Personal and Current Information, Orientation, Mental Control, Logical Memory, Digit Span, Visual Reproduction, and Associate Learning.

WMS Associate Learning Subtest: Test of verbal learning. Paired word-learning task that tests the recall of well-learned verbal associations and retention of new, unfamiliar verbal material.

WMS Logical Memory Scale: A subtest of the WMS which tests the immediate recall of verbal ideas with two prose paragraphs.

reduced short-term verbal recall (Parker and Noble, 1977), subtle deficits in concept formation and mental flexibility, and mild perseververative tendency (MacVane et al., 1982; Grant, 1987) with both amount and frequency of alcohol use. However, other studies have not found any evidence that the quantity of alcohol consumed has an effect on performance on various neuropsychological tests (Parsons, 1986; Walton et al., 1987). A series of studies by Parker et al. (1980, 1981), indicate that small amounts of alcohol taken immediately after a learning session may actually improve memory consolidation, although Jones and Jones (1977), found that learning attempted shortly after alcohol ingestion tends to be compromised.

Chronic Effects

Individuals with chronic alcohol abuse display a wide range and variety of presentations of cognitive disorders, perhaps due to the numerous risk factors that contribute to neuropsychological deficits. As a result, much of the literature on cognitive impairment and chronic alcohol use is contradictory. For example, aging is generally considered a risk factor, but this factor is confounded with duration and intensity of drinking (Carlen et al., 1981; Freund, 1982; Grant, 1987). Gender differences have also been reported; alcoholic men but not women show deficits in visuospatial learning (Fabian et al., 1984), while women show the same kind of response slowing and inaccuracies as men (Glenn and Parsons, 1991).

Chronic alcoholics generally demonstrate a range of cognitive difficulties including mild deficits in visuospatial, perceptual, and graphomotor tasks (Goldstein, 1976; Butters et al., 1977), learning and memory, and tasks which require executive functions including abstraction, planning, and complex problem solving (Oscar-Berman, 1973; Cutting, 1979). Despite this, overall intellectual functioning appears to remain largely uncompromised. Butters et al. (1981) compared chronic alcoholics to matched controls on the Wechsler Adult Intelligence Scale (WAIS), and found no significant differences on overall IQ scores (Full Scale IQ) between the two groups, although scores on the Digit Symbol subtest of the WAIS were significantly lower in the alcoholic group. Additional investigations (Parsons et al., 1972) have noted mildly reduced Performance IQ scores relative to the Verbal IQ scores in chronic alcohol users.

Impairments in visuospatial functions have been some of the most consistently reported deficits demonstrated by long term alcohol users. Tarter (1976) reported that chronic alcoholics were impaired on visuospatial tasks including the WAIS-R Block Design subtest, the Tactual Performance Test, and the Embedded Figures Test. Visuospatial organizational task performance has also been reported as being impaired in these subjects (Parsons and Farr, 1981; Ryan and Butters, 1986). Analysis of the visuospatial impairments of chronic alcoholics suggests that the deficits may be attributed to slowed visual organization and integration (Akshoomoff et al., 1989). In addition, no consistent deficit was found on tasks requiring only perceptuomotor or motor coordination tasks which require no synthesizing or organizational activity (Vivian et al., 1973; Tarter, 1975; Oscar-Berman and Weinstein, 1985).

Cognitive impairments in executive functions have frequently been observed in chronic alcoholics, especially in frontal lobe tasks (Talland, 1965; Parsons, 1975; Tarter, 1976; Walsh, 1985; Ryan and Butters, 1986; Grant, 1987). Chronic alcoholics are characterized by difficulty in maintaining cognitive set, decreased mental flexibility, using overly simplistic problem solving strategies, perseveration, loss of spatial and temporal orientation, and an impaired ability to organize perceptuomotor responses and integrate spatial elements. Several investigations reported poorer performance in chronic alcoholics on the Halstead Category Test as compared to non-drinkers (Fitzhugh et al. 1965; Jones and Parsons, 1971), and on the Wisconsin Card Sorting Test (Tarter, 1973).

While many early studies reported relatively unimpaired memory functions in chronic alcoholics without Wernicke-Korsakoff syndrome, recent studies designed to assess subtle memory impairments have yielded different results. Subtle but consistent short-term memory and learning deficits have been observed by several investigators (Ryan and Butters, 1982, 1986). These impairments become more evident with increasing task difficulty and/or the insertion of a distractor task between learning and recall trials. Some researchers have noted that alcoholic subjects appear to rely on superficial encoding strategies, resulting in a greater than normal number of intrusions appearing throughout successive trials (Weingartner et al., 1971; Kramer et al., 1989). Normal rates of forgetting further implicate encoding rather than retrieval (Becker et al., 1983; Nixon et al., 1987). Ryan and Lewis (1988) suggest that visual learning is perhaps more susceptible to the duration of alcoholism than verbal learning.

Chronic alcohol abuse is selective in the aspects of cognitive functioning it affects. It has been shown that in chronic alcoholics, arithmetic, language, and attention remain relatively unimpaired (Tarter, 1976; Parsons and Farr, 1981; Ryan and Butters, 1986). The severity of cognitive impairment is related to many factors, including intake quantity and/or duration, and age. Pishkin et al. (1985), found that the age at which drinking began was a strong predictor of conceptual level and efficiency. Sanchez-Craig (1980) suggests that binge drinkers may be less prone to cognitive impairment as a result of alcohol than those who are chronic alcoholics. As cognitive alterations in mental flexibility, problem solving skills, short term memory, and learning are exhibited in chronic alcoholics as well as the elderly, some researchers have suggested that alcoholism accelerates aging of the brain (Tarter, 1976; Blusewicz et al., 1977; Graff-Radford et al., 1982).

Speed of performance, the solution of novel and complex tasks, and sensorimotor ability have also been found to be affected in chronic alcoholics. Mergler et al. (1988) found impaired color vision in all heavy drinkers and increasing incidence of the impairment with increased consumption. Visual search and scanning efficiency also seems to be impaired (Kapur and Butters, 1977; Ryan and Butters, 1986; Wilson et al., 1988). Overall slowing of response speed in chronic alcoholics may be partly attributed to these visual scanning problems (Glosser et al., 1977). Goldman (1983) found that chronic alcoholics performed more poorly than control subjects on the Trail Making Test, and the Digit Symbol Test, a composite measure involving speed, learning, and the ability to rapidly come up with a strategy.

Alcohol has been found to have many different structural/physiologic effects on the central nervous system. The toxic effects of alcohol are thought to be the cause of cerebral atrophy among dedicated alcoholics compared to age-matched controls (Harper and Blumbergs, 1982; Ron, 1983; Jernigan et al., 1991). Atrophy has also been linked to duration and intensity of drinking (Kroll et al., 1980; Lusins et al., 1980). However, the degree of cortical atrophy is not a reliable predictor of cognitive impairment (Lishman, 1981; Acker et al., 1984; Grant, 1987). Other cortical anomalies found in the brains of chronic alcoholics include enlarged ventricles, widened spaces between cortical folds, and reduced elaboration of dendrites in the hippocampus and the cerebellum (Lishman, 1981; Ryan and Butters, 1986; Wilkinson, 1987; Jernigan et al., 1991). All measures of regional cerebral blood flow have been found to be relatively reduced in chronic alcoholics (Berglund et al., 1987). Gray matter in the dorsolateral and parietal regions may be especially affected, and white and gray matter abnormalities have been correlated with cognitive deficits (Brust, 1993).

Marijuana

Marijuana remains the most widely abused illicit drug in the United States (National Institutes of Health, 1998). The relative paucity of research in this area is striking, given that nearly 70 million Americans over the age of 12 have tried marijuana at least once, and more than 5 million Americans smoke marijuana at least once a week (National Institutes of Health, 1998). Additionally, the rise in marijuana use that began in the early 1990s among America's junior high and high school students has continued to increase according to NIDA's 1996 Monitoring the Future study (Johnston et al., 1996). Many studies over the years have attempted to assess the residual effects of chronic marijuana use on neuropsychological performance, however, as noted in a recent review (Pope and Yurgelun-Todd, 1996), these studies are subject to many methodologic limitations.

Acute Effects

Although acute marijuana intoxication clearly affects neuropsychological function (Miller, 1974; Fehr and Kalant, 1983), studies of acutely intoxicated subjects do not permit conclusions as to whether marijuana causes residual effects beyond the immediate period of intoxication. In a comprehensive review by Miller (1976), the author noted that for every study of acute neuropsychological effects of marijuana, at least one or more other studies had been published which found no change in cognitive function just after marijuana use. One study (Darley et al., 1973) reported reduced memory efficiency during marijuana use and investigators hypothesized that the deficiency seen in smokers was likely due to impaired attention, or insufficient rehearsal, as opposed to a long term storage deficit. Braff et al. (1981) reported slowed visual processing in subjects intoxicated with marijuana who had also ingested alcohol; no impairment was found in subjects who had only used marijuana.

Chronic Effects

A majority of studies have produced positive findings, but a substantial minority has failed to exhibit residual impairment in cannabis users. Studies finding differences in the traits of heavy marijuana users as compared to non-users (Robins et al., 1970; Mirin et al., 1971; Sharma, 1975; Bourque et al., 1991) are somewhat inconclusive, since any deficits in the former group in social, academic, or occupational function may again reflect simply the effects of frequent acute intoxication rather than residual effects. Conversely, studies failing to show differences between chronic marijuana users and non-users on general measures of social or occupational functioning (Zinberg and Weil, 1970; Comitas, 1976; Pope et al., 1981, 1990) may have missed residual effects of marijuana that would be more readily detectable on direct neuropsychological testing of specific cognitive functions. Additionally, studies of marijuana users with psychiatric disorders, including marijuana users with other forms of substance abuse or dependence, must be excluded, because of the potentially confounding effect of these latter variables. In particular, cannabis dependence is often comorbid with cocaine and alcohol dependence (Miller et al., 1990), and these latter substances clearly affect neuropsychological performance.

These inconsistent results appear likely because of several methodologic limitations. First, the term "residual effect" is ambiguous; this term might describe any of four hypothetical phenomena: a temporary effect caused by persistent drug in the central nervous system (CNS) or acute drug withdrawal; reversible CNS neurotoxicity that persists beyond the period of drug residue or drug withdrawal; irreversible CNS toxicity, in which the CNS does not "heal" even after abstinence; and reduced fund of information, because of reduced learning during chronic intoxication over the years. Most studies do not distinguish between these possible types of residual effects in their analyses.

A survey of several well-known positive studies from the last 20 years illustrates these limitations. In Egypt, Soueif (1975, 1976) found marked differences on testing in 850 male prisoners who had used hashish at least once per month for a year, as compared with 839 nonuser controls. However, it is unclear whether users had access to hashish in the prison and had smoked the drug close to the time of testing. Furthermore, although users and nonusers were matched on age, sex, urban vs rural residence, employment level, and education, they were not matched on other variables, such as use of other drugs or premorbid levels of intelligence. For example, users were somewhat more likely to be illiterate and less likely to have attended high school or college than nonusers. These potential confounding variables compromise interpretation of the findings.

Two Indian studies (Wig and Varma, 1977; Mendhiratta et al., 1978) found marked impairment on neuropsychological testing in long-term heavy users as compared to nonusers, but employed only a 12–48 h abstinence period without uniform supervision of all subjects. Thus, the impairment observed in users might easily have represented temporary effects. These same research groups later published studies of similar design, with various methodological refinements (Mendhiratta et al., 1988; Varma et al., 1988). Although the abstinence period was more carefully supervised in these latter studies, it remained only 12 h in length. This may indicate that the differences found might be best explained as simple drug-residue or drug-withdrawal effects. Interestingly, one of these groups of investigators (Mendhiratta et al., 1988) subsequently examined many of the same subjects whom they had studied ten years earlier (Mendhiratta et al., 1978). On two tests, reaction time and the Bender visuomotor gestalt test, users showed greater deterioration over this 10-yr period than nonusers, providing some evidence for a longer lasting effect. However, users and nonusers were not matched for use of other drugs; for example, 73% of 30 users versus 7% of 15 nonusers reported opiate use.

In a similar longitudinal study, Page et al. (1988) examined a subset of the Costa Rican users previously studied in 1976 by Satz et al. (1976). The original 1976 study had failed to distinguish users from nonusers on a battery of tests, despite the fact that users had smoked many times per day for a mean of 17 yr. However, by 1988, after re-examining a subset of these users and controls, Page et al. found that users were significantly more impaired than nonusers on three of the neuropsychological tests performed (Buschke's Selective Reminding Test, Underlining Test, and Continuous Performance Test). It is of note that testing was performed only 12–24 h after last use, again raising the possibility that the differences observed might be only a short term effect, rather than frank CNS neurotoxicity. By contrast, Rubin and Comitas (1975) employed a 3–4-d period of abstinence, and found very few significant neuropsychological differences between chronic marijuana smokers and non-smokers. However, it is unclear whether these findings, obtained in unskilled Jamaican workers, would generalize to well-educated groups with a comparable degree of marijuana exposure.

Stronger evidence for lingering CNS toxicity comes from the study of Schwartz et al. (1989), who compared "cannabis-dependent" adolescents with nonuser controls and abusers of other drugs. The cannabis-dependent group performed significantly more poorly than either control group on the Wechsler Memory Scale Logical Memory Subtest and the Benton Visual Retention Test, both after 2 d and again after 6 wk of abstinence in a treatment program. The persistence of impairment in this study argues strongly against a mere drug-residue or drug withdrawal effect and raises the ominous possibility of CNS damage. But the very small sample size renders the study vulnerable to a type I error—a false positive finding perhaps because of one or two "outliers" in a group. Block and Ghoneim (1993) compared 144 users to 72 nonusers, using careful measures to minimize confounding variables and to match the groups for premorbid intellectual performance. Again, however, subjects were tested after only 24 h of unsupervised abstinence, so that a temporary effect cannot be excluded.

Among all of the above studies, little consideration is given to the possibility of acute withdrawal effects from marijuana, despite the findings of several investigations which have noted that tolerance may develop with heavy marijuana use, and that a withdrawal syndrome may occur after abrupt discontinuation of the drug (Jones and Benowitz, 1976; Rohr et al., 1989). The withdrawal syndrome is characterized by both physiologic symptoms, such as insomnia, restlessness, and anorexia, and by psychological symptoms, such as irritability, all of which might affect neuropsychological performance (Jones et al., 1981). Only a study comparing users during normal use, immediately after discontinuing use, and again after a more prolonged period of abstinence could assess these effects, and none of the studies employed such a design. Finally, none of the studies appears to have addressed the issue of impaired acquisition of new information over the years.

Summary

In summary, the methodologic limitations of available studies severely limit the conclusions which may be drawn regarding the residual neuropsychological effects of long-term marijuana use. Among those studies with negative findings, many may have been vulnerable to a type II error, because of a failure to include subjects with substantial long-term marijuana exposure. Among the studies with positive findings, all but two employed an abstinence period of 48 h or less, sometimes without supervision. Given the complex and incompletely studied pharmacokinetics of cannabinoids—including such factors as the redistribution of accumulated THC from fat stores back into the circulation, and the possible persistence of THC at receptor sites after its disappearance from the plasma compartment, (Wall and Perez-Reyes, 1981; Seth and Sinha, 1991) it seems likely that a 48-h period may be inadequate to sufficiently clear THC from the CNS. Thus, it is not possible to judge whether these positive findings represent merely a relatively brief drug-residue effect, or a more persistent toxic effect on the CNS. Of the two remaining studies, one (Schwartz et al., 1989) found impairment in 10 users after 6 wk of abstinence, but the small sample size renders this study vulnerable to a false positive finding. The other (Rubin and Comitas, 1975), found few effects after 3–4 d of abstinence, but may be less applicable to an educated American population. Thus, evidence regarding the residual neuropsychological effects of marijuana remains scant and inconclusive. Further, although many of these laboratory studies documented impairment lasting 24–48 h after exposure, none assessed impairment after a period of more than 48 h of abstinence. Clearly, further research, addressing the methodological problems outlined above, is needed to assess the long-term neuropsychological effects of long-term marijuana use.

Hallucinogens

Hallucinogens, also commonly referred to as "psychedelics", have been noted to produce distortions of the visual, auditory, and tactile domains while preserving alertness, attentiveness, memory and orientation (Siegel, 1984). Although the precise effects of hallucinogens depend on both the type and amount of specific drug taken, common CNS effects include dilated pupils, tachycardia, palpitations, and sweating. The most frequently reported psychological symptoms include the intensification of mood, perceptions, and the presence of visual hallucinations. The group of hallucinogens most commonly used in the United States include lysergic acid diethylamide (LSD), indolealkylamines (psilocybin), phenylalkylamines (mescaline), ketamine, and 3,4-methylendioxymethamphetamine (MDMA or "ecstasy"). As use of hallucinogens has not been found to produce physical dependence, most are used episodically. Hallucinogen use in the United States remained relatively constant from the late 1960s to the late 1980s (Pope et al., 1990). However, the National Institute on Drug Abuse (NIDA) reported an increase in LSD use by high school seniors "within the last 12 mo" from 4.8 to 5.6%, from 1988 to 1992. While the magnitude of this rise is slight, it stands in contrast to the abuse of other drugs. For example, the proportion of seniors who had used any cocaine dropped from 7.9 to 3.1% during the same period (Johnston et al., 1996). Thus, the proportion of respondents who reported any use of LSD was almost twice as high as the proportion reporting any cocaine use by high school seniors in 1992. The 1990 NIDA statistics reveal that lifetime prevalence rates for hallucinogens were about the same as those for cocaine, and seven to eight times higher than for heroin. LSD ranked first in the categories of "most intense" and "longest" high among respondents. Between 13 and 17 million individuals in this country have used a hallucinogen at least once (NIDA, 1991).

Acute Effects

Acute adverse effects include brief panic reactions to effects of the drug, which generally respond to verbal reassurance and protection of the individual (Taylor et al., 1970), and psychotic reactions that can last longer than 24 h and may require more intensive management or even hospitalization. As NMDA glutamate receptor antagonists have been reported to induce psychotic symptoms in humans, studies of ketamine have focused on the acute clinical and cognitive effects of the drug. Malhotra et al. (1996) examined the effects of ketamine on free recall and recognition memory in a double-blind placebo-controlled study which included healthy volunteer subjects. Ketamine produced decrements in free recall, recognition memory and attention in all study subjects, and induced a brief psychosis marked by thought disorder and withdrawal-retardation. Findings from this study suggest that NMDA receptors may have a direct role on two types of explicit memory. In a study by Radant and colleagues (1998), investigators administered progressively higher doses of ketamine to healthy male volunteer subjects and assessed oculomotor, cognitive, and symptomatic changes. Measures of verbal recall, recognition memory, and verbal fluency deteriorated significantly after the infusion of ketamine. Additionally, oculomotor abnormalities were also noted after ketamine administration, resulting in reduced pursuit tracking and visual fixation. The investigators concluded that the administration of ketamine induces changes in verbal recall, recognition memory, and verbal fluency which are qualitatively similar to those seen in patients with schizophreniform psychosis. Newcomer et al. (1999) examined the cognitive effects of three fixed steady-state doses of ketamine on healthy male volunteer subjects. Ketamine produced a robust dose-dependent decrease in verbal and nonverbal declarative memory performance, at or below plasma concentrations which caused other clinical symptoms. The authors concluded that increasing NMDA hypofunction is associated with early memory impairments. In a study designed to examine the acute effects of mescaline, investigators administered the drug to normal volunteer subjects (Hermle et al., 1992). Mescaline was found to produce an acute psychotic state three and a half to four hours after ingestion. Performance on a face/non-face decision task was impaired, suggesting a decrease in right hemispheric function. The authors later conducted single photon emission computed tomography (SPECT) studies of regional cerebral blood flow, which indicated that mescaline produced a hyperfrontal pattern with an emphasis on the right hemisphere, a finding which was correlated with mescaline-induced psychotic psychopathology.

Chronic Effects

LSD-induced deficits have been difficult to document with certainty, given the lack of premorbid data and an inability of researchers to control for other substances of abuse (Acord and Barker, 1973). In a study by Cohen and Edwards (1969), investigators examined neurocognitive performance of 30 LSD users and thirty age, sex, and education matched control subjects. Performance on the Trail Making Test A and Ravens Progressive Matrices correlated negatively with the extent of LSD use. It is of note, however, that the investigators did not control for current or past use of other illicit substance. Acord and Barker (1973) compared 15 LSD users to control subjects on several neuropsychological test measures. Users of LSD performed significantly worse on the Trail Making Test B and the Categories subtests of the Reitan battery, and on target location ability on the Tactual Performance Test. Again, the investigators did not control for other illicit substances, although all subjects in the control group denied ever having used LSD. In a study which matched three groups of college seniors for predrug use and Scholastic Aptitude Test (SAT) scores, Culver and King (1974) examined subjects who had no history of marijuana or LSD use, subjects who reported marijuana use but no use of hallucinogens, and subjects who used LSD at least once a month for at least 1 yr. While all neuropsychological test results were within normal limits, the subjects who used LSD scored significantly lower on the Trail Making Tests A and B than subjects in the other two groups. In one study of chronic MDMA users, scores on both the initial and delayed verbal recall subtests and the delayed figural recall subtest of the Wechsler Memory Scale were found to be in the mild to moderately impaired range (Krystal et al., 1992). It is of note that none of these subjects demonstrated any memory deficits on a clinical examination. In a more recent study by Morgan (1998), MDMA users who also used other illicit substances demonstrated worse performance on a matching familiar figures test (MFF20) than polydrug users who had never taken MDMA.

While reductions in neuropsychological performance can be detected in studies of hallucinogen users, it remains unclear what pure "chronic" or long-term effects may be the result of hallucinogen abuse. Nearly all studies reviewed here had small sample sizes, and included subjects who had a total lifetime use of <100 times. Additionally, in most of the studies, investigators failed to control for the use of other illicit drugs, the presence of current or past psychiatric history, and other possible confounding factors, including IQ, handedness, and head trauma. Future investigations should include "pure" hallucinogen users, large sample sizes of well-matched subjects, true "chronic" users, a thorough screening for physical and psychiatric disorders, and a premorbid estimate of cognitive function.

Phencyclidine

Phencyclidine (PCP) is the chief member of a unique category of drugs classified as *N*-methyl-D-aspartate agonist inhibitors that have high abuse potential and severe neurotoxicity at high doses (Zukin and Javitt, 1989). PCP causes pathological changes in the CNS which ultimately result in behavioral and psychological alterations. The resemblance of PCP psychosis to schizophrenia has led to extensive research on abnormalities of PCP receptors in schizophrenic patients. Administration of the drug can induce a full schizophrenic-like syndrome, characterized by alterations in body image, apathy, negativism, and disorganized thinking (Rainey and Crowder, 1975). A psychotic state is often observed after extremely low doses of PCP, although it does not appear to cause significant long lasting brain toxicity (Brust, 1993). Decreased frontal lobe metabolism, a finding often reported in schizophrenia, has been reported in subjects who have taken PCP (Olney et al., 1989). Although the drug has been reported to be a favorite of young people (Lewis et al., 1990), the questionable nature of substances sold as PCP make studies difficult to interpret.

Acute Effects

In a study by Javitt and Zukin (1991), subjects who received subanaesthetic doses of PCP demonstrated impaired attention, perception, and symbolic thinking, similar to what is encountered in schizophrenic patients. Carlin et al. (1986) reported that PCP users showed more "generalized" cognitive impairment than nonusers, however, the subjects were not routinely screened for a history of other drug use, head injury, or learning disability.

Chronic Effects

As PCP's duration of action is dose-related, and symptoms are aggravated by concurrent use of other drugs, the chronic effects of PCP are not well known. The psychotic symptoms, including paranoia, thought disorder, hallucinations and catatonia can last days or weeks after a single dose of PCP, and many chronic users have demonstrated persistent cognitive abnormalities (Fauman et al., 1976). The neurocognitive effects of PCP are difficult to interpret in most users, as nearly all have been found to take other drugs as well, most especially marijuana, alcohol, and cocaine (Lerner and Burns, 1978; Giannini et al., 1987).

Benzodiazepines

Benzodiazepines are the most frequently prescribed medications for the treatment of anxiety and sleep disorders. Classified as sedatives or hypnotics, such medications as valium (diazepam) are commonly used, and Xanax (alprazolam) has recently become a "top ten" drug. Last year, more than 80 million prescriptions for benzodiazepines were filled, and 1 in 10 Americans reported use of a benzodiazepine once or more a year for a medical reason other than insomnia (Miller, 1996). They produce their effects via specific receptors involving gamma aminobutyric acid (GABA), and are thought to depress the activity of the systems that produce arousal or the initiation of behavior. Considered safer and more effective, benzodiazepines have replaced barbiturates in the treatment of both anxiety and insomnia, although their precise mechanism of action is unknown. Some studies have shown that benzodiazepines are effective in the treatment of anxiety and insomnia; other studies have shown they produce pharmacological tolerance and dependence in regular or chronic users that leads to lack of efficacy and adverse consequences.

Acute Effects

The most effective uses of benzodiazepines appear to be short-term in duration. Beyond a few months, the efficacy declines because of the development of tolerance and dependence. Short-term uses include the treatment of alcohol and other drug withdrawals, anxiety, insomnia, and other medical and psychiatric conditions. High doses lead to heavier sedation and can impair both mental sharpness and physical co-ordination. Lower doses are recommended for older individuals and for those with some chronic diseases, since they may be more sensitive to medications and may metabolize them more slowly. It has also been suggested that benzodiazepines can impair the ability to learn and remember new information, although few studies have been published on the acute neurocognitive effects of these drugs.

Johnson and Chernik (1982) examined cognitive functioning and psychomotor performance following the bedtime ingestion of either a benzodiazepine or a placebo. Psychomotor performance was noted to be impaired in the group receiving the benzodiazepine as compared to the placebo group. Hanks et al. (1995) compared cognitive and psychomotor effects of a single dose of lorazepam in normal controls. On tasks including choice reaction time, number vigilance, immediate and delayed word recall, and picture recognition, lorazepam was found to produce marked improvements in the tests of attention and memory. In a more recent study, Bourin et al. (1998) administered alprazolam twice daily for 2 wk to normal control subjects, and compared their neuropsychological performance to a group of volunteers receiving placebo. Although initial performance (the first 3 d) was impaired in the group receiving alprazolam compared to the placebo group, a significant improvement in cognitive performance was reported on d 7, 10, and 14. The neuropsychological measures included the Digit Symbol Substitution Test, the Choice Reaction Time, and the Critical Flicker Fusion test, all of which were improved relative to that of the placebo group. The authors concluded that repeated low doses of alprazolam improved cognitive functions.

Chronic Effects

In contrast to the level of use in the United States, relatively few studies have examined the chronic neurocognitive effects of benzodiazepines. Hendler et al. (1980) examined neuropsychological test performance of abusers of benzodiazepines and narcotics admitted to a chronic pain treatment center. Patients who had abused benzodiazepines demonstrated cognitive alterations on the WAIS, the Wechsler Memory Scale, and the Bender Gestalt Visuomotor test, whereas subjects who abused narcotics did not. In a study by Lucki et al. (1986), investigators examined the cognitive performance of long term users of benzodiazepines (average use 5 yr) who were currently abstinent in relation to that of normal control subjects. No difference between the groups was detected. In order to determine the acute effects of benzodiazepines in the abusers, a subset was reexamined after acute administration of their drug of abuse. Performance on tasks of digit-symbol substitution, and critical flicker fusion were improved relative to their previous "wash out score", while performance on measures of delayed verbal memory was reduced. In another study of long term users, Gorenstein et al. (1994) studied subjects who had abused benzodiazepines for an average of 7–20 yr. Subjects were tested at baseline states and following a single dose of diazepam during chronic use, and at both 3 wk and 10 mo post washout. No acute effects of the drug were noted on psychomotor performance at any time point, suggesting persistence of tolerance. In contrast, memory functions were impaired after the acute dose at each time point. Further studies focusing on the chronic effects of benzodiazepines are clearly warranted.

Opiates

Opiates are made from opium, a white liquid from the poppy plant, and are often referred to as narcotics. Heroin, morphine, methadone and codeine are among some of the most commonly abused opiates. Produced in Mexico and Asia, opiates are reported to be widely available throughout the United States. Heroin was originally developed as a substitute for morphine in an effort to deal with morphine addiction, however, it was quickly recognized that heroin is even more addictive than morphine, and as a result, the drug was made illegal. At the street level, heroin is "cut" with a variety of substances, leading to variation in purity over time and in different areas. Numerous reports have suggested a rise in heroin use in recent years, which has been attributed to young people who are smoking or sniffing rather than injecting the drug. Estimates of the purity of heroin have shown substantial increases between 1984 and 1995 (Drug Enforcement Administration, 1995), which makes smoking and sniffing feasible. The increased purity and the concern about AIDS may be causing the shift from injecting to smoking and sniffing among heroin users. When injected, sniffed or smoked, opiates bind with receptors found in many regions of the brain, with the largest concentrations located in the limbic system. The result is intense euphoria, often referred to as a rush. The rush lasts only briefly and is followed by a couple of hours of a relaxed, contented state. In large doses, opiates can reduce or eliminate respiration. The signs and symptoms of opiate use include euphoria, drowsiness, respiratory depression (which can progress until breathing stops), constricted pupils, and nausea. Withdrawal symptoms include watery eyes, runny nose, yawning, loss of appetite, tremors, panic, chills, sweating, nausea, muscle cramps, and insomnia. Elevations in blood pressure, pulse, respiratory rate, and temperature occur as withdrawal progresses. Symptoms of an opiate overdose include shallow breathing, pinpoint pupils, clammy skin, convulsion, and coma. Despite the recent increase in use, empirical literature on the neurocognitive effects of opiate abuse is sparse.

Acute Effects

In a study designed to examine cognitive and psychomotor effects of opioids, Hanks et al. (1995) administered single doses of morphine, lorazepam, and placebo to 12 volunteer subjects. Cognitive function was assessed using reaction time, number vigilance, immediate and delayed word recall, and the critical flicker fusion test (CFFT). Subjects receiving morphine demonstrated significant impairment after one hour on all memory tests, and scores on the CFFT were reduced for the entire 6-h observation period as compared to the control subjects. The authors concluded that single oral doses of morphine result in minimal impairment of cognitive and psychomotor function. A study by Kerr et al. (1991) used steady-state infusions of morphine to examine changes in cognitive performance and motor control in volunteer subjects. The investigators evaluated performance on encoding and processing of verbal material and verbal recall, during three sequential constant plasma concentrations of morphine and a separate saline infusion day in each subject. Plasma morphine concentrations which approximated the usual therapeutic dose range for analgesia caused significant impairment in the time required to encode and process serially presented verbal information in all subjects. The delayed recall of information presented was significantly impaired 3 h after morphine but not saline infusions.

Chronic Effects

While several studies of the chronic effects of opiates have been published, they often include study populations which are confounded by the presence of other drugs of abuse. For example, in a study by Bruhn and Maage (1975), investigators examined general intelligence and neuropsychological test scores in two groups of drug abusers; although both groups had abused marijuana, amphetamines, and hallucinogens, only one group had abused opiates, although the length of use was unspecified. The authors assumed that differences found between the two groups could be attributed solely to opiate use. No significant differences were found, and general intelligence and all neuropsychological test scores were found to be within normal limits. Rounsaville et al. (1982) compared opiate addicts to both a group of demographically matched normal controls who did not use drugs, and to a group of epileptic patients. While all three groups demonstrated mild impairment on tasks of attention (Trail Making A & B, Digit Symbol Subtest), visual scanning (Visual Search Test), and motor abilities (Grooved Pegboard), no relationship was found between current or past opiate use and neuropsychological performance. In a study by Guerra et al. (1987), investigators compared opiate abusers to a group of normal controls before and after the completion of a 1-wk opiate detoxification program on measures of attention, memory, and verbal fluency. Significant differences were noted between the opiate abusers and the controls at the first time point (prior to detoxification). However, at the re-evaluation, one week after admission to the detoxification program, the opiate abusers showed improvement on most measures, and no significant differences were noted between the groups.

In contrast, a study by Carlin et al. (1986) found lowered scores for opiate abusers as compared to normal control subjects on measures of visuospatial and visuomotor function. A more recent study by Pakesch et al. (1992) compared opiate abusers to normal controls, and found that opiate abusers scored significantly below control subjects on a visual memory recall test (Benton Visual Retention Test). Evidence from these studies indicates that further investigations, which carefully control for the effects of polysubstance abuse, abstinence, duration of opiate use, and other possible confounding factors are indicated.

Cocaine

As recently as 1980, cocaine was believed to be a relatively safe, non-addictive drug associated with few side effects (Grinspoon and Bakalar, 1980). Millions of individuals experimented with the drug, and by 1986, approx 3 million were estimated to abuse cocaine regularly (Adams et al., 1986). The first reports of adverse effects of cocaine were published in the mid to late 1980s; it is therefore somewhat surprising that relatively few studies of the neuropsychological sequelae of cocaine abuse have been published. Cocaine is technically a stimulant, and relevant literature often addresses the neurobiological and clinical-behavioral similarities between cocaine and caffeine (Gold & Miller, 1997). However, cocaine and the other stimulants have been shown to differ in terms of their biochemical effects (Post, 1976), and their predominant sites of action in the brain (Glick, et al., 1987). Moreover, a comparison of recent studies of the neuropsychological effects of different types of stimulants suggests that although some global effects may be demonstrated by all stimulant users, a unique pattern of cognitive deficits has been difficult to identify for cocaine (Herning et al., 1990; Kornetsky et al., 1990; O'Malley & Gawin, 1990; Ardila et al., 1991; O'Malley et al., 1992; Hoff et al., 1996). A review of the neuropsychological effects of cocaine by Berry et al. (1993) reported on the limited number of controlled studies. Overall, studies describe mild to moderate neuropsychological impairment in short-term memory and attentional processing among individuals with chronic heavy cocaine use. Comparative statements about the similarity of neurocognitive outcomes with which cocaine and other types of stimulants are associated are questionable at best.

Acute Effects

While the neurophysiology underlying acute cocaine intoxication is well documented, the neurocognitive profile associated with its acute or chronic use has not been well established. Virtually no controlled studies of the acute effects of cocaine on neuropsychological function have been published to date. This is perhaps in part the result of the "clinical consensus" of many researchers that noticeable clinical differences do not appear in cocaine users until they transition from the well-controlled, initial experimentation phase to the eventual state of uncontrolled use of cocaine that results in abuse (Siegel, 1982; Kleber and Gawin, 1984; Gawin and Kleber, 1985). Still, certain neurophysiological characteristics of acute intoxication are known to result in a change in neurocognitive processing ability. Similar to acute amphetamine use, the effects of acute cocaine intoxication include increased alertness and arousal levels, increased motor activation, and hyperfluency. One study of cortical changes conducted in sleep deprived individuals, found that acute cocaine use was associated with increased vigilance and motor functions (Fischman and Schuster, 1980).

Chronic Effects

Neuropsychological impairment of chronic cocaine users may result from an overstimulation of dopaminergic pathways and subsequent hypoexcitability of these areas when cocaine administration is discontinued. A number of recent investigations have attempted to document the neurocognitive changes associated with chronic cocaine use. O'Malley et al. (1990) utilized a brief neuropsychological test battery to study chronic cocaine abusers who were undergoing inpatient treatment. In this preliminary study, subjects were abstinent from the drug (23 d). They scored significantly lower than controls on short term memory, measured by the Logical Memory Subtest of the Wechsler Memory Scale, abstraction ability, measured by the Category Test, and attention, measured both by the Arithmetic and Digit Symbol Subtests of the WAIS-R and the Neuropsychological Screening Battery (NSB). Unexpectedly, cocaine abusers produced higher average verbal fluency scores as compared to controls subjects. The degree of impairment on short term verbal memory was related to both the amount and recency of cocaine use, suggestive of a direct role of cocaine on cognitive function. The authors concluded that recent abstinence from cocaine is associated with problems in concentration, memory, nonverbal problem solving, and abstraction. In a later study by the same investigators, a more extensive neuropsychological battery was administered to outpatients with a history of cocaine abuse, who had been abstinent for an average of 135 d. These patients were found to perform more poorly than control subjects on measures of Verbal and Performance IQ (measured by the WAIS-R), complex cognitive motor skills (Tactual Performance Test, Performance subtests of the WAIS-R), simple motor skills (Finger Tapping, Grip Strength, Grooved Pegboard), and nonverbal memory (TPT memory and location) (O'Malley et al., 1992). Although the cocaine abusers scores were essentially within normal limits, the authors concluded that similar to alcohol abuse, significant cognitive impairment becomes evident in recently detoxified cocaine abusers. Furthermore, a relatively slow recovery of functions occurs with longer periods of abstinence from the drug. The patterns of deficits noted in these studies suggest that disruptions in attention may recover more quickly than motor impairment, which appear to exhibit a more persistent effect.

A study by Ardila et al. (1991) examined freebase cocaine abusers who had a history of crack use for at least one year but had been abstinent from the drug for an average of approximately one month. The authors found that cocaine abusers scored at least one standard deviation below the mean on measures of short term memory (Wechsler Memory Scale-Logical Memory and Associative Learning Subtests), and attention (WAIS-R Digit Symbol Subtest). When lifetime cocaine use was considered, total use was reported to be inversely related to performance on tasks of attention (Wechsler Memory Scale-Digit Span) and nonverbal memory (Rey-Osterrieth Complex Figure), and proved to be indicative of generalized memory functions (Wechsler Memory Scale-Memory Quotient Score).

Volkow et al. (1988) studied freebase and intravenous (IV) cocaine users, with an average use of six months, within the first 3 d of admission to an inpatient detoxification program. On the Mini Mental Status Exam (MMSE), subjects demonstrated a reduced ability to concentrate, a decreased ability to solve arithmetic problems, and difficulty in performing backward digit span tasks. Additionally, these subjects underwent Positron Emission Tomographic (PET) scanning at admission to the program and demonstrated abnormally decreased blood flow in the fronto-temporal region. Scanning was repeated 10 d after admission and no change in the pattern of blood flow (i.e., improvement) was noted. These imaging findings provide evidence in support of focal cortical changes thought to underlie the neurocognitive deficits exhibited by cocaine abusers (Volkow et al., 1988). Hoff et al. (1996) designed a study to examine these specific brain regions in subjects who had abused cocaine for an average of 3.6 yr and had been abstinent for 24.5 d. They found that compared to normal controls, subjects with a history of cocaine use demonstrated poorer spatial memory but no significant changes in verbal memory, confrontation naming, perceptual motor speed or cognitive flexibility (Trail Making B). The authors concluded that continuous cocaine use may produce a distinctive pattern of neuropsychological test performance with no change on some measures and deterioration on others.

Berry et al. (1993) examined the neuropsychological performance of cocaine abusers three days after admission to an inpatient treatment facility and again 14–18 d post admission. In comparison to control subjects, cocaine abusers who had completed three days of detoxification performed more poorly on visuoconstructional tasks (Rey Osterrieth Complex Figure Copy Condition), verbal and visuospatial memory tasks (Rey Auditory Verbal Learning and Rey Osterrieth Complex Figure Delay Conditions), psychomotor speed (WAIS-R Digit Symbol Subtest) and concentration (Paced Auditory Serial Addition Test). Subjects' scores showed only minor improvement at the second testing session, suggesting that the neurocognitive impairments of chronic cocaine abusers may require lengthy recovery periods. Similarly, a study by Herning et al. (1990) included individuals who had abused cocaine for an average of 3.7 yr, and examined subjects at various points over a three week period of abstinence. The findings indicated deficits in performance that persisted over the period of testing. Specifically, impairments were noted on a Sternberg task for as long as the subjects were tested, with performance worsening throughout the abstinence period. The authors suggest that cognitive deficits in abstinent cocaine abusers may exist for a variety of reasons, including a long-term readjustment in several neurotransmitter systems, an unmasking of a residual functional neurological alteration produced by cocaine use, or an unmasking of a preexisting constitutional cognitive alteration in the cocaine abusers. It was concluded that the decrements observed were most likely caused by a generalized and persistent neurophysiological abnormality which became apparent during abstinence from cocaine.

Summary

In summary, although limited data are available regarding the neurocognitive effects of acute cocaine use, it is evident that individuals experience increased alertness and arousal, and motor activation. Performance on tasks of fluency and simple motor control may be improved during acute cocaine intoxication. The neurocognitive effects of chronic cocaine use are somewhat different, with specific areas of function most often affected including memory, attention, auditory processing, psychomotor speed, and visuospatial/visuoconstructional abilities. It is likely that both duration and amount of abuse contribute to the degree of impairment, and that the period of abstinence required for neurocognitive recovery is dependent on both of these elements. The finding of continued neuropsychological deficits throughout the abstinence period has implications for treatment and subsequent relapse, and is an area which warrants further investigation.

Amphetamine and Other Stimulants

The major amphetamines available in the United States are dextroamphetamine (Dexedrine), methamphetamine, and methylphenidate (Ritalin). Additionally, "designer amphetamines" (which also have hallucinogenic properites) including 3,4 methylene-dioxymethamphetamine (MDMA, also referred to as ecstasy and XTC), 5-methoxy-3,4-methylenedioxyamphetamine (MMDA), and 2,5-dimethoxy4-methylamphetamine (DOM) have become increasingly popular. In general, amphetamines are used to increase performance and induce feelings of euphoria. Amphetamines produce cognitive arousal and counteract sleepiness when used in low doses, however, prolonged use results in tolerance and dependence. Methamphetamine use has been weakly associated with the occurrence of strokes, as a result of spastic occlusion of intracranial arteries (Rothrock et al., 1988). While an early study by Carlin et al. (1978) indicated that even after heavy use, amphetamine abusers did not demonstrate cognitive impairments relative to normal control subjects, more recent studies have reported somewhat different results.

Acute Effects

Little research has been conducted on the acute effects of amphetamine use on neuropsychological functioning. Drachman (1977) administered a single dose of scopolamine to study subjects, and followed this with either a single dose of d-amphetamine or physostigmine (a scopolamine antagonist) in order to examine the effect on memory and cognition. Subjects who received d-amphetamine demonstrated increased alertness but no improvement in cognitive or memory function as compared to the group that received physostigmine. In a double-blind study of d-amphetamine administered intravenously to subjects suffering from depression, researchers found that active drug administration resulted in an increase in verbal free recall but not cued recall (Reus et al., 1979), suggesting specific effects on memory processing. These studies are difficult to interpret, as study subjects were not "naive" prior to the administration of amphetamine.

Chronic Effects

In a study conducted by McKetin and Mattick (1997), an attempt was made to clarify the effect of chronic amphetamine use on neuropsychological functioning. Subjects received a fairly comprehensive neuropsychological test battery, which included measures of general memory function, attention, concentration, general intellectual ability, and reading. Results indicated that severity of amphetamine dependence was associated with poorer performance on memory and attention/concentration measures. In a followup study by the same research group, the authors attempted to clarify the extent of neuropsychological impairment in amphetamine abusers. Amphetamine users were defined as being either high or low dependence users, according to scores achieved on the Severity of Dependence Scale (SDS). The high dependence group performed one-half of a standard deviation worse on measures of verbal memory, attention and concentration, and delayed recall indices of a memory test as compared to control subjects free of drug use (McKetin and Mattick, 1998). In contrast, the low dependence users showed no impairments. Based on negative findings in a choline enzyme study of methamphetamine users, Kish et al. (1999), reported that in very high doses, methamphetamine may acutely impair cognitive function, although specific areas of function are not addressed. It should be noted that "pure" amphetamine users are rare (Darke and Hall, 1995). In general, individuals who use amphetamines also abuse other substances.

Solvents

Volatile organic solvents represent a class of abused compounds with relatively nonspecific, though serious, neurotoxic consequences. Exposure to volatile organic compounds (VOCs) can be achieved either incidentally, as an occupational hazard, or purposefully by concentrating and inhaling products containing the necessary substances. Of all the VOCs, toluene-containing substances seem to have the highest potential for abuse (Sharp et al., 1992). Methyl butyl ketone (MBK), n-hexane, trichloroethylene, methylene chloride (dichloromethane), 1,1,1-trichloroethane, and gasoline are also VOCs of abuse, although it remains to be definitively shown that the latter four actually effect persistent neural damage. These compounds are extremely lipophilic, making them potentially toxic to organs rich in lipids, such as the brain (Sharp & Rosenberg, 1997). Inhalants refer to substances that are sniffed or "huffed" to give the user an immediate head rush or high. They include a diverse group of chemicals that are found in consumer products such as aerosols and cleaning solvents. According to a recent survey by the Substance Abuse and Mental Health Services Administration, inhalant use among all grades has risen steadily since 1991. Nearly 20% of all adolescents report using inhalants at least once in their lives. Current use is highest among eighth graders. Inhalant use can cause a number of physical and emotional problems, and even onetime use can result in death. The primary neurotoxic syndromes with which inhalants are traditionally credited include a general polyneuropathy, ototoxicity, and encephalopathy. Less commonly, a cerebellar ataxic syndrome, parkinsonism, or a myopathy can occur alone or in conjunction with any of the above clinical syndromes (Sharp & Rosenberg, 1997).

The evidence from studies of the neuropsychological and psychiatric consequences of chronic volatile substance abuse is compelling, though not definitive. Inhalant abusers tend to differ from other drug abusers in that they display greater incidents of suicidal and self-directed destructive behavior (Korman et al., 1980). A more recent report suggests a connection between solvent abuse and antisocial personality disorders (Dinwiddie et al., 1987). A single study has shown a correlation between paranoid psychosis and inhalant abuse (Byrne, 1991). However, in each of these reports, other substances of abuse, other medical conditions, or negative life events serve as confounding factors. In addition, it is unclear in any of the studies whether psychiatric symptoms preceded or followed inhalant abuse. Definitive connections between psychiatric disorders and solvent abuse are rare if existent (Ron, 1986).

Acute Effects

Both during and immediately following exposure to solvents, specific cognitive deficits have been noted on tests involving speed, coordination, concentration, memory, and vocabulary (Tsushima and Towne, 1977). The degree of impairment appears directly correlated with duration and intensity of exposure. Anger (1992) reported that tests of attention and monitoring were sensitive to short term exposure, although many of the most sensitive clinical tests had not been used in this type of research.

Chronic Effects

Individuals who suffer chronic workplace solvent exposure often complain of fatigue, memory and concentration difficulties, sleep disturbances, and sensory and motor symptoms involving the extremities (Eskelinen et al., 1986; Bowler et al., 1991). Impairments in visual acuity and color vision have been documented (Mergler et al., 1991), as have certain aspects of attention and memory and response slowing (Anger, 1992; Crossen and Wiens, 1994). One study by Morrow et al. documented impairment on tests of visuospatial function (1990) while a later study by this investigator (1992) revealed deficits in both forward and backward digit span and the acquisition of new information. Studies have also revealed difficulties in reasoning and problem solving (Linz et al., 1986) and executive functions, including reduced spontaneity and impaired planning (Lezak, 1985; Hawkins, 1990) in these individuals. Findings from these studies suggest that the amount of material recalled in individuals who have had chronic exposure to solvents is reduced.

It should be noted that some toxicological studies fail to find convincing evidence that toluene containing compounds cause any persisting neurobehavioral or electrophysiological dysfunction in laboratory animals (Pryor et al., 1983) or in humans (Hayden et al., 1977; Benignus, 1981a,b). Indeed, some chronic toluene abusers have had no persistent cognitive impairment despite having received cumulative doses equivalent to those received by individuals who do display cognitive impairment (Hormes et al., 1986; Rosenberg et al., 1988). This discrepancy suggests that either the abuse histories obtained were inaccurate, or that other factors play a role in resilient individuals. Moreover, there is disagreement within the scientific community as to what criteria should be employed in defining "neurotoxic" substances (Pryor, 1993). Perhaps more so with toluene than with any other VOC, it is unclear just how insalubrious exposure may be.

Conclusion

Neuropsychological assessment has gained increasing popularity over the past several years as its contributions to neuroimaging have become widely recognized. Neuropsychology as a discipline can help to determine the effects of brain insults on cognitive and emotional functioning, provide a description of the extent, scope, and quality of functioning, provide a measure of an individual's potential and recovery course, and provide a calculated estimate of the baseline or premorbid level of functioning. While a single cross-sectional neuropsychological evaluation can offer a measure of an individual's overall cognitive strengths and weaknesses, repeated assessments over time provide an index of change that allow factors such as age, education, treatment interventions, and disease state changes to be evaluated systematically. However, neuropsychological scores cannot be considered in isolation; important background variables, including handedness, cultural background, native language, education, socioeconomic status, and generalized intelligence must be considered in the interpretation of all study results. For example, an individual for whom English is a second language will typically not fare as well on language based tasks normed on English speaking Americans. Tasks that require problem solving are likely to be performed differently by individuals with diverse backgrounds.

While scores from neuropsychological tests should be interpreted in light of IQ and educational levels, the question of normative data poses an interesting problem for researchers. At this time, interpretation of most test results relies on how an individual's performance differs from that of a comparison standard, comprised of normal, non brain damaged control subjects' scores on the same task. Normative data is often limited, as it requires the measure to be administered to a large number of individuals with a stratified sampling strategy. Variations in test scores may reflect sample differences including age, sex, cultural background, and educational level. Additionally, many so-called "normal" subjects which comprise these pools are not properly screened for psychiatric histories, substance abuse, or head trauma. It is therefore imperative for researchers to view these findings carefully, and to keep these variables in mind when planning and executing new studies.

While neuropsychology can inform clinicians and researchers about function in a specific area of the brain during a cognitive task, and can often predict function after an injury or pharmacological treatment, neuropsychological evaluations alone cannot provide absolute distinctions between clinical populations, or provide psychiatric or medical diagnoses. Patterns of neurocognitive function do emerge within clinical and psychiatric populations, however, a neuropsychological exam is not enough to provide definitive diagnostic information. The integration of clinical, functional, and neuropsychological information is a powerful combination that informs the investigator about the individuals' cortical structure, function, and clinical state, and is undoubtedly more accurate and reliable than any of the components alone.

ACKNOWLEDGMENTS

We thank Ms. Ashley Young and Mr. Nathaniel Walker for their invaluable assistance in preparing this chapter. This work was supported in part by a grant from the National Institute of Drug Abuse (NIDA) to Dr. Yurgelun-Todd (1 R01 12483-03).

REFERENCES

Acker, W., Ron, M. A., Lishman, W. A. and Shaw, G. K., A multivariate analysis of psychological, clinical and CT scanning measures in detoxified chronic alcoholics. Br. J. Addict. 79:293–301, 1984.

Acord, L. D. and Barker, D. D., Hallucinogenic drugs and cerebral deficit. J. Nerv. Ment. Dis. 156:281–283, 1973.

Adams, E. H., Gfroerer, J. C., Rouse, B. A. and Kozel, N. J., Trends in prevalence and consequences of cocaine use. Adv. Alcohol Subst. Abuse. 6:49–71, 1986.

Akshoomoff, N., Delis, D. C. and Kiefner, M. G., Block constructions of chronic alcoholic and unilateral brain-damaged patients: a test of the right hemisphere vulnerability hypothesis of alcoholism. Arch. Clin. Neuropsychol. 4:275–281, 1989.

Anger, W. K., Assessment of neurotoxicity in humans. In: Tilson, H. and Mitchell, C. (eds.) Neurotoxicology. New York: Raven Press, 1992.

Ardila, A., Rosselli, M. and Strumwasser, S., Neuropsychological deficits in chronic cocaine abusers. Int. J. Neurosci. 57:73–79, 1991.

Becker, J. T., Butters, N., Hermann, A. and D'Angelo, N., Learning to associate names and faces: impaired acquisition on an ecologically relevant memory task by male alcoholics. J. Nerv. Ment. Dis. 171:617–623, 1983.

Benignus, V. A., Health effects of toluene: a review. Neurotoxicology 2:567–588, 1981a.

Benignus, V. A., Neurobehavioral effects of toluene: a review. Neurobehav. Toxicol. Teratol. 3:407–415, 1981b.

Berglund, M., Hagstadius, S., Risberg, J., Johanson, T. M., Bliding, A. and Mubrin, Z., Normalization of regional cerebral blood flow in alcoholics during the first 7 weeks of abstinence. Acta Psychiatr. Scand. 75:202–208, 1987.

Berry, J., van Gorp, W. G., Herzberg, D. S., Hinkin, C., Boone, K., Steinman, L. and Wilkins, J. N., Neuropsychological deficits in abstinent cocaine abusers: preliminary findings after two weeks of abstinence. Drug Alcohol Depend. 32:231–237, 1993.

Block, R. I. and Ghoneim, M. M., Effects of chronic marijuana use on human cognition. Psychopharmacology (Berl.) 110:219–228, 1993.

Blusewicz, M. J., Dustman, R. E., Schenkenberg, T. and Beck, E. C., Neuropsychological correlates of chronic alcoholism and aging. J. Nerv. Ment. Dis. 165:348–355, 1977.

Bourin, M., Colombel, M. C. and Guitton, B., Alprazolam 0.125 mg twice a day improves aspects of psychometric performance in healthy volunteers. J. Clin. Psychopharmacol. 18:364–372, 1998.

Bourque, L. B., Tashkin, D. P., Clark, V. A. and Schuler, R., Demographic and health characteristics of heavy marijuana smokers in Los Angeles County. Int. J. Addict. 26:739–755, 1991.

Bowler, R. M., Mergler, D., Huel, G., Harrison, R. and Cone, J., Neuropsychological impairment among former microelectronics workers. Neurotoxicology 12:87–103, 1991.

Braff, D. L., Silverton, L., Saccuzzo, D. P. and Janowsky, D. S., Impaired speed of visual information processing in marijuana intoxication. Am. J. Psychiatry 138:613–617, 1981.
Bruhn, P. and Maage, N., Intellectual and neuropsychological functions in young men with heavy and long-term patterns of drug abuse. Am. J. Psychiatry 132:397–401, 1975.
Brust, J. C. M., Neurological aspects of substance abuse. Boston: Butterworth-Heinemann, 1993.
Butters, N., Amnestic Disorders. In: Heilman, K. and Valenstein, E. (eds.) Clinical Neuropsychology. New York, Oxford University Press, pp. 441–477, 1981.
Butters, N., Cermak, L. S., Montgomery, K. and Adinolfi, A., Some comparisons of the memory and visuoperceptive deficits of chronic alcoholics and patients with Korsakoff's disease. Alcohol. Clin. Exp. Res. 1:73–80, 1977.
Byrne, A., Kirby, B., Zibin, T. and Ensminger, S., Psychiatric and neurological effects of chronic solvent abuse. Can. J. Psychiatry 36:735–738, 1991.
Carlen, P. L., Wilkinson, D. A., Wortzman, G., Holgate, R., Cordingley, J., Lee, M. A., Huszar, L., Moddel, G., Singh, R., Kiraly, L. and Rankin, J. G., Cerebral atrophy and functional deficits in alcoholics without clinically apparent liver disease. Neurology 31:377–385, 1981.
Carlin, A.S., Neuropsychological consequences of drug abuse. In: Grant, I. and Adams, K.M. (eds.) Neuropsychological Assessment of Neuropsychiatric Disorders. New York, Oxford University Press, pp. 486–503, 1986.
Carlin, A. S., Stauss, F. F., Adams, K. M. and Grant, I., The prediction of neuropsychological impairment in polydrug abusers. Addict. Behav. 3:5–12, 1978.
Cohen, S. and Edwards, A. E., LSD and organic brain impairment. Drug Dependence 2:1–4, 1969.
Comitas, L., Cannabis and work in Jamaica: a refutation of the amotivational syndrome. Ann. N. Y. Acad. Sci. 282:24–32, 1976.
Crossen, J. R. and Wiens, A. N., Comparison of the Auditory-Verbal Learning Test (AVLT) and California Verbal Learning Test (CVLT) in a sample of normal subjects. J. Clin. Exp. Neuropsychol. 16:190–194, 1994.
Culver, C. M. and King, F. W., Neuropsychological assessment of undergraduate marihuana and LSD users. Arch. Gen. Psychiatry 31:707–711, 1974.
Cutting, J., Differential impairment of memory in Korsakoff's syndrome. Cortex 15:501–506, 1979.
Darke, S. and Hall, W., Levels and correlates of polydrug use among heroin users and regular amphetamine users. Drug Alcohol Depend. 39:231–235, 1995.
Darley, C. F., Tinklenberg, J. R., Roth, W. T., Hollister, L. E. and Atkinson, R. C., Influence of marijuana on storage and retrieval processes in memory. Memory and Cognition 1:196–200, 1973.
Dinwiddie, S. H., Zorumski, C. F. and Rubin, E. H., Psychiatric correlates of chronic solvent abuse. J. Clin. Psychiatry 48:334–337, 1987.
Drachman, D. A., Memory and cognitive function in man: does the cholinergic system have a specific role? Neurology 27:783–790, 1977.
Drug Enforcement Administration, Illegal Drug Price/Purity Report United Sates: January 1992–December 1995.
Eskelinen, L., Luisto, M., Tenkanen, L. and Mattei, O., Neuropsychological methods in the differentiation of organic solvent intoxication from certain neurological conditions. J. Clin. Exp. Neuropsychol. 8:239–256, 1986.
Fabian, M. S., Parsons, O. A. and Sheldon, M. D., Effects of gender and alcoholism on verbal and visual-spatial learning. J. Nerv. Ment. Dis. 172:16–20, 1984.
Fauman, B., Aldinger, G., Fauman, M. and Rosen, P., Psychiatric sequelae of phencyclidine abuse. Clin. Toxicol. 9:529–538, 1976.

Fehr, K. O. and Kalant, H., Cannabis and health hazards: Proceedings of an ARF/WHO scientific meeting on adverse health and behavioral consequences of cannabis use. Toronto, Addiction Research Foundation Press, 1983.

Fischman, M. W. and Schuster, C. R., Cocaine effects in sleep-deprived humans. Psychopharmacology (Berl.) 72:1–8, 1980.

Fitzhugh, L. C., Fitzhugh, K. B. and Reitan, R. M., Adaptive abilities and intellectual functioning of hospitalized alcoholics: further considerations. Q. J. Stud. Alcohol 26:402–411, 1965.

Fox, P. T., Raichle, M. E. and Thach, W. T., Functional mapping of the human cerebellum with positron emission tomography. Proc. Natl. Acad. Sci. USA 82:7462–7466, 1985.

Freund, G., The interaction of chronic alcohol consumption and aging on brain structure and function. Alcohol. Clin. Exp. Res. 6:13–21, 1982.

Frith, C. D., Friston, K. J., Liddle, P. F. and Frackowiak, R. S., A PET study of word finding. Neuropsychologia 29:1137–1148, 1991.

Gawin, F. H. and Kleber, H. D., Cocaine abuse in a treatment population: Patterns and diagnostic distinctions. In: Kozel, N.J. and Adams, E.H. (eds.) Cocaine Use in America: Epidemiologic and Clinical Perspectives., National Institute on Drug Abuse Research Monograph Vol. 61. Washington, D.C., U.S. Govt. Print. Off., DHHS Pub. No. (ADM) 85–1414. pp. 182–192, 1985.

Giannini, A. J., Loiselle, R. H., DiMarzio, L. R. and Giannini, M. C., Augmentation of haloperidol by ascorbic acid in phencyclidine intoxication. Am. J. Psychiatry 144:1207–1209, 1987.

Glenn, S. W. and Parsons, O. A., Impaired efficiency in female alcoholics' neuropsychological performance. J. Clin. Exp. Neuropsychol. 13:895–908, 1991.

Glick, S. D., Hinds, P. A. and Carlson, J. N., Food deprivation and stimulant self-administration in rats: differences between cocaine and d-amphetamine. Psychopharmacology (Berl.) 91:372–374, 1987.

Glosser, G., Butters, N. and Kaplan, E., Visuoperceptual processes in brain damaged patients on the digit symbol substitution test. Int. J. Neurosci. 7:59–66, 1977.

Gold, M. S. and Miller, N. S., Cocaine (and crack): Neurobiology. In: Lowinson, J. H., Ruiz, P., Millman, R. B. and Langrod, J. G. (eds.) Substance abuse: A comprehensive textbook. Baltimore, Williams and Wilkins, pp. 166–180, 1997.

Goldman, M. S., Cognitive impairment in chronic alcoholics. Some cause for optimism. Am. Psychol. 38:1045–1054, 1983.

Goldstein, G., Perceptual and cognitive defecits in alcoholics. In: Goldstein, G. and Neuringer, C. (eds.) Empirical Studies of Alcoholism. Cambridge, MA, Ballinger, pp. 115–151, 1976.

Gorenstein, C., Bernik, M. A. and Pompeia, S., Differential acute psychomotor and cognitive effects of diazepam on long-term benzodiazepine users. Int. Clin. Psychopharmacol. 9:145–153, 1994.

Graff-Radford, N. R., Heaton, R. K., Earnest, M. P. and Rudikoff, J. C., Brain atrophy and neuropsychological impairment in young alcoholics. J. Stud. Alcohol 43:859–868, 1982.

Grant, I., Alcohol and the brain: neuropsychological correlates. J. Consult. Clin. Psychol. 55:310–324, 1987.

Grinspoon, L. and Bakalar, J. B., Drug dependence: Non-narcotic agents. In: Kaplan, H. I., Freedman, A. M., and Sadock, B. J. (eds.) Comprehensive Textbook of Psychiatry. Baltimore, Williams and Wilkins, pp. 1614–1629, 1980.

Guerra, D., Sole, A., Cami, J. and Tobena, A., Neuropsychological performance in opiate addicts after rapid detoxification. Drug Alcohol Depend. 20:261–270, 1987.

Hanks, G. W., O'Neill, W. M., Simpson, P. and Wesnes, K., The cognitive and psychomotor effects of opioid analgesics. II. A randomized controlled trial of single doses of morphine, lorazepam and placebo in healthy subjects. Eur. J. Clin. Pharmacol. 48:455–460, 1995.

Harper, C. G. and Blumbergs, P. C., Brain weights in alcoholics. J. Neurol. Neurosurg. Psychiatry 45:838–840, 1982.

Hawkins, K. A., Occupational neurotoxicology: some neuropsychological issues and challenges. J. Clin. Exp. Neuropsychol. 12:664–680, 1990.

Hayden, J. W., Peterson, R. G. and Bruckner, J. V., Toxicology of toluene (methylbenzene): review of current literature. Clin. Toxicol. 11:549–559, 1977.

Hendler, N., Cimini, C., Ma, T. and Long, D., A comparison of cognitive impairment due to benzodiazepines and to narcotics. Am. J. Psychiatry 137:828–830, 1980.

Hermle, L., Funfgeld, M., Oepen, G., Botsch, H., Borchardt, D., Gouzoulis, E., Fehrenbach, R. A. and Spitzer, M., Mescaline-induced psychopathological, neuropsychological, and neurometabolic effects in normal subjects: experimental psychosis as a tool for psychiatric research. Biol. Psychiatry 32:976–991, 1992.

Herning, R. I., Glover, B. J., Koeppl, B., Weddington, W. and Jaffe, J. H., Cognitive deficits in abstaining cocaine abusers. NIDA Res. Monogr. 101:167–178, 1990.

Hoff, A. L., Riordan, H., Morris, L., Cestaro, V., Wieneke, M., Alpert, R., Wang, G. J. and Volkow, N., Effects of crack cocaine on neurocognitive function. Psychiatry Res. 60:167–176, 1996.

Hormes, J. T., Filley, C. M. and Rosenberg, N. L., Neurologic sequelae of chronic solvent vapor abuse. Neurology 36:698–702, 1986.

Javitt, D. C. and Zukin, S. R., Recent advances in the phencyclidine model of schizophrenia. Am. J. Psychiatry 148:1301–1308, 1991.

Jernigan, T. L., Butters, N., DiTraglia, G., Schafer, K., Smith, T., Irwin, M., Grant, I., Schuckit, M. and Cermak, L. S., Reduced cerebral grey matter observed in alcoholics using magnetic resonance imaging. Alcohol. Clin. Exp. Res. 15:418–427, 1991.

Johnson, L. C. and Chernik, D. A., Sedative-hypnotics and human performance. Psychopharmacology (Berl.) 76:101–113, 1982.

Johnston, L., O'Malley, P. M. and Bachman, J. G., National survey results on drug use from the Monitoring the Future study, 1975–1995. National Institute on Drug Abuse, U.S. Dept. of Health and Human Services., Rockville, MD, 1996.

Jones, B. and Parsons, O. A., Impaired abstracting ability in chronic alcoholics. Arch. Gen. Psychiatry 24:71–75, 1971.

Jones, B. M. and Jones, M. K., Alcohol and memory impairmen in male and female social drinkers. In: Birnbaum, I.M. and Parker, E.S. (eds.) Alcohol and Human Memory. Hillsdale, NJ, Lawrence Earlbaum Associates, pp. 127–141, 1977.

Jones, R. T. and Benowitz, N., The 30-day trip—clinical studies of cannabis tolerance and dependence. In: Braude, M.C. and Szara, S. (eds.) Pharmacology of marihuana., Vol. 2. New York, Raven Press, pp. 627–642, 1976.

Jones, R. T., Benowitz, N. L. and Herning, R. I., Clinical relevance of cannabis tolerance and dependence. J. Clin. Pharmacol. 21:143S–152S, 1981.

Kapur, N. and Butters, N., Visuoperceptive deficits in long-term alcoholics and alcoholics with Korsakoff's psychosis. J. Stud. Alcohol 38:2025–2035, 1977.

Kerr, B., Hill, H., Coda, B., Calogero, M., Chapman, C. R., Hunt, E., Buffington, V. and Mackie, A., Concentration-related effects of morphine on cognition and motor control in human subjects. Neuropsychopharmacology 5:157–166, 1991.

Kish, S. J., Kalasinsky, K. S., Furukawa, Y., Guttman, M., Ang, L., Li, L., Adams, V., Reiber, G., Anthony, R. A., Anderson, W., Smialek, J. and DiStefano, L., Brain choline acetyltransferase activity in chronic, human users of cocaine, methamphetamine, and heroin. Mol. Psychiatry 4:26–32, 1999.

Kleber, H. D. and Gawin, F. H., Cocaine abuse: a review of current and experimental treatments. NIDA Res. Monogr. 50:111–129, 1984.

Kolb, B. and Whishaw, I. Q., Fundamentals of Human Neuropsychology. 3rd Edition. New York, Freeman, 1990.

Korman, M., Trimboli, F. and Semler, I., A comparative evaluation of 162 inhalant users. Addict. Behav. 5:143–152, 1980.

Kornetsky, C., Williams, J. E. and Bird, M., Attentional and motivational effects of psychoactive drugs. NIDA Res. Monogr. 97:177–192, 1990.

Kramer, J. H., Blusewicz, M. J. and Preston, K. A., The premature aging hypothesis: old before its time? J. Consult. Clin. Psychol. 57:257–262, 1989.

Kroll, P., Seigel, R., O'Neill, B. and Edwards, R. P., Cerebral cortical atrophy in alcoholic men. J. Clin. Psychiatry 41:417–421, 1980.

Krystal, J. H., Price, L. H., Opsahl, C., Ricaurte, G. A. and Heninger, G. R., Chronic 3,4-methylenedioxymethamphetamine (MDMA) use: effects on mood and neuropsychological function? Am. J. Drug Alcohol Abuse 18:331–341, 1992.

Kwong, K. K., Belliveau, J. W., Chesler, D. A., Goldberg, I. E., Weisskoff, R. M., Poncelet, B. P., Kennedy, D. N., Hoppel, B. E., Cohen, M. S., Turner, R., Cheng, H.-M., Brady, T. J. and Rosen, B. R., Dynamic magnetic resonance imaging of human brain activity during primary sensory stimulation. Proc. Natl. Acad. Sci. USA 89:5675–5679, 1992.

Lerner, S. and Burns, R., Phencyclidine use among youth: History, epidemiology, and acute chronic intoxication. In: Petersen, R. C. and Stillman, R. C. (eds.) Phencyclidine (PCP) abuse : an appraisal., NIDA Res. Monogr. Vol. 21. Alcohol, Drug Abuse, and Mental Health Administration, National Institute on Drug Abuse, Rockville, MD, pp. 313, 1978.

Lewis, J. E., Lanham, R. A. and Belliveau, T., Contextual neuropsychological toxicology investigation of phencyclidine (PCP) abusers [Abstract]. The Clinical Neuropsychologist 4:303–304, 1990.

Lezak, M. D., Neuropsychological assessment. In: Vinken, P. J., Bruyn, G. W., and Klawans, H. L. (eds.) Handbook of Clinical Neurology. Vol. 45. New York, Elsevier, pp. 515–530, 1985.

Linz, D. H., de Garmo, P. L., Morton, W. E., Wiens, A. N., Coull, B. M. and Maricle, R. A., Organic solvent-induced encephalopathy in industrial painters. J. Occup. Med. 28:119–125, 1986.

Lishman, W. A., Cerebral disorder in alcoholism: syndromes of impairment. Brain 104:1–20, 1981.

Lucki, I., Rickels, K. and Geller, A. M., Chronic use of benzodiazepines and psychomotor and cognitive test performance. Psychopharmacology (Berl.) 88:426–433, 1986.

Lusins, J., Zimberg, S., Smokler, H. and Gurley, K., Alcoholism and cerebral atrophy: a study of 50 patients with CT scan and psychologic testing. Alcohol. Clin. Exp. Res. 4:406–411, 1980.

MacVane, J., Butters, N., Montgomery, K. and Farber, J., Cognitive functioning in men social drinkers; a replication study. J. Stud. Alcohol 43:81–95, 1982.

Malhotra, A. K., Pinals, D. A., Weingartner, H., Sirocco, K., Missar, C. D., Pickar, D. and Breier, A., NMDA receptor function and human cognition: the effects of ketamine in healthy volunteers. Neuropsychopharmacology 14:301–307, 1996.

McKctin, R. and Mattick, R. P., Attention and memory in illicit amphetamine users. Drug Alcohol Depend. 48:235–242, 1997.

McKetin, R. and Mattick, R. P., Attention and memory in illicit amphetamine users: comparison with non-drug-using controls. Drug Alcohol Depend. 50:181–184, 1998.

Mendhiratta, S. S., Wig, N. N. and Verma, S. K., Some psychological correlates of long-term heavy cannabis users. Br. J. Psychiatry 132:482–486, 1978.

Mendhiratta, S. S., Varma, V. K., Dang, R., Malhotra, A. K., Das, K. and Nehra, R., Cannabis and cognitive functions: a re-evaluation study. Br. J. Addict. 83:749–753, 1988.

Mergler, D., Blain, L., Lemaire, J. and Lalande, F., Colour vision impairment and alcohol consumption. Neurotoxicol. Teratol. 10:255–260, 1988.

Mergler, D., Huel, G., Bowler, R., Frenette, B. and Cone, J., Visual dysfunction among former microelectronics assembly workers. Arch. Environ. Health. 46:326–334, 1991.

Mesulam, M. M., Principles of Behavioral Neurology. Philadelphia, F.A. Davis Co, 1985.

Miller, L. L., Marijuana: Effects on human behavior. New York, Academic Press, 1974.
Miller, L. L., Marijuana and human cognition: A review of laboratory investigations. In: Cohen, S. and Stillman, R. C. (eds.) The therapeutic potential of marijuana. New York, Plenum Press, 1976.
Miller, N., Benzodiazepines: Myths and truths., http://www.questpub.com/TT_Mag/1996_3_Sum/ Miller.html, 1996.
Miller, N. S., Gold, M. S. and Klahr, A. L., The diagnosis of alcohol and cannabis dependence (addiction) in cocaine dependence (addiction). Int. J. Addict. 25:735–744, 1990.
Mirin, S. M., Shapiro, L. M., Meyer, R. E., Pillard, R. C. and Fisher, S., Casual versus heavy use of marijuana: a redefinition of the marijuana problem. Am. J. Psychiatry 127:1134–1140, 1971.
Morgan, M. J., Recreational use of "ecstasy" (MDMA) is associated with elevated impulsivity. Neuropsychopharmacology 19:252–264, 1998.
Morrow, L. A., Ryan, C. M., Hodgson, M. J. and Robin, N., Alterations in cognitive and psychological functioning after organic solvent exposure. J. Occup. Med. 32:444–450, 1990.
Morrow, L. A., Steinhauer, S. R. and Hodgson, M. J., Delay in P300 latency in patients with organic solvent exposure. Arch. Neurol. 49:315–320, 1992.
Newcomer, J. W., Farber, N. B., Jevtovic-Todorovic, V., Selke, G., Melson, A. K., Hershey, T., Craft, S. and Olney, J. W., Ketamine-induced NMDA receptor hypofunction as a model of memory impairment and psychosis. Neuropsychopharmacology 20:106–118, 1999.
NIDA, National Household Survey on Drug Abuse: Population Estimates 1990. National Institute on Drug Abuse, U.S. Department of Health and Human Services; U.S. Govt. Printing Office, DHHS Pub. No. (ADM) 91–1732, 1991.
NIH, National Household Survey on Drug Abuse., Vol 1999: National Institutes of Health, National Institute on Drug Abuse. http://165.112.78.61/infofax/marijuana.html, 1998.
Nixon, S. J., Kujawski, A., Parsons, O. A. and Yohman, J. R., Semantic (verbal) and figural memory impairment in alcoholics. J. Clin. Exp. Neuropsychol. 9:311–322, 1987.
Olney, J. W., Labruyere, J. and Price, M. T., Pathological changes induced in cerebrocortical neurons by phencyclidine and related drugs. Science 244:1360–1362, 1989.
O'Malley, S. S. and Gawin, F. H., Abstinence symptomatology and neuropsychological impairment in chronic cocaine abusers. NIDA Res. Monogr. 101:179–190, 1990.
O'Malley, S., Adamse, M., Heaton, R. K. and Gawin, F. H., Neuropsychological impairment in chronic cocaine abusers. Am. J. Drug Alcohol Abuse 18:131–144, 1992.
Oscar-Berman, M., Hypothesis testing and focusing behavior during concept formation by amnesic Korsakoff patients. Neuropsychologia 11:191–198, 1973.
Oscar-Berman, M. and Weinstein, A., Visual processing, memory, and lateralization in alcoholism and aging. Devel. Neuropsychol. 1:99–112, 1985.
Page, J. B., Fletcher, J. and True, W. R., Psychosociocultural perspectives on chronic cannabis use: the Costa Rican follow-up. J. Psychoactive Drugs 20:57–65, 1988.
Pakesch, G., Loimer, N., Grunberger, J., Pfersmann, D., Linzmayer, L. and Mayerhofer, S., Neuropsychological findings and psychiatric symptoms in HIV-1 infected and noninfected drug users. Psychiatry Res. 41:163–177, 1992.
Parker, E. S. and Noble, E. P., Alcohol consumption and cognitive functioning in social drinkers. J. Stud. Alcohol 38:1224–1232, 1977.
Parker, E. S., Birnbaum, I. M., Weingartner, H., Hartley, J. T., Stillman, R. C. and Wyatt, R. J., Retrograde enhancement of human memory with alcohol. Psychopharmacology (Berl.) 69:219–222, 1980.
Parker, E. S., Morihisa, J. M., Wyatt, R. J., Schwartz, B. L., Weingartner, H. and Stillman, R. C., The alcohol facilitation effect on memory: a dose-response study. Psychopharmacology (Berl.) 74:88–92, 1981.

Parks, R. W., Loewenstein, D. A., Dodrill, K. L., Barker, W. W., Yoshii, F., Chang, J. Y., Emran, A., Apicella, A., Sheramata, W. A. and Duara, R., Cerebral metabolic effects of a verbal fluency test: a PET scan study. J. Clin. Exp. Neuropsychol. 10:565–575, 1988.

Parsons, O. A., Brain damage in alcoholics: altered states of unconsciousness. Adv. Exp. Med. Biol. 59:569–584, 1975.

Parsons, O. A., Cognitive functioning in sober social drinkers: a review and critique. J. Stud. Alcohol 47:101–114, 1986.

Parsons, O. A. and Farr, S. D.,The neuropsychology of alcohol and drug use. In: Filskov, S. B. and Boll, T. J. (eds.) Handbook of Clinical Neuropsychology. New York, John Wiley and Sons, pp. 320–365, 1981.

Parsons, O. A., Tarter, R. E. and Edelberg, R., Altered motor control in chronic alcoholics. J. Abnorm. Psychol. 80:308–314, 1972.

Petersen, S. E., Fox, P. T., Posner, M. I., Mintun, M. and Raichle, M. E., Positron emission tomographic studies of the cortical anatomy of single-word processing. Nature 331:585–589, 1988.

Pishkin, V., Lovallo, W. R. and Bourne, L. E., Jr., Chronic alcoholism in males: cognitive deficit as a function of age of onset, age, and duration. Alcohol. Clin. Exp. Res. 9:400–406, 1985.

Pope, H. G., Jr. and Yurgelun-Todd, D., The residual cognitive effects of heavy marijuana use in college students. JAMA 275:521–527, 1996.

Pope, H. G., Jr., Ionescu-Pioggia, M. and Cole, J. O., Drug use and life-style among college undergraduates. Nine years later. Arch. Gen. Psychiatry 38:588–591, 1981.

Pope, H. G., Jr., Ionescu-Pioggia, M., Aizley, H. G. and Varma, D. K., Drug use and life style among college undergraduates in 1989: a comparison with 1969 and 1978. Am. J. Psychiatry 147:998–1001, 1990.

Post, R. M., Comparative psychopharmacology of cocaine and amphetamine. Psychopharmacol. Bull. 12:39–41, 1976.

Pryor, G. T., Persisting neurotoxic consequences of solvent abuse: A developing animal model for toluene-induced neurotoxicity. Drug Abuse Res. Monog. 136:156–166, 1993.

Pryor, G. T., Dickinson, J., Howd, R. A. and Rebert, C. S., Neurobehavioral effects of subchronic exposure of weanling rats to toluene or hexane. Neurobehav. Toxicol. Teratol. 5:47–52, 1983.

Radant, A. D., Bowdle, T. A., Cowley, D. S., Kharasch, E. D. and Roy-Byrne, P. P., Does ketamine-mediated *N*-methyl-D-aspartate receptor antagonism cause schizophrenia-like oculomotor abnormalities? Neuropsychopharmacology 19:434–444, 1998.

Rainey, J. M., Jr. and Crowder, M. K., Prolonged psychosis attributed to phencyclidine: report of three cases. Am. J. Psychiatry 132:1076–1078, 1975.

Reus, V. I., Silberman, E., Post, R. M. and Weingartner, H., d-Amphetamine: effects on memory in a depressed population. Biol. Psychiatry 14:345–356, 1979.

Robins, L. N., Darvish, H. S. and Murphy, G. E., The long-term outcome for adolescent drug users: a follow-up study of 76 users and 146 nonusers. Proc. Annu. Meet. Am. Psychopathol. Assoc., 59:159–180, 1970.

Rohr, J. M., Skowlund, S. W. and Martin, T. E., Withdrawal sequelae to cannabis use. Int. J. Addict. 24:627–631, 1989.

Ron, M. A., The alcoholic brain: CT scan and psychological findings. Psychol. Med. Monogr. Suppl. 3:1–33, 1983.

Ron, M. A., Volatile substance abuse: a review of possible long-term neurological, intellectual and psychiatric sequelae. Br. J. Psychiatry 148:235–246, 1986.

Rosenberg, N. L., Spitz, M. C., Filley, C. M., Davis, K. A. and Schaumburg, H. H., Central nervous system effects of chronic toluene abuse: clinical, brainstem evoked response and magnetic resonance imaging studies. Neurotoxicol. Teratol. 10:489–495, 1988.

Rothrock, J. F., Rubenstein, R. and Lyden, P. D., Ischemic stroke associated with methamphetamine inhalation. Neurology 38:589–592, 1988.

Rounsaville, B. J., Jones, C., Novelly, R. A. and Kleber, H., Neuropsychological functioning in opiate addicts. J. Nerv. Ment. Dis. 170:209–216, 1982.
Rubin, V. and Comitas, L., Psychological assessment. In: Rubin, V. and Comitas, L. (eds.) Ganja in Jamaica: A Medical-Anthropological Study of Chronic Marijuana Use. The Hague, Mouton, pp. 111–119, 1975.
Ryan, C. and Butters, N., Cognitive effects in alcohol abuse. In: Kissin, B. and Begleiter, H. (eds.). Cognitive Effects in Alcohol Abuse. New York, Plenum Press, 1982.
Ryan, C. and Butters, N., Neuropsychology of alcoholism. In: Wedding, D., Horton, A. M., Jr. and Webster, J. S. (eds.) The Neuropsychology Handbook. New York, Springer, pp. 376–410, 1986.
Ryan, J. J. and Lewis, C. V., Comparison of normal controls and recently detoxified alcoholics on the Wechsler Memory Scale-Revised. [Abstract]. Clin. Neuropsychol. 2:173–180, 1988.
Sanchez-Craig, M., Drinking pattern as a determinant of alcoholics' performance on the trail making test. J. Stud. Alcohol 41:1082–1090, 1980.
Satz, P., Fletcher, J. M. and Sutker, L. S., Neuropsychologic, intellectual, and personality correlates of chronic marijuana use in native Costa Ricans. Ann. NY Acad. Sci. 282:266–306, 1976.
Schwartz, R. H., Gruenewald, P. J., Klitzner, M. and Fedio, P., Short-term memory impairment in cannabis-dependent adolescents. Am. J. Dis. Child. 143:1214–1219, 1989.
Seth, R. and Sinha, S., Chemistry and pharmacology of cannabis. Prog. Drug Res. 36:71–115, 1991.
Sharma, B. P., Cannabis and its users in Nepal. Br. J. Psychiatry 127:550–552, 1975.
Sharp, C. W. and Rosenberg, N. L., Inhalants. In: Lowinson, J. H., Ruiz, P., Millman, R. B. and Langrod, J. G. (eds.) Substance Abuse: A Comprehensive Textbook. Baltimore, Williams and Wilkins, pp. 246–263, 1997.
Sharp, C. W., Beauvais, F. and Spence, R. T., Inhalant abuse: a volatile research agenda., Vol 129. Rockville, MD, U.S. Dept. of Health and Human Services Public Health Service National Institutes of Health National Institute on Drug Abuse., 1992.
Siegel, R. K., Cocaine smoking. J. Psychoactive Drugs 14:271–359, 1982.
Siegel, R. K., The natural history of hallucinogens. In: Jacobs, B. (ed.) Hallucinogens: Neurochemical, Behavioral, and Clinical Perspectives., Vol. 1. New York, Raven, pp. 1–19, 1984.
Soueif, M. I., Chronic cannabis users: Further analysis of objective test results. Bull. Narc. 27:1–26, 1975.
Soueif, M. I., Some determinants of psychological deficits associated with chronic cannabis consumption. Bull. Narc. 28:25–42, 1976.
Talland, G. A., Deranged Memory. New York, Academic Press, 1965.
Tarter, R. E., An analysis of cognitive deficits in chronic alcoholics. J. Nerv. Ment. Dis. 157:138–147, 1973.
Tarter, R. E., Brain damage associated with chronic alcoholism. Dis. Nerv. Syst. 36:185–187, 1975.
Tarter, R. E., Neuropsychological investigations of alcoholism. In: Goldstein, G. and Neuringer, C. (eds.) Empirical Studies of Alcoholism. Cambridge, MA, Ballinger, pp. 231–256, 1976.
Taylor, R. L., Maurer, J. I. and Tinklenberg, J. R., Management of "bad trips" in an evolving drug scene. JAMA 213:422–425, 1970.
Tsushima, W. T. and Towne, W. S., Effects of paint sniffing on neuropsychological test performance. J. Abnorm. Psychol. 86:402–407, 1977.
Varma, V. K., Malhotra, A. K., Dang, R., Das, K. and Nehra, R., Cannabis and cognitive functions: a prospective study. Drug Alcohol Depend. 21:147–152, 1988.
Vivian, T. N., Goldstein, G. and Shelly, C., Reaction time and motor speed in chronic alcoholics. Percept. Mot. Skills 36:136–138, 1973.

Volkow, N. D., Mullani, N., Gould, K. L., Adler, S. and Krajewski, K., Cerebral blood flow in chronic cocaine users: a study with positron emission tomography. Br. J. Psychiatry 152:641–648, 1988.

Wall, M. E. and Perez-Reyes, M., The metabolism of delta 9-tetrahydrocannabinol and related cannabinoids in man. J. Clin. Pharmacol. 21:178S–189S, 1981.

Walsh, K. W., Frontal lobe problems. In: Stanley, G. V. and Walsh, K. W. (eds.) Brain Impairment. Proceedings of the 1976 Brain Impairment Workshop. Parkville, Victoria, Australia, 1978.

Walsh, K. W., Understanding Brain Damage. Edinburgh, Churchill-Livingstone, 1985.

Walton, N. H., Bowden, S. C. and Walsh, K. W., Social drinking fails to influence cognitive performance. Proceedings of the 11th annual Brain Impairment conference. Richmond, Victoria, Australia, 1987.

Weingartner, H., Faillace, L. A. and Markley, H. G., Verbal information retention in alcoholics. Q. J. Stud. Alcohol 32:293–303, 1971.

Wig, N. N. and Varma, V. K., Patterns of long-term heavy cannabis use in north India and its effects on cognitive functions: a preliminary report. Drug Alcohol Depend. 2:211–219, 1977.

Wilkinson, A., CT scan and neuropsychological assessments of alcoholism. In: Parsons, O. A., Butters, N., and Nathan, P. E. (eds.) Neuropsychology of Alcoholism: Implications for Diagnosis and Treatment. New York, Guilford Press, pp. 76–102, 1987.

Wilson, J. T., Wiedmann, K. D., Hadley, D. M., Condon, B., Teasdale, G. and Brooks, D. N., Early and late magnetic resonance imaging and neuropsychological outcome after head injury. J. Neurol. Neurosurg. Psychiatry 51:391–396, 1988.

Wise, R., Chollet, F., Hadar, U., Friston, K., Hoffner, E. and Frackowiak, R., Distribution of cortical neural networks involved in word comprehension and word retrieval. Brain 114:1803–1817, 1991.

Zinberg, N. E. and Weil, A. T., A comparison of marijuana users and non-users. Nature 226:119–123, 1970.

Zukin, S. R. and Javitt, D. C., Mechanisms of phencyclidine (PCP)-*n*-methyl-*d*-aspartate (NMDA) receptor interaction: implications for drug abuse research. NIDA Res. Monogr. 95:247–254, 1989.

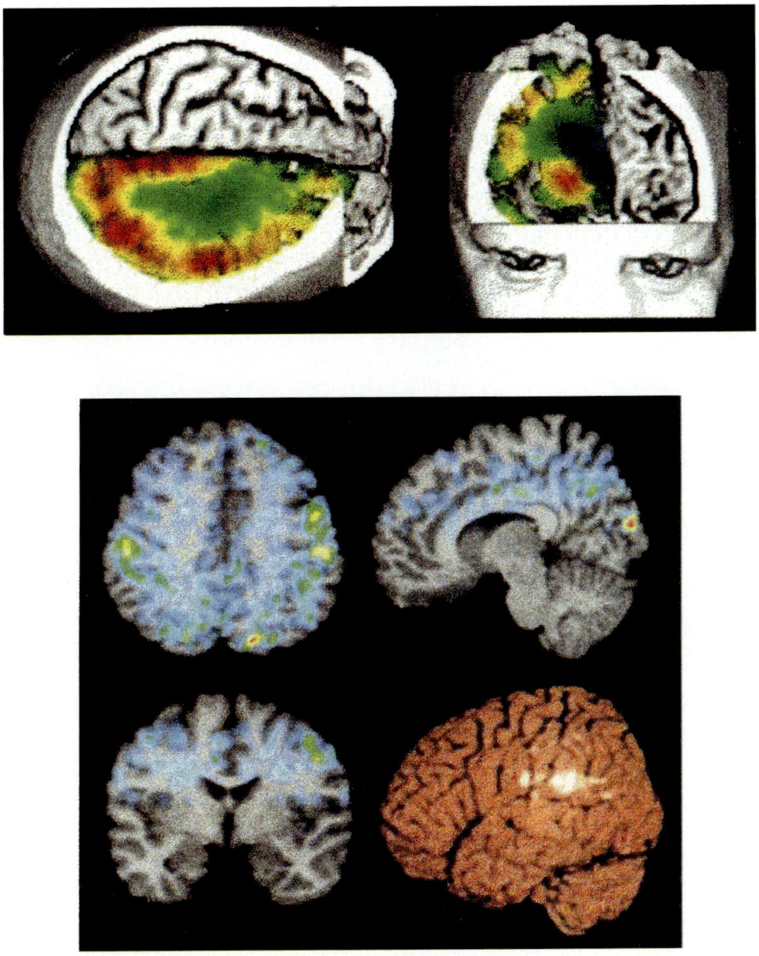

Plate 10. SPECT data overlaid on 3-dimensional MRI renderings of the brain (top). fMRI data (bright pixels) indicating cortical activtions in response to a motor task, interlaced in 3 dimensions with structural MRI data (bottom). *See Chapter 8, Fig. 1, p. 234.*

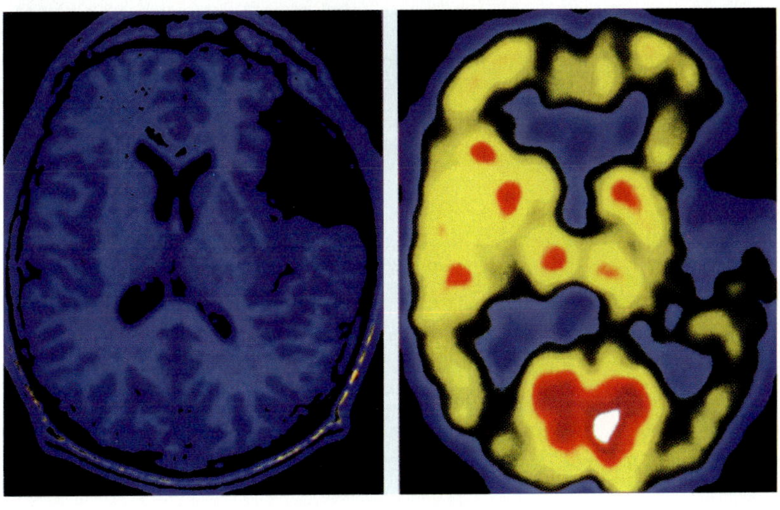

Plate 11. The MRI (left) and PET (right) scans of murder defendant Herbert Weinstein, showing an arachnoid cyst in the frontal lobe. (Reprinted with permission from Diagnostic Imaging, January, 1993). *See Chapter 8, Fig. 2, p. 236.*

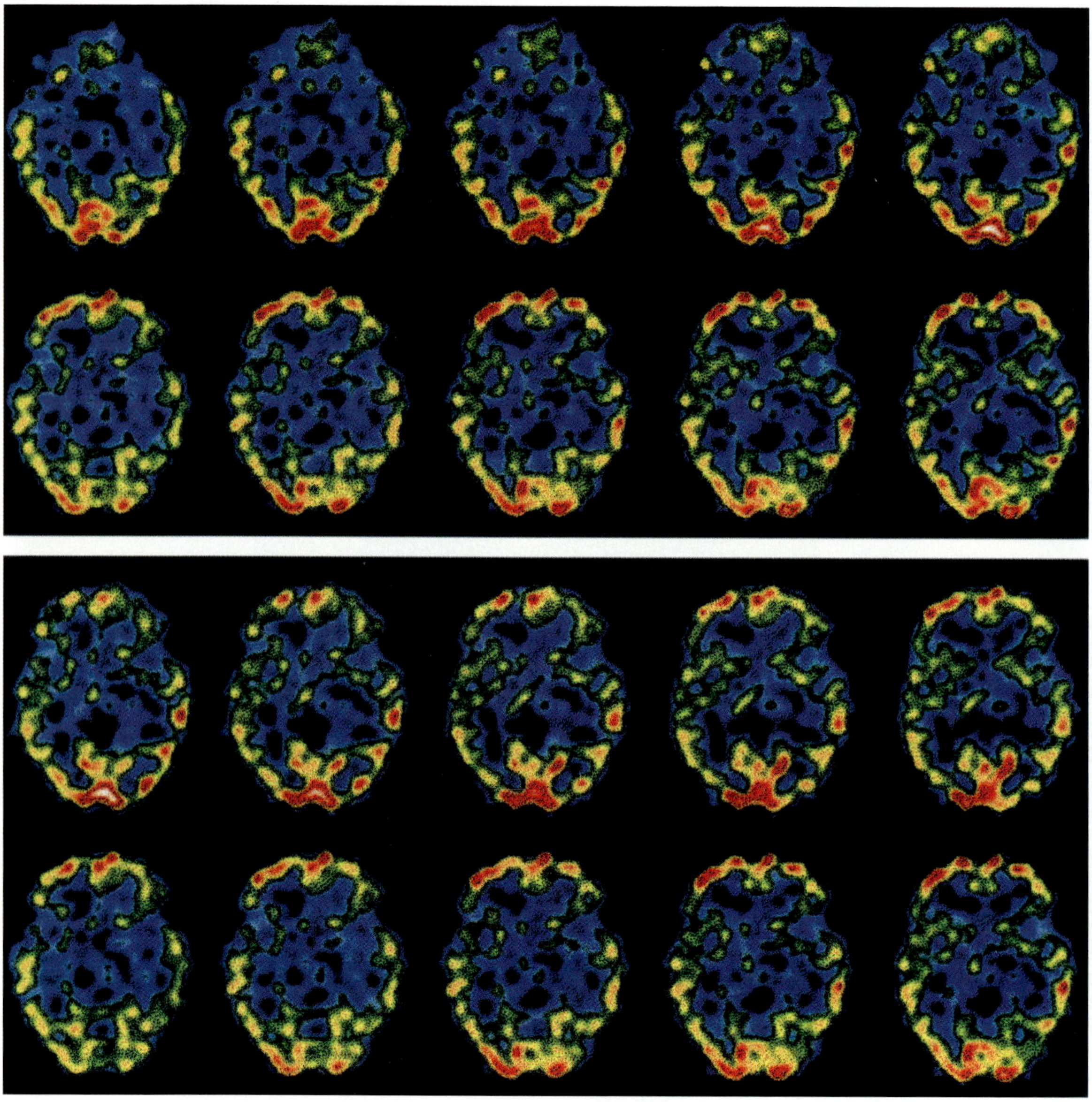

Plate 12. Series of contiguous axial slices from a SPECT blood flow study illustrate how failure to control for the subject's head orientation may give a false impression of "hypofrontality." **(Top)** The upper row of images clearly appears "hypofrontal" (blue/green) relative to the lower row of "normal" (yellow/red) comparison slices. In fact, however, all these images come from the same SPECT study of a single subject. In the upper row of images, the subject's head was rotated back by 5°; in the lower row it is rotated forward by 5° (roughly the width of a finger at the nose). **(Bottom)** Each image volume has been rotated to remove the orientation discrepancy, and neither set shows evidence of "hypofrontality." Care must be taken to ensure proper head orientation, particularly when only a subset of the image volume is presented. *See Chapter 8, Fig. 3, p. 241.*

Chapter 8

Neuroimages as Legal Evidence

Jennifer J. Kulynych, JD, PhD and Douglas W. Jones, PhD

Introduction

Mark Twain once observed, "There is something fascinating about science. One gets such wholesale returns of conjecture out of such a trifling investment of fact."

In his own day, Twain might have been referring to a general tendency to overinterpret experimental results. But Twain's wry comment is equally applicable to a specific, very modern problem of scientific evidence: the increasing use of neuroimaging by psychiatric expert witnesses. In vivo imaging techniques are reanimating the field of psychiatric research, in large part by advancing our theoretical understanding of brain–behavior relationships. Unfortunately, in the courtroom the brain scan has begun to take on the character of a modern-day Rorschach, as testifying clinicians employ neuroimages to render impressionistic judgments about complex mental phenomena. Although the law purports to demand that scientific evidence must meet empirical standards of validity and reliability, courts have been reluctant to invade the special province of the clinician by questioning the scientific basis for psychological interpretations of neuroimaging data.

The views expressed herein are those of the authors alone, and do not reflect official positions of NIH, DHHS, or the Federal Government.

From: *Brain Imaging in Substance Abuse: Research, Clinical, and Forensic Applications*
M. J. Kaufman, ed. © Humana Press Inc., Totowa, New Jersey

This chapter describes the current use of neuroimages as psychiatric evidence in civil and criminal trials, and will identify the limited evidentiary purposes for which brain-scanning techniques are appropriate. The focus will be on determining whether neuroimaging evidence of brain function is relevant to *legal* determinations of criminal intent, cognitive impairment, or insanity. In light of the extensive literature linking substance abuse to crime, the discussion will also consider whether neuroimaging evidence of substance-related neuropathology and brain dysfunction should play a role in the adjudication of crime, or in the sentencing and treatment of substance-abusing criminals.

Because the emphasis here is on an integration of legal and scientific perspectives, a detailed review of neuroimaging methodology or of the neuropsychology and neurophysiology of substance abuse is beyond the scope of this chapter. For further reading in these fields the reader is urged to consult companion chapters in this volume or the many literature reviews on these topics. Throughout this chapter, the term "substance abuse" is used in reference to both alcoholism and drug abuse; the phrase "structural imaging techniques" is used in reference to both CT (computed tomography) and MRI (magnetic resonance imaging); and the phrase "functional imaging techniques" is used to refer predominantly to SPECT (single photon emission computed tomography), PET (positron emission tomography), MRS (magnetic resonance spectroscopy), and fMRI (functional magnetic resonance imaging).

SCIENCE AND THE LAW

The Meaning of "Evidence"

Legal scholars and their fellow academics often warn that a "culture clash" between science and the law is producing dire consequences for the legal system. These commentators maintain that the increasingly scientific nature of many legal problems and the fundamental differences between the legal and the scientific methods lead, ineluctably, to incomprehensible expert testimony, bewildered juries, and a widespread misapplication of scientific research in legal disputes.[1] Admittedly, legal scholarship is sometimes overwrought with hyperbole about the proliferation of "junk science" in the courtroom.[2] Miscommunication can and does occur, however, at the intersection of science and the law, two insular and highly specialized disciplines.

For example, when a lawyer and a scientist use the word "evidence," both are speaking the English language, and the listener might reasonably assume that both have in mind the Webster's definition of the word: evidence as a "sign" or an "indication."[3] Yet the scientist, if queried, would define evidence in terms of the slow accretion of statistically significant findings in support of some general hypothesis. The scientist doesn't really expect to *prove* anything with a single piece of evidence, but rather to *improve* her next attempt to study a research problem.

Not surprisingly, the lawyer has something quite different in mind. Her concept of "evidence" is bound by rigid definitions—definitions that take up two pages of Black's Law Dictionary[4]—and her evidence must shoulder quite a burden: It must help to prove *truth*. Legal evidence is used to demonstrate, to the satisfaction of a judge or jury, the existence of a certain fact or condition, at a specific point in time. The matter to which the evidence is relevant will be adjudicated just once; there will be no chance for replication, follow-up studies, or the "further investigations" that scientists hasten to recommend whenever they are asked to reach a conclusion.

Problems arise when lawyers draw upon scientific evidence to prove legal truths. The scientific literature in a given field often does not yield the type of "evidence" that is needed to resolve a particular legal dispute. Moreover, a field of research may be technologically advanced but methodologically immature, generating exciting hypotheses but few broadly generalizable findings and little normative data. Such is decidedly the case for neuroimaging research, especially when researchers use neuroimaging techniques to study cognition and mental illness.

From the Laboratory to the Courtroom

For the researcher who is unfamiliar with the courtroom, it may be difficult to envision how the adversarial pressures of the legal system distort research, as group data are selectively misapplied in the individual legal case. A brief illustration of this phenomenon is instructive. Consider a hypothetical principal investigator working in the teaching hospital of a major research university. This investigator decides to conduct a typical fMRI activation study with 20 subjects of mixed age, gender, and handedness. The study's experimental condition involves somatosensory stimulation of a subject's fingers, after the subject has ingested a dose of alcohol. Halfway through the study, the research team decides to tweak the scanning parameters and to incorporate the administration of a paramagnetic contrast agent in the study protocol. At the completion of the study, the results are exciting: the amplitude of somatosensory cortical activation is reduced in the alcohol condition.

Yet the raw data are not unequivocally compelling. One of the 20 subjects displays higher absolute values for signal intensity in the targeted cortical region during the control condition. The investigator considers this subject an obvious outlier and drops him from further data analyses. Once the data are massaged, normalized, and the motion effects subtracted with a correction algorithm, the experimental result reaches statistical significance.

The hypothetical investigator submits his paper to a prestigious journal, accompanied by a vivid computer-generated illustration that superimposes a color-coded activation map on a three-dimensional rendering of a human brain (*see* Fig. 1). After several trips through peer review, the core of the investigator's paper becomes dense with qualifiers about the potential confounds in his study, including the small number of subjects, the possibility of gender or lateralization effects, the sensitivity of the data to motion artifacts, the limits of the spatial resolution, and the mid-stream change in the scanning protocol. By contrast, the title of the paper is quite conclusory: "Alcohol Reduces Focal Cortical Activation During fMRI."

As per university policy, the investigator notifies the university's public relations department of his exciting finding. On the eve of journal publication, the investigator's study—and his dramatic illustration depicting the bright foci of activation—are carried in local and national papers, under headlines suggesting that the investigator has discovered a new test for alcoholism. The investigator receives many calls for telephone interviews, but the resulting 30-second stories on evening news and radio programs

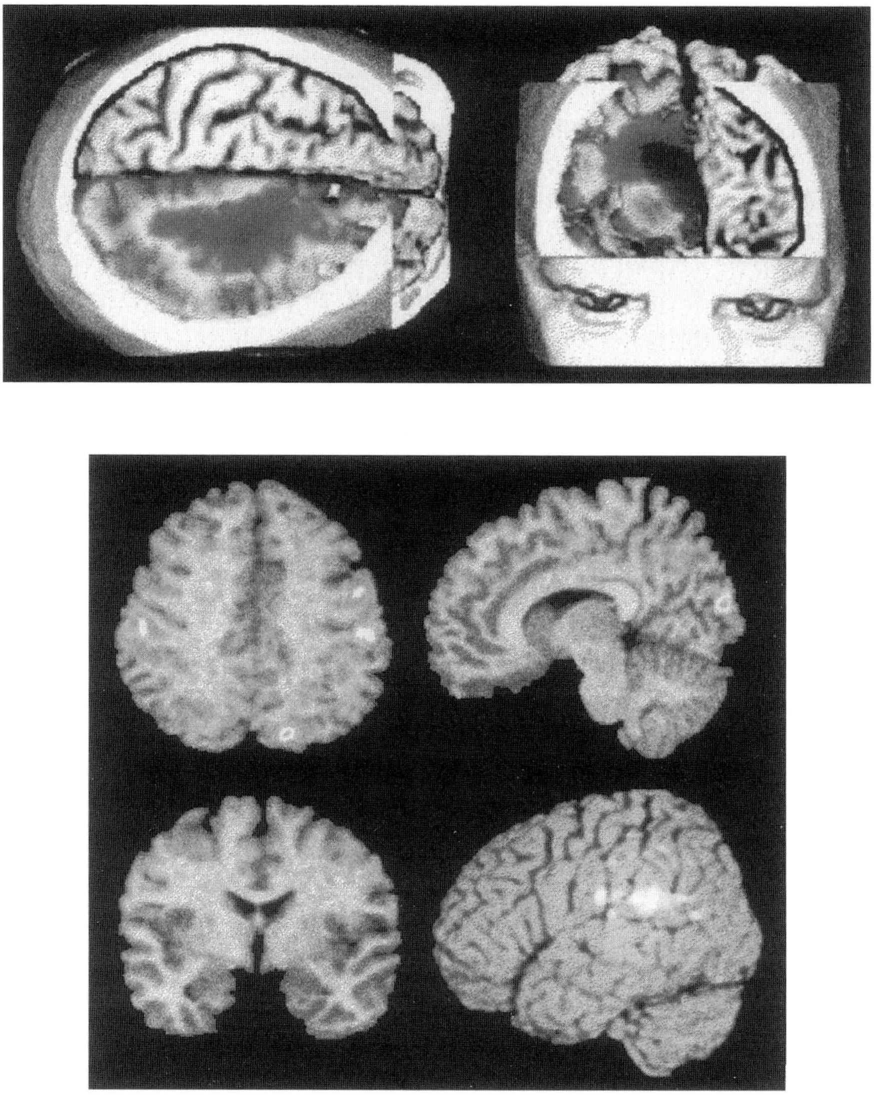

Fig. 1. These illustrations are examples of the manner in which functional data may be overlaid upon a structural image to create a strikingly realistic representation of brain activation. **Top:** SPECT data overlaid on three-dimensional MRI renderings of the brain. **Bottom:** fMRI data (bright or colored pixels), indicating cortical activation in response to a motor task, interlaced in three-dimensions with structural MRI data. The combined volume of data may be resliced, for example, axially (upper left), sagittally (upper right), or coronally (lower left); it may even be digitally rendered to create a pseudo-realistic surface view of cortical activation (lower right). (*See* color plate 10 appearing after p. 230).

omit his measured interpretation of the data in favor of a more arresting sound bite that features the investigator speculating about the potential use of his research to identify cognitive disorders in chronic alcoholics.

Soon thereafter, the investigator receives a phone call from an attorney for the defendant in a controversial murder trial. The defense team is preparing to argue a defense of diminished capacity, and the lawyers want the investigator to scan the defendant's brain using the experimental fMRI protocol. The university urges the investigator to cooperate. When the scan data are analyzed, the defendant's activation values are lower than the average value in the published study, a finding that the investigator knows is meaningless because of the absence of any normative data for focal cortical activation in response to somatosensory stimulation.

Yet at trial the defense team introduces a psychiatric expert witness who will draw the opposite conclusion about the significance of the brain scan. To explain the basis for his clinical opinion that the defendant—whose cognitive functioning is otherwise within normal limits—was unable to form the specific intent to kill the victim, the psychiatrist points to the fMRI images and to the investigator's study as evidence that the defendant has a diminished mental capacity because of an alcohol-related brain impairment. The prosecutor struggles to attack the limited reliability of this testimony, but the "scientific" nature of the psychiatrist's opinion has already created reasonable doubt in the minds of the lay jurors. The hung jury fails to return a verdict, leading to widespread speculation about the impact of the defendant's brain scan on the prosecution's case. Meanwhile, the investigator, well aware of the limitations of his own small study, is disturbed to learn of this alarming misapplication of his research.

The preceding scenario might seem farfetched, but neuroimaging researchers should be aware that attempts to use (and to misuse) neuroimages as legal evidence are becoming increasingly common. For instance, following widespread publicity about his findings, Dr. Daniel Schacter, whose Harvard research team published PET and fMRI studies of "false memories," was surprised to be approached about the potential application of his work in litigation involving evidence of repressed or recovered memories.[5] Interest in the courtroom use of neuroimages actually dates to the early 1980s, when the well-funded defense team for John Hinkley, Jr., introduced a brain scan at Hinkley's trial for the attempted assassination of President Reagan. Hinkley's lawyers recruited both a psychiatrist and NIMH researcher to testify that Hinkley's CT scan, which depicted sulcal "widening," supported a diagnosis of schizophrenia. The court admitted this neuroimaging evidence despite the lack of any foundational testimony to establish that CT scans were a valid and reliable tool for the diagnosis of a mental illness.[6]

Since the Hinkley trial, neuroimaging evidence has played a role in a number of high-profile murder cases, including the California trials of mass murderers Ramon Salcido and Barry Wayne McNamara, and the recent murder trial of the wealthy eccentric John E. Dupont.[7] Yet in most of the criminal cases to date, neuroimages have been introduced only at the post-conviction "penalty phase" of a trial, when evidentiary standards are relaxed and the defendant is permitted to argue any conceivable mitigating grounds for a reduction in sentence.

There is now precedent, however, for the introduction of neuroimaging evidence during the actual trial proper, for the purpose of arguing to a jury that a defendant suffers from an exculpatory brain dysfunction. In 1995 a judge in a New York murder trial ruled admissible a PET scan of the brain of Herbert Weinstein, an advertising executive accused of murdering his wife. The appearance of the scan was unusually dramatic due to the presence of a large, previously undetected arachnoid cyst in Weinstein's frontal

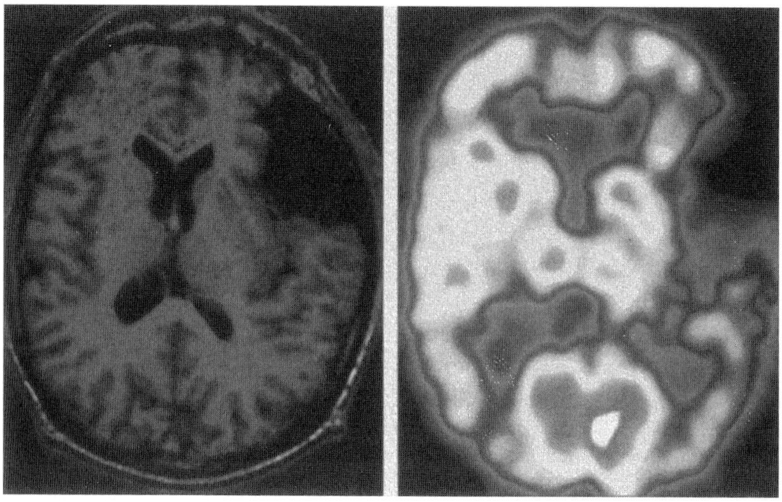

Fig. 2. The MRI and PET scans of murder defendant Herbert Weinstein, showing an arachnoid cyst in Weinstein's frontal lobe. Reprinted with permission from Diagnostic Imaging, January, 1993. ©1993 Miller Freeman, Inc. All rights reserved. (*See* color plate 11 appearing after p. 230).

lobe (Fig. 2). At a pretrial hearing the judge ruled that the defense would be allowed to introduce Weinstein's PET scan, over the objections of prosecution experts who noted that arachnoid cysts are frequently benign, and further, that there is no established correlation between such cysts and criminal behavior.[8]

More recently, the defense attorneys in the embezzlement trial of former United Way executive William Aramony used an MRI scan to argue a "shrinking brain" defense for their client. The gist of the defense argument in this case was that due to his diminished mental capacity, Aramony was unable to form the requisite criminal intent to commit the crime of embezzlement.[9] Both Weinstein and Aramony were permitted to plea bargain for convictions on lesser charges, suggesting that prosecutors in these cases feared that a jury might be unduly persuaded by the visual impact and scientific aura of neuroimaging evidence.

Beyond the risk that brain scans may unduly sway judges and juries, the unnecessary and inappropriate use of neuroimages as evidence may divert scant resources from the publicly funded arm of the criminal justice system, as occurred in 1997 when the Florida Supreme Court ordered a local public defender's office to pay for a PET scan for convicted murderer Johnny Hoskins. The defense neuropsychologist, who had already diagnosed Hoskin's cognitive impairment from the results of neurological and neuropsychological assessment, managed to convince the Florida Supreme Court that a costly PET scan was somehow needed to confirm this diagnosis.[10] Similarly, in 1998 a district court overseeing the trial of Jeremy Strohmeyer—the 18-yr-old college student who allegedly assaulted and strangled a second-grader in the bathroom of a Las Vegas hotel—allotted the defense funds for a CT and MRI. Strohmeyer's defense team reportedly plans to use these images during the guilt phase of his capital murder trial.[11]

Neuroimages as Psychiatric Evidence

The use of neuroimages in criminal cases is still relatively infrequent, although awareness of imaging techniques appears to be spreading among the defense bar, and criminal lawyers have occasionally combined brain scans and evidence of a family history of mental illness in a sort of "genetic" defense to criminal charges.[12] By contrast, plaintiffs in civil cases are far more likely than criminal defendants to rely on SPECT, PET, and MRI scans, especially when the neuropsychological evidence of a plaintiff's cognitive impairment is less than compelling. Neuroimages have been used to buttress claims of brain damage in civil litigation over everything from auto accidents and workman's compensation claims to toxic exposures and mild head injuries.[13]

Used appropriately, imaging data may make an invaluable contribution to the legal fact-finding process. For example, neuroimages are now used to reveal brain damage in cases of child abuse, to determine legal brain death, or to assess and to illustrate brain trauma caused by severe head injuries.[14] In these contexts, a medical witness uses a neuroimage to evaluate or to explain the physiological status of the brain, just as an expert might introduce an X-ray to illustrate an accident victim's broken bone.

Greater cause for concern arises when neuroimages become *psychiatric* evidence, as when an expert witness points to a PET or MRI scan in an attempt to persuade a judge or jury to draw inferences about the subject's mental health, intellect, judgment, or criminal intent. Neuroimaging findings in the areas of cognitive neuroscience and mental illness are essentially group effects of small magnitude; the imaging literature has yet to produce any tests or techniques that are sensitive and specific enough to reliably diagnose cognitive deficits or psychiatric disorders. Reflecting this reality, the Society for Nuclear Medicine has promulgated guidelines that state:

> The use of functional neuroimaging in forensic situations, including criminal, personal injury, product liability, medical malpractice, worker's compensation, and "toxic torts" remains especially controversial… [t]herefore, the appropriateness of findings and conclusions offered in the form of expert testimony, based on (functional imaging studies) in any but the few generally accepted clinical situations is difficult and often impossible to substantiate based on the current level of scientific and clinical knowledge.[15]

With regard to all brain imaging modalities, given the relative immaturity of the science, neuroimaging data for a single individual are not likely to be probative evidence of that individual's cognitive status or volitional state. Unfortunately, neuroimages are most likely to enter the courtroom as psychiatric, not scientific evidence. Under the applicable standards for the admission of scientific evidence (see discussion below), the use of a subject's PET scan or MRI to diagnose mental illness or cognitive impairment is unreliable and should, therefore, be inadmissible at trial. Yet a court will often permit a psychiatric expert witness to render a clinical opinion about mental state or cognitive capacity that is based in part on the results of a brain scan.

This paradoxical result comes about because the law treats psychiatric evidence in a peculiarly deferential fashion. As one commentator who has surveyed forensic mental health professionals observes, if a psychiatric expert diagnoses a plaintiff or defendant with a recognized mental disorder (i.e., a DSM axis I or axis II diagnosis[16]), courts are unwilling to scrutinize the scientific basis for the expert's opinion, and the expert's testimony is likely to go unchallenged.[17] Under current judicial interpretations of the evidence laws of many states, a psychiatric expert may refer to the results of any test or to any outside literature that informs his or her diagnosis, even when such material would otherwise be inadmissible due to its hearsay nature or uncertain reliability. In recent years the Supreme Court has begun to impose a more exacting review upon the scientific evidence presented by expert witnesses, but the application of these new legal standards to psychiatric opinion testimony in state and federal court has been uneven, at best.[18]

Evidentiary Tests for the Admissibility of Expert Scientific Testimony

As a preface to a discussion of scientific testimony, it is important to note that evidence law distinguishes between (1) lay witnesses, who are only permitted to testify to facts of which they have first hand knowledge (or, in some cases, to give opinions based upon personal observation); and (2) experts, who, if qualified by virtue of special knowledge, training or experience, may offer opinions based upon any facts or data that other experts in the same field might reasonably consider. Through the vehicle of an expert witness a party may place evidence before the jury that would otherwise be inadmissible, provided that the party first convinces the court to allow the witness to testify as an expert.[19]

Courts have long evaluated expert testimony under a legal standard known as the *Frye* test. *Frye* originated in 1923, when a federal court of appeals ruled that a psychologist could not testify regarding his use of a primitive polygraph machine to examine a defendant named Alphonse Frye. The court reasoned that the psychologist's testimony was inadmissible because the polygraph machine had not gained general acceptance among psychologists as an instrument for detecting lies.[20] Thereafter, federal and state courts around the country began to invoke the *Frye* principle of "general acceptance" as a threshold test for admitting expert scientific testimony. A witness who purported to testify as an expert would first be required to demonstrate to the court's satisfaction that the theory, test, or instrument upon which the expert based his opinion had been widely adopted within his or her field of expertise.

In 1975, however, the newly adopted Federal Rules of Evidence appeared to revise the *Frye* standard, at least within the federal court system. Rule 702 spoke indirectly to the issue of the *Frye* test, by indicating that an expert witness should be permitted to testify whenever his or her "scientific, technical, or other specialized knowledge" might "assist" the judge or jury. Courts and legal scholars soon disagreed as to whether the "assistance" test of Rule 702 had replaced "general acceptance" with a more stringent standard for expert testimony.

Subsequently, in the case of *Daubert v. Merrell Dow Pharmaceuticals*, the Supreme Court confirmed that the *Frye* test is no longer federal law. Instead, the court announced a new standard for expert scientific testimony. In what has become known as the *Daubert* test, the court held that scientific testimony must be valid, reliable, and relevant to the issues in dispute. The Supreme Court instructed trial court judges to act as "gatekeepers" who would shield the courts from pseudoscience by actively scrutinizing the proposed testimony for indications that the expert's theory or technique has been tested, has a known or potential error rate, has been subject to peer review, and is generally accepted by other experts within the same field.[21]

Many state courts have adopted the federal *Daubert* test; a minority still evaluate the admissibility of expert testimony under the *Frye* standard. Yet even within *Daubert* jurisdictions there remain judges who are uncomfortable with the "gatekeeper" role. These judges have avoided analyzing the scientific bases of expert opinion by categorizing such opinion as "nonscientific" expert testimony (i.e., as "technical or other specialized knowledge" under Rule 702), and by ruling that nonscientific expert testimony is outside the purview of the *Daubert* test.[22] Psychiatric and other forms of "soft" or social science testimony often evade *Daubert* review in this manner. Psychiatric opinion testimony is particularly problematic, because in contrast to past eras when clinical judgments were more obviously subjective, today's clinician is likely to couch his psychiatric opinion in the objective language of neurology and neuropsychiatry.[23]

In the years since the *Daubert* decision, federal circuit courts of appeal have split on the issue of whether trial courts must apply the *Daubert* test to "soft" scientific testimony. The Second, Fourth, Ninth, Tenth, and Eleventh circuits, which encompass a significant number of states, have permitted federal courts to admit expert testimony that does not meet *Daubert*'s standards of validity and reliability. These circuits have evaluated "nonscientific" expert testimony under the "helpfulness" prong of Federal Rule of Evidence 702, which states that a qualified expert may render an opinion if that opinion "will assist the trier of fact to understand the evidence or to determine a fact issue." Conversely, the Fifth and the Eighth circuits have held that all forms of expert testimony must be subjected to a *Daubert*-type scrutiny of the underlying principles and methodology upon which the expert's opinion is based.[24]

As recently as March of 1999, the Supreme Court lent some clarity to the law in this area by ruling in the case of *Kumho Tire, Co., Ltd. v. Carmichael* that the *Daubert* analysis must be applied, albeit in a flexible manner, to all forms of expert testimony.[25] Because the Supreme Court has yet to issue a post-*Kumho* opinion addressing the proper application of *Daubert* to the special case of psychiatric evidence, courts of appeal will likely vary in the degree to which they require trial courts in their circuits to scrutinize the testimony of psychiatric expert witnesses.

In summary, the degree to which a court is likely to scrutinize psychiatric neuroimaging evidence will be determined first by jurisdiction—whether the case is brought in federal court, or in a state court where *Frye* remains in effect—and second, for cases brought in federal court, by the governing circuit. In the future, federal courts in the Fifth and Eight circuits might be expected to subject neuroimaging evidence to a full-fledged *Daubert* analysis of reliability and validity, but the accuracy of this prediction is limited by the tendency for contradictory rulings to occur in an evolving area of the law.

Scientific Uncertainty and the Interpretation of Neuroimaging Data

The extent to which psychiatric neuroimaging evidence meets *Daubert*'s standards for valid and reliable scientific evidence is a critical inquiry. Equally important is the extent to which, under Federal Rule of Evidence 403, psychiatric neuroimaging testimony should be considered inadmissible due to the likelihood that it will confuse, mislead, or distract the jury.[26] Neuroimaging methodologies vary widely, ranging from routine CT, SPECT, and MRI scanning to the more sophisticated PET scans and the largely investigative fMRI techniques. To the uninformed observer, however, each of these imaging modalities creates what science writer Robert Crease has described as the biomedical "illusion of transparency": the impression that an image represents an unmediated snapshot of an underlying biological structure or process.[27] The powerful combination of tomographic or three-dimensional images and complex machinery lends neuroimaging evidence an aura of scientific infallibility, concealing the uncertain relationship between the image, the brain, and the mind.

For the general public, the breadth of what is not yet understood about brain imaging may be obscured by psychiatry's enthusiastic search for a more "scientific" means of diagnosis. A 1997 *New Yorker* magazine piece on the relationship between brain damage and crime illustrates this phenomenon. The author of the article visits a forensic psychiatrist and becomes entranced by a "fascinating" color-coded PET scan, mistakenly believing it to be "a computerized X-ray" of the brain. Subsequent conversations with a psychiatrist and a neurologist who testify on behalf of criminal defendants convince the author that brain imaging may be used to diagnose the organic causes of violent behavior. Completely absent from the article is any appreciation of the exploratory nature of imaging research, or of the fact that imaging techniques are not reliable tests of cognitive impairment or criminal disposition.[28]

Researchers in the imaging field are well aware that the actual image produced by a brain scan is merely a graphical representation of physiological data. Variations in scanning protocols, threshold levels, algorithmic transformations of raw signal data, motion artifacts, and head orientation are all factors that alter the visual appearance of images acquired from scans of the same subject (*see* Fig. 3).[29] Researchers also realize that the normal limits of brain morphology and function have not been precisely defined: according to one published review of the functional neuroimaging literature, little if anything is known about the normal patterns of neuronal activation, or the effects of age, medication, or disease on the neuronal response to stimulation.[30]

Moreover, at present, researchers who study mental processes using functional neuroimaging techniques may only hypothesize that the physiological phenomena that they observe (e.g., blood flow or changes in local arterial deoxyhemoglobin-hemoglobin levels) are directly correlated with neural activity. There remains marked disagreement within the field about the correct interpretation of imaging signal data.[31] Given this dispute about fundamental issues of data interpretation—for example, whether brain signals reflect aerobic or anaerobic neural activity—researchers cannot be certain that their scanning techniques accurately detect and measure brain activation. As a review in the journal *Science* concludes, "[w]ithout a full grasp of how the PET and fMRI signals relate to neuronal activity, neurobiologists worry that they may misinterpret brain images, perhaps missing active brain areas or assigning activity to a larger or different area than is actually activated by a particular stimulus or mental task."[32]

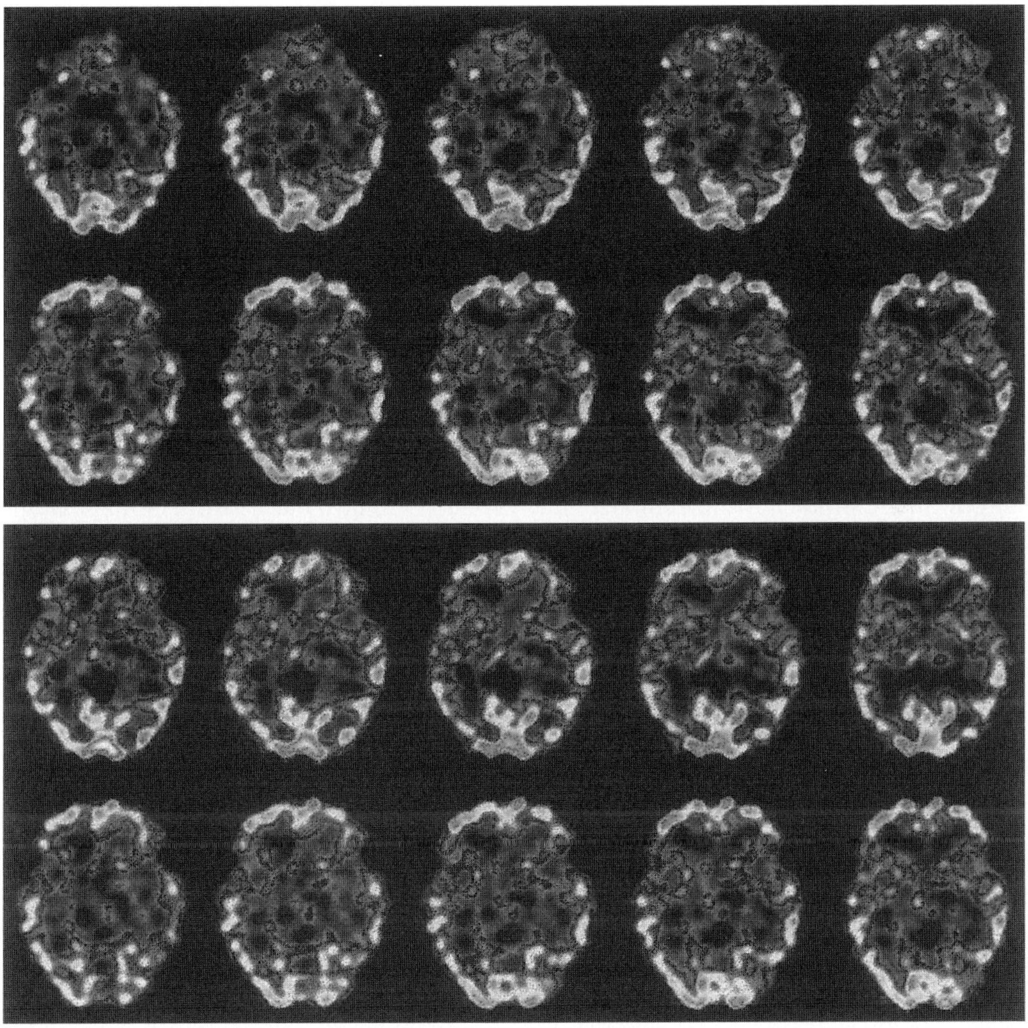

Fig. 3. Series of contiguous axial slices from a SPECT blood flow study illustrate how failure to control for the subject's head orientation may give a false impression of "hypofrontality." **Top:** The upper row of images clearly appears "hypofrontal" (dark or blue/green) relative to the lower row of "normal" (bright or yellow/red) comparison slices. In fact, however, all these images come from the same SPECT study of a single subject. In the upper row of images, the subject's head was rotated back by 5°; in the lower row it is rotated forward by 5° (roughly the width of a finger at the nose). **Bottom:** Each image volume has been rotated to remove the orientation discrepancy, and neither set shows evidence of "hypofrontality." Care must be taken to ensure proper head orientation, particularly when only a subset of the image volume is presented. (*See* color plate 12 appearing after p. 230).

Substance Abuse, Neuroimaging, and Crime

An extensive literature documents the strong association between substance abuse, violence, and crime.[33] Primary findings are that acute intoxication increases the likelihood of criminal or violent behavior, and that chronic substance abuse is prevalent among the criminal population.[34] The relationship between crime and substance abuse appears to hold for male and female offenders and across age groups and ethnicities.[35] Although cocaine, amphetamine, and heroin abuse are recognized correlates of crime, alcohol also appears to be a substantial and perhaps underrecognized predisposing factor to aggressive behavior and violence.[36] Neuropsychological studies and psychiatric research suggest that the association between substance abuse and criminal behavior may be mediated at the neurocognitive level by the disinhibiting or euphorigenic effect of acute intoxication, by cravings or withdrawal-induced delirium or psychosis, or by permanent cognitive impairment resulting from a substance-related dementing illness or amnestic syndrome.[37]

With respect to the application of brain imaging findings in substance abuse to the criminal law, the principal issue is the extent to which neuroimaging is a reliable tool for diagnosing substance-related *cognitive* impairment in the individual case. Findings from structural and functional imaging and neuropsychological studies suggest that chronic substance abuse may produce identifiable neuropathological and neurophysiological abnormalities as well as neuropsychological deficits. Yet these signs are not invariably present in populations of substance abusers, and interpretation of the data is confounded by the common problem of polysubstance abuse among research subjects.[38]

Relevant findings from the alcohol literature may be summarized as follows: Prolonged excessive consumption of alcohol is associated with neuropsychological deficits in tests of executive functioning, cognitive efficiency, memory, and fine motor speed, particularly among alcoholics suffering from Korsakoff's syndrome.[39] Alcohol abuse is also correlated with MRI and CT findings of cortical atrophy.[40]

The drug abuse literature yields fewer conclusive findings. In constrast to alcohol abuse, the neuropsychological sequellae of chronic drug use are not clearly defined, although various cognitive deficits have been identified in populations of substance abusers.[41] Brain imaging may reveal neuropathological changes in cases of substance abuse, as when the vasoconstrictive effects of cocaine ingestion cause stroke, hemorrhage, or seizure, but the brain trauma must be significant for the residual cerebropathology to be visible in MRI or CT.[42] Preliminary PET studies of violent offenders and substance abusers have identified regional metabolic deficits in these overlapping populations.[43] Abnormalities of cerebral activation and metabolism have also been detected in chronic alcoholics and substance abusers using PET and fMRI,[44] although the literature is sparse due to the relatively recent development of fMRI techniques and the costly nature of this research.

In general, when evaluating the brain-behavior research in substance abuse or alcoholism, it is important to keep in mind that there are no reliable quantitative measures of brain morphology or physiology. Neuroimaging findings do not differentiate between chronic substance abusers or alcoholics and normal subjects on an individual basis; nor may neuroimages be used to identify specific cognitive deficits in these populations. Neuroimages are, therefore, neither necessary nor sufficient for a psychiatric expert to render a clinical opinion about the sanity, criminal responsibility, or mental state of an alcoholic or substance-abusing defendant.

Substance Abuse as a Defense to Crime

Although neuroimaging researchers may soon make tremendous strides toward an understanding of the neurological and neuropsychological sequellae of substance abuse, at present, psychiatric neuroimaging evidence should play little if any role in criminal defense. Furthermore, even if neuroimages were to someday prove to be reliable tests for the presence of mental disorders, evidence of a substance-related mental impairment would be relevant to the adjudication of a criminal charge in only two contexts: negation of the mens rea element of specific intent crimes; and the insanity defense.

The criminal law is hostile to a defense based on the voluntary abuse of any intoxicating substance. Thus, proof of voluntary intoxication—no matter how extreme the impairment produced—will not completely exculpate a defendant. "Voluntary" intoxication is broadly defined by case law, and encompasses every circumstance in which a substance is self-administered, even when the act of ingesting the substance appears to be the involuntary result of an addictive craving. The concept of involuntary intoxication, which may serve as a exculpatory defense to most crimes, is reserved for circumstances in which a defendant is coerced into ingesting a substance or in which the defendant suffers an unanticipated pathological reaction to a legal drug.[45]

Many jurisdictions do permit the defense to argue for a conviction on a lesser charge when the evidence shows that the defendant's voluntary intoxication negated the "specific intent" element of a crime. In general terms, most criminal codes differentiate between specific intent crimes, which require proof that the defendant acted with a criminal purpose, and general intent crimes, which merely require proof that the defendant engaged in the criminal act with a reckless or negligent state of mind.[46] To prove murder, for example, the prosecution must show that the defendant had the specific intent to kill the victim. Evidence that a defendant was impaired because of voluntary intoxication may be used to negate the "intent to kill" element of the crime of murder (a specific intent crime), but the same defendant might still be convicted on a charge of manslaughter (a lesser, general intent crime).

Insanity is an affirmative or complete defense to a criminal charge, but for three basic reasons defendants rarely invoke the insanity defense. First, some states no longer permit defendants to present psychiatric evidence for the purpose of claiming innocence by reason of insanity.[47] Second, a defendant who mounts an insanity defense takes a risk by conceding commission of the criminal act and disputing only the issue of criminal responsibility. Third, the defendant bears the burden of proving his own insanity, and the legal test for insanity is exacting. Formulations of the insanity test vary among jurisdictions, but typically the defendant must prove, not only that he suffers from a mental disorder, but also that the disorder rendered him unable to know right from wrong or to conform his conduct to the law.[48]

In cases where a defendant suffers from permanent, substance-related mental impairment, defense attorneys occasionally employ the arcane "settled insanity" defense.[49] The legal concept of settled or "fixed" insanity requires as a threshold matter that a defendant's substance abuse has produced severe, well-documented cognitive impairment or dementia.[50] The defense of settled insanity has been recognized in one form or another in slightly more than half the states in the United States, but the use of this defense is unusual because the evidentiary burden on the defense is great: the defendant must establish not only the existence of a permanent mental or cognitive disorder resulting from substance abuse, but also that the disorder caused the defendant to meet each element of the jurisdiction's insanity test.[51] Additionally, in the federal system the Insanity Defense Reform Act of 1984 has been interpreted by several circuit courts of appeal to provide that a defendant's drug use, irrespective of the cognitive consequences, is not relevant to a determination of sanity in federal court.[52]

Lastly, when a defendant's competence is at issue, courts will often order a cognitive and psychological assessment prior to trial. The legal doctrine of competence to stand trial requires merely that a defendant be able to comprehend the basic nature of court proceedings and to assist defense attorneys in some rudimentary fashion; this is a functional determination and does not turn on the presence or absence of a mental illness or cognitive disorder.[53] A substance-related mental impairment is only relevant to a determination of competence to the extent that the impairment renders a defendant unable to comprehend or to communicate with his attorneys and the court.

Legal Applications of Substance Abuse Imaging Data

The appropriate role for brain imaging evidence in establishing either "settled insanity" or lack of specific intent is unclear. In a legal context, it is cognitive impairment, not brain damage *per se*, that is relevant to the determinative issues of mental state, intent, judgment, and capacity for self-control. Although the imaging literature does contain reports of various structural and functional brain abnormalities among *populations* of substance abusers, by no means are current imaging methodologies diagnostic of particular dementias, psychoses, or amnestic syndromes arising from chronic substance abuse. A psychiatric witness who concludes that a defendant lacked the requisite mens rea for a specific intent crime or was unable to appreciate the wrongfulness of his or her conduct must ground this opinion in the results of cognitive assessment. Unless and until the science of neuroimaging advances far beyond its current state, brain scanning is not a proxy for this cognitive testing.

In the future, neuroimaging might conceivably aid the justice system by informing decisions about parole, probation, or even sentencing for criminal defendants—all contexts in which the evidentiary standards are less stringent than those applied to the adjudication of criminal responsibility. Initial studies of altered brain function in chronic substance abusers suggest that fMRI and MRS techniques could potentially be used to monitor tolerance levels and to evaluate an individual's response to substance abuse treatment, or to detect early signs of substance-related brain dysfunction that predate the onset of clinical symptoms.[54]

The development of such applications will obviously be hampered by the shortage of resources within the criminal justice system for drug treatment, and by the general reluctance of policymakers to recognize the effectiveness of drug treatment as an alternative to incarceration.[55] A further caveat governs the use of neuroimages to predict treatment relapses or future criminal behavior: the American Psychiatric Association has concluded that current medical means of estimating an individual's future dangerousness are so unreliable that psychiatric opinion testimony on such issues should be inadmissible under both *Frye* and the Federal Rules of Evidence.[56]

CONCLUSION

In a recent paper published in *Nature Neuroscience*, Dehaene et al. describe a novel attempt to use neuroimaging as a crude cognitive "test." With almost perfect accuracy, these investigators were able to predict behavior from brain scans by analyzing fMRI signals to determine whether a subject moved his left or his right thumb in response to a visual cue.[57] Somewhat optimistically, Dehaene et al. foresee the eventual use of similar neuroimaging techniques to monitor and assess a wide range of mental phenomena, including cognition, emotion, memory, and judgment.[58]

Without question, neuroimaging techniques offer tremendous promise for the study of addiction and other brain-behavior relationships. At present, however, the scientific literature does not support the use of neuroimages to diagnose specific psychiatric or cognitive disorders in individuals, and courts should regard psychiatric neuroimaging evidence with skepticism. To assist judges in their effort to evaluate the admissibility of neuroimages as evidence, researchers should begin to critique the clinical and legal applications of brain imaging.

Eventually, brain imaging will indeed advance psychiatry, neurology, and neuropsychology toward a more scientific means of diagnosing and treating substance abuse and other mental disorders. As this goal is realized, neuroimaging researchers face an important opportunity to educate lawyers and courts about new technologies, and in so doing, to shape the evolving jurisprudence of scientific evidence.

REFERENCES*

[1]Confronting the New Challenges of Scientific Evidence, Harv. L. Rev., 108:1481 at p. 1484, 1998 (stating that scientific evidence "poses profound challenges for the law," because "most commentators agree that the cultures and purposes of law and science differ in important ways"); S. D. Easton, "Yer Outta Here!": a framework for analyzing the potential exclusion of expert testimony under the federal rules of evidence. U. Rich. L. Rev., 32:1 at p. 4, 1998 (stating "a significant amount of shoddy "science," phony logic, faulty analysis, sleight of hand, and other assorted junk enters the courtroom dressed up in the emperor's clothes of expert testimony") (internal citation omitted); M. G. Farrell, Daubert v. Merrell Dow Pharmaceuticals, Inc.: Epistemology and Legal Process. Cardozo L. Rev. 15:2183, at pp. 2196–2198, 1994 (expressing differring views of the fundamental constructs of law and science); C. B. Meyer, Science and the law: the quest for the neutral expert witness: a view from the trenches. J. Nat. Resources Env. L., 12:35, 1997 (describing the relationship between science and the law as "uneasy and remote" and "a schism").

[2]P. W. Huber, Junk Science in the Courtroom. Val. U. L. Rev., 26:723, 1992 (arguing that courts admit invalid and unreliable scientific evidence).

[3]Webster's New World Dictionary, 3rd Ed., 471, 1988.

[4]Black's Law Dictionary, 5th Ed., at p. 498–499, 1979.

[5]P. J. Hilts, Brain scan shows true colors of memories. San Diego Union-Tribune, Wed., July 10,

*Note: The citation format for this chapter does not follow typical legal conventions for law reviews, journal articles, and cases, to preserve some consistency with other chapters in this monograph.

1996; D. L. Schacter, R. L. Buckner, W. Koutstaal, et al., Late onset of anterior prefrontal activity during true and false recognition: an event-related fMRI study. Neuroimage, 6:259–269, 1997.

[6]A. A. Stone, The trial of John Hinkley. Law, Psychiatry, Morality 77 at p. 86, 1984; S. Taylor Jr., Hinkley's brain is termed normal. N.Y. Times, June 4, 1982, at p. A21 (quoting a prosecution expert who controverted defense testimony that enlarged sulci were evidence of schizophrenia).

[7]S. Emmons, Hunting for brain disorders: attorneys turn to UCI scanner as defense tool. L.A. Times, July 14, 1989, §2 at p. 1; S. Efron, Judge OKs UCI brain scan of Ramon Salcido. L.A. Times, Oct. 12, 1989, at p. B1; J. Rojas-Burke, PET scans advance as tool in insanity defense. J. Nucl. Med., 34:13N–16N, 1993; People v. McNamara, No. CV-88-5343ER (C.D. Cal. 1990), *aff'd*, 923 F.2d 862 (9th Cir.), *cert. denied*, 501 U.S. 1220 (1991); Dupont to be tested for brain malfunction. Bergen Record, Feb. 7, 1996, at p. A6.

[8]591 N.Y.S.2d 715 (Sup. Ct. 1992); R. Sherman, PET brain scan held admissible in murder case. Natl. L. J., Nov. 2, 1992, at p. 10.

[9]R. Chandrasekaran and B. Miller, Aramony's defense strategy called creative but risky. Washington Post, Wed. March 8, 1995, at p. D1.

[10]Hoskins v. Florida, No. 84737 (Fla. Sup. Ct. Oct. 16, 1997; American Bar Association, Ment. Phys. Disabil. L. Rep. 21:727 at p. 728, 1997.

[11]C. Benjamin, Natural-born killer? Las Vegas Rev. J. Sunday, Aug. 30, 1998, at p. A1.

[12]D. Nelkin, After Daubert: the relevance and reliability of genetic information. Cardozo L. Rev., 15:2119 at p. 2120, 1994.

[13]See, e.g., Hose v. Chicago Northwestern Trans. Co., 70 F.3d 968 (8th Cir. 1995) (holding PET scan admissible in plaintiff's toxic exposure suit against employer); Eggar v. Burlington N.R.R., No. CV 89–159-BLG-JFB, 1991 WL 315487 (D. Mont. Dec. 18, 1991); Bushell v. Secretary of Health & Human Serv., No. 91-1270V, 1993 WL 212472 (Fed. Cl. June 3, 1993); R. S. Tikofsky, Predicting outcome in traumatic brain injury: what role for rCBF/SPECT?, J. Nucl. Med., 35:947 at p. 948, 1994 (discussing use of brain imaging in tort cases).

[14]D. R. Smith, Legal recognition of neocortical death, Cornell L. Rev., 71:850 at p. 852, 1986; MRI offers key evidence in abused children. Diagn. Imaging, Mar. 1993 at p. 51; L. D'Agincourt, MRI of brain damage: a malpractice defense. Diagn. Imaging, Mar. 1993, at p. 45.

[15]Society of Nuclear Medicine Brain Imaging Council, Ethical clinical practice of functional brain imaging. J. Nucl. Med., 37:1256 at p. 1259, 1996.

[16]American Psychiatric Association, Diagnostic and Statistical Manual of Mental Disorders.

[17]C. Slobogin, Psychiatric evidence in criminal trials: to junk or not to junk. William and Mary L. Rev. 40:19, 1998.

[18]H. G. Hamilton, the movement from Frye to Daubert: where do the states stand? Jurimetrics J., 38:201 at p. 210 (1998) (listing state-by-state approach to scientific evidence); C. R. Showalter, Distinguishing science from pseudo-science in psychiatry: expert testimony in the post-Daubert era. Va. J. Soc. Policy Law 2:211, 1995.

[19]S. D. Easton. ibid., note 1, pp. 5–6.

[20]Frye v. United States, 923 F. 1013 (D.C. Cir. 1923).

[21]Daubert v. Merrell Dow Pharm., Inc., 509 U.S. 579, at p. 593, 1993.

[22]E. Beecher-Monas, Blinded by Science: How Judges Avoid the Science in Scientific Evidence. Temple L. Rev. 71:55, 1998.

[23]C. Slobogin, ibid., note 17, at p. 8.

[24]For a detailed explanation of Daubert admissibility standard and a review of current state and federal jurisprudence with respect to scientific evidence, see B. Black, Post-Daubert and Joiner caselaw: The good, the bad, and the ugly. SC33 ALI-ABA 145:157, 1998.

[25]119 S.Ct. 1167, 1174, 1999.

[26]Federal Rule 403 states, "Although relevant, evidence may be excluded if its probative value is substantially outweighed by the danger of unfair prejudice, confusion of the issues, or misleading the jury, or by considerations of undue delay, waste of time, or needless presentation of cumulative evidence."

[27]R. P. Crease, Biomedicine in the age of imaging. Science, 261:554, 1993.

[28]M. Gladwell, Damaged. The New Yorker, February 24–March 3, 1997, at pp. 132–146.

[29]P. A. Bandettini and E. C. Wong, Magnetic resonance imaging of human brain function: Principles, practicalities, and possibilities. Neurosurg. Clin. North Am., 8, 345 at p. 371, 1997 (detailing aspects affecting the interpretability of MR images, including physics, physiology, postprocessing, pulse sequences, and hardware); American Academy of Neurology, Report of the Therapeutics and Technology Assessment Subcommittee: Assessment: Positron Emission Tomography. Neurology, 41:163 at p. 167, 1991.

[30]J. M. Levin, M. H. Ross, P. F. Renshaw, Clinical applications of functional MRI in neuropsychiatry. J. Neuropsychiatry Clin. Neurosci. 7:511–522, 1995.

[31]M. Barinaga, What makes brain neurons run? Science, 276:196 at p. 198, 1997.

[32]Ibid.

[33]R. N. Parker, and K. Auerhahn, Alcohol, drugs, and violence. Ann. Rev. Sociol. 24:291–311, 1998; D. S. Lipton and B. D. Johnson, Smack, crack, and score: Two decades of NIDA-funded drugs and crime research at NDRI 1974–1994. Subst. Use Misuse 33:1779–1815, 1998.

[34]D. S. Lipton and B. D. Johnson. ibid., note 33; B. Morentin, L.F. Callado, J.J. Meana. Differences in criminal activity between heroin abusers and subjects without psychiatric disorders: analysis of 578 detainees in Bilbao, Spain. J. Forensic Sci., 43:993–999, 1998; M. E. Denison, A. Paredes, J. B. Booth. Alcohol and cocaine interactions and aggressive behaviors. Recent Dev. Alcohol, 13:283–303, 1997.

[35]J. A. Grunbaum, K. Basenengquist, D. Pandey, Association between violent behaviors and substance abuse among Mexican-American and non-hispanic white high school students. J. Adol. Heath 23:153–159, 1998; A. Valdez, Z. Yin, C. D. Kaplan, A comparison of alcohol, drugs, and aggressive crime among Mexican-American, black, and white male arrestees in Texas. Am. J. Drug Alcohol Abuse, 23:249–265, 1997; B. Spunt, J. H. Brownstein, S. M. Crimmins, S. Langley, Drugs and homicide by women. Subst. Use Misuse 31:825–845, 1996.

[36]J. Chong, Crime indicators for alcohol and drug abuse. Crim. Justice Behav. 25:283–305, 1998.

[37]P. N. Hoaken, P. R. Giancola, R. O. Pihl, Executive cognitive functions as mediators of alcohol-related aggression. Alcohol 33:47–54, 1998; J. C. Brust. Acute neurologic complications of drug and alcohol abuse. Neurol. Clin. 16:503–519, 1998; M. Ingvar, P. H. Ghatan, A. Wirsen-Meurling, et al., Alcohol activates the cerebral reward system in man. J. Stud. Alcohol, 59:258–269, 1998.

[38]M. J. Kaufman, J. M. Levin, J. D. Christensen, P. F. Renshaw, Magnetic resonance studies of substance abuse. Semin. Clin. Neuropsychiatry 1:61–75, 1996; O. F. Dent, M. R. Sulway, G. A. Broe, et al., Alcohol consumption and cognitive performance in a random sample of Australian soldiers who served in the Second World War. BMJ, 314:1655–1657, 1997.

[39]P. N. Hoaken, P. R. Giancola, R. O. Pihl, op. cit. note 37; D. Johnson-Greene, K. Adams, S. Gilman, et al., Effects of abstinence and relapse upon neuropsychological function and cerebral glucose metabolism in severe chronic alcoholism. J. Clin. Exp. Neuropsychol., 19:378–385, 1997; L. W. Welch, A. T. Cunningham, M. J. Eckardt, P. R. Martin, Fine motor speed deficits in alcoholic Korsakoff's syndrome. Alcohol. Clin. Exp. Res., 21:134–139, 1997; S. J. Nixon and D. Bowlby, Evidence of alcohol-related efficiency deficits in an episodic learning task. Alcohol. Clin. Exp. Res., 20:21–24, 1996; J. F. O'Mahoney and B. Doherty, Intellectual impairment among recently abstinent alcohol abusers. Br. J. Clin. Psychol., 35:77–83, 1996.

[40]M. J. Kaufman, J. M. Levin, J. D. Christensen, P. F. Renshaw. op. cit., note 38.

[41]K. I. Bolla, J. L. Cadet, E. D. London. The neuropsychiatry of chronic cocaine abuse. J. Neuropsychiatry Clin. Neurosci., 10:280–289, 1998; M. J. Selby and R. L. Azrin, Neuropsychological functioning in drug abusers. Drug Alcohol Depend., 50:39–45, 1998; R. McKetin and R. P. Mattick. Attention and memory in illicit amphetamine users. Drug Alcohol Depend., 48:235–242, 1997; T. L. Strickland, I. Mena, J. Villaneueva-Meyer, et al., Cerebral perfusion and neuropsychological consequences of chronic cocaine use. J. Neuropsychiatry Clin. Neurosci., 5:419–427, 1993.

[42]T. L. Strickland, B. L. Miller, A. Kowell, R. Stein, Neurobiology of cocaine-induced organic brain impairment: contributions from functional neuroimaging. Neuropsychol. Rev., 8:1–9, 1998.

[43]T. R. Kosten, C. Cheeves, J. Palumbo, et al., Regional cerebral blood flow during acute and chronic abstinence from combined cocaine-alcohol abuse. Drug Alcohol Depend., 50:187–195, 1998; D. Seidenwurm, T. R. Pounds, A. Globus, P. E. Valk. Abnormal temporal lobe metabolism in violent subjects: correlation of imaging and neuropsychiatric findings. Am. J. Neuroradiol., 18:625–631, 1997; A. Raine, D. Phil, J. Stoddard, et al., Prefrontal glucose deficits in murderers lacking psychosocial deprivation. Neuropsychiatry, Neuropsychol. Behav. Neurol., 11:1–7, 1998.

[44]D. Johnson-Greene, K. Adams, S. Gilman, et al. op. cit. L. C. Maas, S. E. Lukas, M. J. Kaufman., et al., Functional magnetic resonance imaging of human brain activation during cue-induced cocaine craving. Am. J. Psychiatry, 155:124–126, 1998.

[45]J. Dressler, Understanding Criminal Law, §24.05 (2d. ed., 1995) (for discussion of legal approach to intoxication and crime).

[46]W. R. LeFave and A. W. Scott Jr., Criminal Law §28, at p. 203, 1972.

[47]Idaho, Montana, and Utah are three such states. For further analysis, see A.M. Levine. Denying the Settled Insanity Defense: Another Necessary Step in Dealing with Drug and Alcohol Abuse. Boston Univ. L. Rev., 78, 75 at p. 79, 1998.

[48]Various tests for legal insanity include the M'Naughten rule, the "irresistable impulse" test, the "product" or Durham test, the federal statutory definition of insanity, and the definition adopted by the American Law Institute's Model Penal Code. For further details, see J. Dressler. op. cit., note 45, at §25, pp. 309–333.

[49]American Bar Association. Case Law Development: Criminal Responsibility. Ment. Phys. Disabil. L. Rep. 20, 662, 1996; Montana v. Englehoff, 518 U.S. 37 at p. 61, 1996 (in which the U.S. Supreme Court held that the constitution does not require a state to permit a defendant the defense of voluntary intoxication).

[50]J. Dressler. op. cit., note 45, at pp. 302–303.

[51]W. R. LeFave and A.W. Scott, Jr. op. cit., note 46; A.M. Levine. op. cit., note 47.

[52]A. M. Levine, ibid., American Bar Association, op. cit., note 49.

[53]American Bar Association, ABA Criminal Justice Standards Committee, ABA Criminal Justice and Mental Health Standards, at p. 174, 1989.

[54]L. C. Maas, S. E. Lukas, M. J. Kaufman et al., op. cit. note 44; M. J. Kaufman, T. Chiu, J. H. Mendelson, et al. Brain alcohol detectability increase with repeated administration in humans: a proton spectroscopy study. Magn. Res. Med., 35:435–440, 1996.

[55]D. S. Lipton and B. D. Johnson. op. cit., note 34.

[56]American Bar Association. op. cit., note 49.

[57]S. Dehaene, G. Le Clec'H, L. Cohen. et al., Inferring behavior from functional brain images. Nature Neurosci., 1:549–550, 1998.

[58]S. Dehaene, G. Le Clec'H, L. Cohen, et al. ibid.; M. Sarter, G. G. Berntson, J. T. Cacioppo, Brain imaging and cognitive neuroscience: toward strong inference in attributing function to structure. Am. J. Psychol., 51:13–21, 1995.

Glossary

abstraction
The ability to formulate conceptual ideas, make generalizations, utilize flexible thinking, apply rules and general principles for problem solving, and be aware of subtle or intrinsic aspects of a problem.

alpha
In electroencephalography, alpha activity comprises brain electrical activity in the range of 8–13 cycles per second (Hz). Alpha activity can be further subdivided into slow and fast bands (8–10 and 11-13 Hz, respectively).

angular momentum
A rotating or spinning object (e.g., the nucleus of an atom) has angular momentum.

Antisocial Personality Disorder (APD)
A mental disorder as defined by the DSM-IV as "a pervasive pattern of disregard for, and violation of, the rights of others that begins in early childhood or early adolescence and continues into adulthood."*

attenuation
In photon detection, some photons (e.g., those originating in the center of the brain or those having to traverse through denser tissues) lose energy and are scattered or absorbed. An attenuation correction must be performed to correct for this effect.

auditory brainstem response
An EEG measure of the sound-induced electrical response through the auditory nerves and brainstem nuclei.

Axis I (of the DSM)
The DSM contains 5 axes that are designed to assist in the evaluation of a patient's mental state, to plan treatment, and to predict outcome. Axis I includes Clinical Disorders and Other Conditions That May be a Focus of Clinical Attention, including substance abuse disorders.

**Diagnostic and Statistical Manual of Mental Disorders*, 4th edition, American Psychiatric Association, Washington, D.C., p. 645, 1994.

Axis II (of the DSM)
An axis of the DSM including personality disorders and mental retardation.

bandpass
A filter that allows energy of a particular frequency or frequency range to be transmitted to recording equipment.

Beck Depression Inventory
A psychiatric test used to assess depressive symptoms.

beta
In electroencephalography, beta activity comprises electrical activity in the range of 14–35 cycles per second (Hz). Beta activity can be further subdivided into slow and fast bands (13.5–19.5 and 20–26 Hz, respectively).

BOLD
Blood oxygen level dependent. This functional MRI technique uses the fact that deoxyhemoglobin concentration is reduced in functionally activated brain regions to magnetically differentiate these regions from other parts of brain.

Boltzmann distribution
The temperature-dependent distribution of atoms in a group of atoms at thermal equilibrium, as specified by the Boltzman constant *(k)*.

box car reference function
A reference function used in functional MRI data analyses, which models brain activation as a simple on–off phenomenon.

CBV
Cerebral blood volume. The vascular volume of brain (mL/g). This quantity can be measured with functional MRI and emission tomography techniques, and is useful in documenting acute or chronic effects of vasoactive drugs.

cognitive set
The ability to understand and maintain guidelines or parameters of assessment measures.

coherence
A measure of correlation between two EEG signals in the frequency domain.

coincidence detection
A system for detecting radionuclide decay in a PET experiment. Two high-energy γ rays are emitted in opposite trajectories during positron-electron collisions. The system only counts decay events registered in diametrically opposed detectors on a very narrow time scale (<10 ns) and discards noncoincident events resulting from random decay events.

collimator
A system for detecting radionuclide decay. A lead block containing many long and narrow holes selects for γ rays of parallel trajectories. γ rays of nonparallel trajectories are absorbed by the lead block and do not contribute to the signal.

concept formation
The ability to utilize abstract thinking and flexibility of thought in order to form ideas.

conduct disorder
A mental disorder as defined by the DSM-IV as "a repetitive and persistent pattern of behavior in which the basic rights of others or major age-appropriate societal norms or rules are violated"*

contrast agent
Any substance that, when administered to a subject, alters image intensity, highlighting tissues or processes of interest. In emission tomography, radionuclides produce contrast, while in magnetic resonance, paramagnetic agents, such as gadoteridol or deoxyhemoglobin, produce contrast.

correlation coefficient analysis
An fMRI data analysis method that derives a correlation coefficient between the activation time course for image pixels and the time course portraying the temporal characteristics of the challenge paradigm (sensory, motor, or cognitive).

cross-tolerance
A state attained after chronic drug use, which is accompanied by a diminished response to a different but closely related drug upon exposure.

Daubert test
This test of scientific expert testimony has replaced the Frye test in the federal court system and requires that expert scientific testimony be valid, reliable, and relevant to the issues in dispute.

daughter nuclei (metastable)
An unstable nucleus in a radionuclide resulting from the nuclear capture of an orbiting electron.

delta
In electroencephalography, delta activity comprises electrical activity less than 4 cycles per second (Hz). Delta activity is normally observed during deeper stages of sleep.

dependence
A state attained after chronic, heavy drug abuse, in which a patient has withdrawal symptoms when drug levels in the blood fall below a threshold concentration.

desynchrony
In electroencephalography, a pattern of activity in which the two hemispheres do not have synchronous waveforms.

distractor task
A task interspersed between other cognitive measures in order to prevent rehearsal.

**Diagnostic and Statistical Manual of Mental Disorders*, 4th edition, American Psychiatric Association, Washington, D.C., p. 85, 1994.

distribution volume
In emission tomography, the ratio of tissue radionuclide to free arterial radionuclide.

double quantum filter
A magnetic resonance spectrum editing technique. This technique permits detection of the inhibitory neurotransmitter γ-aminobutyric acid (GABA) in proton spectra by exploiting the different magnetic couplings of GABA and total creatine (Cr), selectively removing the overlapping Cr resonance.

DRESS
Depth resolved surface coil spectroscopy. This is a magnetic resonance method for obtaining a localized spectrum when using a surface coil.

DSC MRI
Dynamic susceptibility contrast MRI. This fMRI method uses rapid intravenous injections of contrast agents (e.g., gadoteridol) which alter tissue magnetization in proportion to concentration, and allows measurement of cerebral hemodynamic function by tracer kinetic analysis.

DSM
Diagnostic and Statistical Manual of Mental Disorders. This is a set of diagnostic criteria that are used as guidelines for making psychiatric diagnoses.

echo planar
A rapid MR imaging technique in which an entire image plane is acquired following a single radiofrequency (RF) excitation. Echo planar MRI is typically applied in functional MRI studies using BOLD or DSC MRI techniques.

EEG
Electroencephalography. This technique involves sampling of either spontaneous or evoked electrical brain activity to evaluate the activity of neuronal groups.

electromyography
A recording of electrical changes in muscles.

encoding strategy
The process of identifying and labeling incoming stimuli for storage.

event-related potentials (ERPs)
A series of longer-latency voltage fluctuations in the ongoing EEG that are time-locked to sensory, motor, or cognitive events, and are thought to be related to higher levels of cortical processing.

evoked potential
In EEG, an averaged short-latency response to a repeated sensory or cognitive stimulus, providing measures of latency and amplitude. The evoked response may be altered by acute or chronic substance abuse.

executive functions
Functions necessary for appropriate, socially responsible, and effective adult conduct. Includes the ability to apprehend external cues and identify suitable responses.

family history
Pertaining to an individual's predisposition to future alcohol or drug use problems, based on whether a first- or second-degree relative has alcohol or drug use problems.

federal rules of evidence
A group of regulations that concern the use of evidence in federal legal proceedings.

filtered backprojection
A technique used in emission tomographic imaging to reconstruct source images by computing photon paths. Retracings of multiple decay events from multiple projections intersect and are summed to recreate source images.

fMRI
Functional magnetic resonance imaging. A family of techniques that capitalize on the magnetic differences induced by endogenous or exogenous contrast agents (deoxyhemoglobin or gadoteridol, respectively) to map cerebral function and hemodynamics.

Fourier methods
An fMRI data analysis method that assesses frequencies of stimulus switching.

Fourier transform (FT)
This mathematical operation converts time domain information into the frequency domain, by parsing continuous waveforms into discrete peaks of frequency and amplitude data. In electroencephalography, it is used to produce power spectra. In magnetic resonance, the FT converts relaxation information in the form of free induction decay waveforms into image intensities and chemical spectra.

frequency encoding
A method for encoding spatial information in magnetic resonance experiments. A small magnetic gradient is applied during the acquisition of magnetic resonance signals and produces a slightly different magnetic environment (and nuclear spinning frequency) at each point along the gradient, allowing excited spins at different points along the gradient to be spatially localized.

Frye test
A threshold test for admitting scientific expert testimony requiring that the instrument being used to make a case must have "general acceptance" within that expert's field of scientific expertise. The Frye test is no longer federal law, but is still applicable in certain state jurisdictions.

FWHM
Full width at half maximum. A point of radioactivity (emission tomography) or a spectral line (magnetic resonance) produce a signal spread over a small area, with a profile approximating a gaussian curve. The spread of the curve at half its peak height is related to image resolution.

gadolinium
A highly paramagnetic lanthanide metal used as a contrast agent in magnetic resonance imaging; administered to humans in a chelated form.

gamma rays
Radioactive substances emit gamma (γ)-rays or which have energy that is similar to but stronger than x-rays.

gradient
In magnetic resonance, small magnetic gradients (e.g., B_1) can be added to the main magnetic field (e.g., B_0) to produce a pattern of magnetic field differences across two or three dimensions. Each point in space will then have a unique magnetic signature.

half-life
A physical property of a radionuclide which describes its decay from an unstable state having an excess proton to a stable state (via proton to neutron conversion). The rate of decay is exponential.

hematoma
A mass of blood that has leaked from a vessel that may be partly or completely clotted.

heritability index
(H^2) A proportion indicating the degree of variance in phenotype that results from genetic variation.

hyponatremia
A low blood sodium concentration.

hypokalemia
A low blood potassium concentration.

hypsarrhythmia
An EEG pattern characterized by continuous spiking and irregular wave activity.

I.M.
Intramuscular (also i.m.). The administration of a substance via injection into a muscle.

I.N.
Intranasal (also i.n.). The administration of a substance via inhalation or snorting.

I.V.
Intravenous (also i.v.). The administration of a substance into a vein.

insanity defense
A legal defense based on the premise that a defendant cannot be held responsible for a crime if s/he lacked criminal intent (*mens rea*) because of insanity.

ISIS
Image selected in vivo spectroscopy. A localization technique used in magnetic resonance spectroscopy.

Larmor frequency
The resonance frequency of a nucleus in a magnetic field, based on the gyromagnetic ratio (ratio of the magnetic moment to the angular momentum) for the particular nucleus and the applied magnetic field.

MAST
Michigan Alcoholism Screening Test. This is a self-administered questionnaire on alcohol drinking habits used clinically to help determine a diagnosis of alcoholism.

memory consolidation
Progressive strengthening of the memory traces so that information may be stored permanently.

mens rea
The specific intent of doing harm or committing a crime.

monozygotic
Pertaining to a twin birth originating from one fertilized egg. A twin birth from two fertilized eggs is termed dizygotic.

montage
In EEG, the specific arrangement by which electrode pairs are displayed simultaneously in an EEG record. Referential montages compare electrical activity at different electrode sites to an electrode with no cerebral electrical activity. In bipolar montages, both electrodes of the pair are active, and the difference in potential between the two electrodes is displayed.

movement artifact
An artifact induced in an encephalogram (or in other imaging modalities) by subject motion.

MRI
Magnetic resonance imaging.

MRS
Magnetic resonance spectroscopy.

natural abundance
The relative proportion of an isotopic form of an atom of interest in an emission tomographic (radionuclide) or magnetic resonance experiment. Emission tomography takes advantage of the low natural abundance of radionuclides which can thus be exogenously administered to produce selective tissue contrast. Nuclei with high natural abundance [e.g., protons (^{1}H), phosphorus (^{31}P), fluorine (^{19}F), and lithium (^{7}Li)] can be relatively easily studied with magnetic resonance spectroscopy.

NMR
Nuclear magnetic resonance. This includes MRI, MRS, and fMRI techniques.

nuclear magnetic moment (μ)
Each nucleus spins on its axis and this spin generates a magnetic moment, which causes the nucleus to act like a small bar magnet when placed in a magnetic field.

oddball paradigm
In EEG, a task that requires discrimination between a low- and a high-probability stimulus, which differ on some dimension of intensity (e.g., visual intensity) or frequency (e.g., auditory frequency).

paramagnetic
Paramagnetic substances have an odd number of outer shell electrons and are attracted to stronger magnetic fields. In magnetic resonance, paramagnetic substances (e.g., deoxyhemoglobin or gadolinium) can increase the relaxation rates of water, and are useful as contrast agents.

penalty phase
The trial phase occurring after a verdict in which the terms of sentence are established.

perseverative
Continuation or repetition of a behavior after the causative stimulus has been removed, and no such activity is indicated. This may occur in multiple domains, including language, drawing, or writing.

PET
Positron emission tomography. This technique permits in vivo detection of radionuclides. A positron produced during radionuclide decay collides with a neighboring electron, and produces two gamma rays that have opposite trajectories. The two gamma rays are detected with coincidence detection systems.

phase dispersion
In magnetic resonance blood flow experiments, if blood abruptly changes its direction or velocity after phase encoding (e.g., after a stenosis), then the phase of the blood in a voxel may lose coherence, resulting in phase dispersion and signal loss.

phase encoding
A method for encoding spatial information in magnetic resonance experiments. A magnetic gradient is applied after an RF pulse but before collection of the signal, and excited spins at different points along the gradient acquire slightly different phases.

photomultiplier tube
An instrument which converts brief light flashes emitted from crystalline gamma ray detectors in PET/SPECT cameras into electrical pulses.

photon
An elementary amount or quantum of light.

pixel
An area element of a two-dimensional tissue image.

Planck's constant *(h)*
This is a physical constant that describes the radiation energy generated by an oscillating source.

planning
Involves the ability to actively conceptualize a change from an individual's present circumstances, consider alternative situations, and weigh and make decisions.

positron
Radionuclide decay of a nuclear proton into a neutron releases a positron (positively charged electron). The positron, upon collision with an electron, releases two gamma rays of opposite trajectories that are detected in PET studies.

posterior fossa
Pertaining to the back of the brain or head.

power spectrum
In EEG, the energy output across different frequencies during an epoch of spontaneous EEG recording. The power spectrum is obtained by analyzing the EEG signal with a fast Fourier transform.

proton decoupling
A magnetic resonance technique which involves nullifying the magnetic interaction between hydrogen nuclei (protons) and other biologically relevant nuclei in the same molecule, such as carbon or phosphorus nuclei.

proton density image
Gray matter appears brighter than white matter and cerebrospinal fluid is similar to gray matter. These images have a very short TE and a very long TR. A proton density image is similar to a T2-weighted image but has better gray-white matter contrast.

pulse spectroscopy
Acquisition of a magnetic resonance spectrum following single or repeated radiofrequency pulses at a single frequency. This method allows detection of substances in lower concentrations, smaller volumes, or lower MRS sensitivities.

radiotracer
A biologically relevant chemical that has had a radionuclide incorporated into its chemical structure, in order to measure tissue distribution, hemodynamics, or biochemistry.

resonant frequency *(ν)*
The frequency at which energy must be pulsed in order to induce a nucleus to transition between quantized energy states. This frequency is a physical property of each nucleus and is dependent upon the applied magnetic field (B_0).

RF
Radiofrequency. In magnetic resonance, an RF pulse at the Larmor frequency is used to excite magnetized tissue. This tips spins out of their steady–state orientation along the direction of the main magnetic field (B_0) into the transverse plane.

rotating frame of reference
The rotating frame of reference notation subtracts out the rotational component of motion of magnetized tissue (around the main magnetic (B_0) field axis at the Larmor frequency) simplifying the macroscopic description of relaxation behavior (T1 and T2).

S.C.
Subcutaneous (also s.c.). The administration of a substance via injection into the space under the skin.

scatter
In emission tomography, when a photon travels long distances or through dense tissues, it may collide with a nucleus causing it to both lose some of its energy and have its trajectory altered. This increases background noise and reduces image contrast.

sensorimotor ability
Measure of intactness and aptitude of the somatosensory system. Assessments include motor laterality, fine motor coordination, and responses to pain and temperature.

settled insanity
In legal context, a clinically demonstrable cognitive impairment or dementia that is the result of a history of substance abuse.

shift reagent
In magnetic resonance, a chemical which alters the resonance frequency of ions in their vicinity. Shift reagents permit differentiation of resonances from atoms present in intracellular versus extracellular spaces.

spatial orientation
Involves the ability to relate to the position, direction, or movements of objects or points in space.

SPECT
Single photon emission computed tomography. This technique permits in vivo detection of radionuclides, using collimation to detect the radioactive decay of tracer chemicals.

spin angular quantum number (*I*)
Each atomic nucleus has a spin angular momentum quantum number, which takes on half-integer values (e.g. 0, 1/2, 3/2…). Nuclei with nonzero *I* values have a net nuclear magnetic moment and can be studied in a magnetic resonance experiment.

spin–lattice relaxation time (*T*1)
In magnetic resonance, the *T*1 is the time constant that describes the relaxation process of energy exchange between an excited tissue and the environment.

spin–spin relaxation time (*T*2)
In magnetic resonance, the *T*2 is the time constant that describes the relaxation process involving energy exchange between different nuclei in a sample.

Sternberg's memory retrieval task
A continuous performance choice reaction time test that relies on working memory. It is thought that this task is mediated by attentional networks.

surface coil
In magnetic resonance, a circular coil of wire used to excite and/or receive RF signals from a sample. This type of coil is typically used when the region of interest is close to the surface of the brain.

T1-weighted image
A T1-weighted image is one in which the neuroanatomy is well demonstrated. Gray matter appears gray, white matter appears white, and cerebrospinal fluid is dark. These images have a very short TE and a TR roughly half that of brain T1.

T2-weighted image
A T2-weighted image is designed to highlight areas of pathology; gray matter appears dark, white matter appears bright, and cerebrospinal fluid is very bright. These images have a moderate TE and a long TR.

TE
Echo time. In a magnetic resonance spin–echo study, this is the time interval between the first RF pulse and signal sampling, and is a critical determinant of tissue contrast parameters (e.g., T1- or T2-weighted or proton density).

tesla
A unit of magnetic field strength: 1 tesla (T) equals 10,000 gauss (G). The earth possess its own magnetic field that is relatively weak (roughly 0.6 G) compared to the field strengths used in typical clinical magnets (1.5 T = 15,000 G).

theta
In electroencephalography, theta activity comprises electrical activity in the range of 4–8 cycles/s (Hz). Theta activity is normally observed during drowsiness and light stages of sleep.

thought disorder
Often termed mental confusion, this state may include thought blocking, confabulation, loose associations and circumstantiality or tangentiality.

tissue segmentation
A process of separating and quantitating the different types of tissues (gray matter, white matter, cerebrospinal fluid) contributing to voxels or whole brain based on image intensity differences in each of the three tissue types.

tolerance
A biological state attained after chronic drug use, which is accompanied by a diminished response to the drug upon reexposure.

tomography/tomographic
Pertaining to techniques that depict brain structures in three dimensions.

topographic mapping
An EEG technique that provides a comprehensive view of brain electrical activity over the scalp at any time point. Activity in scalp areas between electrodes is interpolated. A power spectrum is calculated, and the voltages are color coded for display.

TR
Repetition time. The time elapsed between radiofrequency pulses in magnetic resonance experiments. TR is important for determining tissue contrast parameters (e.g., T1- or T2-weighted or proton density).

type I error
A false positive statistical finding sometimes due to one or two "outliers" in a group. Studies of small sample size are vulnerable to this type of statistical error.

type II error
A false negative statistical finding.

verbal fluency
Measure of speed and ease of verbal production, assessed by monitoring word producing in uninterrupted strings following a cue.

voxel
A volume element of a three dimensional tissue image.

water suppression
Techniques used in proton (^{1}H) MRS to decrease the water resonance (~80 molar concentration of protons), which otherwise dwarfs resonances of biologically relevant compounds present in concentrations on the order of 10 m*M* (e.g., choline, creatine, or *N*-acetylaspartate).

withdrawal
A state of abnormal mental or physical effects induced by removing an addictive substance from an individual who is dependent on that substance.

Introduction to the Bibliography

Literature searching in the field of substance abuse is a complicated process because important papers are dispersed throughout many journals and many different disciplines. These include medicine, mental health, neurology, neuropsychology, neuroscience, nuclear medicine, pharmacology, physics, physiology, psychiatry, psychology, public health, radiology, substance abuse, and toxicology. For example, the following bibliography includes citations from over 320 different sources, and contains over 1,350 references. Because literature searching is typically accomplished through the use of keyword inputs into computerized search systems, and because keywords can vary between specialties, important references may be missed. Perhaps an even greater problem with today's powerful search engines is executing searches with keywords that are too general. This results in the return of hundreds of "hits," most of which are only peripherally related to the topic of interest.

This bibliography represents an attempt to find and categorize the extant research in substance abuse conducted with the methods described in this book. Most of the citations are from human studies published in peer-reviewed journals. The bibliography is presented in a structured manner to facilitate access to papers of interest, and is categorized by research method and by substance abuse topic. Immediately below is a table of contents outlining the organization of the bibliography, which should be of assistance in helping the reader to locate topics and papers of interest. Within each bibliographic category, references are sorted by publication year and are alphabetized. Some references appear in multiple categories. For example, longitudinal studies that describe findings in multiple states of drug use (e.g., acute withdrawal and early abstinence categories) will appear in both categories, such as the following reference:

> Hemmingsen, R., Vorstrup, S., Clemmesen, L., Holm, S., Tfelt-Hansen, P., Sorensen, A.S., Hansen, C., Sommer, W. and Bolwig, T.G., Cerebral blood flow during delirium tremens and related clinical states studied with xenon-133 inhalation tomography. Am. J. Psychiatry 145:1384–1390, 1988.

Citations for papers in languages other than English, for case reports or abstracts, or for papers using animal models, are indicated with bracketed text following the reference, such as is shown in the next example:

Boroojerdi, B., Hungs, M., Biniek, R. and Noth, J., Subacute encephalopathy with epileptic seizures in a patient with chronic alcoholism. Nervenarzt 69:162–165, 1998. [Case Report] [German]

The time frame for this bibliography is from about 1970 (with a few earlier references included if cited in the book) to about July 1999. I am confident that most of the peer-reviewed literature in the National Library of Medicine database falling within the scope of this book has been included. Use of this bibliography in combination with on-line database systems such as that maintained by the National Library of Medicine (currently located on-line at http://www.ncbi.nlm.nih.gov/PubMed/), which includes abstracts for most journal articles, should facilitate access to the rich and diverse findings in the substance abuse literature. It is my hope that these resources, in combination with the descriptions of imaging methods and findings provided in this monograph, will help the reader to attain a more comprehensive understanding of the brain imaging findings in substance abuse.

—MJK

Bibliography Table of Contents

[1] ERPs include evoked potential and event-related potential studies.

Bibliography

EEG and Evoked Potentials

Alcohol and Alcoholism

Acute Administration

EEG

Davis, P. A., Gibbs, F. A., Davis, H., Jetter, W. W. and Trowbridge, L. S., The effects of alcohol upon the electroencephalogram. Q. J. Stud. Alcohol 1:626–631, 1941.

Engel, G. L. and Rosenbaum, M., Studies of the electroencephalogram in acute alcoholic intoxication. Proc. Cent. Soc. Clin. Res. 17:62–67, 1944.

Docter, R. F., Naitoh, P. and Smith, J. C., Electroencephalographic changes and vigilance behavior during experimentally induced intoxication with alcoholic subjects. Psychosom. Med. 28:605–611, 1966.

Jones, R. T. and Stone, G. C., Psychological studies of marijuana and alcohol in man. Psychopharmacologia 18:108–117, 1970.

Salamy, A. and Williams, H. L., The effects of alcohol on sensory evoked and spontaneous cerebral potentials in man. Electroencephalogr. Clin. Neurophysiol. 35:3–11, 1973.

Peeke, S. C., Callaway, E., Jones, R. T., Stone, G. C. and Doyle, J., Combined effects of alcohol and sleep deprivation in normal young adults. Psychopharmacology (Berl.) 67:279–287, 1980.

Zilm, D. H., Ethanol-induced spontaneous and evoked EEG, heart rate, and respiration rate changes in man. Clin. Toxicol. 18:549–563, 1981.

Cohen, M. J., Schandler, S. L. and Naliboff, B. D., Psychophysiological measures from intoxicated and detoxified alcoholics. J. Stud. Alcohol 44:271–282, 1983.

Pollock, V. E., Volavka, J., Goodwin, D. W., Mednick, S. A., Gabrielli, W. F., Knop, J. and Schulsinger, F., The EEG after alcohol administration in men at risk for alcoholism. Arch. Gen. Psychiatry 40:857–861, 1983.

Lukas, S. E., Mendelson, J. H., Benedikt, R. A. and Jones, B., EEG alpha activity increases during transient episodes of ethanol-induced euphoria. Pharmacol. Biochem. Behav. 25:889–895, 1986.

Christian, J. C., Li, T. K., Norton, J. A., Jr., Propping, P. and Yu, P. L., Alcohol effects on the percentage of beta waves in the electroencephalograms of twins. Genet. Epidemiol. 5:217–224, 1988.

Ehlers, C. L. and Schuckit, M. A., EEG response to ethanol in sons of alcoholics. Psychopharmacol. Bull. 24:434–437, 1988.
Kaplan, R. F., Hesselbrock, V. M., O'Connor, S. and DePalma, N., Behavioral and EEG responses to alcohol in nonalcoholic men with a family history of alcoholism. Prog. Neuropsychopharmacol. Biol. Psychiatry 12:873–885, 1988.
Lukas, S. E. and Mendelson, J. H., Electroencephalographic activity and plasma ACTH during ethanol-induced euphoria. Biol. Psychiatry 23:141–148, 1988.
Pollock, V. E., Gabrielli, W. F., Mednick, S. A. and Goodwin, D. W., EEG identification of subgroups of men at risk for alcoholism? Psychiatry Res. 26:101–104, 1988.
Allen, D. and Lader, M., Interactions of alcohol with amitriptyline, fluoxetine and placebo in normal subjects. Int. Clin. Psychopharmacol. 4 Suppl. 1:7–14, 1989.
Ehlers, C. L., Wall, T. L. and Schuckit, M. A., EEG spectral characteristics following ethanol administration in young men. Electroencephalogr. Clin. Neurophysiol. 73:179–187, 1989.
Lukas, S. E., Mendelson, J. H., Amass, L. and Benedikt, R., Behavioral and EEG studies of acute cocaine administration: comparisons with morphine, amphetamine, pentobarbital, nicotine, ethanol and marijuana. NIDA Res. Monogr. 95:146–151, 1989.
Lukas, S. E., Mendelson, J. H., Woods, B. T., Mello, N. K. and Teoh, S. K., Topographic distribution of EEG alpha activity during ethanol-induced intoxication in women. J. Stud. Alcohol 50:176–185, 1989.
Michel, C. and Battig, K., Separate and combined psychophysiological effects of cigarette smoking and alcohol consumption. Psychopharmacology (Berl.) 97:65–73, 1989.
Tomczak, J. W., Kocur, J. and Sobotka, H., Alcohol intoxication in teenagers using inhalant stupefacients. Pol. J. Pharmacol. Pharm. 41:203–206, 1989.
Ehlers, C. L. and Schuckit, M. A., EEG fast frequency activity in the sons of alcoholics. Biol. Psychiatry 27:631–641, 1990.
Lukas, S. E., Mendelson, J. H., Kouri, E., Bolduc, M. and Amass, L., Ethanol-induced alterations in EEG alpha activity and apparent source of the auditory P300 evoked response potential. Alcohol 7:471–477, 1990.
Ehlers, C. L. and Schuckit, M. A., Evaluation of EEG alpha activity in sons of alcoholics. Neuropsychopharmacology 4:199–205, 1991.
Fujiwara, T., Watanabe, M., Matsuda, K., Senbongi, M., Yagi, K. and Seino, M., Complex partial status epilepticus provoked by ingestion of alcohol: a case report. Epilepsia 32:650–656, 1991. [Case Report]
Bond, A. J., Silveira, J. C. and Lader, M. H., The effects of alprazolam alone and combined with alcohol on central integrative activity. Eur. J. Clin. Pharmacol. 42:495–498, 1992.
Bauer, L. O. and Hesselbrock, V. M., EEG, autonomic and subjective correlates of the risk for alcoholism. J. Stud. Alcohol 54:577–589, 1993.
Cohen, H. L., Porjesz, B. and Begleiter, H., The effects of ethanol on EEG activity in males at risk for alcoholism. Electroencephalogr. Clin. Neurophysiol. 86:368–376, 1993.
Cohen, H. L., Porjesz, B. and Begleiter, H., Ethanol-induced alterations in electroencephalographic activity in adult males. Neuropsychopharmacology 8:365–370, 1993.
Frewer, L. J. and Lader, M., The effects of nefazodone, imipramine and placebo, alone and combined with alcohol, in normal subjects. Int. Clin. Psychopharmacol. 8:13–20, 1993.
Wall, T. L., Gallen, C. C. and Ehlers, C. L., Effects of alcohol on the EEG in Asian men with genetic variations of ALDH2. Biol. Psychiatry 34:91–99, 1993.
Stenberg, G., Sano, M., Rosen, I. and Ingvar, D.H., EEG topography of acute ethanol effects in resting and activated normals. J. Stud. Alcohol 55:645–656, 1994.
Sorbel, J., Morzorati, S., O'Connor, S., Li, T. K. and Christian, J. C., Alcohol effects on the heritability of EEG spectral power. Alcohol. Clin. Exp. Res. 20:1523–1527, 1996.
Volavka, J., Czobor, P., Goodwin, D. W., Gabrielli, W. F. J., Penick, E. C., Mednick, S. A., Jensen, P. and Knop, J., The electroencephalogram after alcohol administration in high-risk

men and the development of alcohol use disorders 10 years later. Arch. Gen. Psychiatry 53:258–263, 1996.

Ehlers, C. L., Havstad, J., Prichard, D. and Theiler, J., Low doses of ethanol reduce evidence for nonlinear structure in brain activity. J. Neurosci. 18:7474–7486, 1998.

O'Connor, S., Sorbel, J., Morzorati, S., Li, T. K. and Christian, J. C., A twin study of genetic influences on the acute adaptation of the EEG to alcohol. Alcohol. Clin. Exp. Res. 23:494–501, 1999.

Sleep EEG

Rouhani, S., Tran, G., Leplaideur, F., Durlach, J. and Poenaru, S., EEG effects of a single low dose of ethanol on afternoon sleep in the nonalcohol-dependent adult. Alcohol 6:87–90, 1989.

Dijk, D. J., Brunner, D. P., Aeschbach, D., Tobler, I. and Borbely, A. A., The effects of ethanol on human sleep EEG power spectra differ from those of benzodiazepine receptor agonists. Neuropsychopharmacology 7:225–232, 1992.

O'Boyle, D. J., Van, F. and Hume, K. I., Effects of alcohol, at two times of day, on EEG-derived indices of physiological arousal. Electroencephalogr. Clin. Neurophysiol. 95:97–107, 1995.

Landolt, H. P., Roth, C., Dijk, D. J. and Borbely, A. A., Late-afternoon ethanol intake affects nocturnal sleep and the sleep EEG in middle-aged men. J. Clin. Psychopharmacol. 16:428–436, 1996.

Kobayashi, T., Misaki, K., Nakagawa, H., Okuda, K., Ota, T., Kanda, I., Isaki, K., Kosino, Y. and Fukuda, H., Alcohol effect on sleep electroencephalography by fast Fourier transformation. Psychiatry Clin. Neurosci. 52:154–155, 1998.

Auditory ERPs

Kopell, B. S., Roth, W. T. and Tinklenberg, J. R., Time course effects of marijuana and ethanol on event related potentials. Psychopharmacology (Berl.) 56:15–20, 1978.

Pfefferbaum, A., Roth, W. T., Tinklenberg, J. R., Rosenbloom, M. J. and Kopell, B. S., The effects of ethanol and meperidine on auditory evoked potentials. Drug Alcohol Depend. 4:371–380, 1979.

Hari, R., Sams, M. and Jarvilehto, T., Effects of small ethanol doses on the auditory evoked transient and sustained potentials in the human EEG. Adv. Exp. Med. Biol. 126:579–587, 1980.

Zilm, D. H., Kaplan, H. L. and Capell, H., Electroencephalographic tolerance and abstinence phenomena during repeated alcohol ingestion by nonalcoholics. Science 212:1175–1177, 1981.

Church, M. W. and Williams, H. L., Dose- and time-dependent effects of ethanol on brain stem auditory evoked responses in young adult males. Electroencephalogr. Clin. Neurophysiol. 54:161–174, 1982.

Elmasian, R., Neville, H., Woods, D., Schuckit, M. and Bloom, F., Event-related brain potentials are different in individuals at high and low risk for developing alcoholism. Proc. Natl. Acad. Sci. USA 79:7900–7903, 1982.

Freedman, R., Waldo, M. C., Adler, L. E., Baker, N., Levin, D. and Deitrich, R., Electrophysiological effects of low dose alcohol on human subjects at high altitude. Alcohol Drug Res. 6:289–297, 1985.

Erwin, C. W., Linnoila, M., Hartwell, J., Erwin, A. and Guthrie, S., Effects of buspirone and diazepam, alone and in combination with alcohol, on skilled performance and evoked potentials. J. Clin. Psychopharmacol. 6:199–209, 1986.

Teo, R. K. and Ferguson, D. A., The acute effects of ethanol on auditory event-related potentials. Psychopharmacology (Berl.) 90:179–184, 1986.

Campbell, K. B. and Lowick, B. M., Ethanol and event-related potentials: the influence of distractor stimuli. Alcohol 4:257–263, 1987.

Allen, D., Baylav, A. and Lader, M., A comparative study of the interaction of alcohol with alpidem, lorazepam and placebo in normal subjects. Int. Clin. Psychopharmacol. 3:327–341, 1988.

Allen, D., Lader, M. and Curran, H. V., A comparative study of the interactions of alcohol with amitriptyline, fluoxetine and placebo in normal subjects. Prog. Neuropsychopharmacol. Biol. Psychiatry 12:63–80, 1988.

Polich, J. and Bloom, F. E., Event-related brain potentials in individuals at high and low risk for developing alcoholism: failure to replicate. Alcohol. Clin. Exp. Res. 12:368–373, 1988.

Schuckit, M. A., Gold, E. O., Croot, K., Finn, P. and Polich, J., P300 latency after ethanol ingestion in sons of alcoholics and in controls. Biol. Psychiatry 24:310–315, 1988.

Lukas, S. E., Mendelson, J. H., Kouri, E., Bolduc, M. and Amass, L., Ethanol-induced alterations in EEG alpha activity and apparent source of the auditory P300 evoked response potential. Alcohol 7:471–477, 1990.

Bond, A. J., Silveira, J. C. and Lader, M. H., The effects of alprazolam alone and combined with alcohol on central integrative activity. Eur. J. Clin. Pharmacol. 42:495–498, 1992.

Murata, K., Araki, S., Tanigawa, T. and Uchida, E., Acute effects of alcohol on cognitive function and central nervous system assessed by auditory event-related potentials. Nippon Eiseigaku Zasshi 47:958–964, 1992.

Jaaskelainen, I. P., Lehtokoski, A., Alho, K., Kujala, T., Pekkonen, E., Sinclair, J. D., Naatanen, R. and Sillanaukee, P., Low dose of ethanol suppresses mismatch negativity of auditory event-related potentials. Alcohol. Clin. Exp. Res. 19:607–610, 1995.

Jaaskelainen, I. P., Pekkonen, E., Alho, K., Sinclair, J. D., Sillanaukee, P. and Naatanen, R., Dose-related effect of alcohol on mismatch negativity and reaction time performance. Alcohol 12:491–495, 1995.

Wall, T. L. and Ehlers, C. L., Acute effects of alcohol on P300 in Asians with different ALDH2 genotypes. Alcohol. Clin. Exp. Res. 19:617–622, 1995.

Hegerl, U., Juckel, G., Schmidt, L. G. and Rommelspacher, H., Serotonergic ethanol effects and auditory evoked dipole activity in alcoholic and healthy subjects. Psychiatry Res. 63:47–55, 1996.

Alexandrov, Y., Sams, M., Lavikainen, J., Reinikainen, K. and Naatanen, R., Differential effects of alcohol on the cortical processing of foreign and native language. Int. J. Psychophysiol. 28:1–10, 1998.

Cohen, H. L., Porjesz, B., Stimus, A. T. and Begleiter, H., Effects of ethanol on temporal recovery of auditory-evoked potentials in individuals at risk for alcoholism. Alcohol. Clin. Exp. Res. 22:945–953, 1998.

Ehlers, C. L., Garcia-Andrade, C., Wall, T. L., Sobel, D. F. and Phillips, E., Determinants of P3 amplitude and response to alcohol in Native American Mission Indians. Neuropsychopharmacology 18:282–292, 1998.

Jaaskelainen, I. P., Hirvonen, J., Kujala, T., Alho, K., Eriksson, C. J., Lehtokoski, A., Pekkonen, E., Sinclair, J. D., Yabe, H., Naatanen, R. and Sillanaukee, P., Effects of naltrexone and ethanol on auditory event-related brain potentials. Alcohol 15:105–111, 1998.

Jaaskelainen, I. P., Schroger, E. and Naatanen, R., Electrophysiological indices of acute effects of ethanol on involuntary attention shifting. Psychopharmacology (Berl.) 141:16–21, 1999.

Visual ERPs

Lewis, E. G., Dustman, R. E. and Beck, E. C., The effect of alcohol on sensory phenomena and cognitive motor tasks. Q. J. Stud. Alcohol 30:618–633, 1969.

Lewis, E. G., Dustman, R. E. and Beck, E. C., The effects of alcohol on visual and somatosensory evoked responses. Electroencephalogr. Clin. Neurophysiol. 28:202–205, 1970.

Roth, W. T., Tinklenberg, J. R. and Kopell, B. S., Ethanol and marihuana effects on event-related potentials in a memory retrieval paradigm. Electroencephalogr. Clin. Neurophysiol. 42:381–388, 1977.

Peeke, S. C., Callaway, E., Jones, R. T., Stone, G. C. and Doyle, J., Combined effects of alcohol and sleep deprivation in normal young adults. Psychopharmacology (Berl.) 67:279–287, 1980.

Zuzewicz, W., Ethyl alcohol effect on the visual evoked potential. Acta. Physiol. Pol. 32:93–98, 1981.

Erwin, C. W., Linnoila, M., Hartwell, J., Erwin, A. and Guthrie, S., Effects of buspirone and diazepam, alone and in combination with alcohol, on skilled performance and evoked potentials. J. Clin. Psychopharmacol. 6:199–209, 1986.

Rohrbaugh, J. W., Stapleton, J. M., Parasuraman, R., Zubovic, E. A., Frowein, H. W., Varner, J. L., Adinoff, B., Lane, E. A., Eckardt, M. J. and Linnoila, M., Dose-related effects of ethanol on visual sustained attention and event-related potentials. Alcohol 4:293–300, 1987.

Pollock, V. E., Volavka, J., Gabrielli, W. F., Mednick, S. A., Knop, J. and Goodwin, D. W., Pattern reversal visual evoked potential among men at risk for alcoholism. Acta Psychiatr. Scand. 78:276–282, 1988.

Pollock, V. E., Volavka, J., Goodwin, D. W., Gabrielli, W. F., Mednick, S. A., Knop, J. and Schulsinger, F., Pattern reversal visual evoked potentials after alcohol administration among men at risk for alcoholism. Psychiatry Res. 26:191–202, 1988.

Schandler, S. L., Cohen, M. J. and McArthur, D. L., Event-related brain potentials in intoxicated and detoxified alcoholics during visuospatial learning. Psychopharmacology (Berl.) 94:275–283, 1988.

Michel, C. and Battig, K., Separate and combined psychophysiological effects of cigarette smoking and alcohol consumption. Psychopharmacology (Berl.) 97:65–73, 1989.

Colrain, I. M., Taylor, J., McLean, S., Buttery, R., Wise, G. and Montgomery, I., Dose dependent effects of alcohol on visual evoked potentials. Psychopharmacology (Berl.) 112:383–388, 1993.

Fowler, B. and Adams, J., Dissociation of the effects of alcohol and amphetamine on inert gas narcosis using reaction time and P300 latency. Aviat. Space Environ. Med. 64:493–499, 1993.

Sommer, W., Leuthold, H. and Hermanutz, M., Covert effects of alcohol revealed by event-related potentials. Percept. Psychophys. 54:127–135, 1993.

Krull, K. R., Smith, L. T. and Parsons, O. A., Simple reaction time event-related potentials: effects of alcohol and diazepam. Prog. Neuropsychopharmacol. Biol. Psychiatry 18:1247–1260, 1994.

Orozco, S., Wall, T. L. and Ehlers, C. L., Influence of alcohol on electrophysiological responses to facial stimuli. Alcohol 18:11–16, 1999.

Quintyn, J. C., Massy, J., Quillard, M. and Brasseur, G., Effects of low alcohol consumption on visual evoked potential, visual field and visual contrast sensitivity. Acta Ophthalmol. Scand. 77:23–26, 1999.

Other ERPs

Lewis, E. G., Dustman, R. E. and Beck, E. C., The effect of alcohol on sensory phenomena and cognitive motor tasks. Q. J. Stud. Alcohol 30:618–633, 1969.

Lewis, E. G., Dustman, R. E. and Beck, E. C., The effects of alcohol on visual and somatosensory evoked responses. Electroencephalogr. Clin. Neurophysiol. 28:202–205, 1970.

Salamy, A. and Williams, H. L., The effects of alcohol on sensory evoked and spontaneous cerebral potentials in man. Electroencephalogr. Clin. Neurophysiol. 35:3–11, 1973.

Zilm, D. H., Ethanol-induced spontaneous and evoked EEG, heart rate, and respiration rate changes in man. Clin. Toxicol. 18:549–563, 1981.

Benzodiazepines and Alcohol

Erwin, C. W., Linnoila, M., Hartwell, J., Erwin, A. and Guthrie, S., Effects of buspirone and diazepam, alone and in combination with alcohol, on skilled performance and evoked potentials. J. Clin. Psychopharmacol. 6:199–209, 1986.

Allen, D., Baylav, A. and Lader, M., A comparative study of the interaction of alcohol with alpidem, lorazepam and placebo in normal subjects. Int. Clin. Psychopharmacol. 3:327–341, 1988.

Bond, A. J., Silveira, J. C. and Lader, M. H., The effects of alprazolam alone and combined with alcohol on central integrative activity. Eur. J. Clin. Pharmacol. 42:495–498, 1992.

Chronic Administration

EEG

Coger, R. W., Dymond, A. M., Serafetinides, E. A., Lowenstam, I. and Pearson, D., EEG signs of brain impairment in alcoholism. Biol. Psychiatry 13:729–739, 1978.

Johannesson, G., Berglund, M. and Ingvar, D. H., Reduction of blood flow in cerebral white matter in alcoholics related to hepatic function. Acta Neurol. Scand. 65:190–202, 1982.

Johannesson, G., Berglund, M. and Ingvar, D. H., EEG abnormalities in chronic alcoholism related to age. Acta Psychiatr. Scand. 65:148–157, 1982.

Cohen, M. J., Schandler, S. L. and Naliboff, B. D., Psychophysiological measures from intoxicated and detoxified alcoholics. J. Stud. Alcohol 44:271–282, 1983.

Saletu, M., Saletu, B., Grunberger, J., Mader, R. and Karobath, M., Clinical symptomatology and computer analyzed EEG before, during and after anxiolytic therapy of alcohol withdrawal patients. Neuropsychobiology 9:119–134, 1983.

Saletu, B., Saletu, M., Grunberger, J. and Mader R., Spontaneous and drug-induced remission of alcoholic organic brain syndrome: clinical, psychometric, and neurophysiological studies. Psychiatry Res. 10:59–75, 1983.

Kaplan, R. F., Glueck, B. C., Hesselbrock, M. N. and Reed, H. B., Jr., Power and coherence analysis of the EEG in hospitalized alcoholics and nonalcoholic controls. J. Stud. Alcohol 46:122–127, 1985.

Schwarz-Ottersbach, E. and Goldberg, L., Activation levels, EEG, and behavioural responses. Int. J. Psychophysiol. 4:7–17, 1986.

Olivennes, A., Comparison of awake electroencephalography tracings of alcoholics and heroin addicts. Study of 2 groups of 70 and 51 patients. Ann. Med. Psychol. (Paris) 145:546–552, 1987. [French]

Hamon, J. F., Camara, P. and Claver, B., Electroencephalogram changes and psychopathologic disorders in 60 cases of chronic palm brandy intoxication. Med. Trop. (Mars.) 52:363–368, 1992. [French]

Holmes, G. L. and Korteling, F., Drug effects on the human EEG. Am. J. EEG Technol. 33:1–26, 1993.

Michael, A., Mirza, K. A., Mukundan, C. R. and Channabasavanna, S. M., Interhemispheric electroencephalographic coherence as a biological marker in alcoholism. Acta Psychiatr. Scand. 87:213–217, 1993.

Jha, S. and Nag, D., Some observations on clinical, cognitive and neurophysiological changes in subjects consuming indigenous alcohol. Indian J. Physiol. Pharmacol. 38:277–280, 1994.

Herning, R. I., Guo, X. and Lange, W. R., The effects of nimodipine on the EEG of substance abusers. Ann. N. Y. Acad. Sci. 765:143–151, 1995.

Braverman, E. R. and Blum, K., Substance use disorder exacerbates brain electrophysiological abnormalities in a psychiatrically-ill population. Clin. Electroencephalogr. 27 (4 Suppl.): 5–27, 1996.

Auditory ERPs

Pfefferbaum, A., Horvath, T. B., Roth, W. T. and Kopell, B. S., Event-related potential changes in chronic alcoholics. Electroencephalogr. Clin. Neurophysiol. 47:637–647, 1979.
Lille, F., Hazemann, P., Massioui, F. E., Lesevre, N. and Dally, S., Effect of chronic alcohol intake and short-term abstinence on early sensory EPs and late 'cognitive' ERPs. Electroencephalogr. Clin. Neurophysiol. Suppl. 40:712–717, 1987.
Branchey, M. H., Buydens-Branchey, L. and Lieber, C. S., P3 in alcoholics with disordered regulation of aggression. Psychiatry Res. 25:49–58, 1988.
Cadaveira, F., Grau, C., Roso, M. and Sanchez-Turet, M., Multimodality exploration of event-related potentials in chronic alcoholics. Alcohol. Clin. Exp. Res. 15:607–611, 1991.
Pfefferbaum, A., Ford, J. M., White, P. M. and Mathalon, D., Event-related potentials in alcoholic men: P3 amplitude reflects family history but not alcohol consumption. Alcohol. Clin. Exp. Res. 15:839–850, 1991.
Cadaveira, F., Roso, M., Grau, C. and Sanchez-Turet, M., Effects of age on event-related potentials in chronic alcoholics: a multimodal study. Neuropsychobiology 25:166–171, 1992.
Glenn, S., Parsons, O. A. and Sinha, R., Assessment of recovery of electrophysiological and neuropsychological functions in chronic alcoholics. Biol. Psychiatry 36:443–452, 1994.
Jha, S. and Nag, D., Some observations on clinical, cognitive and neurophysiological changes in subjects consuming indigenous alcohol. Indian J. Physiol. Pharmacol. 38:277–280, 1994.
Kaseda, Y., Miyazato, Y., Ogura, C., Nakamoto, H., Uema, T., Yamamoto, K. and Ohta, I., Correlation between event-related potentials and MR measurements in chronic alcoholic patients. Jpn. J. Psychiatry Neurol. 48:23–32, 1994.
Fein, G., Biggins, C. A. and MacKay, S., Alcohol abuse and HIV infection have additive effects on frontal cortex function as measured by auditory evoked potential P3A latency. Biol. Psychiatry 37:183–195, 1995.
Herning, R. I., Guo, X. and Lange, W. R., Nimodipine improves information processing in substance abusers. Ann. N. Y. Acad. Sci. 765:152–159, 1995.
Braverman, E. R. and Blum, K., Substance use disorder exacerbates brain electrophysiological abnormalities in a psychiatrically-ill population. Clin. Electroencephalogr. 27 (4 Suppl.): 5–27, 1996.
Fein, G., Biggins, C. and MacKay, S., Cocaine abusers have reduced auditory P50 amplitude and suppression compared to both normal controls and alcoholics. Biol. Psychiatry 39:955–965, 1996.
Hegerl, U., Juckel, G., Schmidt, L. G. and Rommelspacher, H., Serotonergic ethanol effects and auditory evoked dipole activity in alcoholic and healthy subjects. Psychiatry Res. 63:47–55, 1996.
Nicolas, J. M., Estruch, R., Salamero, M., Orteu, N., Fernandez-Sola, J., Sacanella, E. and Urbano-Marquez, A., Brain impairment in well-nourished chronic alcoholics is related to ethanol intake. Ann. Neurol. 41:590–598, 1997.

Visual ERPs

Porjesz, B., Begleiter, H. and Samuelly, I., Cognitive deficits in chronic alcoholics and elderly subjects assessed by evoked brain potentials. Acta Psychiatr. Scand. 62:15–29, 1980.
Ciesielski, K. T., Madden, J. S., Bligh, J. G. and Schopflocher, D., Long-term brain impairment in chronic alcoholics: N2-P3 cognitive potentials in a template-matching memory task. Alcohol Alcohol. 20:403–408, 1985.
Chan, Y. W., McLeod, J. G., Tuck, R. R., Walsh, J. C. and Feary, P. A., Visual evoked responses in chronic alcoholics. J. Neurol. Neurosurg. Psychiatry 49:945–950, 1986.

Schandler, S. L., Cohen, M. J. and McArthur, D. L., Event-related brain potentials in intoxicated and detoxified alcoholics during visuospatial learning. Psychopharmacology (Berl.) 94:275–283, 1988.

Cadaveira, F., Grau, C., Roso, M. and Sanchez-Turet, M., Multimodality exploration of event-related potentials in chronic alcoholics. Alcohol. Clin. Exp. Res. 15:607–611, 1991.

Pfefferbaum, A., Ford, J. M., White, P. M. and Mathalon, D., Event-related potentials in alcoholic men: P3 amplitude reflects family history but not alcohol consumption. Alcohol. Clin. Exp. Res. 15:839–850, 1991.

Cadaveira, F., Roso, M., Grau, C. and Sanchez-Turet, M., Effects of age on event-related potentials in chronic alcoholics: a multimodal study. Neuropsychobiology 25:166–171, 1992.

Glenn, S., Parsons, O. A. and Sinha, R., Assessment of recovery of electrophysiological and neuropsychological functions in chronic alcoholics. Biol. Psychiatry 36:443–452, 1994.

Jha, S. and Nag, D., Some observations on clinical, cognitive and neurophysiological changes in subjects consuming indigenous alcohol. Indian J. Physiol. Pharmacol. 38:277–280, 1994.

Herning, R. I., Guo, X. and Lange, W. R., Nimodipine improves information processing in substance abusers. Ann. N. Y. Acad. Sci. 765:152–159, 1995.

Braverman, E. R. and Blum, K., Substance use disorder exacerbates brain electrophysiological abnormalities in a psychiatrically-ill population. Clin. Electroencephalogr. 27 (4 Suppl.): 5–27, 1996.

Nichols, J. M. and Martin, F., The effect of lorazepam on memory and event-related potentials in heavy and light social drinkers. Psychophysiology 33:446–456, 1996.

Nicolas, J. M., Estruch, R., Salamero, M., Orteu, N., Fernandez-Sola, J., Sacanella, E. and Urbano-Marquez, A., Brain impairment in well-nourished chronic alcoholics is related to ethanol intake. Ann. Neurol. 41:590–598, 1997.

Zhang, X. L., Begleiter, H. and Porjesz, B., Do chronic alcoholics have intact implicit memory? An ERP study. Electroencephalogr. Clin. Neurophysiol. 103:457–473, 1997.

Other ERPs

Lille, F., Hazemann, P., Massioui, F. E., Lesevre, N. and Dally, S., Effect of chronic alcohol intake and short-term abstinence on early sensory EPs and late 'cognitive' ERPs. Electroencephalogr. Clin. Neurophysiol. Suppl. 40:712–717, 1987.

Hazemann, P., Jeftic, M. and Lille, F., Somatosensory evoked potentials in alcoholics and patients occupationally exposed to solvents and lead. Electromyogr. Clin. Neurophysiol. 27:183–187, 1987.

Nichols, J. M. and Martin, F., P300 in heavy social drinkers: the effect of lorazepam. Alcohol 10:269–274, 1993.

Fox, A. M., Michie, P. T., Coltheart, M. and Solowij, N., Memory functioning in social drinkers: a study of event-related potentials. Alcohol Alcohol. 30:303–310, 1995.

Nichols, J. M. and Martin, F., The effect of heavy social drinking on recall and event-related potentials. J. Stud. Alcohol 57:125–135, 1996.

Baguley, I. J., Felmingham, K. L., Lahz, S., Gordan, E., Lazzaro, I. and Schotte, D. E., Alcohol abuse and traumatic brain injury: effect on event-related potentials. Arch. Phys. Med. Rehabil. 78:1248–1253, 1997.

Zhang, X. L., Begleiter, H., Porjesz, B. and Litke, A., Electrophysiological evidence of memory impairment in alcoholic patients. Biol. Psychiatry 42:1157–1171, 1997.

Fallgatter, A. J., Wiesbeck, G. A., Weijers, H. G., Boening, J. and Strik, W. K., Event-related correlates of response suppression as indicators of novelty seeking in alcoholics. Alcohol Alcohol. 33:475–481, 1998.

Special Syndromes Associated with Alcoholism

Hepatic Encephalopathy

Johannesson, G., Berglund, M. and Ingvar, D. H., Reduction of blood flow in cerebral white matter in alcoholics related to hepatic function. Acta Neurol. Scand. 65:190–202, 1982.

Mouradian, M. D. and Penovich, P. E., Spindle coma in benzodiazepine toxicity: case report. Clin. Electroencephalogr. 16:213–218, 1985. [Case Report]

Quero, J. C., Hartmann, I. J., Meulstee, J., Hop, W. C. and Schalm, S. W., The diagnosis of subclinical hepatic encephalopathy in patients with cirrhosis using neuropsychological tests and automated electroencephalogram analysis. Hepatology 24:556–560, 1996.

Boroojerdi, B., Hungs, M., Biniek, R. and Noth, J., Subacute encephalopathy with epileptic seizures in a patient with chronic alcoholism. Nervenarzt 69:162–165, 1998. [Case Report] [German]

Schomerus, H. and Hamster, W., Neuropsychological aspects of portal-systemic encephalopathy. Metab. Brain. Dis. 13:361–377, 1998.

Wernicke and Korsakoff Syndromes

Chan, Y. W., McLeod, J. G., Tuck, R. R., Walsh, J. C. and Feary, P. A., Visual evoked responses in chronic alcoholics. J. Neurol. Neurosurg. Psychiatry 49:945–950, 1986.

Martin, P. R., Loewenstein, R. J., Kaye, W. H., Ebert, M. H., Weingartner, H. and Gillin, J. C., Sleep EEG in Korsakoff's psychosis and Alzheimer's disease. Neurology 36:411–414, 1986.

Blackwood, D. H., St. Clair, D. M., Blackburn, I. M. and Tyrer, G. M., Cognitive brain potentials and psychological deficits in Alzheimer's dementia and Korsakoff's amnesic syndrome. Psychol. Med. 17:349–358, 1987.

Haas, W. and Nickel, B., The value of brainstem auditory evoked potentials in early diagnosis of Wernicke's encephalopathy. Alcohol Alcohol. 26:115–119, 1991.

Joyce, E. M., Rio, D. E., Ruttimann, U. E., Rohrbaugh, J. W., Martin, P. R., Rawlings, R. R. and Eckardt, M. J., Decreased cingulate and precuneate glucose utilization in alcoholic Korsakoff's syndrome. Psychiatry Res. 54:225–239, 1994.

Central Pontine Myelinolysis

Stockard, J. J., Rossiter, V. S., Wiederholt, W. and Kobayashi, R. M., Brain stem auditory-evoked responses in suspected central pontine myelinolysis. Arch. Neurol. 33:726–728, 1976. [Case Report]

Ingram, D. A., Traub, M., Kopelman, P. G., Summers, B. A. and Swash, M., Brain-stem auditory evoked responses in diagnosis of central pontine myelinolysis. J. Neurology 233:23–24, 1986. [Case Report]

Heilemann, H., Skiba, N. and Hillemacher, A., Clinical aspects and electrophysiologic findings in an unusual course of central pontine myelinolysis. Nervenarzt 62:645–647, 1991. [Case Report] [German]

Dieterle, L., Buchler, G. and Pfitzer, F., Central pontine myelinolysis. Dtsch. Med. Wochenschr. 117:332–336, 1992. [Case Report] [German]

Marchiafava-Bignami Disease

Humbert, T., De Guilhermier, P., Maktouf, C., Grasset, G., Lopez, F. M. and Chabrand, P., Marchiafava-Bignami disease. A case studied by structural and functional brain imaging. Eur. Arch. Psychiatry Clin. Neurosci. 242:69–71, 1992. [Case Report]

Withdrawal

EEG

Coger, R. W., Serafetinides, E. A., Dymond, A. M., Lowenstam, I. and Pearson, D., EEG differences between male alcoholics in withdrawal and those stabilized in treatment. Curr. Alcohol. 8:85–96, 1981.

Saletu, M., Saletu, B., Grunberger, J., Mader, R. and Karobath, M., Clinical symptomatology and computer analyzed EEG before, during and after anxiolytic therapy of alcohol withdrawal patients. Neuropsychobiology 9:119–134, 1983.

Schear, H. E., The EEG pattern in delirium tremens. Clin. Electroencephalogr. 16:30–32, 1985. [Case Report]

Spehr, W. and Stemmler, G., Postalcoholic diseases: diagnostic relevance of computerized EEG. Electroencephalogr. Clin. Neurophysiol. 60:106–114, 1985.

Frank, H., Heber, G. and Fritsch, M., Analysis of the EEG of alcoholic patients in the initial phase of abstinence. Nervenarzt 57:730–735, 1986. [German]

Logar, C., Grabmair, W., Reinbacher, N. and Ladurner, G., EEG changes in the withdrawal phase of tranquilizer or drug abuse. EEG EMG Z. Elektroenzephalogr. Verwandte Geb. 17:37–40, 1986. [German]

Krauss, G. L. and Niedermeyer, E., Electroencephalogram and seizures in chronic alcoholism. Electroencephalogr. Clin. Neurophysiol. 78:97–104, 1991.

Ilyuchina, V. A. and Nikitina, L. I., Clinical physiological study of the therapeutic effects of phenytoin in acute alcohol withdrawal and the asthenic-autonomic syndrome in patients with chronic alcoholism. Alcohol 12:511–517, 1995.

Moak, D. H. and Anton, R. F., Alcohol-related seizures and the kindling effect of repeated detoxifications: the influence of cocaine. Alcohol Alcohol. 31:135–143, 1996.

Sullivan, E. V., Marsh, L., Mathalon, D. H., Lim, K. O. and Pfefferbaum, A., Relationship between alcohol withdrawal seizures and temporal lobe white matter volume deficits. Alcohol. Clin. Exp. Res. 20:348–354, 1996.

Sleep EEG

Gillin, J. C., Smith, T. L., Irwin, M., Kripke, D. F. and Schuckit, M., EEG sleep studies in "pure" primary alcoholism during subacute withdrawal: relationships to normal controls, age, and other clinical variables. Biol. Psychiatry 27:477–488, 1990.

Thompson, P. M., Gillin, J. C., Golshan, S. and Irwin, M., Polygraphic sleep measures differentiate alcoholics and stimulant abusers during short-term abstinence. Biol. Psychiatry 38:831–836, 1995.

Auditory ERPs

Romani, A. and Cosi, V., Event-related potentials in chronic alcoholics during withdrawal and abstinence. Neurophysiol. Clin. 19:373–384, 1989.

Hegerl, U., Juckel, G., Schmidt, L. G. and Rommelspacher, H., Serotonergic ethanol effects and auditory evoked dipole activity in alcoholic and healthy subjects. Psychiatry Res. 63:47–55, 1996.

Craving

Fahrion, S. L., Walters, E. D., Coyne, L. and Allen, T., Alterations in EEG amplitude, personality factors, and brain electrical mapping after alpha-theta brainwave training: a controlled case study of an alcoholic in recovery. Alcohol. Clin. Exp. Res. 16:547–552, 1992.

Abstinence

EEG

Zilm, D. H., Huszar, L., Carlen, P. L., Kaplan, H. L. and Wilkinson, D. A., EEG correlates of the alcohol-induced organic brain syndrome in man. Clin. Toxicol. 16:345–358, 1980.

Coger, R. W., Serafetinides, E. A., Dymond, A. M., Lowenstam, I. and Pearson, D., EEG differences between male alcoholics in withdrawal and those stabilized in treatment. Curr. Alcohol. 8:85–96, 1981.

Saletu, M., Saletu, B., Grunberger, J., Mader, R. and Karobath, M., Clinical symptomatology and computer analyzed EEG before, during and after anxiolytic therapy of alcohol withdrawal patients. Neuropsychobiology 9:119–134, 1983.

Kaplan, R. F., Glueck, B. C., Hesselbrock, M. N. and Reed, H. B., Jr., Power and coherence analysis of the EEG in hospitalized alcoholics and nonalcoholic controls. J. Stud. Alcohol 46:122–127, 1985.

Spehr, W. and Stemmler, G., Postalcoholic diseases: diagnostic relevance of computerized EEG. Electroencephalogr. Clin. Neurophysiol. 60:106–114, 1985.

Emmerson, R. Y., Dustman, R. E., Shearer, D. E. and Chamberlin, H. M., EEG, visually evoked and event related potentials in young abstinent alcoholics. Alcohol 4:241–248, 1987.

Pollock, V. E., Schneider, L. S., Zemansky, M. F., Gleason, R. P. and Pawluczyk, S., Topographic quantitative EEG amplitude in recovered alcoholics. Psychiatry Res. 45:25–32, 1992.

Bauer, L. O., Photic driving of EEG alpha activity in recovering cocaine-dependent and alcohol-dependent patients. Am. J. Addict. 3:49–57, 1993.

Bauer, L. O., Vigilance in recovering cocaine-dependent and alcohol-dependent patients: a prospective study. Addict. Behav. 19:599–607, 1994.

Bauer, L. O., Electroencephalographic and autonomic predictors of relapse in alcohol-dependent patients. Alcohol. Clin. Exp. Res. 18:755–760, 1994.

Roemer, R. A., Cornwell, A., Dewart, D., Jackson, P. and Ercegovac, D. V., Quantitative electroencephalographic analyses in cocaine-preferring polysubstance abusers during abstinence. Psychiatry Res. 58:247–257, 1995.

Bauer, L. O., Gross, J. B., Meyer, R. E. and Greenblatt, D. J., Chronic alcohol abuse and the acute sedative and neurophysiologic effects of midazolam. Psychopharmacology (Berl.) 133:293–299, 1997.

Costa, L. and Bauer, L., Quantitative electroencephalographic differences associated with alcohol, cocaine, heroin and dual-substance dependence. Drug Alcohol Depend. 46:87–93, 1997.

Gunther, W., Muller, N., Knesewitsch, P., Haag, C., Trapp, W., Banquet, J. P., Stieg, C. and Alper, K. R., Functional EEG mapping and SPECT in detoxified male alcoholics. Eur. Arch. Psychiatry Clin. Neurosci. 247:128–136, 1997.

Winterer, G., Kloppel, B., Heinz, A., Ziller, M., Dufeu, P., Schmidt, L. G. and Herrmann, W. M., Quantitative EEG (QEEG) predicts relapse in patients with chronic alcoholism and points to a frontally pronounced cerebral disturbance. Psychiatry Res. 78:101–113, 1998.

Sleep EEG

Gillin, J. C., Smith, T. L., Irwin, M., Kripke, D. F. and Schuckit, M., EEG sleep studies in "pure" primary alcoholism during subacute withdrawal: relationships to normal controls, age, and other clinical variables. Biol. Psychiatry 27:477–488, 1990.

Thompson, P. M., Gillin, J. C., Golshan, S. and Irwin, M., Polygraphic sleep measures differentiate alcoholics and stimulant abusers during short-term abstinence. Biol. Psychiatry 38:831–836, 1995.

Auditory ERPs

Lille, F., Hazemann, P., Massioui, F. E., Lesevre, N. and Dally, S., Effect of chronic alcohol intake and short-term abstinence on early sensory EPs and late 'cognitive' ERPs. Electroencephalogr. Clin. Neurophysiol. Suppl. 40:712–717, 1987.

Romani, A. and Cosi, V., Event-related potentials in chronic alcoholics during withdrawal and abstinence. Neurophysiol. Clin. 19:373–384, 1989.

Parsons, O. A., Sinha, R. and Williams, H. L., Relationships between neuropsychological test performance and event-related potentials in alcoholic and nonalcoholic samples. Alcohol. Clin. Exp. Res. 14:746–755, 1990.

Glenn, S., Parsons, O. A. and Sinha, R., Assessment of recovery of electrophysiological and neuropsychological functions in chronic alcoholics. Biol. Psychiatry 36:443–452, 1994.

Biggins, C. A., MacKay, S., Poole, N. and Fein, G., Delayed P3A in abstinent elderly male chronic alcoholics. Alcohol. Clin. Exp. Res. 19:1032–1042, 1995.

Kuruoglu, A. C., Arikan, Z., Vural, G., Karatas, M., Arac, M. and Isik, E., Single photon emission computerised tomography in chronic alcoholism: antisocial personality disorder may be associated with decreased frontal perfusion. Br. J. Psychiatry 169:348–354, 1996.

Biggins, C. A., MacKay, S., Clark, W. and Fein, G., Event-related potential evidence for frontal cortex effects of chronic cocaine dependence. Biol. Psychiatry 42:472–485, 1997.

Visual ERPs

Chan, Y. W., McLeod, J. G., Tuck, R. R., Walsh, J. C. and Feary, P. A., Visual evoked responses in chronic alcoholics. J. Neurol. Neurosurg. Psychiatry 49:945–950, 1986.

Emmerson, R. Y., Dustman, R. E., Shearer, D. E. and Chamberlin, H. M., EEG, visually evoked and event related potentials in young abstinent alcoholics. Alcohol 4:241–248, 1987.

Porjesz, B., Begleiter, H., Bihari, B. and Kissin, B., Event-related brain potentials to high incentive stimuli in abstinent alcoholics. Alcohol 4:283–287, 1987.

Porjesz, B., Begleiter, H., Bihari, B. and Kissin, B., The N2 component of the event-related brain potential in abstinent alcoholics. Electroencephalogr. Clin. Neurophysiol. 66:121–131, 1987.

Schandler, S. L., Cohen, M. J. and McArthur, D. L., Event-related brain potentials in intoxicated and detoxified alcoholics during visuospatial learning. Psychopharmacology (Berl.) 94:275–283, 1988.

Parsons, O. A., Sinha, R. and Williams, H. L., Relationships between neuropsychological test performance and event-related potentials in alcoholic and nonalcoholic samples. Alcohol. Clin. Exp. Res. 14:746–755, 1990.

Glenn, S., Parsons, O. A. and Sinha, R., Assessment of recovery of electrophysiological and neuropsychological functions in chronic alcoholics. Biol. Psychiatry 36:443–452, 1994.

Biggins, C. A., MacKay, S., Poole, N. and Fein, G., Delayed P3A in abstinent elderly male chronic alcoholics. Alcohol. Clin. Exp. Res. 19:1032–1042, 1995.

Bauer, L. O. and Easton, C., Pattern shift visual evoked potentials in abstinent cocaine-dependent, alcohol-dependent, and cross-dependent patients. Drug Alcohol Depend. 40:203–209, 1996.

Bauer, L. O., Gross, J. B., Meyer, R. E. and Greenblatt, D. J., Chronic alcohol abuse and the acute sedative and neurophysiologic effects of midazolam. Psychopharmacology (Berl.) 133:293–299, 1997.

Biggins, C. A., MacKay, S., Clark, W. and Fein, G., Event-related potential evidence for frontal cortex effects of chronic cocaine dependence. Biol. Psychiatry 42:472–485, 1997.

Cohen, H. L., Porjesz, B., Begleiter, H. and Wang, W., Neurophysiological correlates of response production and inhibition in alcoholics. Alcohol. Clin. Exp. Res. 21:1398–1406, 1997.

Other ERPs

Lille, F., Hazemann, P., Massioui, F. E., Lesevre, N. and Dally, S., Effect of chronic alcohol intake and short-term abstinence on early sensory EPs and late 'cognitive' ERPs. Electroencephalogr. Clin. Neurophysiol. Suppl. 40:712–717, 1987.

Bauer, L. O. and Mott, A. E., Differential effects of cocaine, alcohol, and nicotine dependence on olfactory evoked potentials. Drug Alcohol Depend. 42:21–26, 1996.

Zhang, X. L., Begleiter, H. and Projesz, B., Is working memory intact in alcoholics? An ERP study. Psychiatry Res. 75:75–89, 1997.

Family History of Alcoholism

Elmasian, R., Neville, H., Woods, D., Schuckit, M. and Bloom, F., Event-related brain potentials are different in individuals at high and low risk for developing alcoholism. Proc. Natl. Acad. Sci. USA 79:7900–7903, 1982.

Pollock, V. E., Volavka, J., Goodwin, D. W., Mednick, S. A., Gabrielli, W. F., Knop, J. and Schulsinger, F., The EEG after alcohol administration in men at risk for alcoholism. Arch. Gen. Psychiatry 40:857–861, 1983.

Begleiter, H., Porjesz, B., Bihari, B. and Kissin, B., Event-related brain potentials in boys at risk for alcoholism. Science 225:1493–1496, 1984.

Begleiter, H., Porjesz, B. and Bihari, B., Auditory brainstem potentials in sons of alcoholic fathers. Alcohol. Clin. Exp. Res. 11:477–480, 1987.

Begleiter, H., Porjesz, B., Rawlings, R. and Eckardt, M., Auditory recovery function and P3 in boys at high risk for alcoholism. Alcohol 4:315–321, 1987.

Ehlers, C. L. and Schuckit, M. A., EEG response to ethanol in sons of alcoholics. Psychopharmacol. Bull. 24:434–437, 1988.

Kaplan, R. F., Hesselbrock, V. M., O'Connor, S. and DePalma, N., Behavioral and EEG responses to alcohol in nonalcoholic men with a family history of alcoholism. Prog. Neuropsychopharmacol. Biol. Psychiatry 12:873–885, 1988.

Polich, J. and Bloom, F. E., Event-related brain potentials in individuals at high and low risk for developing alcoholism: failure to replicate. Alcohol. Clin. Exp. Res. 12:368–373, 1988.

Polich, J., Burns, T. and Bloom, F. E., P300 and the risk for alcoholism: family history, task difficulty, and gender. Alcohol. Clin. Exp. Res. 12:248–254, 1988.

Polich, J., Haier, R. J., Buchsbaum, M. and Bloom, F. E., Assessment of young men at risk for alcoholism with P300 from a visual discrimination task. J. Stud. Alcohol 49:186–190, 1988.

Pollock, V. E., Gabrielli, W. F., Mednick, S. A. and Goodwin, D. W., EEG identification of subgroups of men at risk for alcoholism? Psychiatry Res. 26:101–104, 1988.

Pollock, V. E., Volavka, J., Gabrielli, W. F., Mednick, S. A., Knop, J. and Goodwin, D. W., Pattern reversal visual evoked potential among men at risk for alcoholism. Acta Psychiatr. Scand. 78:276–282, 1988.

Pollock, V. E., Volavka, J., Goodwin, D. W., Gabrielli, W. F., Mednick, S. A., Knop, J. and Schulsinger, F., Pattern reversal visual evoked potentials after alcohol administration among men at risk for alcoholism. Psychiatry Res. 26:191–202, 1988.

Schuckit, M. A., Gold, E. O., Croot, K., Finn, P. and Polich, J., P300 latency after ethanol ingestion in sons of alcoholics and in controls. Biol. Psychiatry 24:310–315, 1988.

Ehlers, C. L. and Schuckit, M. A., EEG fast frequency activity in the sons of alcoholics. Biol. Psychiatry 27:631–641, 1990.

Porjesz, B. and Begleiter, H., Event-related potentials in individuals at risk for alcoholism. Alcohol 7:465–469, 1990.

Ehlers, C. L. and Schuckit, M. A., Evaluation of EEG alpha activity in sons of alcoholics. Neuropsychopharmacology 4:199–205, 1991.

Pfefferbaum, A., Ford, J. M., White, P. M. and Mathalon, D., Event-related potentials in alcoholic men: P3 amplitude reflects family history but not alcohol consumption. Alcohol. Clin. Exp. Res. 15:839–850, 1991.

Bauer, L. O. and Hesselbrock, V. M., EEG, autonomic and subjective correlates of the risk for alcoholism. J. Stud. Alcohol 54:577–589, 1993.

Cohen, H. L., Porjesz, B. and Begleiter, H., The effects of ethanol on EEG activity in males at risk for alcoholism. Electroencephalogr. Clin. Neurophysiol. 86:368–376, 1993.

Hesselbrock, V., Bauer, L., O'Connor, S. and Gillen, R., Reduced P300 amplitude in relation to family history of alcoholism and antisocial personality disorder among young men at risk for alcoholism. Alcohol Alcohol. Suppl. 2:95–100, 1993.

Bauer, L., Hesselbrock, V. M., O'Connor, S. and Roberts, L., P300 differences between non-alcoholic young men at average and above-average risk for alcoholism: effects of distraction and task modality. Prog. Neuropsychopharmacol. Biol. Psychiatry 18:263–277, 1994.

Bauer, L. O., O'Connor, S. and Hesselbrock, V. M., Frontal P300 decrements in antisocial personality disorder. Alcohol. Clin. Exp. Res. 18:1300–1305, 1994.

O'Connor, S., Bauer, L., Tasman, A. and Hesselbrock, V., Reduced P3 amplitudes are associated with both a family history of alcoholism and antisocial personality disorder. Prog. Neuropsychopharmacol. Biol. Psychiatry 18:1307–1321, 1994.

Polich, J., Pollock, V. E. and Bloom, F. E., Meta-analysis of P300 amplitude from males at risk for alcoholism. Psychol. Bull. 115:55–73, 1994.

Ehlers, C. L., Havstad, J. W. and Schuckit, M. A., EEG dimension in sons of alcoholics. Alcohol. Clin. Exp. Res. 19:992–998, 1995.

Volavka, J., Czobor, P., Goodwin, D. W., Gabrielli, W. F. J., Penick, E. C., Mednick, S. A., Jensen, P. and Knop, J., The electroencephalogram after alcohol administration in high-risk men and the development of alcohol use disorders 10 years later. Arch. Gen. Psychiatry 53:258–263, 1996.

Cohen, H. L., Porjesz, B., Stimus, A. T. and Begleiter, H., Effects of ethanol on temporal recovery of auditory-evoked potentials in individuals at risk for alcoholism. Alcohol. Clin. Exp. Res. 22:945–953, 1998.

Porjesz, B., Begleiter, H., Reich, T., Van Eerdewegh, P., Edenberg, H. J., Foroud, T., Goate, A., Litke, A., Chorlian, D. B., Stimus, A., Rice, J., Blangero, J., Almasy, L., Sorbell, J., Bauer, L. O., Kuperman, S., O'Connor, S. J. and Rohrbaugh, J., Amplitude of visual P3 event-related potential as a phenotypic marker for a predisposition to alcoholism: preliminary results from the COGA Project. Collaborative Study on the Genetics of Alcoholism. Alcohol. Clin. Exp. Res. 22:1317–1323, 1998.

Van der Stelt, O., Geesken, R., Gunning, W. B., Snel, J. and Kok, A., P3 scalp topography to target and novel visual stimuli in children of alcoholics. Alcohol 15:119–136, 1998.

Bauer, L. O. and Hesselbrock, V. M., Subtypes of family history and conduct disorder: effects on P300 during the stroop test. Neuropsychopharmacology 21:51–62, 1999.

Bauer, L. O. and Hesselbrock, V. M., P300 decrements in teenagers with conduct problems: Implications for substance abuse risk and brain development. Biol. Psychiatry 46:263–272, 1999.

Ehlers, C. L., Garcia-Andrade, C., Wall, T. L., Cloutier, D. and Phillips, E., Electroencephalographic responses to alcohol challenge in Native American Mission Indians. Biol. Psychiatry 45:776–787, 1999.

Hill, S. Y., Yuan, H. and Locke, J., Path analysis of P300 amplitude of individuals from families at high and low risk for developing alcoholism. Biol. Psychiatry 45:346–359, 1999.

Genetic Effects

Baseline Studies

Noble, E. P., Berman, S. M., Ozkaragoz, T. Z. and Ritchie, T., Prolonged P300 latency in children with the D_2 dopamine receptor A1 allele. Am. J. Hum. Genet. 54:658–668, 1994.

Johnson, J. P., Muhleman, D., MacMurray, J., Gade, R., Verde, R., Ask, M., Kelley, J. and Comings, D. E., Association between the cannabinoid receptor gene (CNR1) and the P300 event-related potential. Mol. Psychiatry 2:169–171, 1997.

Begleiter, H., Porjesz, B., Reich, T., Edenberg, H. J., Goate, A., Blangero, J., Almasy, L., Foroud, T., Van Eerdewegh, P., Polich, J., Rohrbaugh, J., Kuperman, S., Bauer, L. O., O'Connor, S. J., Chorlian, D. B., Li, T. K., Conneally, P. M., Hesselbrock, V., Rice, J. P., Schuckit, M. A., Cloninger, R., Nurnberger, J. J., Crowe, R. and Bloom, F. E., Quantitative trait loci analysis of human event-related brain potentials: P3 voltage. Electroencephalogr. Clin. Neurophysiol. 108:244–250, 1998.

Acute Alcohol Administration Studies

Propping, P., Genetic control of ethanol action on the central nervous system. An EEG study in twins. Hum. Genet. 35:309–334, 1977.

Propping, P., Kruger, J. and Janah, A., Effect of alcohol on genetically determined variants of the normal electroencephalogram. Psychiatry Res. 2:85–98, 1980.

Christian, J. C., Li, T. K., Norton, J. A. J., Propping, P. and Yu, P. L., Alcohol effects on the percentage of beta waves in the electroencephalograms of twins. Genet. Epidemiol. 5:217–224, 1988.

Wall, T. L., Gallen, C. C. and Ehlers, C. L., Effects of alcohol on the EEG in Asian men with genetic variations of ALDH2. Biol. Psychiatry 34:91–99, 1993.

Wall, T. L. and Ehlers, C. L., Acute effects of alcohol on P300 in Asians with different ALDH2 genotypes. Alcohol. Clin. Exp. Res. 19:617–622, 1995.

Sorbel, J., Morzorati, S., O'Connor, S., Li, T. K. and Christian, J. C., Alcohol effects on the heritability of EEG spectral power. Alcohol. Clin. Exp. Res. 20:1523–1527, 1996.

Ehlers, C. L., Garcia-Andrade, C., Wall, T. L., Sobel, D. F. and Phillips, E., Determinants of P3 amplitude and response to alcohol in Native American Mission Indians. Neuropsychopharmacology 18:282–292, 1998.

Ehlers, C. L., Garcia-Andrade, C., Wall, T. L., Cloutier, D. and Phillips, E., Electroencephalographic responses to alcohol challenge in Native American Mission Indians. Biol. Psychiatry 45:776–787, 1999.

O'Connor, S., Sorbel, J., Morzorati, S., Li, T. K. and Christian, J. C., A twin study of genetic influences on the acute adaptation of the EEG to alcohol. Alcohol. Clin. Exp. Res. 23:494–501, 1999.

Treatment

Saletu, M., Saletu, B., Grunberger, J., Mader, R. and Karobath, M., Clinical symptomatology and computer analyzed EEG before, during and after anxiolytic therapy of alcohol withdrawal patients. Neuropsychobiology 9:119–134, 1983.

Saletu, B., Saletu, M., Grunberger, J. and Mader R., Spontaneous and drug-induced remission of alcoholic organic brain syndrome: clinical, psychometric, and neurophysiological studies. Psychiatry Res. 10:59–75, 1983.

Schwarz-Ottersbach, E. and Goldberg, L., Activation levels, EEG, and behavioural responses. Int. J. Psychophysiol. 4:7–17, 1986.

Fahrion, S. L., Walters, E. D., Coyne, L. and Allen, T., Alterations in EEG amplitude, personality factors, and brain electrical mapping after alpha-theta brainwave training: a controlled case study of an alcoholic in recovery. Alcohol. Clin. Exp. Res. 16:547–552, 1992.

Saletu, B., Saletu, M., Grunberger, J., Frey, R., Anderer, P. and Mader, R., Treatment of the alcoholic organic brain syndrome: double-blind, placebo-controlled clinical, psychometric and electroencephalographic mapping studies with modafinil. Neuropsychobiology 27:26–39, 1993.

Schneider, F., Elbert, T., Heimann, H., Welker, A., Stetter, F., Mattes, R., Birbaumer, N. and Mann, K., Self-regulation of slow cortical potentials in psychiatric patients: alcohol dependency. Biofeedback Self Regul. 18:23–32, 1993.

Herning, R. I., Guo, X. and Lange, W. R., The effects of nimodipine on the EEG of substance abusers. Ann. N. Y. Acad. Sci. 765:143–151, 1995.

Herning, R. I., Guo, X. and Lange, W. R., Nimodipine improves information processing in substance abusers. Ann. N. Y. Acad. Sci. 765:152–159, 1995.

Ilyuchina, V. A. and Nikitina, L. I., Clinical physiological study of the therapeutic effects of phenytoin in acute alcohol withdrawal and the asthenic-autonomic syndrome in patients with chronic alcoholism. Alcohol 12:511–517, 1995.

Prenatal Exposure

Chernick, V., Childiaeva, R. and Ioffe, S., Effects of maternal alcohol intake and smoking on neonatal electroencephalogram and anthropometric measurements. Am. J. Obstet. Gynecol. 146:41–47, 1983.

Loffe, S., Childiaeva, R. and Chernick, V., Prolonged effects of maternal alcohol ingestion on the neonatal electroencephalogram. Pediatrics 74:330–335, 1984.

Ioffe, S. and Chernick, V., Development of the EEG between 30 and 40 weeks gestation in normal and alcohol-exposed infants. Dev. Med. Child Neurol. 30:797–807, 1988.

Scher, M. S., Richardson, G. A., Coble, P. A., Day, N. L. and Stoffer, D. S., The effects of prenatal alcohol and marijuana exposure: disturbances in neonatal sleep cycling and arousal. Pediatr. Res. 24:101–105, 1988.

Ioffe, S. and Chernick, V., Prediction of subsequent motor and mental retardation in newborn infants exposed to alcohol in utero by computerized EEG analysis. Neuropediatrics 21:11–17, 1990.

Mattson, S. N., Riley, E. P., Jernigan, T. L., Ehlers, C. L., Delis, D. C., Jones, K. L., Stern, C., Johnson, K. A., Hesselink, J. R. and Bellugi, U., Fetal alcohol syndrome: a case report of neuropsychological, MRI and EEG assessment of two children. Alcohol. Clin. Exp. Res. 16:1001–1003, 1992. [Case Report]

Kaneko, W. M., Ehlers, C. L., Philips, E. L. and Riley, E. P., Auditory event-related potentials in fetal alcohol syndrome and Down's syndrome children. Alcohol. Clin. Exp. Res. 20:35–42, 1996.

Kaneko, W. M., Phillips, E. L., Riley, E. P. and Ehlers, C. L., EEG findings in fetal alcohol syndrome and Down syndrome children. Electroencephalogr. Clin. Neurophysiol. 98:20–28, 1996.

Scher, M. S., Richardson, G. A., Robles, N., Geva, D., Goldschmidt, L., Dahl, R. E., Sclabassi, R. J. and Day, N. L., Effects of prenatal substance exposure: altered maturation of visual evoked potentials. Pediatr. Neurol. 18:236–243, 1998.

Benzodiazepines and Alcoholism

Saletu, M., Saletu, B., Grunberger, J., Mader, R. and Karobath, M., Clinical symptomatology and computer analyzed EEG before, during and after anxiolytic therapy of alcohol withdrawal patients. Neuropsychobiology 9:119–134, 1983.

Mouradian, M. D. and Penovich, P. E., Spindle coma in benzodiazepine toxicity: case report. Clin. Electroencephalogr. 16:213–218, 1985. [Case Report]

Schwarz-Ottersbach, E. and Goldberg, L., Activation levels, EEG, and behavioural responses. Int. J. Psychophysiol. 4:7–17, 1986.

Bauer, L. O., Gross, J. B., Meyer, R. E. and Greenblatt, D. J., Chronic alcohol abuse and the acute sedative and neurophysiologic effects of midazolam. Psychopharmacology (Berl.) 133:293–299, 1997.

HIV

Fein, G., Biggins, C. A. and MacKay, S., Alcohol abuse and HIV infection have additive effects on frontal cortex function as measured by auditory evoked potential P3A latency. Biol. Psychiatry 37:183–195, 1995.

Methanol

Jameson, H. D. and Kane, R., EEG records during an epidemic of methanol intoxication. Electroencephalogr. Clin. Neurophysiol. 26:112, 1969.

Labay Matias, M. V., Perez Cuesta, P., Hervas Palazon, J., Suau Barcelo, J., Puges Bassols, E., Diaz Garcia, M. and Rul Lan Buades, G., Accidental methanol poisoning in an infant girl. Physiopathology, diagnosis and treatment. An. Esp. Pediatr. 25:271–274, 1986. [Case Report] [Spanish]

Cook, M. R., Bergman, F. J., Cohen, H. D., Gerkovich, M. M., Graham, C., Harris, R. K. and Siemann, L. G., Effects of methanol vapor on human neurobehavioral measures. Res. Rep. Health Eff. Inst. 42:1–45, 1991.

Hamon, J. F., Camara, P. and Claver, B., Electroencephalogram changes and psychopathologic disorders in 60 cases of chronic palm brandy intoxication. Med. Trop. (Mars.) 52:363–368, 1992. [French]

Chuwers, P., Osterloh, J., Kelly, T., D'Alessandro, A., Quinlan, P. and Becker, C., Neurobehavioral effects of low-level methanol vapor exposure in healthy human volunteers. Environ. Res. 71:141–150, 1995.

Reviews

Carlen, P. L. and Wilkinson, D. A., Assessment of neurological dysfunction and recovery in alcoholics: CT scanning and other techniques. Subst. Alcohol Actions Misuse 4:191–197, 1983.

Johnson, J. L., Adinoff, B., Bisserbe, J. C., Martin, P. R., Rio, D., Rohrbaugh, J. W., Zubovic, E. and Eckardt, M. J., Assessment of alcoholism-related organic brain syndromes with positron emission tomography. Alcohol. Clin. Exp. Res. 10:237–240, 1986.

Eckardt, M. J., Rohrbaugh, J. W., Rio, D., Rawlings, R. R. and Coppola, R., Brain imaging in alcoholic patients. Adv. Alcohol. Subst. Abuse 7:59–71, 1988.

Newlin, D. B. and Thomson, J. B., Alcohol challenge with sons of alcoholics: a critical review and analysis. Psychol. Bull. 108:383–402, 1990.

Noldy, N. E. and Carlen, P. L., Acute, withdrawal, and chronic alcohol effects in man: event-related potential and quantitative EEG techniques. Ann. Med. 22:333–339, 1990.

Freedland, E. S. and McMicken, D. B., Alcohol-related seizures, Part I: Pathophysiology, differential diagnosis, and evaluation. J. Emerg. Med. 11:463–473, 1993.

Porjesz, B. and Begleiter, H., Effects of alcohol on electrophysiological activity of the brain. In: Begleiter, H. and Kissin, B. (eds.) Pharmacology of Alcohol and Alcohol Dependence. New York, Oxford University Press, pp. 207–247, 1996.

Krupitsky, E. M. and Grinenko, A. Y., Ketamine psychedelic therapy (KPT): a review of the results of ten years of research. J. Psychoactive Drugs 29:165–183, 1997.

Parsons, O. A. and Nixon, S. J., Cognitive functioning in sober social drinkers: a review of the research since 1986. J. Stud. Alcohol 59:180–190, 1998.

Marijuana

Acute Administration

EEG

Williams, E. G., Himmelsbach, C. K., Wikler, A. and Rubie, D. C., Studies on marihuana and pyrahexyl compound. Public Health Report 61:1059–1085, 1946.

Ames, F., A clinical and metabolic study of acute intoxication with cannabis sativa and its role in the model psychoses. J. Ment. Sci. 104:972–999, 1958.

Hollister, L. E., Sherwood, S. L. and Cavasino, A., Marihuana and the human electroencephalogram. Pharmacol. Res. Commun. 2:305–308, 1970.

Jones, R. T. and Stone, G. C., Psychological studies of marijuana and alcohol in man. Psychopharmacologia 18:108–117, 1970.

Dornbush, R. L., Fink, M. and Freedman, A. M., Marijuana, memory, and perception. Am. J. Psychiatry 128:194–197, 1971.

Tassinari, C. A., Ambrosetto, H. G., Peraita-Adrodos, M. R. and Gastaut, H., Neurophysiological effects of high doses of marihuana in man. Electroencephalogr. Clin. Neurophysiol. 35:404–405, 1973.

Volavka, J., Crown, P., Dornbush, R., Feldstein, S. and Fink, M., EEG, heart rate and mood change ("high") after cannabis. Psychopharmacologia 32:11–25, 1973.

Tassinari, C. A., Ambrosetto, H. G., Peraita-Adrodos, M. R. and Gastaut, H., Effects of marihuana and delta-9-THC at high doses in man: a polygraphic study. Electroencephalogr. Clin. Neurphysiol. 36:94, 1974.

Koukkou, M. and Lehmann, D., Human EEG spectra before and during cannabis hallucinations. Biol. Psychiatry 11:663–677, 1976.

Koukkou, M. and Lehmann, D., Correlations between cannabis-induced psychopathology and EEG before and after drug ingestion. Pharmakopsychiatr. Neuropsychopharmakol. 11:220–227, 1978.

Lukas, S. E., Mendelson, J. H., Amass, L. and Benedikt, R., Behavioral and EEG studies of acute cocaine administration: comparisons with morphine, amphetamine, pentobarbital, nicotine, ethanol and marijuana. NIDA Res. Monogr. 95:146–151, 1989.

Lukas, S. E., Mendelson, J. H. and Benedikt, R., Electroencephalographic correlates of marihuana-induced euphoria. Drug Alcohol Depend. 37:131–140, 1995.

Auditory ERPs

Kopell, B. S., Roth, W. T. and Tinklenberg, J. R., Time course effects of marijuana and ethanol on event-related potentials. Psychopharmacology (Berl.) 56:15–20, 1978.

Solowij, N., Grenyer, B. F., Chesher, G. and Lewis, J., Biopsychosocial changes associated with cessation of cannabis use: a single case study of acute and chronic cognitive effects, withdrawal and treatment. Life Sci. 56:2127–2134, 1995. [Case Report]

Visual ERPs

Roth, W. T., Tinklenberg, J. R. and Kopell, B. S., Ethanol and marihuana effects on event-related potentials in a memory retrieval paradigm. Electroencephalogr. Clin. Neurophysiol. 42:381–388, 1977.

Leweke, M., Kampmann, C., Radwan, M., Dietrich, D. E., Johannes, S., Emrich, H. M. and Munte, T. F., The effects of tetrahydrocannabinol on the recognition of emotionally charged words: an analysis using event-related brain potentials. Neuropsychobiology 37:104–111, 1998.

Chronic Administration

EEG

Jones, R. T., Benowitz, N. L. and Herning, R. I., Clinical relevance of cannabis tolerance and dependence. J. Clin. Pharmacol. 21:143S–152S, 1981.

Struve, F. A., Straumanis, J. J. and Patrick, G., Persistent topographic quantitative EEG sequelae of chronic marihuana use: a replication study and initial discriminant function analysis. Clin. Electroencephalogr. 25:63–75, 1994.

Struve, F. A., Patrick, G., Straumanis, J. J., Fitz-Gerald, M. J. and Manno, J., Possible EEG sequelae of very long duration marihuana use: pilot findings from topographic quantitative EEG analyses of subjects with 15 to 24 years of cumulative daily exposure to THC. Clin. Electroencephalogr. 29:31–36, 1998.

Auditory ERPs

Herning, R. I., Jones, R. T. and Peltzman, D. J., Changes in human event related potentials with prolonged delta-9-tetrahydrocannabinol (THC) use. Electroencephalogr. Clin. Neurophysiol. 47:556–570, 1979.

Pickworth, W. B., Brown, B. S., Hickey, J. E. and Muntaner, C., Effects of self-reported drug use and antisocial behavior on evoked potentials in adolescents. Drug Alcohol Depend. 25:105–110, 1990.

Solowij, N., Michie, P. T. and Fox, A. M., Effects of long-term cannabis use on selective attention: an event-related potential study. Pharmacol. Biochem. Behav. 40:683–688, 1991.

Patrick, G. and Struve, F. A., Brainstem auditory response (BAER) in polydrug abuse. Clin. Electroencephalogr. 25:1–7, 1994.

Herning, R. I., Guo, X. and Lange, W. R., Nimodipine improves information processing in substance abusers. Ann. NY Acad. Sci. 765:152–159, 1995.

Patrick, G., Straumanis, J. J., Struve, F. A., Nixon, F., Fitz-Gerald, M. J., Manno, J. E. and Soucair, M., Auditory and visual P300 event related potentials are not altered in medically and psychiatrically normal chronic marihuana users. Life Sci. 56:2135–2140, 1995.

Solowij, N., Grenyer, B. F., Chesher, G. and Lewis, J., Biopsychosocial changes associated with cessation of cannabis use: a single case study of acute and chronic cognitive effects, withdrawal and treatment. Life Sci. 56:2127–2134, 1995. [Case Report]

Solowij, N., Michie, P. T. and Fox, A. M., Differential impairments of selective attention due to frequency and duration of cannabis use. Biol. Psychiatry 37:731–739, 1995.

Patrick, G., Straumanis, J. J., Struve, F. A., Fitz-Gerald, M. J. and Manno, J. E., Early and middle latency evoked potentials in medically and psychiatrically normal daily marihuana users: a paucity of significant findings. Clin. Electroencephalogr. 28:26–31, 1997.

Visual ERPs

Herning, R. I., Guo, X. and Lange, W. R., Nimodipine improves information processing in substance abusers. Ann. N. Y. Acad. Sci. 765:152–159, 1995.

Patrick, G., Straumanis, J. J., Struve, F. A., Nixon, F., Fitz-Gerald, M. J., Manno, J. E. and Soucair, M., Auditory and visual P300 event related potentials are not altered in medically and psychiatrically normal chronic marihuana users. Life Sci. 56:2135–2140, 1995.

Patrick, G., Straumanis, J. J., Struve, F. A., Fitz-Gerald, M. J. and Manno, J. E., Early and middle latency evoked potentials in medically and psychiatrically normal daily marihuana users: a paucity of significant findings. Clin. Electroencephalogr. 28:26–31, 1997.

Abstinence

Solowij, N., Grenyer, B. F., Chesher, G. and Lewis, J., Biopsychosocial changes associated with cessation of cannabis use: a single case study of acute and chronic cognitive effects, withdrawal and treatment. Life Sci. 56:2127–2134, 1995. [Case Report]

Genetic Study

Johnson, J. P., Muhleman, D., MacMurray, J., Gade, R., Verde, R., Ask, M., Kelley, J. and Comings, D. E., Association between the cannabinoid receptor gene (CNR1) and the P300 event-related potential. Mol. Psychiatry 2:169–171, 1997.

Treatment

Herning, R. I., Guo, X. and Lange, W. R., Nimodipine improves information processing in substance abusers. Ann. N. Y. Acad. Sci. 765:152–159, 1995.

Prenatal Exposure

Scher, M. S., Richardson, G. A., Coble, P. A., Day, N. L. and Stoffer, D. S., The effects of prenatal alcohol and marijuana exposure: disturbances in neonatal sleep cycling and arousal. Pediatr. Res. 24:101–105, 1988.

Dahl, R. E., Scher, M. S., Williamson, D. E., Robles, N. and Day, N., A longitudinal study of prenatal marijuana use. Effects on sleep and arousal at age 3 years. Arch. Pediatr. Adolesc. Med. 149:145–150, 1995.

Scher, M. S., Richardson, G. A., Robles, N., Geva, D., Goldschmidt, L., Dahl, R. E., Sclabassi, R. J. and Day, N. L., Effects of prenatal substance exposure: altered maturation of visual evoked potentials. Pediatr. Neurol. 18:236–243, 1998.

Reviews

Maykut, M. O., Health consequences of acute and chronic marihuana use. Prog. Neuropsychopharmacol. Biol. Psychiatry 9:209–238, 1985.

Wert, R. C. and Raulin, M. L., The chronic cerebral effects of cannabis use. I. Methodological issues and neurological findings. Int. J. Addict. 21:605–628, 1986.

Struve, F. A., Straumanis, J. J., Patrick, G. and Price, L., Topographic mapping of quantitative EEG variables in chronic heavy marihuana users: empirical findings with psychiatric patients. Clin. Electroencephalogr. 20:6–23, 1989.

Hallucinogens

PCP

Stockard, J. J., Werner, S. S., Aalbers, J. A. and Chiappa, K. H., Electroencephalographic findings in phencyclidine intoxication. Arch. Neurol. 33:200–203, 1976. [Case Report]

Shelburne, S. A. J. and McLaurin, R. L., The effects of phencyclidine on visually evoked potentials of rhesus monkeys. Electroencephalogr. Clin. Neurophysiol. 43:95–98, 1977. [Nonhuman Primate]

Fariello, R. G. and Black, J. A., Pseudoperiodic bilateral EEG paroxysms in a case of phencyclidine intoxication. J. Clin. Psychiatry 39:579–581, 1978. [Case Report]

Fitch, W., McGeorge, A. P. and MacKenzie, E. T., Anaesthesia for studies of the cerebral circulation: a comparison of phencyclidine and althesin in the baboon. Br. J. Anaesth. 50:985–991, 1978. [Nonhuman Primate]

Matsuzaki, M. and Dowling, K. C., Effects of phencyclidine (PCP) on the visual evoked potentials in the rhesus monkey. Brain Res. Bull. 10:33–38, 1983. [Nonhuman Primate]

Matsuzaki, M. and Dowling, K. C., Phencyclidine (PCP): effects on auditory evoked potentials in the rhesus monkey. Brain Res. Bull. 13:155–161, 1984. [Nonhuman Primate]

Matsuzaki, M. and Dowling, K. C., Phencyclidine (PCP): effects of acute and chronic administration on EEG activities in the rhesus monkey. Electroencephalogr. Clin. Neurophysiol. 60:356–366, 1985. [Nonhuman Primate]

Ketamine

Weber, M., Laxenaire, M. C., Fays, J., Hottier, M. C. and Cozette, P., Electro-clinical features of short-term anaesthesia. (author's transl). Rev. Electroencephalogr. Neurophysiol. Clin. 7:38–44, 1977.

White, P. F., Schuttler, J., Shafer, A., Stanski, D. R., Horai, Y. and Trevor, A. J., Comparative pharmacology of the ketamine isomers. Studies in volunteers. Br. J. Anaesth. 57:197–203, 1985.

Hou, W. Y., Lee, W. Y., Lin, S. M., Liu, C. C., Susceto, L., Sun, W. Z. and Lin, S. Y., The effects of ketamine, propofol and nitrous oxide on visual evoked potential during fentanyl anesthesia. Ma Tsui Hsueh Tsa Chi 31:97–102, 1993.

Engelhardt, W., Stahl, K., Marouche, A., Hartung, E. and Dierks, T., Ketamine racemate versus S-(+)-ketamine with or without antagonism with physostigmine. A quantitative EEG study on volunteers. Anaesthesist 43 Suppl. 2:S76–82, 1994. [German]

Schwender, D., Faber-Zullig, E., Fett, W., Klasing, S., Finsterer, U., Poppel, E. and Peter, K., Mid-latency auditory evoked potentials in humans during anesthesia with S (+) ketamine: a double-blind, randomized comparison with racemic ketamine. Anesth. Analg. 78:267–274, 1994.

Krupitsky, E. M. and Grinenko, A. Y., Ketamine psychedelic therapy (KPT): a review of the results of ten years of research. J. Psychoactive Drugs 29:165–183, 1997.

Langeron, O., Lille, F., Zerhouni, O., Orliaguet, G., Saillant, G., Riou, B. and Coriat, P., Comparison of the effects of ketamine-midazolam with those of fentanyl- midazolam on cortical somatosensory evoked potentials during major spine surgery. Br. J. Anaesth. 78:701–706, 1997.
Plourde, G., Baribeau, J. and Bonhomme, V., Ketamine increases the amplitude of the 40-Hz auditory steady-state response in humans. Br. J. Anaesth. 78:524–529, 1997.
van Berckel, B. N., Oranje, B., van Ree, J. M., Verbaten, M. N. and Kahn, R. S., The effects of low dose ketamine on sensory gating, neuroendocrine secretion and behavior in healthy human subjects. Psychopharmacology (Berl.) 137:271–281, 1998.

MDMA and MDE

Gouzoulis, E., Steiger, A., Ensslin, M., Kovar, A. and Hermle, L., Sleep EEG effects of 3,4-methylenedioxyethamphetamine (MDE; "eve") in healthy volunteers. Biol. Psychiatry 32:1108–1117, 1992.
Allen, R. P., McCann, U. D. and Ricaurte, G. A., Persistent effects of (+/-)3,4-methylenedioxy-methamphetamine (MDMA, "ecstasy") on human sleep. Sleep 16:560–564, 1993.
Dafters, R. I., Duffy, F., O'Donnell, P. J. and Bouquet, C., Level of use of 3,4-methylenedioxy-methamphetamine (MDMA or Ecstasy) in humans correlates with EEG power and coherence. Psychopharmacology (Berl.) 145:82–90, 1999.

LSD

Fink, M., EEG and human psychopharmacology. Annu. Rev. Pharmacol. 9:241–258, 1969.
Abraham, H. D. and Duffy, F. H., Stable quantitative EEG difference in post-LSD visual disorder by split-half analysis: evidence for disinhibition. Psychiatry Res. 67:173–187, 1996.

Anabolic Steroids

Frankle, M. A., Eichberg, R. and Zachariah, S. B., Anabolic androgenic steroids and a stroke in an athlete: case report. Arch. Phys. Med. Rehabil. 69:632–633, 1988. [Case Report]

Unspecified

Pickworth, W. B., Brown, B. S., Hickey, J. E. and Muntaner, C., Effects of self-reported drug use and antisocial behavior on evoked potentials in adolescents. Drug Alcohol Depend. 25:105–110, 1990.

Benzodiazepines

Acute Administration

EEG

Montagu, J. D., Effects of diazepam on the EEG in man. Eur. J. Pharmacol. 17:167–170, 1972.
Brown, C. R., Sarnquist, F. H., Canup, C. A. and Pedley, T. A., Clinical, electroencephalographic, and pharmacokinetic studies of a water-soluble benzodiazepine, midazolam maleate. Anesthesiology 50:467–470, 1979.
Hendler, N., Cimini, C., Ma, T. and Long, D., A comparison of cognitive impairment due to benzodiazepines and to narcotics. Am. J. Psychiatry 137:828–830, 1980.
Guterman, B., Sebastian, P. and Sodha, N., Recovery from alpha coma after lorazepam overdose. Clin. Electroencephalogr. 12:205–208, 1981. [Case Report]
Bond, A., Lader, M. and Shrotriya, R., Comparative effects of a repeated dose regime of diazepam and buspirone on subjective ratings, psychological tests and the EEG. Eur. J. Clin. Pharmacol. 24:463–467, 1983.
Laurian, S., Gaillard, J. M., Le, P. K. and Schopf, J., Effects of a benzodiazepine antagonist on the diazepam-induced electrical brain activity modifications. Neuropsychobiology 11:55–58, 1984.

Mizuki, Y., Hamasaki, J., Hirano, H., Miyoshi, A., Yamada, M. and Inanaga, K., Effects of centrally acting drugs on the frontal midline theta activity in man. Jpn. J. Psychiatry Neurol. 40:647–653, 1986.

Forster, A., Juge, O., Louis, M. and Nahory, A., Effects of a specific benzodiazepine antagonist (RO 15-1788) on cerebral blood flow. Anesth. Analg. 66:309–313, 1987.

Greenblatt, D. J., Ehrenberg, B. L., Gunderman, J., Locniskar, A., Scavone, J. M., Harmatz, J. S. and Shader, R. I., Pharmacokinetic and electroencephalographic study of intravenous diazepam, midazolam, and placebo. Clin. Pharmacol. Ther. 45:356–365, 1989.

Blom, M. W., Bartel, P. R., de Sommers, K., Van der Meyden, C. H. and Becker, P. J., The effects of alprazolam, quazepam and diazepam on saccadic eye movements, parameters of psychomotor function and the EEG. Fundam. Clin. Pharmacol. 4:653–661, 1990.

Breimer, L. T., Hennis, P. J., Burm, A. G., Danhof, M., Bovill, J. G., Spierdijk, J. and Vletter, A. A., Quantification of the EEG effect of midazolam by aperiodic analysis in volunteers. Pharmacokinetic/pharmacodynamic modelling. Clin. Pharmacokinet. 18:245–253, 1990.

Buhrer, M., Maitre, P. O., Hung, O. and Stanski, D. R., Electroencephalographic effects of benzodiazepines. I. Choosing an electroencephalographic parameter to measure the effect of midazolam on the central nervous system. Clin. Pharmacol. Ther. 48:544–554, 1990.

Breimer, L. T., Burm, A. G., Danhof, M., Hennis, P. J., Vletter, A. A., de Voogt, J. W., Spierdijk, J. and Bovill, J. G., Pharmacokinetic-pharmacodynamic modelling of the interaction between flumazenil and midazolam in volunteers by aperiodic EEG analysis. Clin. Pharmacokinet. 20:497–508, 1991.

Bond, A. J., Silveira, J. C. and Lader, M. H., The effects of alprazolam alone and combined with alcohol on central integrative activity. Eur. J. Clin. Pharmacol. 42:495–498, 1992.

Engelhardt, W., Friess, K., Hartung, E., Sold, M. and Dierks, T., EEG and auditory evoked potential P300 compared with psychometric tests in assessing vigilance after benzodiazepine sedation and antagonism. Br. J. Anaesth. 69:75–80, 1992.

Muraoka, M., Tada, K., Nogami, Y., Ishikawa, K. and Nagoya, T., Residual effects of repeated administration of triazolam and nitrazepam in healthy volunteers. Neuropsychobiology 25:134–139, 1992.

Link, C. G., Leigh, T. J. and Dennison, J. K., The effects of BRL 46470A, a novel 5-HT3 receptor antagonist, and lorazepam on psychometric performance and the EEG. Br. J. Clin. Pharmacol. 35:395–399, 1993.

Van Steveninck, A. L., Mandema, J. W., Tuk, B., Van Dijk, J. G., Schoemaker, H. C., Danhof, M. and Cohen, A. F., A comparison of the concentration-effect relationships of midazolam for EEG-derived parameters and saccadic peak velocity. Br. J. Clin. Pharmacol. 36:109–115, 1993.

Greenblatt, D. J., Harmatz, J. S., Gouthro, T. A., Locke, J. and Shader, R. I., Distinguishing a benzodiazepine agonist (triazolam) from a nonagonist anxiolytic (buspirone) by electroencephalography: kinetic-dynamic studies. Clin. Pharmacol. Ther. 56:100–111, 1994.

Kinoshita, T., Michel, C. M., Yagyu, T., Lehmann, D. and Saito, M., Diazepam and sulpiride effects on frequency domain EEG source locations. Neuropsychobiology 30:126–131, 1994.

Fiset, P., Lemmens, H. L., Egan, T. E., Shafer, S. L. and Stanski, D. R., Pharmacodynamic modeling of the electroencephalographic effects of flumazenil in healthy volunteers sedated with midazolam. Clin. Pharmacol. Ther. 58:567–582, 1995.

Michel, C. M., Pascual-Marqui, R. D., Strik, W. K., Koenig, T. and Lehmann, D., Frequency domain source localization shows state-dependent diazepam effects in 47-channel EEG. J. Neural. Transm. Gen. Sect. 99:157–171, 1995.

Bauer, L. O., Gross, J. B., Meyer, R. E. and Greenblatt, D. J., Chronic alcohol abuse and the acute sedative and neurophysiologic effects of midazolam. Psychopharmacology (Berl.) 133:293–299, 1997.

Feshchenko, V. A., Veselis, R. A. and Reinsel, R. A., Comparison of the EEG effects of midazolam, thiopental, and propofol: the role of underlying oscillatory systems. Neuropsychobiology 35:211–220, 1997.

Sierra, J. C., Luna-Villegas, G., Buela-Casal, G. and Fernandez-Guardiola, A., The assessment of residual effects of a single dose of diazepam on visually-defined EEG patterns. J. Psychopharmacol. 11:367–372, 1997.

Sleep EEG

Tan, X., Uchida, S., Matsuura, M., Nishihara, K., Iguchi, Y. and Kojima, T., Benzodiazepine effects on human sleep EEG spectra: a comparison of triazolam and flunitrazepam. Life Sci. 63:675–684, 1998.

Auditory ERPs

Herrmann, W. M., Hofmann, W. and Kubicki, S., Psychotropic drug induced changes in auditory averaged evoked potentials: results of a double-blind trial using an objective fully automated AEP analysis method. Int. J. Clin. Pharmacol. Ther. Toxicol. 19:56–62, 1981.

Laurian, S., Gaillard, J. M., Le, P. K. and Schopf, J., Effects of a benzodiazepine antagonist on the diazepam-induced electrical brain activity modifications. Neuropsychobiology 11:55–58, 1984.

Adams, D. A., McClelland, R. J., Houston, H. G. and Gamble, W. G., The effects of diazepam on the auditory brain stem responses. Br. J. Audiol. 19:277–280, 1985.

Erwin, C. W., Linnoila, M., Hartwell, J., Erwin, A. and Guthrie, S., Effects of buspirone and diazepam, alone and in combination with alcohol, on skilled performance and evoked potentials. J. Clin. Psychopharmacol. 6:199–209, 1986.

Loughnan, B. L., Sebel, P. S., Thomas, D., Rutherfoord, C. F. and Rogers, H., Evoked potentials following diazepam or fentanyl. Anaesthesia 42:195–198, 1987.

Allen, D., Baylav, A. and Lader, M., A comparative study of the interaction of alcohol with alpidem, lorazepam and placebo in normal subjects. Int. Clin. Psychopharmacol. 3:327–341, 1988.

Milligan, K. R., Lumsden, J., Howard, R. C., Howe, J. P. and Dundee, J. W., Use of auditory evoked responses as a measure of recovery from benzodiazepine sedation. J. R. Soc. Med. 82:595–597, 1989.

Shinotoh, H., Iyo, M., Yamada, T., Inoue, O., Suzuki, K., Itoh, T., Fukuda, H., Yamasaki, T., Tateno, Y. and Hirayama, K., Detection of benzodiazepine receptor occupancy in the human brain by positron emission tomography. Psychopharmacology (Berl.) 99:202–207, 1989.

Noldy, N. E., Neiman, J., el-Nesr, B. and Carlen, P. L., Late auditory evoked potentials: a method for monitoring drug effects on the central nervous system. Neuropsychobiology 23:48–52, 1990.

Rockstroh, B., Elbert, T., Lutzenberger, W. and Altenmuller, E., Effects of the anticonvulsant benzodiazepine clonazepam on event-related brain potentials in humans. Electroencephalogr. Clin. Neurophysiol. 78:142–149, 1991.

Bond, A. J., Silveira, J. C. and Lader, M. H., The effects of alprazolam alone and combined with alcohol on central integrative activity. Eur. J. Clin. Pharmacol. 42:495–498, 1992.

Engelhardt, W., Friess, K., Hartung, E., Sold, M. and Dierks, T., EEG and auditory evoked potential P300 compared with psychometric tests in assessing vigilance after benzodiazepine sedation and antagonism. Br. J. Anaesth. 69:75–80, 1992.

Schwender, D., Klasing, S., Madler, C., Poppel, E. and Peter, K., Effects of benzodiazepines on mid-latency auditory evoked potentials. Can. J. Anaesth. 40:1148–1154, 1993.

Semlitsch, H. V., Anderer, P. and Saletu, B., Acute effects of the anxiolytics suriclone and alprazolam on cognitive information processing utilizing topographic mapping of event-related brain potentials (P300) in healthy subjects. Eur. J. Clin. Pharmacol. 49:183–191, 1995.

Unrug, A., van Luijtelaar, E. L., Coles, M. G. and Coenen, A. M., Event-related potentials in a passive and active auditory condition: effects of diazepam and buspirone on slow wave positivity. Biol. Psychol. 46:101–111, 1997.

Nakagome, K., Ichikawa, I., Kanno, O., Akaho, R., Suzuki, M., Takazawa, S., Watanabe, H. and Kazamatsuri, H., Overnight effects of triazolam on cognitive function: an event-related potentials study. Neuropsychobiology 38:232–240, 1998.

VISUAL ERPs

Ebe, M., Meier-Ewert, K. H. and Broughton, R., Effects of intravenous diazepam (valium) upon evoked potentials of photosensitive epileptic and normal subjects. Electroencephalogr. Clin. Neurophysiol. 27:429–435, 1969.

Boker, T. and Heinze, H. J., Influence of diazepam on visual pattern-evoked potentials with due regard to nonstationary effects. Methodological problems. Neuropsychobiology 11:207–212, 1984.

Loughnan, B. L., Sebel, P. S., Thomas, D., Rutherfoord, C. F. and Rogers, H., Evoked potentials following diazepam or fentanyl. Anaesthesia 42:195–198, 1987.

Rockstroh, B., Elbert, T., Lutzenberger, W. and Altenmuller, E., Effects of the anticonvulsant benzodiazepine clonazepam on event-related brain potentials in humans. Electroencephalogr. Clin. Neurophysiol. 78:142–149, 1991.

Krull, K. R., Smith, L. T. and Parsons, O. A., Simple reaction time event-related potentials: effects of alcohol and diazepam. Prog. Neuropsychopharmacol. Biol. Psychiatry 18:1247–1260, 1994.

Pang, E. and Fowler, B., Discriminating the effects of triazolam on stimulus and response processing by means of reaction time and P300 latency. Psychopharmacology (Berl.) 115:509–515, 1994.

Nichols, J. M. and Martin, F., The effect of lorazepam on memory and event-related potentials in heavy and light social drinkers. Psychophysiology 33:446–456, 1996.

Bauer, L. O., Gross, J. B., Meyer, R. E. and Greenblatt, D. J., Chronic alcohol abuse and the acute sedative and neurophysiologic effects of midazolam. Psychopharmacology (Berl.) 133:293–299, 1997.

OTHER ERPs

Loughnan, B. L., Sebel, P. S., Thomas, D., Rutherfoord, C. F. and Rogers, H., Evoked potentials following diazepam or fentanyl. Anaesthesia 42:195–198, 1987.

Rockstroh, B., Elbert, T., Lutzenberger, W. and Altenmuller, E., Effects of the anticonvulsant benzodiazepine clonazepam on event-related brain potentials in humans. Electroencephalogr. Clin. Neurophysiol. 78:142–149, 1991.

van Leeuwen, T. H., Verbaten, M. N., Koelega, H. S., Kenemans, J. L. and Slangen, J. L., Effects of bromazepam on single-trial event-related potentials in a visual vigilance task. Psychopharmacology (Berl.) 106:555–564, 1992.

Coulthard, P. and Rood, J. P., Midazolam and somatosensory evoked potentials. Br. J. Oral Maxillofac. Surg. 31:28–31, 1993.

Nichols, J. M. and Martin, F., P300 in heavy social drinkers: the effect of lorazepam. Alcohol 10:269–274, 1993.

Lauer, K., Munshi, C. and Larson, S., The effect of midazolam on median nerve somatosensory evoked potentials. J. Clin. Monit. 10:181–184, 1994.

Nichols, J. M. and Martin, F., The effect of lorazepam on memory and event-related potentials in heavy and light social drinkers. Psychophysiology 33:446–456, 1996.

Nichols, J. M. and Martin, F., The effect of heavy social drinking on recall and event-related potentials. J. Stud. Alcohol 57:125–135, 1996.

Langeron, O., Lille, F., Zerhouni, O., Orliaguet, G., Saillant, G., Riou, B. and Coriat, P., Comparison of the effects of ketamine-midazolam with those of fentanyl- midazolam on cortical somatosensory evoked potentials during major spine surgery. Br. J. Anaesth. 78:701–706, 1997.

Curran, H. V., Pooviboonsuk, P., Dalton, J. A. and Lader, M. H., Differentiating the effects of centrally acting drugs on arousal and memory: an event-related potential study of scopolamine, lorazepam and diphenhydramine. Psychopharmacology (Berl.) 135:27–36, 1998.

Effects in Social Drinking Populations

Nichols, J. M. and Martin, F., P300 in heavy social drinkers: the effect of lorazepam. Alcohol 10:269–274, 1993.

Nichols, J. M. and Martin, F., The effect of lorazepam on memory and event-related potentials in heavy and light social drinkers. Psychophysiology 33:446–456, 1996.

Nichols, J. M. and Martin, F., The effect of heavy social drinking on recall and event-related potentials. J. Stud. Alcohol 57:125–135, 1996.

Benzodiazepines in Alcoholics

Saletu, M., Saletu, B., Grunberger, J., Mader, R. and Karobath, M., Clinical symptomatology and computer analyzed EEG before, during and after anxiolytic therapy of alcohol withdrawal patients. Neuropsychobiology 9:119–134, 1983.

Mouradian, M. D. and Penovich, P. E., Spindle coma in benzodiazepine toxicity: case report. Clin. Electroencephalogr. 16:213–218, 1985. [Case Report]

Schwarz-Ottersbach, E. and Goldberg, L., Activation levels, EEG, and behavioural responses. Int. J. Psychophysiol. 4:7–17, 1986.

Bauer, L. O., Gross, J. B., Meyer, R. E. and Greenblatt, D. J., Chronic alcohol abuse and the acute sedative and neurophysiologic effects of midazolam. Psychopharmacology (Berl.) 133:293–299, 1997.

Withdrawal

Hallstrom, C. and Lader, M., Benzodiazepine withdrawal phenomena. Int. Pharmacopsychiatry 16:235–244, 1981.

Petursson, H. and Lader, M. H., Withdrawal from long-term benzodiazepine treatment. Br. Med. J. (Clin. Res. Ed.) 283:643–635, 1981.

Manmaru, S. and Matsuura, M., Two kinds of spatiotemporal EEG changes after discontinuation of benzodiazepine, medazepam. Jpn. J. Psychiatry Neurol. 44:85–90, 1990.

Reviews

Fink, M., EEG and human psychopharmacology. Annu. Rev. Pharmacol. 9:241–258, 1969.

Lader, M., Benzodiazepine dependence. Prog. Neuropsychopharmacol. Biol. Psychiatry 8:85–95, 1984.

Barbiturates

Fink, M., Shapiro, D. M. and Itil, T. M., EEG profiles of fenfluramine, amobarbital and dextroamphetamine in normal volunteers. Psychopharmacologia 22:369–383, 1971.

Frowein, H. W., Gaillard, A. W. and Varey, C. A., EP components, visual processing stages, and the effect of a barbiturate. Biol. Psychol. 13:239–249, 1981.

Logar, C., Grabmair, W., Reinbacher, N. and Ladurner, G., EEG changes in the withdrawal phase of tranquilizer or drug abuse. EEG EMG Z. Elektroenzephalogr. Verwandte Geb. 17:37–40, 1986. [German]

McPherson, R. W., Sell, B. and Traystman, R. J., Effects of thiopental, fentanyl, and etomidate on upper extremity somatosensory evoked potentials in humans. Anesthesiology 65:584–589, 1986.

Mizuki, Y., Hamasaki, J., Hirano, H., Miyoshi, A., Yamada, M. and Inanaga, K., Effects of centrally acting drugs on the frontal midline theta activity in man. Jpn. J. Psychiatry Neurol. 40:647–653, 1986.

Schwarz-Ottersbach, E. and Goldberg, L., Activation levels, EEG, and behavioural responses. Int. J. Psychophysiol. 4:7–17, 1986.

Lukas, S. E., Mendelson, J. H., Amass, L. and Benedikt, R., Behavioral and EEG studies of acute cocaine administration: comparisons with morphine, amphetamine, pentobarbital, nicotine, ethanol and marijuana. NIDA Res. Monogr. 95:146–151, 1989.

Feshchenko, V. A., Veselis, R. A. and Reinsel, R. A., Comparison of the EEG effects of midazolam, thiopental, and propofol: the role of underlying oscillatory systems. Neuropsychobiology 35:211–220, 1997.

Fowler, B. and Mitchell, I., Biological determinants of P300: the effects of a barbiturate on latency and amplitude. Biol. Psychol. 46:113–124, 1997.

Heroin and Opiates

Heroin

Acute Administration

Lewis, S. A., Oswald, I., Evans, J. I., Akindele, M. O. and Tompsett, S. L., Heroin and human sleep. Electroencephalogr. Clin. Neurophysiol. 28:374–381, 1970.

Volavka, J., Zaks, A., Roubicek, J. and Fink, M., Electrographic effects of diacetylmorphine (heroin) and naloxone in man. Neuropharmacology 9:587–593, 1970.

Volavka, J., Zaks, A., Roubicek, J. and Fink, M., Acute EEG effects of heroin and naloxone. Electroencephalogr. Clin. Neurophysiol. 165, 1971.

Volavka, J., Levine, R., Feldstein, S. and Fink, M., Short-term effects of heroin in man. Is EEG related to behavior? Arch. Gen. Psychiatry 30:677–681, 1974.

Chronic Administration

Feinstein, B., EEG findings in heroin addicts during induction and maintenance on methadone. Electroencephalogr. Clin. Neurophysiol. 39:96–99, 1975.

Olivennes, A., Comparison of awake electroencephalography tracings of alcoholics and heroin addicts. Study of 2 groups of 70 and 51 patients. Ann. Med. Psychol. (Paris) 145:546–552, 1987. [French]

Shufman, E., Perl, E., Cohen, M., Dickman, M., Gandaku, D., Adler, D., Veler, A., Bar-Hamburger, R. and Ginath, Y., Electro-encephalography spectral analysis of heroin addicts compared with abstainers and normal controls. Isr. J. Psychiatry Relat. Sci. 33:196–206, 1996.

Withdrawal

Howe, R. C., Hegge, F. W. and Phillips, J. L., Acute heroin abstinence in man: I. Changes in behavior and sleep. Drug Alcohol Depend. 5:341–356, 1980a.

Howe, R. C., Hegge, F. W. and Phillips, J. L., Acute heroin abstinence in man: II. Alterations in rapid eye movement (REM) sleep. Drug Alcohol Depend. 6:149–161, 1980b.

Howe, R. C., Phillips, J. L. and Hegge, F. W., Acute heroin abstinence in man. III. Effect upon waking and slow wave sleep. Drug Alcohol Depend. 6:247–262, 1980c.

Howe, R. C., Phillips, J. L. and Hegge, F. W., Acute heroin abstinence in man: IV. Sleep—waking state contingencies. Drug Alcohol Depend. 7:163–176, 1981.

Abstinence

Gritz, E. R., Shiffman, S. M., Jarvik, M. E., Haber, J., Dymond, A. M., Coger, R., Charuvastra, V. and Schlesinger, J., Physiological and psychological effects of methadone in man. Arch. Gen. Psychiatry 32:237–242, 1975.

Kouri, E. M., Lukas, S. E. and Mendelson, J. H., P300 assessment of opiate and cocaine users: effects of detoxification and buprenorphine treatment. Biol. Psychiatry 40:617–628, 1996.

Shufman, E., Perl, E., Cohen, M., Dickman, M., Gandaku, D., Adler, D., Veler, A., Bar-Hamburger, R. and Ginath, Y., Electro-encephalography spectral analysis of heroin addicts compared with abstainers and normal controls. Isr. J. Psychiatry Relat. Sci. 33:196–206, 1996.

Costa, L. and Bauer, L., Quantitative electroencephalographic differences associated with alcohol, cocaine, heroin and dual-substance dependence. Drug Alcohol Depend. 46:87–93, 1997.

Bauer, L. O., Effects of chronic opioid dependence and HIV-1 infection on pattern shift visual evoked potentials. Drug Alcohol Depend. 50:147–155, 1998.

Treatment

Feinstein, B., EEG findings in heroin addicts during induction and maintenance on methadone. Electroencephalogr. Clin. Neurophysiol. 39:96–99, 1975.

Gritz, E. R., Shiffman, S. M., Jarvik, M. E., Haber, J., Dymond, A. M., Coger, R., Charuvastra, V. and Schlesinger, J., Physiological and psychological effects of methadone in man. Arch. Gen. Psychiatry 32:237–242, 1975.

Kay, D. C., Human sleep and EEG through a cycle of methadone dependence. Electroencephalogr. Clin. Neurophysiol. 35–43, 1975.

Kay, D. C., Pickworth, W. B., Neidert, G. L., Falcone, D., Fishman, P. M. and Othmer, E., Opioid effects on computer-derived sleep and EEG parameters in nondependent human addicts. Sleep 2:175–191, 1979.

Herning, R. I., Guo, X. and Lange, W. R., The effects of nimodipine on the EEG of substance abusers. Ann. N. Y. Acad. Sci. 765:143–151, 1995.

Herning, R. I., Guo, X. and Lange, W. R., Nimodipine improves information processing in substance abusers. Ann. N. Y. Acad. Sci. 765:152–159, 1995.

Kouri, E. M., Lukas, S. E. and Mendelson, J. H., P300 assessment of opiate and cocaine users: effects of detoxification and buprenorphine treatment. Biol. Psychiatry 40:617–628, 1996.

Staedt, J., Wassmuth, F., Stoppe, G., Hajak, G., Rodenbeck, A., Poser, W. and Ruther, E., Effects of chronic treatment with methadone and naltrexone on sleep in addicts. Eur. Arch. Psychiatry Clin. Neurosci. 246:305–309, 1996.

Prenatal Exposure

Guo, X., Spencer, J. W., Suess, P. E., Hickey, J. E., Better, W. E. and Herning, R. I., Cognitive brain potential alterations in boys exposed to opiates: in utero and lifestyle comparisons. Addict. Behav. 19:429–441, 1994.

Morphine

Kay, D. C., Human sleep during chronic morphine intoxication. Psychopharmacologia 44:117–124, 1975.

Kay, D. C., Pickworth, W. B., Neidert, G. L., Falcone, D., Fishman, P. M. and Othmer, E., Opioid effects on computer-derived sleep and EEG parameters in nondependent human addicts. Sleep 2:175–191, 1979.

Matejcek, M., Pokorny, R., Ferber, G. and Klee, H., Effect of morphine on the electroencephalogram and other physiological and behavioral parameters. Neuropsychobiology 19:202–211, 1988.

Lukas, S. E., Mendelson, J. H., Amass, L. and Benedikt, R., Behavioral and EEG studies of acute cocaine administration: comparisons with morphine, amphetamine, pentobarbital, nicotine, ethanol and marijuana. NIDA Res. Monogr. 95:146–151, 1989.

Schwender, D., Rimkus, T., Haessler, R., Klasing, S., Poppel, E. and Peter, K., Effects of increasing doses of alfentanil, fentanyl and morphine on mid-latency auditory evoked potentials. Br. J. Anaesth. 71:622–628, 1993.

Phillips, R. L., Herning, R. and London, E. D., Morphine effects on the spontaneous electroencephalogram in polydrug abusers: correlations with subjective self-reports. Neuropsychopharmacology 10:171–181, 1994.

Fentanyl

Velasco, M., Velasco, F., Castaneda, R. and Lee, M., Effect of fentanyl and naloxone on the P300 auditory potential. Neuropharmacology 23:931–938, 1984.

Velasco, M., Velasco, F., Castaneda, R. and Sanchez, R., Effect of fentanyl and naloxone on human somatic and auditory-evoked potential components. Neuropharmacology 23:359–366, 1984.

McPherson, R. W., Sell, B. and Traystman, R. J., Effects of thiopental, fentanyl, and etomidate on upper extremity somatosensory evoked potentials in humans. Anesthesiology 65:584–589, 1986.

Loughnan, B. L., Sebel, P. S., Thomas, D., Rutherfoord, C. F. and Rogers, H., Evoked potentials following diazepam or fentanyl. Anaesthesia 42:195–198, 1987.

Thurner, F., Schramm, J. and Pasch, T., Effect of fentanyl and enflurane on sensory evoked potentials in the human in basic flunitrazepam/N2O anesthesia. Anaesthesist 36:548–554, 1987. [German]

Scott, J. C., Cooke, J. E. and Stanski, D. R., Electroencephalographic quantitation of opioid effect: comparative pharmacodynamics of fentanyl and sufentanil. Anesthesiology 74:34–42, 1991.

Inoue, T., Kawasaki, H., Shiraishi, S. and Takasaki, M., Effects of high-dose fentanyl anesthesia on auditory brain stem responses. Masui 41:1414–1418, 1992. [Japanese]

Hou, W. Y., Lee, W. Y., Lin, S. M., Liu, C. C., Susceto, L., Sun, W. Z. and Lin, S. Y., The effects of ketamine, propofol and nitrous oxide on visual evoked potential during fentanyl anesthesia. Ma Tsui Hsueh Tsa Chi 31:97–102, 1993.

Schwender, D., Rimkus, T., Haessler, R., Klasing, S., Poppel, E. and Peter, K., Effects of increasing doses of alfentanil, fentanyl and morphine on mid- latency auditory evoked potentials. Br. J. Anaesth. 71:622–628, 1993.

Lemmens, H. J., Dyck, J. B., Shafer, S. L. and Stanski, D. R., Pharmacokinetic-pharmacodynamic modeling in drug development: application to the investigational opioid trefentanil. Clin. Pharmacol. Ther. 56:261–271, 1994.

Langeron, O., Lille, F., Zerhouni, O., Orliaguet, G., Saillant, G., Riou, B. and Coriat, P., Comparison of the effects of ketamine-midazolam with those of fentanyl- midazolam on cortical somatosensory evoked potentials during major spine surgery. Br. J. Anaesth. 78:701–706, 1997.

Other Opiates

Pfefferbaum, A., Roth, W. T., Tinklenberg, J. R., Rosenbloom, M. J. and Kopell, B. S., The effects of ethanol and meperidine on auditory evoked potentials. Drug Alcohol Depend. 4:371–380, 1979.

Bromm, B., Meier, W. and Scharein, E., Pre-stimulus/post-stimulus relations in EEG spectra and their modulations by an opioid and an antidepressant. Electroencephalogr. Clin. Neurophysiol. 73:188–197, 1989.

Scott, J. C., Cooke, J. E. and Stanski, D. R., Electroencephalographic quantitation of opioid effect: comparative pharmacodynamics of fentanyl and sufentanil. Anesthesiology 74:34–42, 1991.

Lemmens, H. J., Egan, T. D., Fiset, P. and Stanski, D. R., Pharmacokinetic/dynamic assessment in drug development: application to the investigational opioid mirfentanil. Anesth. Analg. 80:1206–1211, 1995.

Schwender, D., Weninger, E., Schnatmann, N., Mulzer, S., Klasing, S. and Peter, K., Acoustic evoked potentials mid-latency following anesthesia with sufentanil. Anaesthesist 44:478–482, 1995. [German]

Cocaine

Acute Administration

EEG

Herning, R. I., Jones, R. T., Hooker, W. D., Mendelson, J. and Blackwell, L., Cocaine increases EEG beta: a replication and extension of Hans Berger's historic experiments. Electroencephalogr. Clin. Neurophysiol. 60:470–477, 1985.

Lukas, S. E., Mendelson, J. H., Amass, L. and Benedikt, R., Behavioral and EEG studies of acute cocaine administration: comparisons with morphine, amphetamine, pentobarbital, nicotine, ethanol and marijuana. NIDA Res. Monogr. 95:146–151, 1989.

Conway, E. E., Jr., Mezey, A. P. and Powers, K., Status epilepticus following the oral ingestion of cocaine in an infant. Pediatr. Emerg. Care 6:189–190, 1990. [Case Report]

Pascual-Leone, A., Dhuna, A., Altafullah, I. and Anderson, D. C., Cocaine-induced seizures. Neurology 40:404–407, 1990.

Herning, R. I., Glover, B. J., Koeppl, B., Phillips, R. L. and London, E. D., Cocaine-induced increases in EEG alpha and beta activity: evidence for reduced cortical processing. Neuropsychopharmacology 11:1–9, 1994.

Rothman, R. B., Gorelick, D. A., Baumann, M. H., Guo, X. Y., Herning, R. I., Pickworth, W. B., Gendron, T. M., Koeppl, B., Thomson, L. E., 3rd and Henningfield, J. E., Lack of evidence for context-dependent cocaine-induced sensitization in humans: preliminary studies. Pharmacol. Biochem. Behav. 49:583–588, 1994.

Sleep EEG

Watson, R., Bakos, L., Compton, P. and Gawin, F., Cocaine use and withdrawal: the effect on sleep and mood. Am. J. Drug Alcohol Abuse 18:21–28, 1992.

Auditory ERPs

Herning, R. I., Jones, R. T., Hooker, W. D. and Tulunay, F. C., Information processing components of the auditory event related potential are reduced by cocaine. Psychopharmacology (Berl.) 87:178–185, 1985.

Herning, R. I., Hooker, W. D. and Jones, R. T., Cocaine effects on electroencephalographic cognitive event-related potentials and performance. Electroencephalogr. Clin. Neurophysiol. 66:34–42, 1987.

Herning, R. I., Glover, B. J. and Guo, X., Effects of cocaine on P3B in cocaine abusers. Neuropsychobiology 30:132–142, 1994.

Chronic Administration

EEG

Pascual-Leone, A., Dhuna, A., Altafullah, I. and Anderson, D. C., Cocaine-induced seizures. Neurology 40:404–407, 1990.

Dhuna, A., Pascual-Leone, A. and Langendorf, F., Chronic, habitual cocaine abuse and kindling-induced epilepsy: a case report. Epilepsia 32:890–894, 1991. [Case Report]

Braverman, E. R. and Blum, K., Substance use disorder exacerbates brain electrophysiological abnormalities in a psychiatrically-ill population. Clin. Electroencephalogr. 27 (4 Suppl.): 5–27, 1996.

Moak, D. H. and Anton, R. F., Alcohol-related seizures and the kindling effect of repeated detoxifications: the influence of cocaine. Alcohol Alcohol. 31:135–143, 1996.

Costa, L. and Bauer, L., Quantitative electroencephalographic differences associated with alcohol, cocaine, heroin and dual-substance dependence. Drug Alcohol Depend. 46:87–93, 1997.

Auditory ERPs

Pickworth, W. B., Brown, B. S., Hickey, J. E. and Muntaner, C., Effects of self-reported drug use and antisocial behavior on evoked potentials in adolescents. Drug Alcohol Depend. 25:105–110, 1990.

Braverman, E. R. and Blum, K., Substance use disorder exacerbates brain electrophysiological abnormalities in a psychiatrically-ill population. Clin. Electroencephalogr. 27 (4 Suppl.): 5–27, 1996.

Kouri, E. M., Lukas, S. E. and Mendelson, J. H., P300 assessment of opiate and cocaine users: effects of detoxification and buprenorphine treatment. Biol. Psychiatry 40:617-628, 1996.

Visual ERPs

Braverman, E. R. and Blum, K., Substance use disorder exacerbates brain electrophysiological abnormalities in a psychiatrically-ill population. Clin. Electroencephalogr. 27 (4 Suppl.): 5–27, 1996.

Withdrawal

EEG

Alper, K. R., Chabot, R. J., Kim, A. H., Prichep, L. S. and John, E. R., Quantitative EEG correlates of crack cocaine dependence. Psychiatry Res. 35:95–105, 1990.

Bauer, L. O., Vigilance in recovering cocaine-dependent and alcohol-dependent patients: a prospective study. Addict. Behav. 19:599–607, 1994.

Bauer, L. O. and Kranzler, H. R., Electroencephalographic activity and mood in cocaine-dependent outpatients: effects of cocaine cue exposure. Biol. Psychiatry 36:189–197, 1994.

Noldy, N. E., Santos, C. V., Politzer, N., Blair, R. D. and Carlen, P. L., Quantitative EEG changes in cocaine withdrawal: evidence for long-term CNS effects. Neuropsychobiology 30:189–196, 1994.

Moak, D. H. and Anton, R. F., Alcohol-related seizures and the kindling effect of repeated detoxifications: the influence of cocaine. Alcohol Alcohol. 31:135–143, 1996.

Herning, R. I., Guo, X., Better, W. E., Weinhold, L. L., Lange, W. R., Cadet, J. L. and Gorelick, D. A., Neurophysiological signs of cocaine dependence: increased electroencephalogram beta during withdrawal. Biol. Psychiatry 41:1087–1094, 1997.

Sleep EEG

Kowatch, R. A., Schnoll, S. S., Knisely, J. S., Green, D. and Elswick, R. K., Electroencephalographic sleep and mood during cocaine withdrawal. J. Addict. Dis. 11:21–45, 1992.

Thompson, P. M., Gillin, J. C., Golshan, S. and Irwin, M., Polygraphic sleep measures differentiate alcoholics and stimulant abusers during short-term abstinence. Biol. Psychiatry 38:831–836, 1995.

Auditory ERPs

Bauer, L. O., Vigilance in recovering cocaine-dependent and alcohol-dependent patients: a prospective study. Addict. Behav. 19:599–607, 1994.

Noldy, N. E. and Carlen, P. L., Event-related potential changes in cocaine withdrawal: evidence for long-term cognitive effects. Neuropsychobiology 36:53–56, 1997.

Craving

Bauer, L. O. and Kranzler, H. R., Electroencephalographic activity and mood in cocaine-dependent outpatients: effects of cocaine cue exposure. Biol. Psychiatry 36:189–197, 1994.

Hersh, D., Bauer, L. O. and Kranzler, H. R., Carbamazepine and cocaine-cue reactivity. Drug Alcohol Depend. 39:213–221, 1995.

Liu, X., Vaupel, D. B., Gran, S. and London, E. D., Effect of cocaine-related environmental stimuli on the spontaneous electroencephalogram in polydrug abusers. Neuropsychopharmacology 19:10–17, 1998.

Abstinence

EEG

Alper, K. R., Chabot, R. J., Kim, A. H., Prichep, L. S. and John, E. R., Quantitative EEG correlates of crack cocaine dependence. Psychiatry Res. 35:95–105, 1990.

Bauer, L. O., Photic driving of EEG alpha activity in recovering cocaine-dependent and alcohol-dependent patients. Am. J. Addict. 3:49–57, 1993.

Bauer, L. O., Vigilance in recovering cocaine-dependent and alcohol-dependent patients: a prospective study. Addict. Behav. 19:599–607, 1994.

Bauer, L. O. and Kranzler, H. R., Electroencephalographic activity and mood in cocaine-dependent outpatients: effects of cocaine cue exposure. Biol. Psychiatry 36:189–197, 1994.

Noldy, N. E., Santos, C. V., Politzer, N., Blair, R. D. and Carlen, P. L., Quantitative EEG changes in cocaine withdrawal: evidence for long-term CNS effects. Neuropsychobiology 30:189–196, 1994.

Roemer, R. A., Cornwell, A., Dewart, D., Jackson, P. and Ercegovac, D. V., Quantitative electroencephalographic analyses in cocaine-preferring polysubstance abusers during abstinence. Psychiatry Res. 58:247–257, 1995.

Prichep, L. S., Alper, K. R., Kowalik, S., Merkin, H., Tom, M., John, E. R. and Rosenthal, M. S., Quantitative electroencephalographic characteristics of crack cocaine dependence. Biol. Psychiatry 40:986–993, 1996.

Costa, L. and Bauer, L., Quantitative electroencephalographic differences associated with alcohol, cocaine, heroin and dual-substance dependence. Drug Alcohol Depend. 46:87–93, 1997.

Herning, R. I., Guo, X., Better, W. E., Weinhold, L. L., Lange, W. R., Cadet, J. L. and Gorelick, D. A., Neurophysiological signs of cocaine dependence: increased electroencephalogram beta during withdrawal. Biol. Psychiatry 41:1087–1094, 1997.

Alper, K. R., Prichep, L. S., Kowalik, S., Rosenthal, M. S. and John, E. R., Persistent QEEG abnormality in crack cocaine users at 6 months of drug abstinence. Neuropsychopharmacology 19:1–9, 1998.

Prichep, L. S., Alper, K. R., Kowalik, S. C., Vaysblat, L. S., Merkin, H. A., Tom, M., John, E. R. and Rosenthal, M. S., Prediction of treatment outcome in cocaine dependent males using quantitative EEG. Drug Alcohol Depend. 54:35–43, 1999.

Sleep EEG

Kowatch, R. A., Schnoll, S. S., Knisely, J. S., Green, D. and Elswick, R. K., Electroencephalographic sleep and mood during cocaine withdrawal. J. Addict. Dis. 11:21–45, 1992.

Auditory ERPs

Bauer, L. O., Vigilance in recovering cocaine-dependent and alcohol-dependent patients: a prospective study. Addict. Behav. 19:599–607, 1994.

Fein, G., Biggins, C. and MacKay, S., Cocaine abusers have reduced auditory P50 amplitude and suppression compared to both normal controls and alcoholics. Biol. Psychiatry 39:955–965, 1996.

Kouri, E. M., Lukas, S. E. and Mendelson, J. H., P300 assessment of opiate and cocaine users: effects of detoxification and buprenorphine treatment. Biol. Psychiatry 40:617–628, 1996.

Biggins, C. A., MacKay, S., Clark, W. and Fein, G., Event-related potential evidence for frontal cortex effects of chronic cocaine dependence. Biol. Psychiatry 42:472–485, 1997.

Visual ERPs

Bauer, L. O. and Easton, C., Pattern shift visual evoked potentials in abstinent cocaine-dependent, alcohol-dependent, and cross-dependent patients. Drug Alcohol Depend. 40:203–209, 1996.

Bauer, L. O., Frontal P300 decrements, childhood conduct disorder, family history, and the prediction of relapse among abstinent cocaine abusers. Drug Alcohol Depend. 44:1–10, 1997.

Biggins, C. A., MacKay, S., Clark, W. and Fein, G., Event-related potential evidence for frontal cortex effects of chronic cocaine dependence. Biol. Psychiatry 42:472–485, 1997.

Other ERPs

Bauer, L. O. and Mott, A. E., Differential effects of cocaine, alcohol, and nicotine dependence on olfactory evoked potentials. Drug Alcohol Depend. 42:21–26, 1996.

Treatment

EEG

Herning, R. I., Guo, X. and Lange, W. R., The effects of nimodipine on the EEG of substance abusers. Ann. N. Y. Acad. Sci. 765:143–151, 1995.

Hersh, D., Bauer, L. O. and Kranzler, H. R., Carbamazepine and cocaine-cue reactivity. Drug Alcohol Depend. 39:213–221, 1995.

Easton, C. J. and Bauer, L. O., Beneficial effects of thiamine on recognition memory and P300 in abstinent cocaine-dependent patients. Psychiatry Res. 70:165–174, 1997.

Auditory ERPs

Herning, R. I., Guo, X. and Lange, W. R., Nimodipine improves information processing in substance abusers. Ann. N. Y. Acad. Sci. 765:152–159, 1995.

Kouri, E. M., Lukas, S. E. and Mendelson, J. H., P300 assessment of opiate and cocaine users: effects of detoxification and buprenorphine treatment. Biol. Psychiatry 40:617–628, 1996.

Brandt, M. E., Visual and auditory evoked phase resetting of the alpha EEG. Int. J. Psychophysiol. 26:285–298, 1997.

Prenatal Exposure

EEG

Doberczak, T. M., Shanzer, S., Senie, R. T. and Kandall, S. R., Neonatal neurologic and electroencephalographic effects of intrauterine cocaine exposure. J. Pediatr. 13:354–358, 1988.

Konkol, R. J., Tikofsky, R. S., Wells, R., Hellman, R. S., Nemeth, P., Walsh, D. J., Heimler, R. and Sty, J. R., Normal high-resolution cerebral 99mTc-HMPAO SPECT scans in symptomatic neonates exposed to cocaine. J. Child Neurol. 9:278–283, 1994.

Prichep, L. S., Kowalik, S. C., Alper, K. and de Jesus, C., Quantitative EEG characteristics of children exposed in utero to cocaine. Clin. Electroencephalogr. 26:166–172, 1995.

Sleep EEG

Legido, A., Clancy, R. R., Spitzer, A. R. and Finnegan, L. P., Electroencephalographic and behavioral-state studies in infants of cocaine-addicted mothers. Am. J. Dis. Child. 146:748–752, 1992.

Visual ERPs

Hansen, R. L., Struthers, J. M. and Gospe, S. M. J., Visual evoked potentials and visual processing in stimulant drug-exposed infants. Dev. Med. Child Neurol. 35:798–805, 1993.

Reviews

Pascual-Leone, A., Dhuna, A. and Anderson, D. C., Longterm neurological complications of chronic, habitual cocaine abuse. Neurotoxicology 12:393–400, 1991.

Bauer, L. O., Psychomotor and electroencephalographic sequelae of cocaine dependence. In: Neurotoxicity and Neuropathology Associated with Cocaine Abuse. Majewska, MD (ed.), NIDA Res. Mono. Vol. 163, Rockville, MD, pp. 66–93, 1996.

Cadet, J. L. and Bolla, K. I., Chronic cocaine use as a neuropsychiatric syndrome: a model for debate. Synapse 22:28–34, 1996.

Prichep, L. S., Alper, K., Kowalik, S. C. and Rosenthal, M., Neurometric QEEG studies of crack cocaine dependence and treatment outcome. J. Addict. Dis. 15:39–53, 1996.

Lukas, S. E. and Renshaw, P. F.: Cocaine Effects on Brain Function. In: Cocaine Abuse: Behavior, Pharmacology, and Clinical Applications, S. T. Higgins and J. L. Katz, (eds.) Academic Press, San Diego, CA, pp. 265–287, 1998.

Strickland, T. L., Miller, B. L., Kowell, A. and Stein, R., Neurobiology of cocaine-induced organic brain impairment: contributions from functional neuroimaging. Neuropsychol. Rev. 8:1–9, 1998.

Amphetamine and Other Stimulants

Acute Administration

EEG

Fink, M., Shapiro, D. M. and Itil, T. M., EEG profiles of fenfluramine, amobarbital and dextroamphetamine in normal volunteers. Psychopharmacologia 22:369–383, 1971.

Hamilton, M. J., Smith, P. R. and Peck, A. W., Effects of bupropion, nomifensine and dexamphetamine on performance, subjective feelings, autonomic variables and electroencephalogram in healthy volunteers. Br. J. Clin. Pharmacol. 15:367–374, 1983.

Lukas, S. E., Mendelson, J. H., Amass, L. and Benedikt, R., Behavioral and EEG studies of acute cocaine administration: comparisons with morphine, amphetamine, pentobarbital, nicotine, ethanol and marijuana. NIDA Res. Monogr. 95:146–151, 1989.

Saletu, B., Barbanoj, M. J., Anderer, P., Sieghart, W. and Grunberger, J., Clinical-pharmacological study with the two isomers (d-, l-) of fenfluramine and its comparison with chlorpromazine and d-amphetamine: blood levels, EEG mapping and safety evaluation. Methods Find. Exp. Clin. Pharmacol. 15:291–312, 1993.

Caldwell, J. A., Caldwell, J. L., Crowley, J. S. and Jones, H. D., Sustaining helicopter pilot performance with Dexedrine during periods of sleep deprivation. Aviat. Space Environ. Med. 66:930–937, 1995.

Slattum, P. W., Venitz, J. and Barr, W. H., Comparison of methods for the assessment of central nervous system stimulant response after dextroamphetamine administration to healthy male volunteers. J. Clin. Pharmacol. 36:1039–1050, 1996.

Sleep EEG

Saletu, B., Frey, R., Krupka, M., Anderer, P., Grunberger, J. and Barbanoj, M. J., Differential effects of the new central adrenergic agonist modafinil and d-amphetamine on sleep and early morning behaviour in elderlies. Arzneimittelforschung 39:1268–1273, 1989.

Saletu, B., Frey, R., Krupka, M., Anderer, P., Grunberger, J. and Barbanoj, M. J., Differential effects of a new central adrenergic agonist—modafinil—and D-amphetamine on sleep and early morning behaviour in young healthy volunteers. Int. J. Clin. Pharmacol. Res. 9:183–195, 1989.

Thompson, P. M., Gillin, J. C., Golshan, S. and Irwin, M., Polygraphic sleep measures differentiate alcoholics and stimulant abusers during short-term abstinence. Biol. Psychiatry 38:831–836, 1995.

Auditory ERPs

Herrmann, W. M., Hofmann, W. and Kubicki, S., Psychotropic drug induced changes in auditory averaged evoked potentials: results of a double-blind trial using an objective fully automated AEP analysis method. Int. J. Clin. Pharmacol. Ther. Toxicol. 19:56–62, 1981.

McKetin, R., Ward, P. B., Catts, S. V., Mattick, R. P. and Bell, J. R., Changes in auditory selective attention and event-related potentials following oral administration of D-amphetamine in humans. Neuropsychopharmacology 21:380–390, 1999.

Visual ERPs

Fowler, B. and Adams, J., Dissociation of the effects of alcohol and amphetamine on inert gas narcosis using reaction time and P300 latency. Aviat. Space Environ. Med. 64:493–499, 1993.

Chronic Administration

Pickworth, W. B., Brown, B. S., Hickey, J. E. and Muntaner, C., Effects of self-reported drug use and antisocial behavior on evoked potentials in adolescents. Drug Alcohol Depend. 25:105–110, 1990.

Khattab, N. Y. and Amer, G., Undetected neuropsychophysiological sequelae of khat chewing in standard aviation medical examination. Aviat. Space Environ. Med. 66:739–744, 1995.

Thompson, P. M., Gillin, J. C., Golshan, S. and Irwin, M., Polygraphic sleep measures differentiate alcoholics and stimulant abusers during short-term abstinence. Biol. Psychiatry 38:831–836, 1995.

McKetin, R. and Solowij, N., Event-related potential indices of auditory selective attention in dependent amphetamine users. Biol. Psychiatry 45:1488–1497, 1999.

Prenatal Exposure

Hansen, R. L., Struthers, J. M. and Gospe, S. M. J., Visual evoked potentials and visual processing in stimulant drug-exposed infants. Dev. Med. Child Neurol. 35:798–805, 1993.

Methamphetamine

Weiss, S. R., Raskind, R., Morganstern, N. L., Pytlyk, P. J. and Baiz, T. C., Intracerebral and subarachnoid hemorrhage following use of methamphetamine ("speed"). Int. Surg. 53:123–127, 1970. [Case Report]

Iwanami, A., Kato, N. and Nakatani, Y., P300 in methamphetamine psychosis. Biol. Psychiatry 30:726–730, 1991.

Iwanami, A., Suga, I., Kaneko, T., Sugiyama, A. and Nakatani, Y., P300 component of event-related potentials in methamphetamine psychosis and schizophrenia. Prog. Neuropsychopharmacol. Biol. Psychiatry 18:465–475, 1994.

Iwanami, A., Kanamori, R., Suga, I., Kaneko, T. and Kamijima, K., Reduced attention-related negative potentials in methamphetamine psychosis. J. Nerv. Ment. Dis. 183:693–697, 1995.

Iwanami, A., Kuroki, N., Iritani, S., Isono, H., Okajima, Y. and Kamijima, K., P3a of event-related potential in chronic methamphetamine dependence. J. Nerv. Ment. Dis. 186:746–751, 1998.

Methylphenidate

Coons, H. W., Peloquin, L. J., Klorman, R., Bauer, L. O., Ryan, R. M., Perlmutter, R. A. and Salzman, L. F., Effect of methylphenidate on young adult's vigilance and event-related potentials. Electroencephalogr. Clin. Neurophysiol. 51:373–387, 1981.

Klorman, R., Bauer, L. O., Coons, H. W., Lewis, J. L., Peloquin, J., Perlmutter, R. A., Ryan, R. M., Salzman, L. F. and Strauss, J., Enhancing effects of methylphenidate on normal young adults' cognitive processes. Psychopharmacol. Bull. 20:3–9, 1984.

Strauss, J., Lewis, J. L., Klorman, R., Peloquin, L. J., Perlmutter, R. A. and Salzman, L. F., Effects of methylphenidate on young adults' performance and event-related potentials in a vigilance and a paired-associates learning test. Psychophysiology 21:609–621, 1984.

Naylor, H., Halliday, R. and Callaway, E., The effect of methylphenidate on information processing. Psychopharmacology (Berl.) 86:90–95, 1985.

Mizuki, Y., Hamasaki, J., Hirano, H., Miyoshi, A., Yamada, M. and Inanaga, K., Effects of centrally acting drugs on the frontal midline theta activity in man. Jpn. J. Psychiatry Neurol. 40:647–653, 1986.

Peloquin, L. J. and Klorman, R., Effects of methylphenidate on normal children's mood, event-related potentials, and performance in memory scanning and vigilance. J. Abnorm. Psychol. 95:88–98, 1986.

Oken, B. S., Kishiyama, S. S. and Salinsky, M. C., Pharmacologically induced changes in arousal: effects on behavioral and electrophysiologic measures of alertness and attention. Electroencephalogr. Clin. Neurophysiol. 95:359–371, 1995.

Review

Klorman, R. and Brumaghim, J. T., Stimulant drugs and ERPs. Electroencephalogr. Clin. Neurophysiol. Suppl. 42:135–141, 1991.

Solvents and Toluene

Acute Administration

Pierce, C. H., Becker, C. E., Tozer, T. N., Owen, D. J. and So, Y., Modeling the acute neurotoxicity of styrene. J. Occup. Environ. Med. 40:230–240, 1998.

Chronic Administration

EEG

Knox, J. W. and Nelson, J. R., Permanent encephalopathy from toluene inhalation. N. Engl. J. Med. 275:1494–1496, 1966. [Case Report]

King, M. D., Neurological sequelae of toluene abuse. Hum. Toxicol. 1:281–287, 1982.

Hormes, J. T., Filley, C. M. and Rosenberg, N. L., Neurologic sequelae of chronic solvent vapor abuse. Neurology 36:698–702, 1986.

Tomczak, J. W., Kocur, J. and Sobotka, H., Alcohol intoxication in teenagers using inhalant stupefacients. Pol. J. Pharmacol. Pharm. 41:203–206, 1989.

Ottelio, C., Giagheddu, M. and Marrosu, F., Altered EEG pattern in aromatic hydrocarbon intoxication: a case report. Acta Neurol. (Napoli) 15:357–362, 1993. [Case Report]

Auditory ERPs

Metrick, S. A. and Brenner, R. P., Abnormal brainstem auditory evoked potentials in chronic paint sniffers. Ann. Neurol. 12:553–556, 1982. [Case Report]

Lazar, R. B., Ho, S. U., Melen, O. and Daghestani, A. N., Multifocal central nervous system damage caused by toluene abuse. Neurology 33:1337–1340, 1983. [Case Report]

Hormes, J. T., Filley, C. M. and Rosenberg, N. L., Neurologic sequelae of chronic solvent vapor abuse. Neurology 36:698–702, 1986.

Rosenberg, N. L., Spitz, M. C., Filley, C. M., Davis, K. A. and Schaumburg, H. H., Central nervous system effects of chronic toluene abuse—clinical, brainstem evoked response and magnetic resonance imaging studies. Neurotoxicol. Teratol. 10:489–495, 1988.

Morrow, L. A., Steinhauer, S. R. and Hodgson, M. J., Delay in P300 latency in patients with organic solvent exposure. Arch. Neurol. 49:315–320, 1992.

Occupational Exposure

EEG

Seppalainen, A. M., Husman, K. and Martenson, C., Neurophysiological effects of long-term exposure to a mixture of organic solvents. Scand. J. Work Environ. Health 4:304–314, 1978.

Biscaldi, G. P., Mingardi, M., Pollini, G., Moglia, A. and Bossi, M. C., Acute toluene poisoning. Electroneurophysiological and vestibular investigations. Toxicol. Eur. Res. 3:271–273, 1981.

Arai, K., Tokumaru, Y., Yagishita, T., Hirayama, K. and Iwasaki, I., Chronic toluene intoxication and hyperkinesie volitionnelle. No To Shinkei 38:1181–1186, 1986. [Case Report] [Japanese]

Orbaek, P., Rosen, I. and Svensson, K., Power spectrum analysis of EEG at diagnosis and follow up of patients with solvent induced chronic toxic encephalopathy. Br. J. Ind. Med. 45:476–482, 1988.

Szyrocka-Szwed, K., Evaluation of the nervous system with reference to the bioelectric activity of the brain and neural conduction in workers exposed to organic solvents. Med. Pr. 40:342–349, 1989. [Polish]

Tomczak, J. W., Kocur, J. and Sobotka, H., Alcohol intoxication in teenagers using inhalant stupefacients. Pol. J. Pharmacol. Pharm. 41:203–206, 1989.

Indulski, J. A., Sinczuk-Walczak, H., Szymczak, M. and Wesolowski, W., Neurological and neurophysiological examinations of workers occupationally exposed to organic solvent mixtures used in the paint and varnish production. Int. J. Occup. Med. Environ. Health 9:235–244, 1996.

Lindgren, M., Osterberg, K., Orbaek, P. and Rosen, I., Solvent-induced toxic encephalopathy: electrophysiological data in relation to neuropsychological findings. J. Clin. Exp. Neuropsychol. 19:772–783, 1997.

Auditory ERPs

Morrow, L. A., Steinhauer, S. R. and Hodgson, M. J., Delay in P300 latency in patients with organic solvent exposure. Arch. Neurol. 49:315–320, 1992.

Vrca, A., Karacic, V., Bozicevic, D., Bozikov, V. and Malinar, M., Brainstem auditory evoked potentials in individuals exposed to long- term low concentrations of toluene. Am. J. Ind. Med. 30:62–66, 1996.

Vrca, A., Bozicevic, D., Bozikov, V., Fuchs, R. and Malinar, M., Brain stem evoked potentials and visual evoked potentials in relation to the length of occupational exposure to low levels of toluene. Acta Med. Croatica 51:215–219, 1997.

Steinhauer, S. R., Morrow, L. A., Condray, R. and Dougherty, G. G., Event-related potentials in workers with ongoing occupational exposure. Biol. Psychiatry 42:854–858, 1997.

Visual ERPs

Urban, P. and Lukas, E., Visual evoked potentials in rotogravure printers exposed to toluene. Br. J. Ind. Med. 47:819–823, 1990.

Vrca, A., Bozicevic, D., Karacic, V., Fuchs, R., Prpic-Majic, D. and Malinar, M., Visual evoked potentials in individuals exposed to long-term low concentrations of toluene. Arch. Toxicol. 69:337–340, 1995.

Indulski, J. A., Sinczuk-Walczak, H., Szymczak, M. and Wesolowski, W., Neurological and neurophysiological examinations of workers occupationally exposed to organic solvent mixtures used in the paint and varnish production. Int. J. Occup. Med. Environ. Health 9:235–244, 1996.

Vrca, A., Bozicevic, D., Bozikov, V., Fuchs, R. and Malinar, M., Brain stem evoked potentials and visual evoked potentials in relation to the length of occupational exposure to low levels of toluene. Acta Med. Croatica 51:215–219, 1997.

Vrca, A., Karacic, V., Bozicevic, D., Fuchs, R. and Malinar, M., Cognitive evoked potentials VEP P300 persons occupationally exposed to low concentrations of toluene. Arh. Hig. Rada. Toksikol. 48:277–285, 1997.

OTHER ERPS

Hazemann, P., Jeftic, M. and Lille, F., Somatosensory evoked potentials in alcoholics and patients occupationally exposed to solvents and lead. Electromyogr. Clin. Neurophysiol. 27:183–187, 1987.

Morrow, L. A., Steinhauer, S. R. and Condray, R., Predictors of involvement in P300 latency in solvent-exposed adults. Neuropsychiatry Neuropsychol. Behav. Neurol. 11:146–150, 1998.

Hageman, G., van der Hoek, J., van Hout, M., van der Laan, G., Steur, E. J., de Bruin, W. and Herholz, K., Parkinsonism, pyramidal signs, polyneuropathy, and cognitive decline after long-term occupational solvent exposure. J. Neurology 246:198–206, 1999. [Case Report]

Review

Winneke, G., Acute behavioral effects of exposure to some organic solvents—psychophysiological aspects. Acta Neurol. Scand. Suppl. 92:117–129, 1982.

Yamanouchi, N., Okada, S. I., Kodama, K. and Sato, T., Central nervous system impairment caused by chronic solvent abuse—a review of Japanese studies on the clinical and neuroimaging aspects. Addiction Biol. 3:15–27, 1998.

Polydrug Abuse

EEG

Grant, I. and Judd, L. L., Neuropsychological and EEG disturbances in polydrug users. Am. J. Psychiatry 133:1039–1042, 1976.

Tomczak, J. W., Kocur, J. and Sobotka, H., Alcohol intoxication in teenagers using inhalant stupefacients. Pol. J. Pharmacol. Pharm. 41:203–206, 1989.

Herning, R. I., Glover, B. J., Koeppl, B., Phillips, R. L. and London, E. D., Cocaine-induced increases in EEG alpha and beta activity: evidence for reduced cortical processing. Neuropsychopharmacology 11:1–9, 1994.

Herning, R. I., Guo, X. and Lange, W. R., The effects of nimodipine on the EEG of substance abusers. Ann. N. Y. Acad. Sci. 765:143–151, 1995.

Braverman, E. R. and Blum, K., Substance use disorder exacerbates brain electrophysiological abnormalities in a psychiatrically-ill population. Clin. Electroencephalogr. 27 (4 Suppl.): 5–27, 1996.

Moak, D. H. and Anton, R. F., Alcohol-related seizures and the kindling effect of repeated detoxifications: the influence of cocaine. Alcohol Alcohol. 31:135–143, 1996.

AUDITORY ERPS

Pickworth, W. B., Brown, B. S., Hickey, J. E. and Muntaner, C., Effects of self-reported drug use and antisocial behavior on evoked potentials in adolescents. Drug Alcohol Depend. 25:105–110, 1990.

Patrick, G. and Struve, F. A., Brainstem auditory response (BAER) in polydrug abuse. Clin. Electroencephalogr. 25:1–7, 1994.

Herning, R. I., Guo, X. and Lange, W. R., Nimodipine improves information processing in substance abusers. Ann. NY Acad. Sci. 765:152–159, 1995.

Braverman, E. R. and Blum, K., Substance use disorder exacerbates brain electrophysiological abnormalities in a psychiatrically-ill population. Clin. Electroencephalogr. 27 (4 Suppl.): 5–27, 1996.

Biggins, C. A., MacKay, S., Clark, W. and Fein, G., Event-related potential evidence for frontal cortex effects of chronic cocaine dependence. Biol. Psychiatry 42:472–485, 1997.

VISUAL ERPs

Bauer, L. O. and Easton, C., Pattern shift visual evoked potentials in abstinent cocaine-dependent, alcohol-dependent, and cross-dependent patients. Drug Alcohol Depend. 40:203–209, 1996.

Braverman, E. R. and Blum, K., Substance use disorder exacerbates brain electrophysiological abnormalities in a psychiatrically-ill population. Clin. Electroencephalogr. 27 (4 Suppl.): 5–27, 1996.

Biggins, C. A., MacKay, S., Clark, W. and Fein, G., Event-related potential evidence for frontal cortex effects of chronic cocaine dependence. Biol. Psychiatry 42:472–485, 1997.

Abstinence

Roemer, R. A., Cornwell, A., Dewart, D., Jackson, P. and Ercegovac, D. V., Quantitative electroencephalographic analyses in cocaine-preferring polysubstance abusers during abstinence. Psychiatry Res. 58:247–257, 1995.

Kouri, E. M., Lukas, S. E. and Mendelson, J. H., P300 assessment of opiate and cocaine users: effects of detoxification and buprenorphine treatment. Biol. Psychiatry 40:617–628, 1996.

Costa, L. and Bauer, L., Quantitative electroencephalographic differences associated with alcohol, cocaine, heroin and dual-substance dependence. Drug Alcohol Depend. 46:87–93, 1997.

Family History of Polydrug Abuse

Brigham, J., Herning, R. I. and Moss, H. B., Event-related potentials and alpha synchronization in preadolescent boys at risk for psychoactive substance use. Biol. Psychiatry 37:834–846, 1995.

Brigham, J., Moss, H. B., Murrelle, E. L., Kirisci, L. and Spinelli, J. S., Event-related potential negative shift in sons of polysubstance- and alcohol-use disorder fathers. Psychiatry Res. 73:133–146, 1997.

Treatment

Herning, R. I., Guo, X. and Lange, W. R., The effects of nimodipine on the EEG of substance abusers. Ann. N. Y. Acad. Sci. 765:143–151, 1995.

Herning, R. I., Guo, X. and Lange, W. R., Nimodipine improves information processing in substance abusers. Ann. N. Y. Acad. Sci. 765:152–159, 1995.

Kouri, E. M., Lukas, S. E. and Mendelson, J. H., P300 assessment of opiate and cocaine users: effects of detoxification and buprenorphine treatment. Biol. Psychiatry 40:617–628, 1996.

Prenatal Exposure

Scher, M. S., Richardson, G. A., Robles, N., Geva, D., Goldschmidt, L., Dahl, R. E., Sclabassi, R. J. and Day, N. L., Effects of prenatal substance exposure: altered maturation of visual evoked potentials. Pediatr. Neurol. 18:236–243, 1998.

EMISSION TOMOGRAPHY

Alcohol and Alcoholism

Acute Administration

METABOLISM

Hine, C. H., Shick, A. F., Margolis, L., Burbridge, T. N. and Simon, A., Effects of alcohol in small doses and tetraethylthiuramdisulphide (Antabuse) on cerebral blood flow and cerebral metabolism. J. Pharmacol. Exp. Ther. 106:253–260, 1952.

Battey, L. L., Heyman, A. and Patterson, J. L., Effects of ethyl alcohol on cerebral blood flow and metabolism. JAMA 152:6–10, 1953.

de Wit, H., Metz, J., Wagner, N. and Cooper, M., Behavioral and subjective effects of ethanol: relationship to cerebral metabolism using PET. Alcohol. Clin. Exp. Res. 14:482–489, 1990.

Volkow, N. D., Hitzemann, R., Wolf, A. P., Logan, J., Fowler, J. S., Christman, D., Dewey, S. L., Schlyer, D., Burr, G., Vitkun, S. and Hirschowitz, J., Acute effects of ethanol on regional brain glucose metabolism and transport. Psychiatry Res. 35:39–48, 1990.

Heinz, A., Higley, J. D., Gorey, J. G., Saunders, R. C., Jones, D. W., Hommer, D., Zajicek, K., Suomi, S. J., Lesch, K. P., Weinberger, D. R. and Linnoila, M., In vivo association between alcohol intoxication, aggression, and serotonin transporter availability in nonhuman primates. Am. J. Psychiatry 155:1023–1028, 1998. [Nonhuman primate].

Haier, R. J., Schandler, S. L., MacLachlan, A., Soderling, E., Buchsbaum, M. S. and Cohen, M. J., Alcohol induced changes in regional cerebral glucose metabolic rate during divided attention. Person. Individ. Diff. 26:425–439, 1999.

Perfusion

Hine, C. H., Shick, A. F., Margolis, L., Burbridge, T. N. and Simon, A., Effects of alcohol in small doses and tetraethylthiuramdisulphide (Antabuse) on cerebral blood flow and cerebral metabolism. J. Pharmacol. Exp. Ther. 106:253–260, 1952.

Battey, L. L., Heyman, A. and Patterson, J. L., Effects of ethyl alcohol on cerebral blood flow and metabolism. JAMA 152:6–10, 1953.

Newlin, D. B., Golden, C. J., Quaife, M. and Graber, B., Effect of alcohol ingestion on regional cerebral blood flow. Int. J. Neurosci. 17:145–150, 1982.

Mathew, R. J. and Wilson, W. H., Regional cerebral blood flow changes associated with ethanol intoxication. Stroke 17:1156–1159, 1986.

Volkow, N. D., Mullani, N., Gould, L., Adler, S. S., Guynn, R. W., Overall, J. E. and Dewey, S., Effects of acute alcohol intoxication on cerebral blood flow measured with PET. Psychiatry Res. 24:201–209, 1988.

Berglund, M., Prohovnik, I. and Risberg, J., Regional cerebral blood flow during alcoholic blackout. Psychiatry Res. 27:49–54, 1989. [Case Report]

Fujiwara, T., Watanabe, M., Matsuda, K., Senbongi, M., Yagi, K. and Seino, M., Complex partial status epilepticus provoked by ingestion of alcohol: a case report. Epilepsia 32:650–656, 1991. [Case Report]

Sano, M., Wendt, P. E., Wirsen, A., Stenberg, G., Risberg, J. and Ingvar, D. H., Acute effects of alcohol on regional cerebral blood flow in man. J. Stud. Alcohol 54:369–375, 1993.

Schwartz, J. A., Speed, N. M., Gross, M. D., Lucey, M. R., Bazakis, A. M., Hariharan, M. and Beresford, T. P., Acute effects of alcohol administration on regional cerebral blood flow: the role of acetate. Alcohol. Clin. Exp. Res. 17:1119–1123, 1993.

Tiihonen, J., Kuikka, J., Hakola, P., Paanila, J., Airaksinen, J., Eronen, M. and Hallikainen, T., Acute ethanol-induced changes in cerebral blood flow. Am. J. Psychiatry 151:1505–1508, 1994.

Wendt, P. E., Risberg, J., Stenberg, G., Rosen, I. and Ingvar, D. H., Ethanol reduces asymmetry of visual rCBF responses. J. Cereb. Blood Flow Metab. 14:963–973, 1994.

Boecker, H., Wills, A. J., Ceballos-Baumann, A., Samuel, M., Thompson, P. D., Findley, L. J. and Brooks, D. J., The effect of ethanol on alcohol-responsive essential tremor: a positron emission tomography study. Ann. Neurol. 39:650–658, 1996.

Ingvar, M., Ghatan, P. H., Wirsen-Meurling, A., Risberg, J., Von Heijne, G., Stone-Elander, S. and Ingvar, D. H., Alcohol activates the cerebral reward system in man. J. Stud. Alcohol 59:258–269, 1998.

Benzodiazepine Receptors

Pauli, S., Liljequist, S., Farde, L., Swahn, C. G., Halldin, C., Litton, J. E. and Sedvall, G., PET analysis of alcohol interaction with the brain disposition of [^{11}C]flumazenil. Psychopharmacology (Berl.) 107:180–185, 1992.

Farde, L., Pauli, S., Litton, J. E., Halldin, C., Neiman, J. and Sedvall, G., PET-determination of benzodiazepine receptor binding in studies on alcoholism. EXS 71:143–153, 1994.

Alcohol-Cocaine Interaction

Fowler, J. S., Volkow, N. D., Logan, J., MacGregor, R. R., Wang, G. J. and Wolf, A. P., Alcohol intoxication does not change [^{11}C]cocaine pharmacokinetics in human brain and heart. Synapse 12:228–235, 1992.

Chronic Administration

Metabolism

Samson, Y., Baron, J.-C., Feline, A., Bories, J. and Crouzel, C., Local cerebral glucose utilisation in chronic alcoholics: a positron tomographic study. J. Neurol. Neurosurg. Psychiatry 49:1165–1170, 1986.

Sachs, H., Russell, J. A., Christman, D. R. and Cook, B., Alteration of regional cerebral glucose metabolic rate in non-Korsakoff chronic alcoholism. Arch. Neurol. 44:1242–1251, 1987.

Wik, G., Borg, S., Sjogren, I., Wiesel, F. A., Blomqvist, G., Borg, J., Greitz, T., Nyback, H., Sedvall, G., Stone-Elander, S. and Widen, L., PET determination of regional cerebral glucose metabolism in alcohol-dependent men and healthy controls using ^{11}C-glucose. Acta Psychiatr. Scand. 78:234–241, 1988.

Martin, P. R., Rio, D., Adinoff, B., Johnson, J. L., Bisserbe, J. C., Rawlings, R. R., Rohrbaugh, J. W., Stapleton, J. M. and Eckardt, M. J., Regional cerebral glucose utilization in chronic organic mental disorders associated with alcoholism. J. Neuropsychiatry Clin. Neurosci. 4:159–167, 1992.

Volkow, N. D., Hitzemann, R., Wang, G. J., Fowler, J. S., Burr, G., Pascani, K., Dewey, S. L. and Wolf, A. P., Decreased brain metabolism in neurologically intact healthy alcoholics. Am. J. Psychiatry 149:1016–1022, 1992.

Wang, G. J., Volkow, N. D., Hitzemann, R., Oster, Z. H., Roque, C. and Cestaro, V., Brain imaging of an alcoholic with MRI, SPECT, and PET. Am. J. Physiol. Imaging 7:194–198, 1992. [Case Report]

Adams, K. M., Gilman, S., Koeppe, R. A., Kluin, K. J., Brunberg, J. A., Dede, D., Berent, S. and Kroll, P. D., Neuropsychological deficits are correlated with frontal hypometabolism in positron emission tomography studies of older alcoholic patients. Alcohol. Clin. Exp. Res. 17:205–210, 1993.

Wang, G. J., Volkow, N. D., Roque, C. T., Cestaro, V. L., Hitzemann, R. J., Cantos, E. L., Levy, A. V. and Dhawan, A. P., Functional importance of ventricular enlargement and cortical atrophy in healthy subjects and alcoholics as assessed with PET, MR imaging, and neuropsychologic testing. Radiology 186:59–65, 1993.

Welch, L. W., Nimmerrichter, A., Kessler, R., King, D., Hoehn, R., Margolin, R. and Martin, P. R., Severe global amnesia presenting as Wernicke-Korsakoff syndrome but resulting from atypical lesions. Psychol. Med. 26:421–425, 1996. [Case Report]

Hommer, D., Andreasen, P., Rio, D., Williams, W., Ruttimann, U., Momenan, R., Zametkin, A., Rawlings, R. and Linnoila, M., Effects of m-chlorophenylpiperazine on regional brain glucose utilization: a positron emission tomographic comparison of alcoholic and control subjects. J. Neurosci. 17:2796–2806, 1997.

Adams, K. M., Gilman, S., Johnson-Greene, D., Koeppe, R. A., Junck, L., Kluin, K. J., Martorello, S., Johnson, M. J., Heumann, M. and Hill, E., The significance of family history status in relation to neuropsychological test performance and cerebral glucose metabolism studied with positron emission tomography in older alcoholic patients. Alcohol. Clin. Exp. Res. 22:105–110, 1998.

Dao-Castellana, M. H., Samson, Y., Legault, F., Martinot, J. L., Aubin, H. J., Crouzel, C., Feldman, L., Barrucand, D., Rancurel, G., Feline, A. and Syrota, A., Frontal dysfunction in neurologically normal chronic alcoholic subjects: metabolic and neuropsychological findings. Psychol. Med. 28:1039–1048, 1998.

Wang, G. J., Volkow, N. D., Fowler, J. S., Pappas, N. R., Wong, C. T., Pascani, K., Felder, C. A. and Hitzemann, R. J., Regional cerebral metabolism in female alcoholics of moderate severity does not differ from that of controls. Alcohol. Clin. Exp. Res. 22:1850-1854, 1998.

Perfusion

Berglund, M. and Ingvar, D. H., Cerebral blood flow and its regional distribution in alcoholism and in Korsakoff's psychosis. J. Stud. Alcohol 37:586–597, 1976.

Berglund, M. and Sonesson B., Personality impairment in alcoholism. Its relation to regional cerebral blood flow and psychometric performance. J. Stud. Alcohol 37:298–310, 1976.

Rogers, R. L., Meyer, J. S., Shaw, T. G. and Mortel, K. F., Reductions in regional cerebral blood flow associated with chronic consumption of alcohol. J. Am. Geriatr. Soc. 31:540–543, 1983.

Hata, T., Meyer, J. S., Tanahashi, N., Ishikawa, Y., Imai, A., Shinohara, T., Velez, M., Fann, W. E., Kandula, P. and Sakai, F., Three-dimensional mapping of local cerebral perfusion in alcoholic encephalopathy with and without Wernicke-Korsakoff syndrome. J. Cereb. Blood Flow Metab. 7:35–44, 1987.

Dally, S., Luft, A., Ponsin, J. C., Girre, C., Mamo, H. and Fournier, E., Abnormal pattern of cerebral blood flow distribution in young alcohol addicts. Br. J. Addict. 83:105–109, 1988.

Melgaard, B., Henrikson, L., Ahlgren, P., Danielsen, U. T., Sorensen, H. and Paulson, O. B., Regional cerebral blood flow in chronic alcoholics measured by single photon emission computerized tomography. Acta Neurol. Scand. 82:87–93, 1990.

Erbas, B., Bekdik, C., Erbengi, G., Enunlu, T., Aytac, S., Kumbasar, H. and Dogan, Y., Regional cerebral blood flow changes in chronic alcoholism using Tc-99m HMPAO SPECT: comparison with CT parameters. Clin. Nucl. Med. 17:123–127, 1992.

Wang, G. J., Volkow, N. D., Hitzemann, R., Oster, Z. H., Roque, C. and Cestaro, V., Brain imaging of an alcoholic with MRI, SPECT, and PET. Am. J. Physiol. Imaging 7:194–198, 1992. [Case Report]

Nicolas, J. M., Catafau, A. M., Estruch, R., Lomena, F. J., Salamero, M., Herranz, R., Monforte, R., Cardenal, C. and Urbano-Marquez, A., Regional cerebral blood flow-SPECT in chronic alcoholism: relation to neuropsychological testing. J. Nucl. Med. 34:1452–1459, 1993.

Denays, R., Tondeur, M., Noel, P. and Ham, H. R., Bilateral cerebral mediofrontal hypoactivity in Tc-99m HMPAO SPECT imaging. Clin. Nucl. Med. 19:873–876, 1994.

Kuruoglu, A. C., Arikan, Z., Vural, G., Karatas, M., Arac, M. and Isik, E., Single photon emission computerised tomography in chronic alcoholism. Antisocial personality disorder may be associated with decreased frontal perfusion. Br. J. Psychiatry 169:348–354, 1996.

Heinz, A., Ragan, P., Jones, D. W., Hommer, D., Williams, W., Knable, M. B., Gorey, J. G., Doty, L., Geyer, C., Lee, K. S., Coppola, R., Weinberger, D. R. and Linnoila, M., Reduced central serotonin transporters in alcoholism. Am. J. Psychiatry 155:1544–1549, 1998.

Drug Challenge/Receptor Binding Studies

Benzodiazepines

Litton, J. E., Neiman, J., Pauli, S., Farde, L., Hindmarsh, T., Halldin, C. and Sedvall, G., PET analysis of [^{11}C]flumazenil binding to benzodiazepine receptors in chronic alcohol-dependent men and healthy controls. Psychiatry Res. 50:1–13, 1993.

Volkow, N. D., Wang, G. J., Hitzemann, R., Fowler, J. S., Wolf, A. P., Pappas, N., Biegon, A. and Dewey, S. L., Decreased cerebral response to inhibitory neurotransmission in alcoholics. Am. J. Psychiatry 150:417–422, 1993.

Farde, L., Pauli, S., Litton, J. E., Halldin, C., Neiman, J. and Sedvall, G., PET-determination of benzodiazepine receptor binding in studies on alcoholism. EXS 71:143–153, 1994.

Volkow, N. D., Wang, G. J., Begleiter, H., Hitzemann, R., Pappas, N., Burr, G., Pascani, K., Wong, C., Fowler, J. S. and Wolf, A. P., Regional brain metabolic response to lorazepam in subjects at risk for alcoholism. Alcohol. Clin. Exp. Res. 19:510–516, 1995.

Gilman, S., Koeppe, R. A., Adams, K., Johnson-Greene, D., Junck, L., Kluin, K. J., Brunberg, J., Martorello, S. and Lohman, M., Positron emission tomographic studies of cerebral benzodiazepine-receptor binding in chronic alcoholics. Ann. Neurol. 40:163–171, 1996.

Volkow, N. D., Wang, G. J., Overall, J. E., Hitzemann, R., Fowler, J. S., Pappas, N., Frecska, E. and Piscani, K., Regional brain metabolic response to lorazepam in alcoholics during early and late alcohol detoxification. Alcohol. Clin. Exp. Res. 21:1278–1284, 1997.

Abi-Dargham, A., Krystal, J., Anjilvel, S., Scanley, B. E., Zoghbi, S., Baldwin, R. M., Rajeevan, N., Ellis, S., Petrakis, I. L., Seibyl, J. P., Charney, D. S., Laruelle, M. and Innis, R. B., Alterations of benzodiazepine receptors in Type II alcoholic subjects measured with SPECT and [^{123}I]Iomazenil. Am. J. Psychiatry 155:1550–1555, 1998.

Lingford-Hughes, A. R., Acton, P. D., Gacinovic, S., Suckling, J., Busatto, G. F., Boddington, S. J., Bullmore, E., Woodruff, P. W., Costa, D. C., Pilowsky, L. S., Ell, P. J., Marshall, E. J. and Kerwin, R. W., Reduced levels of GABA-benzodiazepine receptor in alcohol dependency in the absence of grey matter atrophy. Br. J. Psychiatry 173:116–122, 1998.

Amines

Hietala, J., West, C., Syvalahti, E., Nagren, K., Lehikoinen, P., Sonninen, P. and Ruotsalainen, U., Striatal D_2 dopamine receptor binding characteristics in vivo in patients with alcohol dependence. Psychopharmacology (Berl.) 116:285–290, 1994.

Tiihonen, J., Kuikka, J., Bergstrom, K., Hakola, P., Karhu, J., Ryynanen, O. P. and Fohr, J., Altered striatal dopamine re-uptake site densities in habitually violent and non-violent alcoholics. Nat. Med. 1:654–657, 1995.

Volkow, N. D., Wang, G. J., Fowler, J. S., Logan, J., Hitzemann, R., Ding, Y. S., Pappas, N., Shea, C. and Piscani, K., Decreases in dopamine receptors but not in dopamine transporters in alcoholics. Alcohol. Clin. Exp. Res. 20:1594–1598, 1996.

Tiihonen, J., Kuikka, J. T., Bergstrom, K. A., Karhu, J., Viinamaki, H., Lehtonen, J., Hallikainen, T., Yang, J. and Hakola, P., Single-photon emission tomography imaging of monoamine transporters in impulsive violent behaviour. Eur. J. Nucl. Med. 24:1253–1260, 1997.

Gilman, S., Koeppe, R. A., Adams, K. M., Junck, L., Kluin, K. J., Johnson-Greene, D., Martorello, S., Heumann, M. and Bandekar, R., Decreased striatal monoaminergic terminals in severe chronic alcoholism demonstrated with (+)[^{11}C]dihydrotetrabenazine and positron emission tomography. Ann. Neurol. 44:326–333, 1998.

Heinz, A., Ragan, P., Jones, D. W., Hommer, D., Williams, W., Knable, M. B., Gorey, J. G., Doty, L., Geyer, C., Lee, K. S., Coppola, R., Weinberger, D. R. and Linnoila, M., Reduced central serotonin transporters in alcoholism. Am. J. Psychiatry 155:1544–1549, 1998.

Kuikka, J. T., Tiihonen, J., Bergstrom, K. A., Karhu, J., Rasanen, P. and Eronen, M., Abnormal structure of human striatal dopamine re-uptake sites in habitually violent alcoholic offenders: a fractal analysis. Neurosci. Lett. 253:195–197, 1998.

Tiihonen, J., Vilkman, H., Rasanen, P., Ryynanen, O. P., Hakko, H., Bergman, J., Hamalainen, T., Laakso, A., Haaparanta-Solin, M., Solin, O., Kuoppamaki, M., Syvalahti, E. and Hietala, J., Striatal presynaptic dopamine function in type 1 alcoholics measured with positron emission tomography. Mol. Psychiatry 3:156–161, 1998.

Special Syndromes Associated with Alcoholism

Hepatic Encephalopathy

Johannesson, G., Berglund, M. and Ingvar, D. H., Reduction of blood flow in cerebral white matter in alcoholics related to hepatic function. Acta Neurol. Scand. 65:190–202, 1982.

Valmier, J., Touchon, J., Zanca, M., Fauchere, V., Bories, P. and Baldy-Moulinier, M., Correlations between cerebral grey matter flow and hepatic histology in alcoholism. Eur. Neurol. 25:428–435, 1986.

Lockwood, A. H., Murphy, B. W., Donnelly, K. Z., Mahl, T. C. and Perini, S., Positron-emission tomographic localization of abnormalities of brain metabolism in patients with minimal hepatic encephalopathy. Hepatology 18:1061–1068, 1993.

Wernicke & Korsakoff Syndromes

Metabolism

Fazio, F., Perani, D., Gilardi, M. C., Colombo, F., Cappa, S. F., Vallar, G., Bettinardi, V., Paulesu, E., Alberoni, M., Bressi, S., Franceschi, M. and Lenzi, G. L., Metabolic impairment in human amnesia: a PET study of memory networks. J. Cereb. Blood Flow Metab. 12:353–358, 1992.

Martin, P. R., Rio, D., Adinoff, B., Johnson, J. L., Bisserbe, J. C., Rawlings, R. R., Rohrbaugh, J. W., Stapleton, J. M. and Eckardt, M. J., Regional cerebral glucose utilization in chronic organic mental disorders associated with alcoholism. J. Neuropsychiatry Clin. Neurosci. 4:159–167, 1992.

Joyce, E. M., Rio, D. E., Ruttimann, U. E., Rohrbaugh, J. W., Martin, P. R., Rawlings, R. R. and Eckardt, M. J., Decreased cingulate and precuneate glucose utilization in alcoholic Korsakoff's syndrome. Psychiatry Res. 54:225–239, 1994.

Welch, L. W., Nimmerrichter, A., Kessler, R., King, D., Hoehn, R., Margolin, R. and Martin, P. R., Severe global amnesia presenting as Wernicke-Korsakoff syndrome but resulting from atypical lesions. Psychol. Med. 26:421–425, 1996.

Perfusion

Berglund, M. and Ingvar, D. H., Cerebral blood flow and its regional distribution in alcoholism and in Korsakoff's psychosis. J. Stud. Alcohol 37:586–597, 1976.

Rogers, R. L., Meyer, J. S., Shaw, T. G. and Mortel, K. F., Reductions in regional cerebral blood flow associated with chronic consumption of alcohol. J. Am. Geriatr. Soc. 31:540–543, 1983.

Meyer, J. S., Tanahashi, N., Ishikawa, Y., Hata, T., Velez, M., Fann, W. E., Kandula, P., Mortel, K. F. and Rogers, R. L., Cerebral atrophy and hypoperfusion improve during treatment of Wernicke-Korsakoff syndrome. J. Cereb. Blood Flow Metab. 5:376–385, 1985.

Sharp, P., Gemmell, H., Cherryman, G., Besson, J., Crawford, J. and Smith, F., Application of iodine-123-labeled isopropylamphetamine imaging to the study of dementia. J. Nucl. Med. 27:761–768, 1986.

Hata, T., Meyer, J. S., Tanahashi, N., Ishikawa, Y., Imai, A., Shinohara, T., Velez, M., Fann, W. E., Kandula, P. and Sakai, F., Three-dimensional mapping of local cerebral perfusion in alcoholic encephalopathy with and without Wernicke-Korsakoff syndrome. J. Cereb. Blood Flow Metab. 7:35–44, 1987.

Hunter, R., McLuskie, R., Wyper, D., Patterson, J., Christie, J. E., Brooks, D. N., McCulloch, J., Fink, G. and Goodwin, G. M., The pattern of function-related regional cerebral blood flow investigated by single photon emission tomography with ^{99m}Tc-HMPAO in patients with presenile Alzheimer's disease and Korsakoff's psychosis. Psychol. Med. 19:847–855, 1989.

Moffoot, A., O'Carroll, R.E., Murray, C., Dougall, N., Ebmeier, K. and Goodwin, G.M., Clonidine infusion increases uptake of ^{99m}Tc-Exametazime in anterior cingulate cortex in Korsakoff's psychosis. Psychol. Med. 24:53–61, 1994.

Benson, D. F., Djenderedjian, A., Miller, B. L., Pachana, N. A., Chang, L., Itti, L. and Mena, I., Neural basis of confabulation. Neurology 46:1239–1243, 1996. [Case Report]

Matsuda, K., Yamaji, S., Ishii, K., Sasaki, M., Sakamoto, S., Kitagaki, H., Imamura, T. and Mori, E., Regional cerebral blood flow and oxygen metabolism in a patient with Korsakoff syndrome. Ann. Nucl. Med. 11:33–35, 1997. [Case Report]

Marchiafava-Bignami Syndrome

Namba, Y., Bando, M., Takeda, K., Iwata, M. and Mannen, T., Marchiafava-Bignami disease with symptoms of the motor impersistence and unilateral hemispatial neglect. Rinsho Shinkeigaku 31:632–635, 1991. [Case Report] [Japanese]

Humbert, T., De Guilhermier, P., Maktouf, C., Grasset, G., Lopez, F. M. and Chabrand, P., Marchiafava-Bignami disease. A case studied by structural and functional brain imaging. Eur. Arch. Psychiatry Clin. Neurosci. 242:69–71, 1992. [Case Report]

Kamaki, M., Kawamura, M., Moriya, H. and Hirayama, K., "Crossed homonymous hemianopia" and "crossed left hemispatial neglect" in a case of Marchiafava-Bignami disease. J. Neurol. Neurosurg. Psychiatry 56:1027–1032, 1993. [Case Report]

Pappata, S., Chabriat, H., Levasseur, M., Legault-Demare, F. and Baron, J. C., Marchiafava-Bignami disease with dementia: severe cerebral metabolic depression revealed by PET. J. Neural. Transm. Park. Dis. Dement. Sect. 8:131–137, 1994. [Case Report]

Logak, M., Feve, A., Samson, Y., Guillard, A., Rancurel, G., Contribution of position emission tomography in a case of Marchiafava Bignami disease: Morel's laminar sclerosis? Rev. Neurol. (Paris) 152:47–50, 1996. [Case Report] [French]

Ferracci, F., Conte, F., Gentile, M., Candeago, R., Foscolo, L., Bendini, M. and Fassetta, G., Marchiafava-Bignami disease: computed tomographic scan, ^{99m}Tc HMPAO-SPECT, and FLAIR MRI findings in a patient with subcortical aphasia, alexia, bilateral agraphia, and left-handed deficit of constructional ability. Arch. Neurol. 56:107–110, 1999. [Case Report]

Cerebellar Degeneration

Gilman, S., Adams, K., Koeppe, R. A., Berent, S., Kluin, K. J., Modell, J. G., Kroll, P. and Brunberg, J. A., Cerebellar and frontal hypometabolism in alcoholic cerebellar degeneration studied with positron emission tomography. Ann. Neurol. 28:775–785, 1990.

Withdrawal

Berglund, M. and Risberg, J., Regional cerebral blood flow during alcohol withdrawal. Arch. Gen. Psychiatry 38:351–355, 1981.

Hemmingsen, R., Vorstrup, S., Clemmesen, L., Holm, S., Tfelt-Hansen, P., Sorensen, A. S., Hansen, C., Sommer, W. and Bolwig, T. G., Cerebral blood flow during delirium tremens and related clinical states studied with xenon-133 inhalation tomography. Am. J. Psychiatry 145:1384–1390, 1988.

Caspari, D., Trabert, W., Heinz, G., Lion, N., Henkes, H. and Huber, G., The pattern of regional cerebral blood flow during alcohol withdrawal—a single photon emission tomography study with ^{99m}Tc-HMPAO. Acta Psychiatr. Scand. 87:414–417, 1993.

Shih, W. J. and Hyatt, M., Volume and surface three-dimensional displays of Tc-99m HMPAO brain SPECT imaging in a chronic hypnosedative abuser. Clin. Nucl. Med. 18:506–509, 1993. [Case Report]

Welch, L. W., Nimmerrichter, A., Kessler, R., King, D., Hoehn, R., Margolin, R. and Martin, P. R., Severe global amnesia presenting as Wernicke-Korsakoff syndrome but resulting from atypical lesions. Psychol. Med. 26:421–425, 1996. [Case Report]

Tutus, A., Kugu, N., Sofuoglu, S., Nardali, M., Simsek, A., Karaaslan, F. and Gonul, A. S., Transient frontal hypoperfusion in Tc-99m hexamethylpropyleneamineoxime single photon emission computed tomography imaging during alcohol withdrawal. Biol. Psychiatry 43:923–928, 1998.

Laine, T. P. J., Ahonen, A., Torniainen, P., Heikkila, J., Pyhtinen, J., Rasanen, P., Niemela, O. and Hillbom, M., Dopamine transporters increase in human brain after alcohol withdrawal. Mol. Psychiatry 4:189–191, 1999.

Laine, T. P. J., Ahonen, A., Rasanen, P. and Tiihonen, J., Dopamine transporter availability and depressive symptoms during alcohol withdrawal. Psychiatry Res. 90:153–157, 1999.

Craving

Modell, J. G. and Mountz, J. M., Focal cerebral blood flow change during craving for alcohol measured by SPECT. J. Neuropsychiatry Clin. Neurosci. 7:15–22, 1995.

Abstinence

Metabolism

Adams, K. M., Gilman, S., Koeppe, R. A., Kluin, K. J., Brunberg, J. A., Dede, D., Berent, S. and Kroll, P. D., Neuropsychological deficits are correlated with frontal hypometabolism in positron emission tomography studies of older alcoholic patients. Alcohol. Clin. Exp. Res. 17:205–210, 1993.

Volkow, N. D., Wang, G. J., Hitzemann, R., Fowler, J. S., Overall, J. E., Burr, G. and Wolf, A. P., Recovery of brain glucose metabolism in detoxified alcoholics. Am. J. Psychiatry 151:178–183, 1994.

Johnson-Greene, D., Adams, K. M., Gilman, S., Koeppe, R. A., Junck, L., Kluin, K. J., Martorello, S. and Heumann, M., Effects of abstinence and relapse upon neuropsychological function and cerebral glucose metabolism in severe chronic alcoholism. J. Clin. Exp. Neuropsychol. 19:378–385, 1997.

Perfusion

Berglund, M., Bliding, G., Bliding, A. and Risberg, J., Reversibility of cerebral dysfunction in alcoholism during the first seven weeks of abstinence—a regional cerebral blood flow study. Acta Psychiatr. Scand. Suppl. 286:119–127, 1980.

Ishikawa, Y., Meyer, J. S., Tanahashi, N., Hata, T., Velez, M., Fann, W. E., Kandula, P., Motel, K. F. and Rogers, R. L., Abstinence improves cerebral perfusion and brain volume in alcoholic neurotoxicity without Wernicke-Korsakoff syndrome. J. Cereb. Blood Flow Metab. 6:86–94, 1986.

Berglund, M., Hagstadius, S., Risberg, J., Johanson, T. M., Bliding, A. and Mubrin, Z., Normalization of regional cerebral blood flow in alcoholics during the first 7 weeks of abstinence. Acta Psychiatr. Scand. 75:202–208, 1987.

Hemmingsen, R., Vorstrup, S., Clemmesen, L., Holm, S., Tfelt-Hansen, P., Sorensen, A. S., Hansen, C., Sommer, W. and Bolwig, T. G., Cerebral blood flow during delirium tremens and related clinical states studied with xenon-133 inhalation tomography. Am. J. Psychiatry 145:1384–1390, 1988.

Mampunza, S., Verbanck, P., Verhas, M., Martin, P., Paternot, J., LeBon, O., Kornreich, C., Den Bulk, A. and Pelc, I., Cerebral blood flow in just detoxified alcohol dependent patients: a 99m Tc-HMPAO-SPECT study. Acta Neurol. Belg. 95:164–169, 1995.

Dupont, R. M., Rourke, S. B., Grant, I., Lehr, P. P., Reed, R. J., Challakere, K., Lamoureux, G. and Halpern, S., Single photon emission computed tomography with iodoamphetamine-123 and neuropsychological studies in long-term abstinent alcoholics. Psychiatry Res. 67:99–111, 1996.

Gunther, W., Muller, N., Knesewitsch, P., Haag, C., Trapp, W., Banquet, J. P., Stieg, C. and Alper, K. R., Functional EEG mapping and SPECT in detoxified male alcoholics. Eur. Arch. Psychiatry Clin. Neurosci. 247:128–136, 1997.

Kosten, T. R., Cheeves, C., Palumbo, J., Seibyl, J. P., Price, L. H. and Woods, S. W., Regional cerebral blood flow during acute and chronic abstinence from combined cocaine-alcohol abuse. Drug Alcohol Depend. 50:187–195, 1998.

George, M. S., Teneback, C. C., Malcolm, R. J., Moore, J., Stallings, L. E., Spicer, K. M., Anton, R. F. and Ballenger, J. C., Multiple previous alcohol detoxifications are associated with decreased medial temporal and paralimbic function in the postwithdrawal period. Alcohol. Clin. Exp. Res. 23:1077–1084, 1999.

Receptor Levels

Laine, T. P. J., Ahonen, A., Torniainen, P., Heikkila, J., Pyhtinen, J., Rasanen, P., Niemela, O. and Hillbom, M., Dopamine transporters increase in human brain after alcohol withdrawal. Mol. Psychiatry 4:189–191, 1999.

Laine, T. P. J., Ahonen, A., Rasanen, P. and Tiihonen, J., Dopamine transporter availability and depressive symptoms during alcohol withdrawal. Psychiatry Res. 90:153–157, 1999.

Family History of Alcoholism

Volkow, N. D., Wang, G. J., Begleiter, H., Hitzemann, R., Pappas, N., Burr, G., Pascani, K., Wong, C., Fowler, J. S. and Wolf, A. P., Regional brain metabolic response to lorazepam in subjects at risk for alcoholism. Alcohol. Clin. Exp. Res. 19:510–516, 1995.

Adams, K. M., Gilman, S., Johnson-Greene, D., Koeppe, R. A., Junck, L., Kluin, K. J., Martorello, S., Johnson, M. J., Heumann, M. and Hill, E., The significance of family history status in relation to neuropsychological test performance and cerebral glucose metabolism studied with positron emission tomography in older alcoholic patients. Alcohol. Clin. Exp. Res. 22:105–110, 1998.

Treatment

Moffoot, A., O'Carroll, R. E., Murray, C., Dougall, N., Ebmeier, K. and Goodwin, G. M., Clonidine infusion increases uptake of ^{99m}Tc-Exametazime in anterior cingulate cortex in Korsakoff's psychosis. Psychol. Med. 24:53–61, 1994.

Gilman, S., Adams, K. M., Johnson-Greene, D., Koeppe, R. A., Junck, L., Kluin, K. J., Martorello, S., Heumann, M. and Hill, E., Effects of disulfiram on positron emission tomography and neuropsychological studies in severe chronic alcoholism. Alcohol. Clin. Exp. Res. 20:1456–1461, 1996.

Catafau, A. M., Etcheberrigaray, A., Perez de los Cobos, J., Estorch, M., Guardia, J., Flotats, A., Berna, L., Mari, C., Casas, M. and Carrio, I., Regional cerebral blood flow changes in chronic alcoholic patients induced by naltrexone challenge during detoxification. J. Nucl. Med. 40:19–24, 1999.

Reviews

Johnson, J. L., Adinoff, B., Bisserbe, J. C., Martin, P. R., Rio, D., Rohrbaugh, J. W., Zubovic, E. and Eckardt, M. J., Assessment of alcoholism-related organic brain syndromes with positron emission tomography. Alcohol. Clin. Exp. Res. 10:237–240, 1986.

Eckardt, M. J., Rohrbaugh, J. W., Rio, D., Rawlings, R. R. and Coppola, R., Brain imaging in alcoholic patients. Adv. Alcohol. Subst. Abuse 7:59–71, 1988.

Eckardt, M. J., Rohrbaugh, J. W., Rio, D. E. and Martin, P. R., Positron emission tomography as a technique for studying the chronic effects of alcohol on the human brain. Ann. Med. 22:341–345, 1990.

Mathew, R. J. and Wilson, W. H., Substance abuse and cerebral blood flow. Am. J. Psychiatry 148:292–305, 1991.

O'Carroll, R., Neuropsychological and neuroimaging aspects of latent hepatic encephalopathy (LHE). Alcohol Alcohol. Suppl. 2:191–195, 1993.

Heinz, A., Schmidt, L. G. and Reischies, F. M., Anhedonia in schizophrenic, depressed, or alcohol-dependent patients—neurobiological correlates. Pharmacopsychiatry 27 Suppl. 1:7–10, 1994.

Amen, D. G., Yantis, S., Trudeau, J., Stubblefield, M. S. and Halverstadt, J. S., Visualizing the firestorms in the brain: an inside look at the clinical and physiological connections between drugs and violence using brain SPECT imaging. J. Psychoactive Drugs 29:307–319, 1997.

Gatley, S. J. and Volkow, N. D., Addiction and imaging of the living human brain. Drug Alcohol Depend. 51:97–108, 1998.

Roebuck, T. M., Mattson, S. N. and Riley, E. P., A review of the neuroanatomical findings in children with fetal alcohol syndrome or prenatal exposure to alcohol. Alcohol. Clin. Exp. Res. 22:339–344, 1998.

Marijuana

Acute Administration

Mathew, R. J., Wilson, W. H. and Tant, S. R., Acute changes in cerebral blood flow associated with marijuana smoking. Acta Psychiatr. Scand. 79:118–128, 1989.

Volkow, N. D., Gillespie, H., Mullani, N., Tancredi, L., Grant, C., Ivanovic, M. and Hollister, L., Cerebellar metabolic activation by delta-9-tetrahydro-cannabinol in human brain: a study with positron emission tomography and ^{18}F-2-fluoro-2-deoxyglucose. Psychiatry Res. 40:69–78, 1991.

Mathew, R. J., Wilson, W. H., Humphreys, D. F., Lowe, J. V. and Wiethe, K. E., Regional cerebral blood flow after marijuana smoking. J. Cereb. Blood Flow Metab. 12:750–758, 1992.

Mathew, R. J. and Wilson, W. H., Acute changes in cerebral blood flow after smoking marijuana. Life Sci. 52:757–767, 1993.

Volkow, N. D., Gillespie, H., Mullani, N., Tancredi, L., Grant, C., Valentine, A. and Hollister, L., Brain glucose metabolism in chronic marijuana users at baseline and during marijuana intoxication. Psychiatry Res. 67:29–38, 1996.

Mathew, R. J., Wilson, W. H., Coleman, R. E., Turkington, T. G. and DeGrado, T. R., Marijuana intoxication and brain activation in marijuana smokers. Life Sci. 60:2075–2089, 1997.

Mathew, R. J., Wilson, W. H., Turkington, T. G. and Coleman, R. E., Cerebellar activity and disturbed time sense after THC. Brain Res. 797:183–189, 1998.

Gatley, S. J., Lan, R., Volkow, N. D., Pappas, N., King, P., Wong, C. T., Gifford, A. N., Pyatt, B., Dewey, S. L. and Makriyannis. A., Imaging the brain marijuana receptor: development of a radioligand that binds to cannabinoid CB1 receptors in vivo. J. Neurochem. 70:417–423, 1998. [Nonhuman Primate]

Chronic Administration

Mathew, R. J., Tant, S. and Burger, C., Regional cerebral blood flow in marijuana smokers. Br. J. Addict. 81:567–571, 1986.

Tunving, K., Thulin, S. O., Risberg, J. and Warkentin, S., Regional cerebral blood flow in long-term heavy cannabis use. Psychiatry Res. 17:15–21, 1986.

Volkow, N. D., Gillespie, H., Mullani, N., Tancredi, L., Grant, C., Valentine, A. and Hollister, L., Brain glucose metabolism in chronic marijuana users at baseline and during marijuana intoxication. Psychiatry Res. 67:29–38, 1996.

Amen, D. G. and Waugh, M., High resolution brain SPECT imaging of marijuana smokers with AD/HD. J. Psychoactive Drugs 30:209–214, 1998.

Hallucinogens

PCP

Fitch, W., McGeorge, A. P. and MacKenzie, E. T., Anaesthesia for studies of the cerebral circulation: a comparison of phencyclidine and althesin in the baboon. Br. J. Anaesth. 50:985–991, 1978. [Nonhuman Primate]

Wu, J. C., Buchsbaum, M. S. and Bunney, W. E., Positron emission tomography study of phencyclidine users as a possible drug model of schizophrenia. Yakubutsu Seishin Kodo 11:47–48, 1991.

Ketamine

Rockoff, M. A., Naughton, K. V., Shapiro, H. M., Ingvar, M., Ray, K. F., Gagnon, R. L. and Marshall, L. F., Cerebral circulatory and metabolic responses to intravenously administered lorazepam. Anesthesiology 53:215–218, 1980. [Nonhuman Primate]

Dormehl, I., Redelinghuys, F., Hugo, N., Oliver, D. and Pilloy, W., The baboon model under anesthesia for in vivo cerebral blood flow studies using single photon emission computed tomographic (SPECT) techniques. J. Med. Primatol. 21:270–274, 1992. [Nonhuman Primate]

Hartvig, P., Valtysson, J., Lindner, K. J., Kristensen, J., Karlsten, R., Gustafsson, L. L., Persson, J., Svensson, J. O., Oye, I., Antoni, G., Westerberg, G. and Langstrom, B., Central nervous system effects of subdissociative doses of (S)-ketamine are related to plasma and brain concentrations measured with positron emission tomography in healthy volunteers. Clin. Pharmacol. Ther. 58:165–173, 1995.

Breier, A., Malhotra, A. K., Pinals, D. A., Weisenfeld, N. I. and Pickar, D., Association of ketamine-induced psychosis with focal activation of the prefrontal cortex in healthy volunteers. Am. J. Psychiatry 154:805–811, 1997.

Vollenweider, F. X., Leenders, K. L., Oye, I., Hell, D. and Angst, J., Differential psychopathology and patterns of cerebral glucose utilisation produced by (S)- and (R)-ketamine in healthy volunteers using positron emission tomography (PET). Eur. Neuropsychopharmacol. 7:25–38, 1997.

Vollenweider, F. X., Leenders, K. L., Scharfetter, C., Antonini, A., Maguire, P., Missimer, J. and Angst, J., Metabolic hyperfrontality and psychopathology in the ketamine model of psychosis using positron emission tomography (PET) and [^{18}F]fluorodeoxyglucose (FDG). Eur. Neuropsychopharmacol. 7:9–24, 1997.

Breier, A., Adler, C. M., Weisenfeld, N., Su, T. P., Elman, I., Picken, L., Malhotra, A. K. and Pickar, D., Effects of NMDA antagonism on striatal dopamine release in healthy subjects: application of a novel PET approach. Synapse 29:142–147, 1998.

Smith, G. S., Schloesser, R., Brodie, J. D., Dewey, S. L., Logan, J., Vitkun, S. A., Simkowitz, P., Hurley, A., Cooper, T., Volkow, N. D. and Cancro, R., Glutamate modulation of dopamine measured in vivo with positron emission tomography (PET) and ^{11}C-raclopride in normal human subjects. Neuropsychopharmacology 18:18–25, 1998.

Newcomer, J. W., Farber, N. B., Jevtovic-Todorovic, V., Selke, G., Melson, A. K., Hershey, T., Craft, S. and Olney, J. W., Ketamine-induced NMDA receptor hypofunction as a model of memory impairment and psychosis. Neuropsychopharmacology 20:106–118, 1999.

MDMA and MDE

Scheffel, U., Szabo, Z., Mathews, W. B., Finley, P. A., Dannals, R. F., Ravert, H. T., Szabo, K., Yuan, J. and Ricaurte, G. A., In vivo detection of short- and long-term MDMA neurotoxicity—a positron emission tomography study in the living baboon brain. Synapse 29:183–192, 1998. [Nonhuman Primate]

McCann, U. D., Szabo, Z., Scheffel, U., Dannals, R. F. and Ricaurte, G. A., Positron emission tomographic evidence of toxic effect of MDMA ("Ecstasy") on brain serotonin neurons in human beings. Lancet 352(9138):1433–1437, 1998.

Schreckenberger, M., Gouzoulis-Mayfrank, E., Sabri, O., Arning, C., Tuttass, T., Schulz, G., Kaiser, H. J., Wagenknecht, G., Sass, H. and Bull, U., Investigations on the effect of "ecstasy" on cerebral glucose metabolism: an 18-FDG PET study. Nuklearmedizin 37:262–267, 1998. [German]

Gouzoulis-Mayfrank, E., Schreckenberger, M., Sabri, O., Arning, C., Thelen, B., Spitzer, M., Kovar, K.-A., Hermle, L., Bull, U. and Sass, H., Neurometabolic effects of psilocybin, 3,4-methylenedioxyethylamphetamine (MDE) and d-methamphetamine in healthy volunteers. A double-blind, placebo-controlled PET study with [^{18}F]FDG. Neuropsychopharmacology 20:565–581, 1999.

Semple, D. M., Ebmeier, K. P., Glabus, M. F., O'Carroll, R. E. and Johnstone, E. C., Reduced *in vivo* binding to the serotonin transporter in the cerebral cortex of MDMA ('ecstasy') users. Br. J. Psychiatry 175:63–69, 1999.

Psilocybin

Vollenweider, F. X., Leenders, K. L., Scharfetter, C., Maguire, P., Stadelmann, O. and Angst, J., Positron emission tomography and fluorodeoxyglucose studies of metabolic hyperfrontality and psychopathology in the psilocybin model of psychosis. Neuropsychopharmacology 16:357–372, 1997.

Vollenweider, F. X., Vontobel, P., Hell, D. and Leenders, K. L., 5-HT modulation of dopamine release in basal ganglia in psilocybin- induced psychosis in man—A PET study with [^{11}C]raclopride. Neuropsychopharmacology 20:424–433, 1999.

Gouzoulis-Mayfrank, E., Schreckenberger, M., Sabri, O., Arning, C., Thelen, B., Spitzer, M., Kovar, K.-A., Hermle, L., Bull, U. and Sass, H., Neurometabolic effects of psilocybin, 3,4-methylenedioxyethylamphetamine (MDE) and d-methamphetamine in healthy volunteers. A double-blind, placebo-controlled PET study with [^{18}F]FDG. Neuropsychopharmacology 20:565–581, 1999.

Mescaline

Oepen, G., Fuenfgeld, M., Harrington, A., Hermle, L. and Botsch, H., Right hemisphere involvement in mescaline-induced psychosis. Psychiatry Res. 29:335–336, 1989.

Hermle, L., Funfgeld, M., Oepen, G., Botsch, H., Borchardt, D., Gouzoulis, E., Fehrenbach, R. A. and Spitzer, M., Mescaline-induced psychopathological, neuropsychological, and neurometabolic effects in normal subjects: experimental psychosis as a tool for psychiatric research. Biol. Psychiatry 32:976–991, 1992.

Hermle, L., Gouzoulis-Mayfrank, E. and Spitzer, M., Blood flow and cerebral laterality in the mescaline model of psychosis. Pharmacopsychiatry 31 Suppl. 2:85–91, 1998.

Reviews

Mathew, R. J. and Wilson, W. H., Substance abuse and cerebral blood flow. Am. J. Psychiatry 148:292–305, 1991.

Gatley, S. J. and Volkow, N. D., Addiction and imaging of the living human brain. Drug Alcohol Depend. 51:97–108, 1998.

Benzodiazepines

Acute Administration

Metabolism

Rockoff, M. A., Naughton, K. V., Shapiro, H. M., Ingvar, M., Ray, K. F., Gagnon, R. L. and Marshall, L. F., Cerebral circulatory and metabolic responses to intravenously administered lorazepam. Anesthesiology 53:215–218, 1980.

Buchsbaum, M. S., Wu, J., Haier, R., Hazlett, E., Ball, R., Katz, M., Sokolski, K., Lagunas-Solar, M. and Langer, D., Positron emission tomography assessment of effects of benzodiazepines on regional glucose metabolic rate in patients with anxiety disorder. Life Sci. 40:2393–2400, 1987.

de Wit, H., Metz, J., Wagner, N. and Cooper, M., Effects of diazepam on cerebral metabolism and mood in normal volunteers. Neuropsychopharmacology 5:33–41, 1991.

Volkow, N. D., Wang, G. J., Hitzemann, R., Fowler, J. S., Pappas, N., Lowrimore, P., Burr, G., Pascani, K., Overall, J. and Wolf, A. P., Depression of thalamic metabolism by lorazepam is associated with sleepiness. Neuropsychopharmacology 12:123–132, 1995.

Wang, G. J., Volkow, N. D., Overall, J., Hitzemann, R. J., Pappas, N., Pascani, K. and Fowler, J. S., Reproducibility of regional brain metabolic responses to lorazepam. J. Nucl. Med. 37:1609–1613, 1996.

Wang, G. J., Volkow, N. D., Fowler, J. S., Hitzemann, R. J., Pappas, N. R. and Netusil, N., Evaluation of gender difference in regional brain metabolic responses to lorazepam. Psychiatry Res. 82:37–46, 1998.

Wang, G. J., Volkow, N. D., Levy, A. V., Felder, C. A., Fowler, J. S., Pappas, N. R., Hitzemann, R. J. and Wong, C. T., Measuring reproducibility of regional brain metabolic responses to lorazepam using statistical parametric maps. J. Nucl. Med. 40:715–720, 1999.

Perfusion

Rockoff, M. A., Naughton, K. V., Shapiro, H. M., Ingvar, M., Ray, K. F., Gagnon, R. L. and Marshall, L. F., Cerebral circulatory and metabolic responses to intravenously administered lorazepam. Anesthesiology 53:215–218, 1980.

Forster, A., Juge, O. and Morel, D., Effects of midazolam on cerebral hemodynamics and cerebral vasomotor responsiveness to carbon dioxide. J. Cereb. Blood Flow Metab. 3:246–249, 1983.

Mathew, R. J., Wilson, W. H. and Daniel, D. G., The effect of nonsedating doses of diazepam on regional cerebral blood flow. Biol. Psychiatry 20:1109–1116, 1985.

Forster, A., Juge, O., Louis, M. and Nahory, A., Effects of a specific benzodiazepine antagonist (RO 15-1788) on cerebral blood flow. Anesth. Analg. 66:309–313, 1987.

Wolf, J., Friberg, L., Jensen, J., Hansen, P. B., Andersen, A. R. and Lassen, N. A., The effect of the benzodiazepine antagonist flumazenil on regional cerebral blood flow in human volunteers. Acta Anaesthesiol. Scand. 34:628–631, 1990.

Roy-Byrne, P., Fleishaker, J., Arnett, C., Dubach, M., Stewart, J., Radant, A., Veith, R. and Graham, M., Effects of acute and chronic alprazolam treatment on cerebral blood flow, memory, sedation, and plasma catecholamines. Neuropsychopharmacology 8:161–169, 1993.

Matthew, E., Andreason, P., Pettigrew, K., Carson, R. E., Herscovitch, P., Cohen, R., King, C., Johanson, C. E., Greenblatt, D. J. and Paul, S. M., Benzodiazepine receptors mediate regional blood flow changes in the living human brain. Proc. Natl. Acad. Sci. U. S. A. 92:2775–2779, 1995.

Veselis, R. A., Reinsel, R. A., Beattie, B. J., Mawlawi, O. R., Feshchenko, V. A., DiResta, G. R., Larson, S. M. and Blasberg, R. G., Midazolam changes cerebral blood flow in discrete brain regions: an H2(15)O positron emission tomography study. Anesthesiology 87:1106–1117, 1997.

Receptors and Distribution

Shinotoh, H., Iyo, M., Yamada, T., Inoue, O., Suzuki, K., Itoh, T., Fukuda, H., Yamasaki, T., Tateno, Y. and Hirayama, K., Detection of benzodiazepine receptor occupancy in the human brain by positron emission tomography. Psychopharmacology (Berl.) 99:202–207, 1989.

Dewey, S. L., Smith, G. S., Logan, J., Brodie, J. D., Yu, D. W., Ferrieri, R. A., King, P. T., MacGregor, R. R., Martin, T. P., Wolf, A. P., Volkow, N. D., Fowler, J. S. and Meller, E., GABAergic inhibition of endogenous dopamine release measured in vivo with ^{11}C-raclopride and positron emission tomography. J. Neurosci. 12:3773–3780, 1992 [Nonhuman Primate].

Laruelle, M., Abi-Dargham, A., Rattner, Z., al-Tikriti, M. S., Zea-Ponce, Y., Zoghbi, S. S., Charney, D. S., Price, J., Frost, J. J., Hoffer, P. B., Baldwin, R. and Innis, R., Single photon emission tomography measurement of benzodiazepine receptor number and affinity in primate brain: a constant infusion paradigm with [^{123}I]iomazenil. Eur. J. Pharmacol. 230:119–123, 1993. [Nonhuman Primate]

Sybirska, E., Seibyl, J. P., Bremner, J. D., Baldwin, R. M., al-Tikriti, M. S., Bradberry, C., Malison, R. T., Zea-Ponce, Y., Zoghbi, S., During, M., Woods, S., Hoffer, P., Charney, D. and Innis, R., [^{123}I]iomazenil SPECT imaging demonstrates significant benzodiazepine receptor reserve in human and nonhuman primate brain. Neuropharmacology 32:671–680, 1993.

Suhara, T., Inoue, O., Kobayashi, K., Satoh, T. and Tateno, Y., An acute effect of triazolam on muscarinic cholinergic receptor binding in the human brain measured by positron emission tomography. Psychopharmacology (Berl.) 113:311–317, 1994.

Fujita, M., Woods, S. W., Verhoeff, N. P., Abi-Dargham, A., Baldwin, R. M., Zoghbi, S. S., Soares, J. C., Jatlow, P. A., Krystal, J. H., Rajeevan, N., Charney, D. S., Seibyl, J. P. and Innis, R. B., Changes of benzodiazepine receptors during chronic benzodiazepine administration in humans. Eur. J. Pharmacol. 368:161–172, 1999.

Benzodiazepines and Alcoholism

Litton, J. E., Neiman, J., Pauli, S., Farde, L., Hindmarsh, T., Halldin, C. and Sedvall, G., PET analysis of [^{11}C]flumazenil binding to benzodiazepine receptors in chronic alcohol-dependent men and healthy controls. Psychiatry Res. 50:1–13, 1993.

Volkow, N. D., Wang, G. J., Hitzemann, R., Fowler, J. S., Wolf, A. P., Pappas, N., Biegon, A. and Dewey, S. L., Decreased cerebral response to inhibitory neurotransmission in alcoholics. Am. J. Psychiatry 150:417–422, 1993.

Farde, L., Pauli, S., Litton, J. E., Halldin, C., Neiman, J. and Sedvall, G., PET-determination of benzodiazepine receptor binding in studies on alcoholism. EXS 71:143–153, 1994.

Volkow, N. D., Wang, G. J., Begleiter, H., Hitzemann, R., Pappas, N., Burr, G., Pascani, K., Wong, C., Fowler, J. S. and Wolf, A. P., Regional brain metabolic response to lorazepam in subjects at risk for alcoholism. Alcohol. Clin. Exp. Res. 19:510–516, 1995.

Gilman, S., Adams, K. M., Johnson-Greene, D., Koeppe, R. A., Junck, L., Kluin, K. J., Martorello, S., Heumann, M. and Hill, E., Effects of disulfiram on positron emission tomography and neuropsychological studies in severe chronic alcoholism. Alcohol. Clin. Exp. Res. 20:1456–1461, 1996.

Gilman, S., Koeppe, R. A., Adams, K., Johnson-Greene, D., Junck, L., Kluin, K. J., Brunberg, J., Martorello, S. and Lohman, M., Positron emission tomographic studies of cerebral benzodiazepine-receptor binding in chronic alcoholics. Ann. Neurol. 40:163–171, 1996.

Welch, L. W., Nimmerrichter, A., Kessler, R., King, D., Hoehn, R., Margolin, R. and Martin, P. R., Severe global amnesia presenting as Wernicke-Korsakoff syndrome but resulting from atypical lesions. Psychol. Med. 26:421–425, 1996. [Case Report]

Volkow, N. D., Wang, G. J., Overall, J. E., Hitzemann, R., Fowler, J. S., Pappas, N., Frecska, E. and Piscani, K., Regional brain metabolic response to lorazepam in alcoholics during early and late alcohol detoxification. Alcohol. Clin. Exp. Res. 21:1278–1284, 1997.

Benzodiazepines and Cocaine

Volkow, N. D., Wang, G. J., Fowler, J. S., Hitzemann, R., Gatley, S. J., Dewey, S. S. and Pappas, N., Enhanced sensitivity to benzodiazepines in active cocaine-abusing subjects: a PET study. Am. J. Psychiatry 155:200–206, 1998.

Dewey, S. L., Morgan, A. E., Ashby, C. R., Jr., Horan, B., Kushner, S. A., Logan, J., Volkow, N. D., Fowler, J. S., Gardner, E. L. and Brodie, J. D., A novel strategy for the treatment of cocaine addiction. Synapse 30:119–129, 1998. [Nonhuman Primate]

Chronic Administration

Roy-Byrne, P., Fleishaker, J., Arnett, C., Dubach, M., Stewart, J., Radant, A., Veith, R. and Graham, M., Effects of acute and chronic alprazolam treatment on cerebral blood flow, memory, sedation, and plasma catecholamines. Neuropsychopharmacology 8:161–169, 1993.

Shih, W. J. and Hyatt, M., Volume and surface three-dimensional displays of Tc-99m HMPAO brain SPECT imaging in a chronic hypnosedative abuser. Clin. Nucl. Med. 18:506–509, 1993. [Case Report]

Fujita, M., Woods, S. W., Verhoeff, N. P., Abi-Dargham, A., Baldwin, R. M., Zoghbi, S. S., Soares, J. C., Jatlow, P. A., Krystal, J. H., Rajeevan, N., Charney, D. S., Seibyl, J. P. and Innis, R. B., Changes of benzodiazepine receptors during chronic benzodiazepine administration in humans. Eur. J. Pharmacol. 368:161–172, 1999.

Reviews

Mathew, R. J. and Wilson, W. H., Substance abuse and cerebral blood flow. Am. J. Psychiatry 148:292–305, 1991.

Gatley, S. J. and Volkow, N. D., Addiction and imaging of the living human brain. Drug Alcohol Depend. 51:97–108, 1998.

Barbiturates

Dormehl, I., Redelinghuys, F., Hugo, N., Oliver, D. and Pilloy, W., The baboon model under anesthesia for in vivo cerebral blood flow studies using single photon emission computed tomographic (SPECT) techniques. J. Med. Primatol. 21:270–274, 1992. [Nonhuman Primate]

Heroin and Opiates

Acute Administration

Metabolism

London, E. D., Broussolle, E. P., Links, J. M., Wong, D. F., Cascella, N. G., Dannals, R. F., Sano, M., Herning, R., Snyder, F. R., Rippetoe, L. R., Toung, T. J. K., Jaffe, J. H. and Wagner, H. N., Jr., Morphine-induced metabolic changes in human brain. Studies with positron emission tomography and [fluorine 18]fluorodeoxyglucose. Arch. Gen. Psychiatry 47:73–81, 1990.

Walsh, S. L., Gibson, S. F., Jasinski, D. R., Stapleton, J. M., Phillips, R. L., Dannals, R. F., Schmidt, J., Preston, K. L., Grayson, R., Bigelow, G. E., Sullivan, J. T., Contoreggi, C. and London, E. D., Buprenorphine reduces cerebral glucose metabolism in poly drug users. Neuropsychopharmacology 10:157–170, 1994.

Firestone, L. L., Gyulai, F., Mintun, M., Adler, L. J., Urso, K. and Winter, P. M., Human brain activity response to fentanyl imaged by positron emission tomography. Anesth. Analg. 82:1247–1251, 1996.

Perfusion

Adler, L. J., Gyulai, F. E., Diehl, D. J., Mintun, M. A., Winter, P. M. and Firestone, L. L., Regional brain activity changes associated with fentanyl analgesia elucidated by positron emission tomography. Anesth. Analg. 84:120–126, 1997.

Schlaepfer, T. E., Strain, E. C., Greenberg, B. D., Preston, K. L., Lancaster, E., Bigelow, G. E., Barta, P. E. and Pearlson, G. D., Site of opioid action in the human brain: mu and kappa agonists' subjective and cerebral blood flow effects. Am. J. Psychiatry 155:470–473, 1998.

Sell, L. A., Morris, J., Bearn, J., Frackowiak, R. S., Friston, K. J. and Dolan, R. J., Activation of reward circuitry in human opiate addicts. Eur. J. Neurosci. 11:1042–1048, 1999.

Receptor Levels

Hartvig, P., Bergstrom, K., Lindberg, B., Lundberg, P. O., Lundqvist, H., Langstrom, B., Svard, H. and Rane, A., Kinetics of ^{11}C-labeled opiates in the brain of rhesus monkeys. J. Pharmacol. Exp. Ther. 230:250–255, 1984. [Nonhuman Primate]

Carson, R. E., Channing, M. A., Blasberg, R. G., Dunn, B. B., Cohen, R. M., Rice, K. C. and Herscovitch, P., Comparison of bolus and infusion methods for receptor quantitation: application to [^{18}F]cyclofoxy and positron emission tomography. J. Cereb. Blood Flow Metab. 13:24–42, 1993. [Nonhuman primate]

Zubieta, J.-K., Gorelick, D. A., Stauffer, R., Ravert, H. T., Dannals, R. F. and Frost, J. J., Increased mu opioid receptor binding detected by PET in cocaine-dependent men is associated with cocaine craving. Nat. Med. 2:1225–1229, 1996.

Smith, Y. R., Zubieta, J. K., del Carmen, M. G., Dannals, R. F., Ravert, H. T., Zacur, H. A. and Frost, J. J., Brain opioid receptor measurements by positron emission tomography in normal cycling women: relationship to luteinizing hormone pulsatility and gonadal steroid hormones. J. Clin. Endocrinol. Metab. 83:4498–4505, 1998.

Schadrack, J., Willoch, F., Platzer, S., Bartenstein, P., Mahal, B., Dworzak, D., Wester, H. J., Zieglgansberger, W. and Tolle, T. R., Opioid receptors in the human cerebellum: evidence from [^{11}C]diprenorphine PET, mRNA expression and autoradiography. Neuroreport 10:619–624, 1999.

Zubieta, J. K., Dannals, R. F. and Frost, J. J., Gender and age influences on human brain mu-opioid receptor binding measured by PET. Am. J. Psychiatry 156:842–848, 1999.

Chronic Administration

Metabolism

Volkow, N. D., Valentine, A. and Kulkarni, M., Radiological and neurological changes in the drug abuse patient: a study with MRI. J. Neuroradiol. 15:288–293, 1988.

London, E. D., Margolin, R. A., Wong, D. F., Links, J., La France, N. D., Cascella, N. G., Broussolle, E. P. M., Wagner, H. N., Jr., Snyder, F. R. and Jasinski, D. R., Cerebral glucose utilization in human heroin addicts: Case reports from a positron emission tomographic study. Res. Comm. Subst. Abuse 10:141–144, 1989. [Case Report]

Perfusion

Jensen, R., Olsen, T. S. and Winther, B. B., Severe non-occlusive ischemic stroke in young heroin addicts. Acta Neurol. Scand. 81:354–357, 1990. [Case Report]

Holman, B. L., Carvalho, P. A., Mendelson, J., Teoh, S. K., Nardin, R., Hallgring, E., Hebben, N. and Johnson, K. A., Brain perfusion is abnormal in cocaine-dependent polydrug users: a study using technetium-99m-HMPAO and ASPECT. J. Nucl. Med. 32:1206–1210, 1991.

Levin, J. M., Holman, B. L., Mendelson, J. H., Teoh, S. K., Garada, B., Johnson, K. A. and Springer, S., Gender differences in cerebral perfusion in cocaine abuse: ^{99m}Tc-HMPAO SPECT study of drug abusing women J. Nucl. Med. 35:1902–1909, 1994.

Krystal, J. H., Woods, S. W., Kosten, T. R., Rosen, M. I., Seibyl, J. P., van Dyck, C. C., Price, L. H., Zubal, I. G., Hoffer, P. B. and Charney, D. S., Opiate dependence and withdrawal: preliminary assessment using single photon emission computerized tomography (SPECT). Am. J. Drug Alcohol Abuse 21:47–63, 1995.

Levin, J. M., Mendelson, J. H., Holman, B. L., Teoh, S. K., Garada, B., Schwartz, R. B. and Mello, N. K., Improved regional cerebral blood flow in chronic cocaine polydrug users treated with buprenorphine. J. Nucl. Med. 36:1211–1215, 1995.

Cohen, R. M., Andreason, P. J., Doudet, D. J., Carson, R. E. and Sunderland, T., Opiate receptor avidity and cerebral blood flow in Alzheimer's disease. J. Neurol. Sci. 148:171–180, 1997.

Sex Differences

Levin, J. M., Holman, B. L., Mendelson, J. H., Teoh, S. K., Garada, B., Johnson, K. A. and Springer, S., Gender differences in cerebral perfusion in cocaine abuse: ^{99m}Tc-HMPAO SPECT study of drug abusing women J. Nucl. Med. 35:1902–1909, 1994.

Zubieta, J. K., Dannals, R. F. and Frost, J. J., Gender and age influences on human brain mu-opioid receptor binding measured by PET. Am. J. Psychiatry 156:842–848, 1999.

Withdrawal

van Dyck, C. H., Rosen, M. I., Thomas, H. M., McMahon, T. J., Wallace, E. A., O'Connor, P. G., Sullivan, M., Krystal, J. H., Hoffer, P. B., Woods, S. W. and Kosten, T. R., SPECT regional cerebral blood flow alterations in naltrexone-precipitated withdrawal from buprenorphine. Psychiatry Res. 55:181–191, 1994.

Krystal, J. H., Woods, S. W., Kosten, T. R., Rosen, M. I., Seibyl, J. P., van Dyck, C. C., Price, L. H., Zubal, I. G., Hoffer, P. B. and Charney, D. S., Opiate dependence and withdrawal: preliminary assessment using single photon emission computerized tomography (SPECT). Am. J. Drug Alcohol Abuse 21:47–63, 1995.

Christensen, J. D., Kaufman, M. J., Levin, J. M., Mendelson, J. H., Holman, B. L., Cohen, B. M. and Renshaw, P. F., Abnormal cerebral metabolism in polydrug abusers during early withdrawal: a ^{31}P MR spectroscopy study. Magn. Reson. Med. 35:658–663, 1996.

Rose, J. S., Branchey, M., Buydens-Branchey, L., Stapleton, J. M., Chasten, K., Werrell, A. and Maayan, M. L., Cerebral perfusion in early and late opiate withdrawal: a technetium-99m-HMPAO SPECT study. Psychiatry Res. 67:39–47, 1996.

Wang, G. J., Volkow, N. D., Fowler, J. S., Logan, J., Abumrad, N. N., Hitzemann, R. J., Pappas, N. S. and Pascani, K., Dopamine D_2 receptor availability in opiate-dependent subjects before and after naloxone-precipitated withdrawal. Neuropsychopharmacology 16:174–182, 1997.

Danos, P., Kasper, S., Grunwald, F., Klemm, E., Krappel, C., Broich, K., Hoflich, G., Overbeck, B., Biersack, H. J. and Moller, H. J., Pathological regional cerebral blood flow in opiate-dependent patients during withdrawal: a HMPAO-SPECT study. Neuropsychobiology 37:194–199, 1998.

Craving

Zubieta, J.-K., Gorelick, D. A., Stauffer, R., Ravert, H. T., Dannals, R. F. and Frost, J. J., Increased mu opioid receptor binding detected by PET in cocaine-dependent men is associated with cocaine craving. Nat. Med. 2:1225–1229, 1996.

Weinstein, A., Feldtkeller, B., Malizia, A., Wilson, S., Bailey, J. and Nutt, D. J., Integrating the cognitive and physiological aspects of craving. J. Psychopharmacol. 12:31–38, 1998.

Abstinence

Rose, J. S., Branchey, M., Buydens-Branchey, L., Stapleton, J. M., Chasten, K., Werrell, A. and Maayan, M. L., Cerebral perfusion in early and late opiate withdrawal: a technetium-99m-HMPAO SPECT study. Psychiatry Res. 67:39–47, 1996.

Gerra, G., Calbiani, B., Zaimovic, A., Sartori, R., Ugolotti, G., Ippolito, L., Delsignore, R., Rustichelli, P. and Fontanesi, B., Regional cerebral blood flow and comorbid diagnosis in abstinent opioid addicts. Psychiatry Res. 83:117–126, 1998.

Treatment

Holman, B. L., Mendelson, J., Garada, B., Teoh, S. K., Hallgring, E., Johnson, K. A. and Mello, N. K., Regional cerebral blood flow improves with treatment in chronic cocaine polydrug users. J. Nucl. Med. 34:723–727, 1993.

Levin, J. M., Mendelson, J. H., Holman, B. L., Teoh, S. K., Garada, B., Schwartz, R. B. and Mello, N. K., Improved regional cerebral blood flow in chronic cocaine polydrug users treated with buprenorphine. J. Nucl. Med. 36:1211–1215, 1995.

HIV

Woods, S. W., O'Malley, S. S., Martini, B. L., McDougle, C. J., Price, L. H., Krystal, J. H., Hoffer, P. B. and Kosten, T. R., SPECT regional cerebral blood flow and neuropsychological testing in non-demented HIV-positive drug abusers. Prog. Neuropsychopharmacol. Biol. Psychiatry 15:649–662, 1991.

Holman, B. L., Garada, B., Johnson, K. A., Mendelson, J. H., Hallgring, E., Teoh, S. K., Worth, J. and Navia, B., A comparison of brain perfusion SPECT in cocaine abuse and AIDS dementia complex. J. Nucl. Med. 33:1312–1315, 1992.

Reviews

Mathew, R. J. and Wilson, W. H., Substance abuse and cerebral blood flow. Am. J. Psychiatry 148:292–305, 1991.

Ernst, M. and London, E. D., Brain imaging studies of drug abuse—therapeutic implications. Sem. Neurosci. 9:120–130, 1997.

Gatley, S. J. and Volkow, N. D., Addiction and imaging of the living human brain. Drug Alcohol Depend. 51:97–108, 1998.

Cocaine

Acute Administration

Receptor Effects and Distribution

Fowler, J. S., Volkow, N. D., Wolf, A. P., Dewey, S. L., Schlyer, D. J., Macgregor, R. R., Hitzemann, R., Logan, J., Bendriem, B., Gatley, S. J. and Christman, D., Mapping cocaine binding sites in human and baboon brain in vivo. Synapse 4:371–377, 1989.

Logan, J., Fowler, J. S., Volkow, N. D., Wolf, A. P., Dewey, S. L., Schlyer, D. J., MacGregor, R. R., Hitzemann, R., Bendriem, B., Gatley, S. J. and Christman, D., Graphical analysis of reversible radioligand binding from time-activity measurements applied to [N-^{11}C-methyl]-(-)-cocaine PET studies in human subjects. J. Cereb. Blood Flow Metab. 10:740–747, 1990.

Laruelle, M., Wallace, E., Seibyl, J. P., Baldwin, R. M., Zea-Ponce, Y., Zoghbi, S. S., Neumeyer, J. L., Charney, D. S., Hoffer, P. B. and Innis, R. B., Graphical, kinetic, and equilibrium analyses of in vivo [^{123}I] β-CIT binding to dopamine transporters in healthy human subjects. J. Cereb. Blood Flow Metab. 14:982–994, 1994.

Malison, R. T., Best, S. E., Wallace, E. A., McCance, E., Laruelle, M., Zoghbi, S. S., Baldwin, R. M., Seibyl, J. S., Hoffer, P. B., Price, L. H., Kosten, T. R. and Innis, R. B., Euphorigenic doses of cocaine reduce [^{123}I]β-CIT SPECT measures of dopamine transporter availability in human cocaine addicts. Psychopharmacology (Berl.) 122:358–362, 1995.

Volkow, N. D., Ding, Y.-S., Fowler, J. S., Wang, G.-J., Logan, J., Gatley, J. S., Dewey, S., Ashby, C., Liebermann, J., Hitzemann, R. and Wolf, A. P., Is methylphenidate like cocaine? Studies on their pharmacokinetics and distribution in the human brain. Arch. Gen. Psychiatry 52:456–463, 1995.

Wang, G. J., Volkow, N. D., Logan, J., Fowler, J. S., Schlyer, D., MacGregor, R. R., Hitzemann, R. J., Gjedde, A. and Wolf, A. P., Serotonin 5-HT2 receptor availability in chronic cocaine abusers. Life Sci. 56:PL299–PL303, 1995.

Volkow, N. D., Wang, G. J., Fowler, J. S., Gatley, S. J., Ding, Y. S., Logan, J., Dewey, S. L., Hitzemann, R. and Lieberman, J., Relationship between psychostimulant-induced "high" and dopamine transporter occupancy. Proc. Natl. Acad. Sci. U. S. A. 93:10388–10392, 1996.

Logan, J., Volkow, N. D., Fowler, J. S., Wang, G. J., Fischman, M. W., Foltin, R. W., Abumrad, N. N., Vitkun, S., Gatley, S. J., Pappas, N., Hitzemann, R. and Shea, C. E., Concentration and occupancy of dopamine transporters in cocaine abusers with [^{11}C]cocaine and PET. Synapse 27:347–356, 1997.

Mach, R. H., Nader, M. A., Ehrenkaufer, R. L., Line, S. W., Smith, C. R., Gage, H. D. and Morton, T. E., Use of positron emission tomography to study the dynamics of psychostimulant-induced dopamine release. Pharmacol. Biochem. Behav. 57:477–486, 1997. [Nonhuman Primate]

Schlaepfer, T. E., Pearlson, G. D., Wong, D. F., Marenco, S., Dannals, R. F., PET study of competition between intravenous cocaine and [^{11}C]raclopride at dopamine receptors in human subjects. Am. J. Psychiatry 54:1209–1213, 1997.

Volkow, N. D., Wang, G. J., Fischman, M. W., Foltin, R. W., Fowler, J. S., Abumrad, N. N., Vitkun, S., Logan, J., Gatley, S. J., Pappas, N., Hitzemann, R. and Shea, C. E., Relationship between subjective effects of cocaine and dopamine transporter occupancy. Nature 386:827–830, 1997.

Telang, F. W., Volkow, N. D., Levy, A., Logan, J., Fowler, J. S., Felder, C., Wong, C. and Wang, G. J., Distribution of tracer levels of cocaine in the human brain as assessed with averaged [^{11}C]cocaine images. Synapse 31:290–296, 1999.

Villemagne, V. L., Rothman, R. B., Yokoi, F., Rice, K. C., Matecka, D., Dannals, R. F. and Wong, D. F., Doses of GBR12909 that suppress cocaine self-administration in non-human primates substantially occupy dopamine transporters as measured by [^{11}C] WIN35,428 PET scans. Synapse 32:44–50, 1999. [Nonhuman Primate]

Villemagne, V. L., Wong, D. F., Yokoi, F., Stephane, M., Rice, K. C., Matecka, D., Clough, D. J., Dannals, R. F. and Rothman, R. B., GBR12909 attenuates amphetamine-induced striatal dopamine release as measured by [(^{11})C]raclopride continuous infusion PET scans. Synapse 33:268–273, 1999. [Nonhuman Primate]

Volkow, N. D., Fowler, J. S., Gatley, S. J., Dewey, S. L., Wang, G. J., Logan, J., Ding, Y. S., Franceschi, D., Gifford, A., Morgan, A., Pappas, N. and King, P., Comparable changes in synaptic dopamine induced by methylphenidate and by cocaine in the baboon brain. Synapse 31:59–66, 1999. [Nonhuman Primate]

Alcohol–Cocaine Interaction

Fowler, J. S., Volkow, N. D., Logan, J., MacGregor, R. R., Wang, G. J. and Wolf, A. P., Alcohol intoxication does not change [^{11}C]cocaine pharmacokinetics in human brain and heart. Synapse 12:228–235, 1992.

Fentanyl–Cocaine Interaction

Bergstrom, K. A., Jolkkonen, J., Kuikka, J. T., Akerman, K. K., Viinamaki, H., Airaksinen, O., Lansimies, E. and Tiihonen, J., Fentanyl decreases β-CIT binding to the dopamine transporter. Synapse 29:413–415, 1998. [Case Report]

Metabolism

Gatley, S. J., MacGregor, R. R., Fowler, J. S., Wolf, A. P., Dewey, S. L. and Schlyer, D. J., Rapid stereoselective hydrolysis of (+)-cocaine in baboon plasma prevents its uptake in the brain: implications for behavioral studies. J. Neurochem. 54:720–723, 1990. [Nonhuman Primate]

London, E. D., Cascella, N. G., Wong, D. F., Phillips, R. L., Dannals, R. F., Links, J. M., Herning, R., Grayson, R., Jaffe, J. H. and Wagner, H. N., Jr., Cocaine-induced reduction of glucose utilization in human brain. A study using positron emission tomography and [fluorine 18]-fluorodeoxyglucose Arch. Gen. Psychiatry 47:567–574, 1990.

Morgan, M. J., Cascella, N. G., Stapleton, J. M., Phillips, R. L., Yung, B. C., Wong, D. F., Shaya, E. K. and London, E. D., Sensitivity to subjective effects of cocaine in drug abusers: relationship to cerebral ventricle size. Am. J. Psychiatry 150:1712–1717, 1993.

Lyons, D., Friedman, D. P., Nader, M. A. and Porrino, L. J., Cocaine alters cerebral metabolism within the ventral striatum and limbic cortex of monkeys. J. Neurosci. 16:1230–1238, 1996. [Nonhuman Primate]

Bartzokis, G., Beckson, M., Newton, T., Mandelkern, M., Mintz, J., Foster, J. A., Ling, W. and Bridge, T. P., Selegiline effects on cocaine-induced changes in medial temporal lobe metabolism and subjective ratings of euphoria. Neuropsychopharmacology 20:582–590, 1999.

PERFUSION

Pearlson, G. D., Jeffery, P. J., Harris, G. J., Ross, C. A., Fischman, M. W. and Camargo, E. E., Correlation of acute cocaine-induced changes in local cerebral blood flow with subjective effects. Am. J. Psychiatry 150:495–497, 1993.

Mena, I., Giombetti, R. J., Miller, B. L., Garrett, K., Villanueva-Meyer, J., Mody, C. and Goldberg, M. A., Cerebral blood flow changes with acute cocaine intoxication: Clinical correlations with SPECT, CT and MRI. In: Imaging Techniques in Medications Development: Preclinical and Clinical Aspects, Sorer, H. and Rapaka,, R. S. (eds.) U.S. Dept. of Health and Human Services, Rockville, MD, pp. 161–173, 1994.

Mathew, R. J., Wilson, W. H., Lowe, J. V. and Humphries, D., Acute changes in cranial blood flow after cocaine hydrochloride. Biol. Psychiatry 40:609–616, 1996.

Wallace, E. A., Wisniewski, G., Zubal, G., vanDyck, C. H., Pfau, S. E., Smith, E. O., Rosen, M. I., Sullivan, M. C., Woods, S. W. and Kosten, T. R., Acute cocaine effects on absolute cerebral blood flow. Psychopharmacology (Berl.) 128:17–20, 1996.

Chen, Y. C., Galpern, W. R., Brownell, A. L., Matthews, R. T., Bogdanov, M., Isacson, O., Keltner, J. R., Beal, M. F., Rosen, B. R. and Jenkins, B. G., Detection of dopaminergic neurotransmitter activity using pharmacologic MRI: correlation with PET, microdialysis, and behavioral data. Magn. Reson. Med. 38:389–398, 1997. [Rodent]

Gottschalk, P. C. H., Van Heertum, R. L., Perera, G. M., Pozniakoff, T. A., Moeller, J. R., Young, W. L., Volkow, N. D., Foltin, R. W. and Fischman, M. W., Cerebral blood flow response to IV cocaine in humans: Quantitative xenon-133-SPECT studies. In: Problems of Drug Dependence 1996: Proceedings of the 58th Annual Scientific Meeting, The College on Problems of Drug Dependence, Inc., Harris, L. S. (ed.) U.S. Dept. of Health and Human Services, Washington, D.C., NIH Pub. No. 97-4236, pp. 117, 1997. [Abstract]

Johnson, B., Lamki, L., Barron, B., Spiga, R., Chen, R., Meisch, R. and Khilnani, N., Brain blood flow abnormalities associated with oral cocaine use. Ir. J. Psych. Med. 14:72–73, 1997. [Case Report]

Johnson, B., Lamki, L., Fang, B., Barron, B., Wagner, L., Wells, L., Kenny, P., Overton, D., Dhother, S., Abramson, D., Chen, R. and Kramer, L., Demonstration of dose-dependent global and regional cocaine-induced reductions in brain blood flow using a novel approach to quantitative single photon emission computerized tomography. Neuropsychopharmacology 18:377–384, 1998.

Johnson, B., Barron, B., Fang, B., Lamki, L., Wagner, L., Wells, L., Kenny, P., Overton, D., Dhother, S., Abramson, D., Chen, R. and Kramer, L., Isradipine prevents global and regional cocaine-induced changes in brain blood flow: a preliminary study. Psychopharmacology (Berl.) 136:335–341, 1998.

Chronic Administration

METABOLISM

Baxter, L. R., Jr., Schwartz, J. M., Phelps, M. E., Mazziotta, J. C., Barrio, J., Rawson, R. A., Engel, J., Guze, B. H., Selin, C. and Sumida, R., Localization of neurochemical effects of cocaine and other stimulants in the human brain J. Clin. Psychiatry 49 Suppl.:23–26, 1988.

Volkow, N., Fowler, J., Wolf, A., Hitzemann, R., Dewey, S., Bendriem, B., Alpert, R. and Hoff, A., Changes in brain glucose metabolism in cocaine dependence and withdrawal. Am. J. Psychiatry 148:621–626, 1991.

Volkow, N. D., Fowler, J. S., Wang, G. J., Hitzemann, R., Logan, J., Schlyer, D. J., Dewey, S. L. and Wolf, A. P., Decreased dopamine D_2 receptor availability is associated with reduced frontal metabolism in cocaine abusers. Synapse 14:169–177, 1993.

Stapleton, J. M., Morgan, M. J., Phillips, R. L., Wong, D. F., Yung, B. C., Shaya, E. K., Dannals, R. F., Liu, X., Grayson, R. L. and London, E. D., Cerebral glucose utilization in polysubstance abuse. Neuropsychopharmacology 13:21–31, 1995.

Volkow, N. D., Wang, G. J., Fowler, J. S., Hitzemann, R., Gatley, S. J., Dewey, S. S. and Pappas, N., Enhanced sensitivity to benzodiazepines in active cocaine-abusing subjects: a PET study. Am. J. Psychiatry 155:200–206, 1998.

Perfusion

Volkow, N. D., Mullani, N., Gould, K. L., Adler, S. and Krajewski, K., Cerebral blood flow in chronic cocaine users: a study with positron emission tomography. Br. J. Psychiatry 152:641–648, 1988.

Volkow, N. D., Valentine, A. and Kulkarni, M., Radiological and neurological changes in the drug abuse patient: a study with MRI. J. Neuroradiol. 15:288–293, 1988. [Case Report]

Tumeh, S. S., Nagel, J. S., English, R. J., Moore, M. and Holman, B. L., Cerebral abnormalities in cocaine abusers: demonstration by SPECT perfusion brain scintigraphy. Work in progress. Radiology 176:821–824, 1990.

Holman, B. L., Carvalho, P. A., Mendelson, J., Teoh, S. K., Nardin, R., Hallgring, E., Hebben, N. and Johnson, K. A., Brain perfusion is abnormal in cocaine-dependent polydrug users: a study using technetium-99m-HMPAO and ASPECT. J. Nucl. Med. 32:1206–1210, 1991.

Holman, B. L., Garada, B., Johnson, K. A., Mendelson, J. H., Hallgring, E., Teoh, S. K., Worth, J. and Navia, B., A comparison of brain perfusion SPECT in cocaine abuse and AIDS dementia complex. J. Nucl. Med. 33:1312–1315, 1992.

Miller, B. L., Mena, I., Giombetti, R., Villanueva-Meyer, J. and Djenderedjian, A. H., Neuropsychiatric effects of cocaine: SPECT measurements. J. Addict. Dis. 11:47–58, 1992.

Weber, D. A., Franceschi, D., Ivanovic, M., Atkins, H. L., Cabahug, C., Wong, C. T. C. and Susskind, H., SPECT and planar brain imaging in crack abuse: Iodine-123-iodoamphetamine uptake and localization. J. Nucl. Med. 34:899–907, 1993.

Levin, J. M., Holman, B. L., Mendelson, J. H., Teoh, S. K., Garada, B., Johnson, K. A. and Springer, S., Gender differences in cerebral perfusion in cocaine abuse: ^{99m}Tc-HMPAO SPECT study of drug abusing women J. Nucl. Med. 35:1902–1909, 1994.

Levin, J. M., Mendelson, J. H., Holman, B. L., Teoh, S. K., Garada, B., Schwartz, R. B. and Mello, N. K., Improved regional cerebral blood flow in chronic cocaine polydrug users treated with buprenorphine. J. Nucl. Med. 36:1211–1215, 1995.

Christensen, J. D., Kaufman, M. J., Levin, J. M., Mendelson, J. H., Holman, B. L., Cohen, B. M. and Renshaw, P. F., Abnormal cerebral metabolism in polydrug abusers during early withdrawal: A ^{31}P MR spectroscopy study. Magn. Reson. Med. 35:658–663, 1996.

LaMonaca, G., Donatelli, A. and Katz, J. L., A case of mutism subsequent to cocaine abuse. J. Subst. Abuse Treat. 17:109–112, 1999. [Case Report]

Sex Differences

Levin, J. M., Holman, B. L., Mendelson, J. H., Teoh, S. K., Garada, B., Johnson, K. A. and Springer, S., Gender differences in cerebral perfusion in cocaine abuse: ^{99m}Tc-HMPAO SPECT study of drug abusing women J. Nucl. Med. 35:1902–1909, 1994.

Receptor/Transporter Effects

Volkow, N. D., Fowler, J. S., Wolf, A. P., Schlyer, D., Shiue, C. Y., Alpert, R., Dewey, S. L., Logan, J., Bendriem, B., Christman, D., Hitzemann, R. and Henn, F., Effects of chronic cocaine abuse on postsynaptic dopamine receptors. Am. J. Psychiatry 147:719–724, 1990.

Volkow, N. D., Fowler, J. S., Wang, G. J., Hitzemann, R., Logan, J., Schlyer, D. J., Dewey, S. L. and Wolf, A. P., Decreased dopamine D_2 receptor availability is associated with reduced frontal metabolism in cocaine abusers. Synapse 14:169–177, 1993.

Volkow, N. D., Wang, G. J., Fowler, J. S., Logan, J., Hitzemannn, R., Gatley, S. J., MacGregor, R. R. and Wolf, A. P., Cocaine uptake is decreased in the brain of detoxified cocaine abusers. Neuropsychopharmacology 14:159–168, 1996.

Zubieta, J.-K., Gorelick, D. A., Stauffer, R., Ravert, H. T., Dannals, R. F. and Frost, J. J., Increased mu opioid receptor binding detected by PET in cocaine-dependent men is associated with cocaine craving. Nat. Med. 2:1225–1229, 1996.

Logan, J., Volkow, N. D., Fowler, J. S., Wang, G. J., Fischman, M. W., Foltin, R. W., Abumrad, N. N., Vitkun, S., Gatley, S. J., Pappas, N., Hitzemann, R. and Shea, C. E., Concentration and occupancy of dopamine transporters in cocaine abusers with [^{11}C]cocaine and PET. Synapse 27:347–356, 1997.

Volkow, N. D., Wang, G. J., Fowler, J. S., Logan, J., Gatley, S. J., Hitzemann, R., Chen, A. D., Dewey, S. L. and Pappas, N., Decreased striatal dopaminergic responsiveness in detoxified cocaine-dependent subjects. Nature 386:830–833, 1997.

Wang, G. J., Volkow, N. D., Fowler, J. S., Fischman, M., Foltin, R., Abumrad, N. N., Logan, J. and Pappas, N. R., Cocaine abusers do not show loss of dopamine transporters with age. Life Sci. 61:1059–1065, 1997.

Malison, R. T., McCance, E., Carpenter, L. L., Baldwin, R. M., Seibyl, J. P., Price, L. H., Kosten, T. R. and Innis, R. B., [^{123}I]β-CIT SPECT imaging of dopamine transporter availability after mazindol administration in human cocaine addicts. Psychopharmacology (Berl.) 137:321–325, 1998.

Withdrawal

Volkow, N., Fowler, J., Wolf, A., Hitzemann, R., Dewey, S., Bendriem, B., Alpert, R. and Hoff, A., Changes in brain glucose metabolism in cocaine dependence and withdrawal. Am. J. Psychiatry 148:621–626, 1991.

Volkow, N. D., Hitzemann, R., Fowler, J. S. and Wolf, A. P., Regional brain metabolic activity during different stages of cocaine withdrawal. J. Nucl. Med. 32:960, 1991. [Abstract]

Christensen, J. D., Kaufman, M. J., Levin, J. M., Mendelson, J. H., Holman, B. L., Cohen, B. M. and Renshaw, P. F., Abnormal cerebral metabolism in polydrug abusers during early withdrawal: A ^{31}P MR spectroscopy study. Magn. Reson. Med. 35:658–663, 1996.

Wu, J. C., Bell, K., Najafi, A., Widmark, C., Keator, D., Tang, C., Klein, E., Bunney, B. G., Fallon, J. and Bunney, W. E., Decreasing striatal 6-FDOPA uptake with increasing duration of cocaine withdrawal. Neuropsychopharmacology 17:402–409, 1997.

Kosten, T. R., Cheeves, C., Palumbo, J., Seibyl, J. P., Price, L. H. and Woods, S. W., Regional cerebral blood flow during acute and chronic abstinence from combined cocaine-alcohol abuse. Drug Alcohol Depend. 50:187–195, 1998.

Craving

Grant, S., London, E. D., Newlin, D. B., Villemagne, V. L., Liu, X., Contoreggi, C., Phillips, R. L., Kimes, A. S. and Margolin, A., Activation of memory circuits during cue-elicited cocaine craving. Proc. Natl. Acad. Sci. U.S.A. 93:12040–12045, 1996.

Zubieta, J.-K., Gorelick, D. A., Stauffer, R., Ravert, H. T., Dannals, R. F. and Frost, J. J., Increased mu opioid receptor binding detected by PET in cocaine-dependent men is associated with cocaine craving. Nat. Med. 2:1225–1229, 1996.

Liu, X., Vaupel, D. B., Gran, S. and London, E. D., Effect of cocaine-related environmental stimuli on the spontaneous electroencephalogram in polydrug abusers. Neuropsychopharmacology 19:10–17, 1998.

Childress, A. R., Mozley, P. D., McElgin, W., Fitzgerald, J., Reivich, M. and O'Brien, C. P., Limbic activation during cue-induced cocaine craving. Am. J. Psychiatry 156:11–18, 1999.

Wang, G. J., Volkow, N. D., Fowler, J. S., Cervany, P., Hitzemann, R. J., Pappas, N. R., Wong, C. T. and Felder, C., Regional brain metabolic activation during craving elicited by recall of previous drug experiences. Life Sci. 64:775–784, 1999.

Abstinence

Volkow, N., Hitzemann, R., Wang, G., Fowler, J., Wolf, A., Dewey, S. and Handlesman, L., Long-term frontal brain metabolic changes in cocaine abusers. Synapse 11:184–190, 1992.

Strickland, T. L., Mena, I., Villanueva-Meyer, J., Miller, B. L., Cummings, J., Mehringer, C. M., Satz, P. and Myers, H., Cerebral perfusion and neuropsychological consequences of chronic cocaine use. J. Neuropsychiatry Clin. Neurosci. 5:419–427, 1993.

Malison, R. T., Best, S. E., Zoghbi, S., Zea-Ponce, Y., Baldwin, R. M., Charney, D., Hoffer, P., Seibyl, J. P., Price, L. H., Kosten, T. R. and Innis, R. B., SPECT imaging of dopamine transporters during sustained cocaine abstinence with [^{123}I]β-CIT. J. Nucl. Med. 37:44P, 1996. [Abstract]

Volkow, N. D., Wang, G. J., Fowler, J. S., Logan, J., Hitzemannn, R., Gatley, S. J., MacGregor, R. R. and Wolf, A. P., Cocaine uptake is decreased in the brain of detoxified cocaine abusers. Neuropsychopharmacology 14:159–168, 1996.

Wu, J. C., Bell, K., Najafi, A., Widmark, C., Keator, D., Tang, C., Klein, E., Bunney, B. G., Fallon, J. and Bunney, W. E., Decreasing striatal 6-FDOPA uptake with increasing duration of cocaine withdrawal. Neuropsychopharmacology 17:402–409, 1997.

Bowers, M. B., Jr., Malison, R. T., Seibyl, J. P. and Kosten, T. R., Plasma homovanillic acid and the dopamine transporter during cocaine withdrawal. Biol. Psychiatry 43:278–281, 1998.

Kosten, T. R., Cheeves, C., Palumbo, J., Seibyl, J. P., Price, L. H. and Woods, S. W., Regional cerebral blood flow during acute and chronic abstinence from combined cocaine-alcohol abuse. Drug Alcohol Depend. 50:187–195, 1998.

Malison, R. T., Best, S. E., van Dyck, C. H., McCance, E. F., Wallace, E. A., Laruelle, M., Baldwin, R. M., Seibyl, J. P., Price, L. H., Kosten, T. R. and Innis, R. B., Elevated striatal dopamine transporters during acute cocaine abstinence as measured by [^{123}I]β-CIT SPECT. Am. J. Psychiatry 155:832–834, 1998.

Treatment

Holman, B. L., Mendelson, J., Garada, B., Teoh, S. K., Hallgring, E., Johnson, K. A. and Mello, N. K., Regional cerebral blood flow improves with treatment in chronic cocaine polydrug users. J. Nucl. Med. 34:723–727, 1993.

Levin, J. M., Mendelson, J. H., Holman, B. L., Teoh, S. K., Garada, B., Schwartz, R. B. and Mello, N. K., Improved regional cerebral blood flow in chronic cocaine polydrug users treated with buprenorphine. J. Nucl. Med. 36:1211–1215, 1995.

Dewey, S. L., Morgan, A. E., Ashby, C. R., Jr., Horan, B., Kushner, S. A., Logan, J., Volkow, N. D., Fowler, J. S., Gardner, E. L. and Brodie, J. D., A novel strategy for the treatment of cocaine addiction. Synapse 30:119–129, 1998. [Nonhuman Primate]

Johnson, B., Barron, B., Fang, B., Lamki, L., Wagner, L., Wells, L., Kenny, P., Overton, D., Dhother, S., Abramson, D., Chen, R. and Kramer, L., Isradipine prevents global and regional cocaine-induced changes in brain blood flow: a preliminary study. Psychopharmacology (Berl.) 136:335–341, 1998.

Bartzokis, G., Beckson, M., Newton, T., Mandelkern, M., Mintz, J., Foster, J. A., Ling, W. and Bridge, T. P., Selegiline effects on cocaine-induced changes in medial temporal lobe metabolism and subjective ratings of euphoria. Neuropsychopharmacology 20:582–590, 1999.

Prenatal Exposure

Konkol, R. J., Tikofsky, R. S., Wells, R., Hellman, R. S., Nemeth, P., Walsh, D. J., Heimler, R. and Sty, J. R., Normal high-resolution cerebral ^{99m}Tc-HMPAO SPECT scans in symptomatic neonates exposed to cocaine. J. Child Neurol. 9:278–283, 1994.

Reviews

Mathew, R. J. and Wilson, W. H., Substance abuse and cerebral blood flow. Am. J. Psychiatry 148:292–305, 1991.

Woods, S. W., Regional cerebral blood flow imaging with SPECT in psychiatric disease: focus on schizophrenia, anxiety disorders, and substance abuse. J. Clin. Psychiatry 53 Suppl.:20–25, 1992.

Lago, J. A. and Kosten, T. R., Stimulant withdrawal. Addiction 89:1477–1481, 1994.

Levin, J. M. and Kaufman, M. J., Functional studies in substance abuse: imaging and beyond. J. Nucl. Med. 36:1298–1300, 1995.

Cadet, J. L. and Bolla, K. I., Chronic cocaine use as a neuropsychiatric syndrome: a model for debate. Synapse 22:28–34, 1996.

Volkow, N. D., Ding, Y. S., Fowler, J. S. and Wang, G. J., Cocaine addiction: hypothesis derived from imaging studies with PET. J. Addict. Dis. 15:55–71, 1996.

Ernst, M. and London, E. D., Brain imaging studies of drug abuse—therapeutic implications. Sem. Neurosci. 9:120–130, 1997.

Gatley, S. J. and Volkow, N. D., Addiction and imaging of the living human brain. Drug Alcohol Depend. 51:97–108, 1998.

Strickland, T. L., Miller, B. L., Kowell, A. and Stein, R., Neurobiology of cocaine-induced organic brain impairment: contributions from functional neuroimaging. Neuropsychol. Rev. 8:1–9, 1998.

Wong, D. F., Ricaurte, G., Grunder, G., Rothman, R., Naidu, S., Singer, H., Harris, J., Yokoi, F., Villemagne, V., Szymanski, S., Gjedde, A. and Kuhar, M., Dopamine transporter changes in neuropsychiatric disorders. Adv. Pharmacol. 42:219–223, 1998.

Amphetamine and Other Stimulants

Acute Administration

Metabolism

Wolkin, A., Angrist, B., Wolf, A., Brodie, J., Wolkin, B., Jaeger, J., Cancro, R. and Rotrosen, J., Effects of amphetamine on local cerebral metabolism in normal and schizophrenic subjects as determined by positron emission tomography. Psychopharmacology (Berl.) 92:241–246, 1987.

Ernst, M., Zametkin, A. J., Matochik, J., Schmidt, M., Jons, P. H., Liebenauer, L. L., Hardy, K. K. and Cohen, R. M., Intravenous dextroamphetamine and brain glucose metabolism. Neuropsychopharmacology 17:391–401, 1997.

Vollenweider, F. X., Maguire, R. P., Leenders, K. L., Mathys, K. and Angst, J., Effects of high amphetamine dose on mood and cerebral glucose metabolism in normal volunteers using positron emission tomography. Psychiatry Res. 83:149–162, 1998.

Perfusion

Berglund, M., Risberg, J., Regional cerebral blood flow in a case of amphetamine intoxication. Psychopharmacology (Berl.) 70:219–221, 1980. [Case Report]

Mathew, R. J. and Wilson, W. H., Dextroamphetamine-induced changes in regional cerebral blood flow. Psychopharmacology (Berl.) 87:298–302, 1985.

Kahn, D. A., Prohovnik, I., Lucas, L. R. and Sackeim, H. A., Dissociated effects of amphetamine on arousal and cortical blood flow in humans. Biol. Psychiatry 25:755–767, 1989.

Mathew, R. J. and Wilson, W. H., Changes in cerebral blood flow and mental state after amphetamine challenge in schizophrenic patients. Neuropsychobiology 21:117–123, 1989.

Mattay, V. S., Berman, K. F., Ostrem, J. L., Esposito, G., Van Horn, J. D., Bigelow, L. B. and Weinberger, D. R., Dextroamphetamine enhances "neural network-specific" physiological signals: a positron-emission tomography rCBF study. J. Neurosci. 16:4816–4822, 1996.

Chen, Y. C., Galpern, W. R., Brownell, A. L., Matthews, R. T., Bogdanov, M., Isacson, O., Keltner, J. R., Beal, M. F., Rosen, B. R. and Jenkins, B. G., Detection of dopaminergic neurotransmitter activity using pharmacologic MRI: correlation with PET, microdialysis, and behavioral data. Magn. Reson. Med. 38:389–398, 1997. [Rodent]

Neurotransmitter Changes

Dewey, S. L., Logan, J., Wolf, A. P., Brodie, J. D., Angrist, B., Fowler, J. S. and Volkow, N. D., Amphetamine induced decreases in (^{18}F)-N-methylspiroperidol binding in the baboon brain using positron emission tomography (PET). Synapse 7:324–327, 1991. [Nonhuman Primate]

Dewey, S. L., Smith, G. S., Logan, J., Brodie, J. D., Fowler, J. S. and Wolf, A. P., Striatal binding of the PET ligand ^{11}C-raclopride is altered by drugs that modify synaptic dopamine levels. Synapse 13:350–356, 1993. [Nonhuman Primate]

Laruelle, M., Abi-Dargham, A., van Dyck, C. H., Rosenblatt, W., Zea-Ponce, Y., Zoghbi, S. S., Baldwin, R. M., Charney, D. S., Hoffer, P. B., Kung, H. F. and Innis, R. B., SPECT imaging of striatal dopamine release after amphetamine challenge. J. Nucl. Med. 36:1182–1190, 1995.

Laruelle, M., Abi-Dargham, A., van Dyck, C. H., Gil, R., D'Souza, C. D., Erdos, J., McCance, E., Rosenblatt, W., Fingado, C., Zoghbi, S. S., Baldwin, R. M., Seibyl, J. P., Krystal, J. H., Charney, D. S. and Innis, R. B., Single photon emission computerized tomography imaging of amphetamine-induced dopamine release in drug-free schizophrenic subjects. Proc. Natl. Acad. Sci. USA 93:9235–9240, 1996.

Breier, A., Su, T. P., Saunders, R., Carson, R. E., Kolachana, B. S., de Bartolomeis, A., Weinberger, D. R., Weisenfeld, N., Malhotra, A. K., Eckelman, W. C. and Pickar, D., Schizophrenia is associated with elevated amphetamine-induced synaptic dopamine concentrations: evidence from a novel positron emission tomography method. Proc. Natl. Acad. Sci. USA 94:2569–2574, 1997.

Carson, R. E., Breier, A., de Bartolomeis, A., Saunders, R. C., Su, T. P., Schmall, B., Der, M. G., Pickar, D. and Eckelman, W. C., Quantification of amphetamine-induced changes in [^{11}C] raclopride binding with continuous infusion. J. Cereb. Blood Flow Metab. 17:437–447, 1997. [Nonhuman Primate]

Hartvig, P., Torstenson, R., Tedroff, J., Watanabe, Y., Fasth, K. J., Bjurling, P. and Langstrom B., Amphetamine effects on dopamine release and synthesis rate studied in the Rhesus monkey brain by positron emission tomography. J. Neural. Transm. 104:329–339, 1997. [Nonhuman Primate]

Laruelle, M., Iyer, R. N., al-Tikriti, M. S., Zea-Ponce, Y., Malison, R., Zoghbi, S. S., Baldwin, R. M., Kung, H. F., Charney, D. S., Hoffer, P. B., Innis, R. B. and Bradberry, C. W., Microdialysis and SPECT measurements of amphetamine-induced dopamine release in nonhuman primates. Synapse 25:1–14, 1997. [Nonhuman Primate]

Mach, R. H., Nader, M. A., Ehrenkaufer, R. L., Line, S. W., Smith, C. R., Gage, H. D. and Morton, T. E., Use of positron emission tomography to study the dynamics of psychostimulant-induced dopamine release. Pharmacol. Biochem. Behav. 57:477–486, 1997. [Nonhuman Primate]

Melega, W. P., Raleigh, M. J., Stout, D. B., Lacan, G., Huang, S. C. and Phelps, M. E., Recovery of striatal dopamine function after acute amphetamine- and methamphetamine-induced neurotoxicity in the vervet monkey. Brain Res. 766:113–120, 1997. [Nonhuman Primate]

Tibbo, P., Silverstone, P. H., McEwan, A. J., Scott, J., Joshua, A. and Golberg, K., A single photon emission computed tomography scan study of striatal dopamine D_2 receptor binding with ^{123}I-epidepride in patients with schizophrenia and controls. J. Psychiatry Neurosci. 22:39–45, 1997.

Abi-Dargham, A., Gil, R., Krystal, J., Baldwin, R. M., Seibyl, J. P., Bowers, M., van Dyck, C. H., Charney, D. S., Innis, R. B. and Laruelle, M., Increased striatal dopamine transmission in schizophrenia: confirmation in a second cohort. Am. J. Psychiatry 155:761–767, 1998.

Kegeles, L. S., Zea-Ponce, Y., Abi-Dargham, A., Rodenhiser, J., Wang, T., Weiss, R., Van Heertum, R. L., Mann, J. J. and Laruelle, M., Stability of [^{123}I]IBZM SPECT measurement of amphetamine-induced striatal dopamine release in humans. Synapse 31:302–308, 1999.

Malison, R., Mechanic, K., Klumpp, H., Baldwin, R., Kosten, T., Seibyl, J. and Innis, R., Reduced amphetamine-stimulated dopamine release in cocaine addicts as measured by [^{123}I]IBZM SPECT. J. Nucl. Med. 40:110P, 1999. [Abstract]

Villemagne, V. L., Wong, D. F., Yokoi, F., Stephane, M., Rice, K. C., Matecka, D., Clough, D. J., Dannals, R. F. and Rothman, R. B., GBR12909 attenuates amphetamine-induced striatal dopamine release as measured by [(^{11})C]raclopride continuous infusion PET scans. Synapse 33:268–273, 1999. [Nonhuman Primate]

Chronic Administration

Ohta, H., Komibuchi, T., Nishino, I., Enomoto, Y. and Miyata, M., Brain perfusion abnormalities in a thinner and amphetamine abuser detected by I-123 IMP scintigraphy. Ann. Nucl. Med. 6:273–275, 1992. [Case Report]

Kao, C. H., Wang, S. J. and Yeh, S. H., Presentation of regional cerebral blood flow in amphetamine abusers by 99Tcm-HMPAO brain SPECT. Nucl. Med. Commun. 15:94–98, 1994.

Melega, W. P., Quintana, J., Raleigh, M. J., Stout, D. B., Yu, D. C., Lin, K. P., Huang, S. C. and Phelps, M. E., 6-[^{18}F]fluoro-L-DOPA-PET studies show partial reversibility of long-term effects of chronic amphetamine in monkeys. Synapse 22:63–69, 1996. [Nonhuman Primate]

Melega, W. P., Raleigh, M. J., Stout, D. B., Huang, S. C. and Phelps, M. E., Ethological and 6-[^{18}F]fluoro-L-DOPA-PET profiles of long-term vulnerability to chronic amphetamine. Behav. Brain Res. 84:259–268, 1997. [Nonhuman Primate]

Ginovart, N., Farde, L., Halldin, C. and Swahn, C. G., Changes in striatal D_2-receptor density following chronic treatment with amphetamine as assessed with PET in nonhuman primates. Synapse 31:154–162, 1999. [Nonhuman Primate]

Reviews

Mathew, R. J. and Wilson, W. H., Substance abuse and cerebral blood flow. Am. J. Psychiatry 148:292–305, 1991.

Lago, J. A. and Kosten, T. R., Stimulant withdrawal. Addiction 89:1477–1481, 1994.

Gatley, S. J. and Volkow, N. D., Addiction and imaging of the living human brain. Drug Alcohol Depend. 51:97–108, 1998.

Methamphetamine

Iyo, M., Nishio, M., Itoh, T., Fukuda, H., Suzuki, K., Yamasaki, T., Fukui, S. and Tateno, Y., Dopamine D_2 and serotonin S2 receptors in susceptibility to methamphetamine psychosis detected by positron emission tomography. Psychiatry Res. 50:217–231, 1993.

Iyo, M., Namba, H., Yanagisawa, M., Hirai, S., Yui, N. and Fukui, S., Abnormal cerebral perfusion in chronic methamphetamine abusers: a study using 99MTc-HMPAO and SPECT. Prog. Neuropsychopharmacol. Biol. Psychiatry 21:789–796, 1997.

Mach, R. H., Nader, M. A., Ehrenkaufer, R. L., Line, S. W., Smith, C. R., Gage, H. D. and Morton, T. E., Use of positron emission tomography to study the dynamics of psychostimulant-induced dopamine release. Pharmacol. Biochem. Behav. 57:477–486, 1997. [Nonhuman Primate]

Melega, W. P., Raleigh, M. J., Stout, D. B., Lacan, G., Huang, S. C. and Phelps, M. E., Recovery of striatal dopamine function after acute amphetamine- and methamphetamine-induced neurotoxicity in the vervet monkey. Brain Res. 766:113–120, 1997. [Nonhuman Primate]

McCann, U. D., Wong, D. F., Yokoi, F., Villemagne, V., Dannals, R. F. and Ricaurte, G. A., Reduced striatal dopamine transporter density in abstinent methamphetamine and methcathinone users: evidence from positron emission tomography studies with [^{11}C]WIN-35,428. J. Neurosci. 18:8417–8422, 1998.

Melega, W. P., Lacan, G., Harvey, D. C., Huang, S. C. and Phelps M. E., Dizocilpine and reduced body temperature do not prevent methamphetamine-induced neurotoxicity in the vervet monkey: [^{11}C]WIN 35,428—positron emission tomography studies. Neurosci. Lett. 258:17–20, 1998. [Nonhuman Primate]

Villemagne, V., Yuan, J., Wong, D. F., Dannals, R. F., Hatzidimitriou, G., Mathews, W. B., Ravert, H. T., Musachio, J., McCann, U. D. and Ricaurte, G. A., Brain dopamine neurotoxicity in baboons treated with doses of methamphetamine comparable to those recreationally abused by humans: evidence from [^{11}C]WIN-35,428 positron emission tomography studies and direct in vitro determinations. J. Neurosci. 18:419–427, 1998. [Nonhuman Primate]

Gouzoulis-Mayfrank, E., Schreckenberger, M., Sabri, O., Arning, C., Thelen, B., Spitzer, M., Kovar, K.-A., Hermle, L., Bull, U. and Sass, H., Neurometabolic effects of psilocybin, 3,4-methylenedioxyethylamphetamine (MDE) and d-methamphetamine in healthy volunteers. A double-blind, placebo-controlled PET study with [^{18}F]FDG. Neuropsychopharmacology 20:565–581, 1999.

Methcathinone

McCann, U. D., Wong, D. F., Yokoi, F., Villemagne, V., Dannals, R. F. and Ricaurte, G. A., Reduced striatal dopamine transporter density in abstinent methamphetamine and methcathinone users: evidence from positron emission tomography studies with [^{11}C]WIN-35,428. J. Neurosci. 18:8417–8422, 1998.

Methylphenidate

Volkow, N. D., Wang, G. J., Fowler, J. S., Logan, J., Schyler, D., Hitzemann, R., Lieberman, J., Angrist, B., Pappas, N., MacGregor, R., Burr, G., Cooper, T. and Wolf, A. P., Imaging endogenous dopamine competition with [^{11}C] raclopride in the human brain. Synapse 16:255–262, 1994.

Wang, G. J., Volkow, N. D., Fowler, J. S., Ferrieri, R., Schlyer, D. J., Alexoff, D., Pappas, N., Lieberman, J., King, P., Warner, D., Wong, C., Hitzemann, R. J. and Wolf, A. P., Methylphenidate decreases regional cerebral blood flow in normal human subjects. Life Sci. 54:PL143–PL146, 1994.

Volkow, N. D., Ding, Y.-S., Fowler, J. S., Wang, G.-J., Logan, J., Gatley, J. S., Dewey, S., Ashby, C., Liebermann, J., Hitzemann, R. and Wolf, A. P., Is methylphenidate like cocaine? Studies on their pharmacokinetics and distribution in the human brain. Arch. Gen. Psychiatry 52:456–463, 1995.

Volkow, N. D., Wang, G. J., Fowler, J. S., Gatley, S. J., Ding, Y. S., Logan, J., Dewey, S. L., Hitzemann, R. and Lieberman, J., Relationship between psychostimulant-induced "high" and dopamine transporter occupancy. Proc. Natl. Acad. Sci. USA 93:10388–10392, 1996.

Volkow, N. D., Wang, G. J., Gatley, S. J., Fowler, J. S., Ding, Y. S., Logan, J., Hitzemann, R., Angrist, B. and Lieberman, J., Temporal relationships between the pharmacokinetics of methylphenidate in the human brain and its behavioral and cardiovascular effects. Psychopharmacology (Berl.) 123:26–33, 1996.

Booij, J., Korn, P., Linszen, D. H. and van Royen, E. A., Assessment of endogenous dopamine release by methylphenidate challenge using iodine-123 iodobenzamide single-photon emission tomography. Eur. J. Nucl. Med. 24:674–677, 1997.

Mach, R. H., Nader, M. A., Ehrenkaufer, R. L., Line, S. W., Smith, C. R., Gage, H. D. and Morton, T. E., Use of positron emission tomography to study the dynamics of psychostimulant-induced dopamine release. Pharmacol. Biochem. Behav. 57:477–486, 1997. [Nonhuman Primate]

Volkow, N. D., Wang, G. J., Fowler, J. S., Logan, J., Angrist, B., Hitzemann, R., Lieberman, J. and Pappas, N., Effects of methylphenidate on regional brain glucose metabolism in humans: relationship to dopamine D_2 receptors. Am. J. Psychiatry 154:50–55, 1997.

Volkow, N. D., Wang, G. J., Fowler, J. S., Logan, J., Gatley, S. J., Hitzemann, R., Chen, A. D., Dewey, S. L. and Pappas, N., Decreased striatal dopaminergic responsiveness in detoxified cocaine-dependent subjects. Nature 386:830–833, 1997.

Volkow, N. D., Wang, G. J., Fowler, J. S., Hitzemann, R. J., Gatley, J., Ding, Y. S., Wong, C. and Pappas, N. R., Differences in regional brain metabolic responses between single and repeated doses of methylphenidate. Psychiatry Res. 83:29–36, 1998.

Volkow, N. D., Wang, G. J., Fowler, J. S., Gatley, S. J., Logan, J., Ding, Y. S., Hitzemann, R. and Pappas, N., Dopamine transporter occupancies in the human brain induced by therapeutic doses of oral methylphenidate. Am. J. Psychiatry 155:1325–1331, 1998.

Volkow, N. D., Wang, G. J., Fowler, J. S., Hitzemann, R., Angrist, B., Gatley, S. J., Logan, J., Ding, Y. S. and Pappas, N., Association of methylphenidate-induced craving with changes in right striato-orbitofrontal metabolism in cocaine abusers: implications in addiction. Am. J. Psychiatry 156:19–26, 1999.

Volkow, N. D., Wang, G. J., Fowler, J. S., Gatley, S. J., Logan, J., Ding, Y. S., Dewey, S. L., Hitzemann, R., Gifford, A. N. and Pappas, N. R., Blockade of striatal dopamine transporters by intravenous methylphenidate is not sufficient to induce self-reports of "High". J. Pharmacol. Exp. Ther. 288:14–20, 1999.

Volkow, N. D., Fowler, J. S., Gatley, S. J., Dewey, S. L., Wang, G. J., Logan, J., Ding, Y. S., Franceschi, D., Gifford, A., Morgan, A., Pappas, N. and King, P., Comparable changes in synaptic dopamine induced by methylphenidate and by cocaine in the baboon brain. Synapse 31:59–66, 1999. [Nonhuman Primate]

Review

Gatley, S. J. and Volkow, N. D., Addiction and imaging of the living human brain. Drug Alcohol Depend. 51:97–108, 1998.

Solvents and Toluene

Acute Administration

Mathew, R. J., Wilson, W. H. and Tant, S. R., Regional cerebral blood flow changes associated with amyl nitrite inhalation. Br. J. Addict. 84:293–299, 1989.

Edling, C., Hellman, B., Arvidson, B., Johansson, G., Andersson, J., Hartvig, P., Valind, S. and Langstrom, B., Positron emission tomography studies of healthy volunteers—no effects on the dopamine terminals and synthesis after short-term exposure to toluene. Hum. Exp. Toxicol. 16:171–176, 1997.

Chronic Administration

Hagstadius, S., Orbaek, P., Risberg, J. and Lindgren, M., Regional cerebral blood flow at the time of diagnosis of chronic toxic encephalopathy induced by organic-solvent exposure and after the cessation of exposure. Scand. J. Work Environ. Health 15:130–135, 1989.

Ohta, H., Komibuchi, T., Nishino, I., Enomoto, Y. and Miyata, M., Brain perfusion abnormalities in a thinner and amphetamine abuser detected by I-123 IMP scintigraphy. Ann. Nucl. Med. 6:273–275, 1992. [Case Report]

Hirai, H. and Ikeuchi, Y., MRI of chronic toluene intoxication. Rinsho Shinkeigaku 33:552–555, 1993. [Case Report] [Japanese]

Heuser, G., Mena, I. and Alamos, F., NeuroSPECT findings in patients exposed to neurotoxic chemicals. Toxicol. Ind. Health 10:561–571, 1994.

Terashi, H., Nagata, K., Satoh, Y., Hirata, Y. and Hatazawa, J., Hippocampal hypoperfusion underlying dementia due to chronic toluene intoxication. Rinsho Shinkeigaku 37:1010–1013, 1997. [Case Report] [Japanese]

Pelegrin, C., Ceballos, C., Baringo, T., Poza, A. and Carrero, P., Secondary encephalopathy due to exposure to organic solvents: psychopathological, neuropsychological and neuroimaging findings. An. Med. Interna 15:91–94, 1998. [Case Report] [Spanish]

Ryu, Y. H., Lee, J. D., Yoon, P. H., Jeon, P., Kim, D. I. and Shin, D. W., Cerebral perfusion impairment in a patient with toluene abuse. J. Nucl. Med. 39:632–633, 1998. [Case Report]

Kitabayashi, Y., Ueda, H., Matsuda, M., Narumoto, J., Kobayashi, T. and Fukui, K., A case report of organic solvent abuse with amotivational syndrome. Nihon Arukoru Yakubutsu Igakkai Zasshi 34:130–137, 1999. [Case Report] [Japanese]

Occupational Exposure

Arlien-Soborg, P., Henriksen, L., Gade, A., Gyldensted, C. and Paulson, O. B., Cerebral blood flow in chronic toxic encephalopathy in house painters exposed to organic solvents. Acta Neurol. Scand. 66:34–41, 1982.

Maximilian, V. A., Risberg, J., Prohovnik, I., Rehnstrom, S. and Haeger-Aronsen, B., Regional cerebral blood flow and verbal memory after chronic exposure to organic solvents. Brain Cogn. 1:196–205, 1982.

Risberg, J. and Hagstadius, S., Effects on the regional cerebral blood flow of long-term exposure to organic solvents. Acta Psychiatr. Scand. Suppl. 303:92–99, 1983.

Callender, T. J., Morrow, L., Subramanian, K., Duhon, D. and Ristovu, M., Three-dimensional brain metabolic imaging in patients with toxic encephalopathy. Environ. Res. 60:295–319, 1993.

Edling, C., Hellman, B., Arvidson, B., Andersson, J., Hartvig, P., Lilja, A., Valind, S. and Langstrom, B., Do organic solvents induce changes in the dopaminergic system? Positron emission tomography studies of occupationally exposed subjects. Int. Arch. Occup. Environ. Health 70:180–186, 1997.

Hageman, G., van der Hoek, J., van Hout, M., van der Laan, G., Steur, E.J., de Bruin, W. and Herholz, K., Parkinsonism, pyramidal signs, polyneuropathy, and cognitive decline after long-term occupational solvent exposure. J. Neurology 246:198–206, 1999. [Case Report]

Review

Mathew, R. J. and Wilson, W. H., Substance abuse and cerebral blood flow. Am. J. Psychiatry 148:292–305, 1991.

Yamanouchi, N., Okada, S.-I., Kodama, K. and Sato, T., Central nervous system impairment caused by chronic solvent abuse—a review of Japanese studies on the clinical and neuroimaging aspects. Addiction Biol. 3:15–27, 1998.

Polydrug Abuse

Volkow, N. D., Valentine, A. and Kulkarni, M., Radiological and neurological changes in the drug abuse patient: a study with MRI. J. Neuroradiol. 15:288–293, 1988. [Case Report]

Tumeh, S. S., Nagel, J. S., English, R. J., Moore, M. and Holman, B. L., Cerebral abnormalities in cocaine abusers: demonstration by SPECT perfusion brain scintigraphy. Work in progress. Radiology 176:821–824, 1990.

Holman, B. L., Carvalho, P. A., Mendelson, J., Teoh, S. K., Nardin, R., Hallgring, E., Hebben, N. and Johnson, K. A., Brain perfusion is abnormal in cocaine-dependent polydrug users: a study using technetium-99m-HMPAO and ASPECT. J. Nucl. Med. 32:1206–1210, 1991.

Woods, S. W., O'Malley, S. S., Martini, B. L., McDougle, C. J., Price, L. H., Krystal, J. H., Hoffer, P. B. and Kosten, T. R., SPECT regional cerebral blood flow and neuropsychological testing in non-demented HIV-positive drug abusers. Prog. Neuropsychopharmacol. Biol. Psychiatry 15:649–662, 1991.

Holman, B. L., Mendelson, J., Garada, B., Teoh, S. K., Hallgring, E., Johnson, K. A. and Mello, N. K., Regional cerebral blood flow improves with treatment in chronic cocaine polydrug users. J. Nucl. Med. 34:723–727, 1993.

Morgan, M. J., Cascella, N. G., Stapleton, J. M., Phillips, R. L., Yung, B. C., Wong, D. F., Shaya, E. K. and London, E. D., Sensitivity to subjective effects of cocaine in drug abusers: relationship to cerebral ventricle size. Am. J. Psychiatry 150:1712–1717, 1993.

Levin, J. M., Holman, B. L., Mendelson, J. H., Teoh, S. K., Garada, B., Johnson, K. A. and Springer, S., Gender differences in cerebral perfusion in cocaine abuse: ^{99m}Tc-HMPAO SPECT study of drug abusing women J. Nucl. Med. 35:1902–1909, 1994.

Levin, J. M., Mendelson, J. H., Holman, B. L., Teoh, S. K., Garada, B., Schwartz, R. B. and Mello, N. K., Improved regional cerebral blood flow in chronic cocaine polydrug users treated with buprenorphine. J. Nucl. Med. 36:1211–1215, 1995.

Stapleton, J. M., Morgan, M. J., Phillips, R. L., Wong, D. F., Yung, B. C., Shaya, E. K., Dannals, R. F., Liu, X., Grayson, R. L. and London, E. D., Cerebral glucose utilization in polysubstance abuse. Neuropsychopharmacology 13:21–31, 1995.

Christensen, J. D., Kaufman, M. J., Levin, J. M., Mendelson, J. H., Holman, B. L., Cohen, B. M. and Renshaw, P. F., Abnormal cerebral metabolism in polydrug abusers during early withdrawal: A ^{31}P MR spectroscopy study. Magn. Reson. Med. 35:658–663, 1996.

Kosten, T. R., Cheeves, C., Palumbo, J., Seibyl, J. P., Price, L. H. and Woods, S. W., Regional cerebral blood flow during acute and chronic abstinence from combined cocaine-alcohol abuse. Drug Alcohol Depend. 50:187–195, 1998.

MAGNETIC RESONANCE

Alcohol and Alcoholism

Acute Administration

RELAXOMETRY

Besson, J. A. O., Glen, A. I. M., Foreman, E. I., MacDonald, A., Smith, F. W., Hutchison, J. M. S., Mallard, J. R. and Ashcroft, G. W., Nuclear magnetic resonance observations in alcoholic cerebral disorder and the role of vasopressin. Lancet 2:923–924, 1981.

Mander, A. J., Smith, M. A., Kean, D. M., Chick, J., Douglas, R. H., Rehman, A. U., Weppner, G. J. and Best, J. J., Brain water measured in volunteers after alcohol and vasopressin. Lancet 2:1075, 1985.

Logsdail, S., Miller, D., Macmanus, D., Johnson, G., Lolin, Y. and O'Gorman, P., The effect of moderate blood alcohol levels on T1 and T2 relaxation times in the brains of normal volunteers. Magn. Reson. Med. 4:378–379, 1987.

Thomsen, H., Kaatsch, H. J. and Asmus, R., Magnetic resonance imaging of the brain during alcohol absorption and elimination—a study of the "rising tide phenomenon". Blutalkohol 31:178–185, 1994.

Imaging

Friedman, D. I., Aravapalli, S. R. and Shende, M. C., Visual pathway hemorrhage associated with alcohol-induced coagulopathy. J. Neuroophthalmol. 16:124–133, 1996. [Case Report]

Spectroscopy

Hetherington, H. P., Rowley, H., Peterson, K., Boska, M., Diamond, I. and Weiner, M. W., The kinetics of alcohol uptake in human brain and blood by volume selective ^{1}H MRS. Society of Magnetic Resonance in Medicine, Eighth Scientific Meeting, Amsterdam, The Netherlands, p. 370, 1989. [Abstract]

Hanstock, C. C., Rothman, D. L., Shulman, R. G., Novotny, E. J., Jr., Petroff, O. A. and Prichard, J. W., Measurement of ethanol in the human brain using NMR spectroscopy. J. Stud. Alcohol 51:104–107, 1990.

Mendelson, J. H., Woods, B. T., Chiu, T. M., Mello, N. K., Lukas, S. E., Teoh, S. K., Sintavanarong, P., Cochin, J., Hopkins, M. A. and Dobrosielski, M., In vivo proton magnetic resonance spectroscopy of alcohol in human brain. Alcohol 7:443–447, 1990.

Lukas, S. E., Dobrosielski, M., Chiu, T. M., Woods, B. T., Teoh, S. K. and Mendelson, J. H., A nonferrous instrumental joystick device for recording behavioral responses during magnetic resonance imaging and spectroscopy. Pharmacol. Biochem. Behav. 46:781–785, 1993.

Spielman, D. M., Glover, G. H., Macovski, A. and Pfefferbaum, A., Magnetic resonance spectroscopic imaging of ethanol in the human brain: a feasibility study. Alcohol. Clin. Exp. Res. 17:1072–1077, 1993.

Chiu, T.-M., Mendelson, J. H., Woods, B. T., Teoh, S. K., Levisohn, L. and Mello, N. K., In vivo proton magnetic resonance spectroscopy detection of human alcohol tolerance. Magn. Reson. Med. 32:511–516, 1994.

Kaufman, M. J., Chiu, T. M., Mendelson, J. H., Woods, B. T., Mello, N. K., Lukas, S. E., Fivel, P. A. and Wighton, L. G., In vivo proton magnetic resonance spectroscopy of alcohol in rhesus monkey brain. Magn. Reson. Imaging 12:1245–1253, 1994. [Nonhuman Primate]

Schauss, G., Schild, H., Urban, R., Bunke, J., Riepert, T., Grebe, P., Kersjes, W., Schunk, K. and Thelen, M., ^{1}H-MR spectroscopic imaging: an approach to evaluating alcohol breakdown in the brain. Rofo Fortschr. Geb. Rontgenstr. Neuen Bildgeb. Verfahr 160:493–499, 1994. [German]

Kaufman, M. J., Chiu, T.-M., Mendelson, J. H., Woods, B. T., Teoh, S. K., Eros-Sarnyai, M., Mercer, G. and Mello, N. K., Brain alcohol detectability increase with repeated administration in humans: a proton spectroscopy study. Magn. Reson. Med. 35:435–440, 1996.

Meyerhoff, D. J., Rooney, W. D., Tokumitsu, T. and Weiner, M. W., Evidence of multiple ethanol pools in the brain: an in vivo proton magnetization transfer study. Alcohol. Clin. Exp. Res. 20:1283–1288, 1996. [Rodent]

Meyerhoff, D. J., Ethanol in human brain: relaxation and magnetization transfer. International Society for Magnetic Resonance in Medicine, Sixth Scientific Meeting and Exhibition. Sydney, Australia, p. 193, 1998. [Abstract]

Functional MRI

Levin, J. M., Ross, M. H., Mendelson, J. H., Kaufman, M. J., Lange, N., Maas, L. C., Mello, N. K., Cohen, B. M. and Renshaw, P. F., Reduction in BOLD fMRI response to primary visual stimulation following alcohol ingestion. Psychiatry Res. 82:135–146, 1998.

Chronic Administration

RELAXOMETRY

Besson, J. A. O., Glen, A. I. M., Foreman, E. I., MacDonald, A., Smith, F. W., Hutchison, J. M. S., Mallard, J. R. and Ashcroft, G. W., Nuclear magnetic resonance observations in alcoholic cerebral disorder and the role of vasopressin. Lancet 2:923–924, 1981.

Smith, M. A., Chick, J., Kean, D. M., Douglas, R. H., Singer, A., Kendell, R. E. and Best, J. J., Brain water in chronic alcoholic patients measured by magnetic resonance imaging. Lancet 1:1273–1274, 1985.

Schroth, G., Naegele, T., Klose, U., Mann, K. and Petersen, D., Reversible brain shrinkage in abstinent alcoholics, measured by MRI. Neuroradiology 30:385–389, 1988.

Smith, M. A., Chick, J. D., Engleman, H. M., Kean, D. M., Mander, A. J., Douglas, R. H. and Best, J. J., Brain hydration during alcohol withdrawal in alcoholics measured by magnetic resonance imaging. Drug Alcohol Depend. 21:25–28, 1988.

Chick, J. D., Smith, M. A., Engleman, H. M., Kean, D. M., Mander, A. J., Douglas, R. H. and Best, J. J., Magnetic resonance imaging of the brain in alcoholics: cerebral atrophy, lifetime alcohol consumption, and cognitive deficits. Alcohol. Clin. Exp. Res. 13:512–518, 1989.

Mander, A. J., Young, A., Chick, J. D. and Best, J. J., The relationship of cerebral atrophy and T_1 in alcoholics: an MRI study. Drug Alcohol Depend. 24:57–59, 1989.

Mander, A. J., Young, A., Chick, J. D., Ridgway, J. and Best, J. J., NMR T_1 relaxation time of the brain during alcohol withdrawal and its lack of relationship with symptom severity. Br. J. Addict. 84:669–672, 1989.

Mann, K., Opitz, H., Petersen, D., Schroth, G. and Heimann, H., Intracranial CSF volumetry in alcoholics: studies with MRI and CT. Psychiatry Res. 29:277–279, 1989.

Agartz, I., Saaf, J., Wahlund, L. O. and Wetterberg, L., T_1 and T_2 relaxation time estimates and brain measures during withdrawal in alcoholic men. Drug Alcohol Depend. 29:157–169, 1991.

Bergman, H., Engelbrektson, K., Fransson, A., Herlitz, K., Hindmarsh, T. and Neiman, J., Alcohol-induced cognitive impairment is reversible. Neuropsychological tests but not MRT show improvement after abstinence. Lakartidningen 95:4228,4231–4236, 1998. [Swedish]

IMAGING

Ventricular Enlargement

Mann, K., Opitz, H., Petersen, D., Schroth, G. and Heimann, H., Intracranial CSF volumetry in alcoholics: studies with MRI and CT. Psychiatry Res. 29:277–279, 1989.

Zipursky, R. B., Lim, K. C. and Pfefferbaum, A., MRI study of brain changes with short-term abstinence from alcohol. Alcohol. Clin. Exp. Res. 13:664–666, 1989.

Jernigan, T. L., Butters, N., DiTraglia, G., Schafer, K., Smith, T., Irwin, M., Grant, I., Schuckit, M. and Cermak, L. S., Reduced cerebral grey matter observed in alcoholics using magnetic resonance imaging. Alcohol. Clin. Exp. Res. 15:418–427, 1991.

Kroft, C. L., Gescuk, B., Woods, B. T., Mello, N. K., Weiss, R. D. and Mendelson, J. H., Brain ventricular size in female alcoholics: an MRI study. Alcohol 8:31–34, 1991.

Hayakawa, K., Kumagai, H., Suzuki, Y., Furusawa, N., Haga, T., Hoshi, T., Fujiwara, Y. and Yamaguchi, K., MR imaging of chronic alcoholism. Acta Radiol. 33:201–206, 1992.

Pfefferbaum, A., Lim, K. O., Zipursky, R. B., Mathalon, D. H., Rosenbloom, M. J., Lane, B., Ha, C. N. and Sullivan, E. V., Brain gray and white matter volume loss accelerates with aging in chronic alcoholics: a quantitative MRI study. Alcohol. Clin. Exp. Res. 16:1078–1089, 1992.

Shear, P. K., Butters, N., Jernigan, T. L., DiTraglia, G. M., Irwin, M., Schuckit, M. A. and Cermak, L. S., Olfactory loss in alcoholics: correlations with cortical and subcortical MRI indices. Alcohol 9:247–255, 1992.

Wang, G. J., Volkow, N. D., Hitzemann, R., Oster, Z. H., Roque, C. and Cestaro, V., Brain imaging of an alcoholic with MRI, SPECT, and PET. Am. J. Physiol. Imaging 7:194–198, 1992. [Case Report]

Litton, J.-E., Neiman, J., Pauli, S., Farde, L., Hindmarsh, T., Halldin, C. and Sedvall, G., PET analysis of [^{11}C]Flumazenil binding to benzodiazepine receptors in chronic alcohol-dependent men and healthy controls. Psychiatry Res. 50:1–13, 1993.

Pfefferbaum, A., Sullivan, E. V., Rosenbloom, M. J., Shear, P. K., Mathalon, D. H. and Lim, K. O., Increase in brain cerebrospinal fluid volume is greater in older than in younger alcoholic patients: a replication study and CT/MRI comparison. Psychiatry Res. 50:257–274, 1993.

Wang, G. J., Volkow, N. D., Roque, C. T., Cestaro, V. L., Hitzemann, R. J., Cantos, E. L., Levy, A. V. and Dhawan, A. P., Functional importance of ventricular enlargement and cortical atrophy in healthy subjects and alcoholics as assessed with PET, MR imaging, and neuropsychologic testing. Radiology 186:59–65, 1993.

Kaseda, Y., Miyazato, Y., Ogura, C., Nakamoto, H., Uema, T., Yamamoto, K. and Ohta, I., Correlation between event-related potentials and MR measurements in chronic alcoholic patients. Jpn. J. Psychiatry Neurol. 48:23–32, 1994.

Di Sclafani, V., Ezekiel, F., Meyerhoff, D. J., MacKay, S., Dillon, W. P., Weiner, M. W. and Fein, G., Brain atrophy and cognitive function in older abstinent alcoholic men. Alcohol. Clin. Exp. Res. 19:1121–1126, 1995.

Pfefferbaum, A., Sullivan, E. V., Mathalon, D. H., Shear, P. K., Rosenbloom, M. J. and Lim, K. O., Longitudinal changes in magnetic resonance imaging brain volumes in abstinent and relapsed alcoholics. Alcohol. Clin. Exp. Res. 19:1177–1191, 1995.

Sullivan, E. V., Marsh, L., Mathalon, D. H., Lim, K. O. and Pfefferbaum, A., Anterior hippocampal volume deficits in nonamnesic, aging chronic alcoholics. Alcohol. Clin. Exp. Res. 19:110–122, 1995.

Sullivan, E. V., Marsh, L., Mathalon, D. H., Lim, K. O. and Pfefferbaum, A., Relationship between alcohol withdrawal seizures and temporal lobe white matter volume deficits. Alcohol. Clin. Exp. Res. 20:348–354, 1996.

Pfefferbaum, A., Sullivan, E. V., Mathalon, D. H. and Lim, K. O., Frontal lobe volume loss observed with magnetic resonance imaging in older chronic alcoholics. Alcohol. Clin. Exp. Res. 21:521–529, 1997.

Sullivan, E. V., Mathalon, D. H., Lim, K. O., Marsh, L. and Pfefferbaum, A., Patterns of regional cortical dysmorphology distinguishing schizophrenia and chronic alcoholism. Biol. Psychiatry 43:118–131, 1998.

Cortical Atrophy/Sulcal Enlargement

Mander, A. J., Young, A., Chick, J. D. and Best, J. J., The relationship of cerebral atrophy and T1 in alcoholics: an MRI study. Drug Alcohol Depend. 24:57–59, 1989.

Ditraglia, G. M., Press, D. S., Butters, N., Jernigan, T. L., Cermak, L. S., Velin, R. A., Shear, P. K., Irwin, M. and Schuckit, M., Assessment of olfactory deficits in detoxified alcoholics. Alcohol 8:109–115, 1991.

Jernigan, T. L., Butters, N., DiTraglia, G., Schafer, K., Smith, T., Irwin, M., Grant, I., Schuckit, M. and Cermak, L. S., Reduced cerebral grey matter observed in alcoholics using magnetic resonance imaging. Alcohol. Clin. Exp. Res. 15:418–427, 1991.

Blansjaar, B. A., Vielvoye, G. J., van Dijk, J. G. and Rijnders, R. J., Similar brain lesions in alcoholics and Korsakoff patients: MRI, psychometric and clinical findings. Clin. Neurol. Neurosurg. 94:197–203, 1992.

Hayakawa, K., Kumagai, H., Suzuki, Y., Furusawa, N., Haga, T., Hoshi, T., Fujiwara, Y. and Yamaguchi, K., MR imaging of chronic alcoholism. Acta Radiol. 33:201–206, 1992.

Pfefferbaum, A., Lim, K. O., Zipursky, R. B., Mathalon, D. H., Rosenbloom, M. J., Lane, B., Ha, C. N. and Sullivan, E. V., Brain gray and white matter volume loss accelerates with aging in chronic alcoholics: a quantitative MRI study. Alcohol. Clin. Exp. Res. 16:1078–1089, 1992.

Shear, P. K., Butters, N., Jernigan, T. L., DiTraglia, G. M., Irwin, M., Schuckit, M. A. and Cermak, L. S., Olfactory loss in alcoholics: correlations with cortical and subcortical MRI indices. Alcohol 9:247–255, 1992.

Wang, G. J., Volkow, N. D., Hitzemann, R., Oster, Z. H., Roque, C. and Cestaro, V., Brain imaging of an alcoholic with MRI, SPECT, and PET. Am. J. Physiol. Imaging 7:194–198, 1992. [Case Report]

Adams, K. M., Gilman, S., Koeppe, R. A., Kluin, K. J., Brunberg, J. A., Dede, D., Berent, S. and Kroll, P. D., Neuropsychological deficits are correlated with frontal hypometabolism in positron emission tomography studies of older alcoholic patients. Alcohol. Clin. Exp. Res. 17:205–210, 1993.

Pfefferbaum, A., Sullivan, E. V., Rosenbloom, M. J., Shear, P. K., Mathalon, D. H. and Lim, K. O., Increase in brain cerebrospinal fluid volume is greater in older than in younger alcoholic patients: a replication study and CT/MRI comparison. Psychiatry Res. 50:257–274, 1993.

Wang, G. J., Volkow, N. D., Roque, C. T., Cestaro, V. L., Hitzemann, R. J., Cantos, E. L., Levy, A. V. and Dhawan, A. P., Functional importance of ventricular enlargement and cortical atrophy in healthy subjects and alcoholics as assessed with PET, MR imaging, and neuropsychologic testing. Radiology 186:59–65, 1993.

Kaseda, Y., Miyazato, Y., Ogura, C., Nakamoto, H., Uema, T., Yamamoto, K. and Ohta, I., Correlation between event-related potentials and MR measurements in chronic alcoholic patients. Jpn. J. Psychiatry Neurol. 48:23–32, 1994.

Di Sclafani, V., Ezekiel, F., Meyerhoff, D. J., MacKay, S., Dillon, W. P., Weiner, M. W. and Fein, G., Brain atrophy and cognitive function in older abstinent alcoholic men. Alcohol. Clin. Exp. Res. 19:1121–1126, 1995.

Pfefferbaum, A., Sullivan, E. V., Mathalon, D. H., Shear, P. K., Rosenbloom, M. J. and Lim, K. O., Longitudinal changes in magnetic resonance imaging brain volumes in abstinent and relapsed alcoholics. Alcohol. Clin. Exp. Res. 19:1177–1191, 1995.

Sullivan, E. V., Marsh, L., Mathalon, D. H., Lim, K. O. and Pfefferbaum, A., Anterior hippocampal volume deficits in nonamnesic, aging chronic alcoholics. Alcohol. Clin. Exp. Res. 19:110–122, 1995.

Bigler, E. D., Blatter, D. D., Johnson, S. C., Anderson, C. V., Russo, A. A., Gale, S. D., Ryser, D. K., MacNamara, S. E. and Bailey, B. J., Traumatic brain injury, alcohol and quantitative neuroimaging: preliminary findings. Brain Inj. 10:197–206, 1996.

Sullivan, E. V., Marsh, L., Mathalon, D. H., Lim, K. O. and Pfefferbaum, A., Relationship between alcohol withdrawal seizures and temporal lobe white matter volume deficits. Alcohol. Clin. Exp. Res. 20:348–354, 1996.

Pfefferbaum, A., Sullivan, E. V., Mathalon, D. H. and Lim, K. O., Frontal lobe volume loss observed with magnetic resonance imaging in older chronic alcoholics. Alcohol. Clin. Exp. Res. 21:521–529, 1997.

Boroojerdi, B., Hungs, M., Biniek, R. and Noth, J., Subacute encephalopathy with epileptic seizures in a patient with chronic alcoholism. Nervenarzt 69:162–165, 1998. [German]

Sullivan, E. V., Mathalon, D. H., Lim, K. O., Marsh, L. and Pfefferbaum, A., Patterns of regional cortical dysmorphology distinguishing schizophrenia and chronic alcoholism. Biol. Psychiatry 43:118–131, 1998.

Agartz, I., Momenan, R., Rawlings, R. R., Kerich, M. J. and Hommer, D. W., Hippocampal volume in patients with alcohol dependence. Arch. Gen. Psychiatry 56:356–363, 1999.

Corpus Callosum Abnormalities

Hommer, D., Momenan, R., Rawlings, R., Ragan, P., Williams, W., Rio, D. and Eckardt, M., Decreased corpus callosum size among alcoholic women. Arch. Neurol. 53:359–363, 1996.

Pfefferbaum, A., Lim, K. O., Desmond, J. E. and Sullivan, E. V., Thinning of the corpus callosum in older alcoholic men: a magnetic resonance imaging study. Alcohol. Clin. Exp. Res. 20:752–757, 1996.

Estruch, R., Nicolas, J. M., Salamero, M., Aragon, C., Sacanella, E., Fernandez-Sola, J. and Urbano-Marquez, A., Atrophy of the corpus callosum in chronic alcoholism. J. Neurol. Sci. 146:145–151, 1997.

White Matter Abnormalities

Gallucci, M., Amicarelli, I., Rossi, A., Stratta, P., Masciocchi, C., Zobel, B. B., Casacchia, M. and Passariello, R., MR imaging of white matter lesions in uncomplicated chronic alcoholism. J. Comput. Assist. Tomogr. 13:395–398, 1989.

Ostertun, B., Dewes, W., Hanisch, E. and Harder, T., MR tomography and computer tomography of alcohol-induced brain tissue changes. Rofo Fortschr. Geb. Rontgenstr. Neuen Bildgeb. Verfahr 152:87–90, 1990. [German]

Hayakawa, K., Kumagai, H., Suzuki, Y., Furusawa, N., Haga, T., Hoshi, T., Fujiwara, Y. and Yamaguchi, K., MR imaging of chronic alcoholism. Acta Radiol. 33:201–206, 1992.

Meyerhoff, D. J., MacKay, S., Sappey-Marinier, D., Deicken, R., Calabrese, G., Dillon, W. P., Weiner, M. W. and Fein, G., Effects of chronic alcohol abuse and HIV infection on brain phosphorus metabolites. Alcohol. Clin. Exp. Res. 19:685–692, 1995.

Cerebellar Abnormalities

Okudaira, K., Endo, S., Saito, A., Nagano, K., Masaoka, A. and Kaneko, Y., Clinical course and MRI findings of two cases of alcoholic cerebellar degeneration. Arukoru Kenkyuto Yakubutsu Ison 23:170–175, 1988. [Case Report] [Japanese]

Blansjaar, B. A., Vielvoye, G. J., van Dijk, J. G. and Rijnders, R. J., Similar brain lesions in alcoholics and Korsakoff patients: MRI, psychometric and clinical findings. Clin. Neurol. Neurosurg. 94:197–203, 1992.

Hayakawa, K., Kumagai, H., Suzuki, Y., Furusawa, N., Haga, T., Hoshi, T., Fujiwara, Y. and Yamaguchi, K., MR imaging of chronic alcoholism. Acta Radiol. 33:201–206, 1992.

Aasly, J., Storsaeter, O., Nilsen, G., Smevik, O. and Rinck, P., Minor structural brain changes in young drug abusers. A magnetic resonance study. Acta Neurol. Scand. 87:210–214, 1993.

Tsuchiya, K., Watabiki, S., Shiojiri, T., Matsumoto, A., and Tsukagoshi, H., Alcoholic cerebellar degeneration with pyramidal sign—in relation to alcoholic myelopathy. No To Shinkei 45:169–175, 1993. [Japanese]

Davila, M. D., Shear, P. K., Lane, B., Sullivan, E. V. and Pfefferbaum, A., Mamillary body and cerebellar shrinkage in chronic alcoholics: an MRI and neuropsychological study. Neuropsychology 8:433–444, 1994.

Shear, P. K., Sullivan, E. V., Lane, B. and Pfefferbaum, A., Mammillary body and cerebellar shrinkage in chronic alcoholics with and without amnesia. Alcohol. Clin. Exp. Res. 20:1489–1495, 1996.

Seitz, D., Widmann, U., Seeger, U., Nagele, T., Klose, U., Mann, K. and Grodd, W., Localized proton magnetic resonance spectroscopy of the cerebellum in detoxifying alcoholics. Alcohol. Clin. Exp. Res. 23:158–163, 1999.

Spectroscopy

MacKay, S., Meyerhoff, D. J., Dillon, W. P., Weiner, M. W. and Fein, G., Alteration of brain phospholipid metabolites in cocaine-dependent polysubstance abusers. Biol. Psychiatry 34:261–264, 1993.

Meyerhoff, D. J., MacKay, S., Sappey-Marinier, D., Deicken, R., Calabrese, G., Dillon, W. P., Weiner, M. W. and Fein, G., Effects of chronic alcohol abuse and HIV infection on brain phosphorus metabolites. Alcohol. Clin. Exp. Res. 19:685–692, 1995.

Jagannathan, N. R., Desai, N. G. and Raghunathan, P., Brain metabolite changes in alcoholism: an in vivo proton magnetic resonance spectroscopy (MRS) study. Magn. Reson. Imaging 14:553–557, 1996.

Meyerhoff, D. J., Bloomer, C., Salas, G., Schuff, N., Norman, D., Weiner, M. W. and Fein, G., Cortical metabolite alterations in recently abstinent cocaine and cocaine/alcohol dependent subjects. International Society for Magnetic Resonance in Medicine Sixth Scientific Meeting and Exhibition. Sydney, Australia, p. 1715, 1998. [Abstract]

Behar, K. L., Rothman, D. L., Petersen, K. F., Hooten, M., Delaney, R., Petroff, O. A., Shulman, G. I., Navarro, V., Petrakis, I. L., Charney, D. S. and Krystal, J. H., Preliminary evidence of low cortical GABA levels in localized ^{1}H-MR spectra of alcohol-dependent and hepatic encephalopathy patients. Am. J. Psychiatry 156:952–954, 1999.

Seitz, D., Widmann, U., Seeger, U., Nagele, T., Klose, U., Mann, K. and Grodd, W., Localized proton magnetic resonance spectroscopy of the cerebellum in detoxifying alcoholics. Alcohol. Clin. Exp. Res. 23:158–163, 1999.

Aging

Hayakawa, K., Kumagai, H., Suzuki, Y., Furusawa, N., Haga, T., Hoshi, T., Fujiwara, Y. and Yamaguchi, K., MR imaging of chronic alcoholism. Acta Radiol. 33:201–206, 1992.

Pfefferbaum, A., Lim, K. O., Zipursky, R. B., Mathalon, D. H., Rosenbloom, M. J., Lane, B., Ha, C. N. and Sullivan, E. V., Brain gray and white matter volume loss accelerates with aging in chronic alcoholics: a quantitative MRI study. Alcohol. Clin. Exp. Res. 16:1078–1089, 1992.

Adams, K. M., Gilman, S., Koeppe, R. A., Kluin, K. J., Brunberg, J. A., Dede, D., Berent, S. and Kroll, P. D., Neuropsychological deficits are correlated with frontal hypometabolism in positron emission tomography studies of older alcoholic patients. Alcohol. Clin. Exp. Res. 17:205–210, 1993.

Pfefferbaum, A., Sullivan, E. V., Rosenbloom, M. J., Shear, P. K., Mathalon, D. H. and Lim, K. O., Increase in brain cerebrospinal fluid volume is greater in older than in younger alcoholic patients: a replication study and CT/MRI comparison. Psychiatry Res. 50:257–274, 1993.

Di Sclafani, V., Ezekiel, F., Meyerhoff, D. J., MacKay, S., Dillon, W. P., Weiner, M. W. and Fein, G., Brain atrophy and cognitive function in older abstinent alcoholic men. Alcohol. Clin. Exp. Res. 19:1121–1126, 1995.

Sullivan, E. V., Marsh, L., Mathalon, D. H., Lim, K. O. and Pfefferbaum, A., Anterior hippocampal volume deficits in nonamnesic, aging chronic alcoholics. Alcohol. Clin. Exp. Res. 19:110–122, 1995.

Pfefferbaum, A., Lim, K. O., Desmond, J. E. and Sullivan, E. V., Thinning of the corpus callosum in older alcoholic men: a magnetic resonance imaging study. Alcohol. Clin. Exp. Res. 20:752–757, 1996.

Sullivan, E. V., Marsh, L., Mathalon, D. H., Lim, K. O. and Pfefferbaum, A., Relationship between alcohol withdrawal seizures and temporal lobe white matter volume deficits. Alcohol. Clin. Exp. Res. 20:348–354, 1996.

Pfefferbaum, A., Sullivan, E. V., Mathalon, D. H. and Lim, K. O., Frontal lobe volume loss observed with magnetic resonance imaging in older chronic alcoholics. Alcohol. Clin. Exp. Res. 21:521–529, 1997.

Pfefferbaum, A., Sullivan, E. V., Rosenbloom, M. J., Mathalon, D. H. and Lim, K. O., A controlled study of cortical gray matter and ventricular changes in alcoholic men over a 5-year interval. Arch. Gen. Psychiatry 55:905–912, 1998.

Withdrawal

Mander, A. J., Weppner, G. J., Chick, J. D., Morton, J. J. and Best, J. J., An NMR study of cerebral oedema and its biological correlates during withdrawal from alcohol. Alcohol Alcohol. 23:97–102, 1988.

Smith, M. A., Chick, J. D., Engleman, H. M., Kean, D. M., Mander, A. J., Douglas, R. H. and Best, J. J., Brain hydration during alcohol withdrawal in alcoholics measured by magnetic resonance imaging. Drug Alcohol Depend. 21:25–28, 1988.

Mander, A. J., Young, A., Chick, J. D., Ridgway, J. and Best, J. J., NMR T_1 relaxation time of the brain during alcohol withdrawal and its lack of relationship with symptom severity. Br. J. Addict. 84:669–672, 1989.

Agartz, I., Saaf, J., Wahlund, L. O. and Wetterberg, L., T_1 and T_2 relaxation time estimates and brain measures during withdrawal in alcoholic men. Drug Alcohol Depend. 29:157–169, 1991.

Sullivan, E. V., Marsh, L., Mathalon, D. H., Lim, K. O. and Pfefferbaum, A., Relationship between alcohol withdrawal seizures and temporal lobe white matter volume deficits. Alcohol. Clin. Exp. Res. 20:348–354, 1996.

Abstinence/Relapse

Schroth, G., Naegele, T., Klose, U., Mann, K. and Petersen, D., Reversible brain shrinkage in abstinent alcoholics, measured by MRI. Neuroradiology 30:385–389, 1988.

Mann, K., Opitz, H., Petersen, D., Schroth, G. and Heimann, H., Intracranial CSF volumetry in alcoholics: studies with MRI and CT. Psychiatry Res. 29:277–279, 1989.

Zipursky, R. B., Lim, K. C. and Pfefferbaum, A., MRI study of brain changes with short-term abstinence from alcohol. Alcohol. Clin. Exp. Res. 13:664–666, 1989.

Kroft, C. L., Gescuk, B., Woods, B. T., Mello, N. K., Weiss, R. D. and Mendelson, J. H., Brain ventricular size in female alcoholics: an MRI study. Alcohol 8:31–34, 1991.

Shear, P. K., Jernigan, T. L. and Butters, N., Volumetric magnetic resonance imaging quantification of longitudinal brain changes in abstinent alcoholics. Alcohol. Clin. Exp. Res. 18:172–176, 1994.

Di Sclafani, V., Ezekiel, F., Meyerhoff, D. J., MacKay, S., Dillon, W. P., Weiner, M. W. and Fein, G., Brain atrophy and cognitive function in older abstinent alcoholic men. Alcohol. Clin. Exp. Res. 19:1121–1126, 1995.

Martin, P. R., Gibbs, S. J., Nimmerrichter, A. A., Riddle, W. R., Welch, L. W. and Willcott, M. R., Brain proton magnetic resonance spectroscopy studies in recently abstinent alcoholics. Alcohol. Clin. Exp. Res. 19:1078–1082, 1995.

Pfefferbaum, A., Sullivan, E. V., Mathalon, D. H., Shear, P. K., Rosenbloom, M. J. and Lim, K. O., Longitudinal changes in magnetic resonance imaging brain volumes in abstinent and relapsed alcoholics. Alcohol. Clin. Exp. Res. 19:1177–1191, 1995.

Bergman, H., Engelbrektson, K., Fransson, A., Herlitz, K., Hindmarsh, T. and Neiman, J., Alcohol-induced cognitive impairment is reversible. Neuropsychological tests but not MRT show improvement after abstinence. Lakartidningen 95:4228, 4231–4236, 1998. [Swedish]

Disclafani, V., Truran, D. L., Bloomer, C., Toloushams, M., Clark, H. W., Norman, D., Hannauer, D. and Fein, G., Abstinent chronic crack-cocaine and crack-cocaine/alcohol abusers evidence normal hippocampal volumes on MRI despite persistent cognitive impairments. Addiction Biol. 3:261–270, 1998.

Pfefferbaum, A., Sullivan, E. V., Rosenbloom, M. J., Mathalon, D. H. and Lim, K. O., A controlled study of cortical gray matter and ventricular changes in alcoholic men over a 5-year interval. Arch. Gen. Psychiatry 55:905–912, 1998.

Special Syndromes Associated with Alcoholism

Hepatic Encephalopathy

Imaging

Moore, J. W., Dunk, A. A., Crawford, J. R., Deans, H., Besson, J. A., De Lacey, G., Sinclair, T. S., Mowat, N. A. and Brunt, P. W., Neuropsychological deficits and morphological MRI brain scan abnormalities in apparently healthy non-encephalopathic patients with cirrhosis. A controlled study. J. Hepatology 9:319–325, 1989.

Zeneroli, M. L., Cioni, G., Crisi, G., Vezzelli, C. and Ventura, E., Globus pallidus alterations and brain atrophy in liver cirrhosis patients with encephalopathy: an MR imaging study. Magn. Reson. Imaging 9:295–302, 1991.

Barthauer, L., Tarter, R., Hirsch, W. and Van, T. D., Brain morphologic characteristics of cirrhotic alcoholics and cirrhotic nonalcoholics: an MRI study Alcohol. Clin. Exp. Res. 16:982–985, 1992.

Bourgeois, S. and Telerman-Toppet, N., Reversible spastic triparesis with hyperammonemia. Acta Neurol. Belg. 92:41–44, 1992. [Case Report] [French]

Kulisevsky, J., Pujol, J., Balanzo, J., Junque, C., Deus, J., Capdevilla, A. and Villanueva, C., Pallidal hyperintensity on magnetic resonance imaging in cirrhotic patients: clinical correlations. Hepatology 16:1382–1388, 1992.

Pujol, A., Pujol, J., Graus, F., Rimola, A., Peri, J., Mercader, J. M., Garcia-Pagan, J. C., Bosch, J., Rodes, J. and Tolosa, E., Hyperintense globus pallidus on T_1-weighted MRI in cirrhotic patients is associated with severity of liver failure. Neurology 43:65–69, 1993.

Kulisevsky, J., Pujol, J., Junque, C., Deus, J., Balanzo, J. and Capdevila, A., MRI pallidal hyperintensity and brain atrophy in cirrhotic patients: two different MRI patterns of clinical deterioration? Neurology 43:2570–2573, 1993.

Thuluvath, P. J., Edwin, D., Yue, N. C., deVilliers, C., Hochman, S. and Klein, A., Increased signals seen in globus pallidus in T1-weighted magnetic resonance imaging in cirrhotics are not suggestive of chronic hepatic encephalopathy. Hepatology 21:440–442, 1995.

Krieger, S., Jauss, M., Jansen, O., Theilmann, L., Geissler, M. and Krieger, D., Neuropsychiatric profile and hyperintense globus pallidus on T_1-weighted magnetic resonance images in liver cirrhosis. Gastroenterology 111:147–155, 1996.

Vymazal, J., Babis, M., Brooks, R. A., Filip, K., Dezortova, M., Hrncarkova, H. and Hajek, M., T_1 and T_2 alterations in the brains of patients with hepatic cirrhosis. AJNR Am. J. Neuroradiol. 17:333–336, 1996.

Geissler, A., Lock, G., Frund, R., Held, P., Hollerbach, S., Andus, T., Scholmerich, J., Feuerbach, S. and Holstege, A., Cerebral abnormalities in patients with cirrhosis detected by proton magnetic resonance spectroscopy and magnetic resonance imaging. Hepatology 25:48–54, 1997.

Maeda, H., Sato, M., Yoshikawa, A., Kimura, M., Sonomura, T., Terada, M. and Kishi, K., Brain MR imaging in patients with hepatic cirrhosis: relationship between high intensity signal in basal ganglia on T_1-weighted images and elemental concentrations in brain. Neuroradiology 39:546–550, 1997.

Boroojerdi, B., Hungs, M., Biniek, R. and Noth, J., Subacute encephalopathy with epileptic seizures in a patient with chronic alcoholism. Nervenarzt 69:162–165, 1998. [Case Report] [German]

Iwasa, M., Kinosada, Y., Watanabe, S., Furuta, M., Yuda, H., Kawamura, N., Nakayabu, M., Esaki, A., Sato, T., Deguchi, T., Nakatsuka, A. and Adachi, Y., Hepatic cirrhosis: magnetisation transfer contrast in the globus pallidus. Neuroradiology 40:145–149, 1998.

Spectroscopy

Kreis, R., Farrow, N. A. and Ross, B. D., Diagnosis of hepatic encephalopathy by proton magnetic resonance spectroscopy. Lancet 336:635–636, 1990.

Kreis, R., Ross, B. D., Farrow, N. A. and Ackerman, Z., Metabolic disorders of the brain in chronic hepatic encephalopathy detected with H-1 MR spectroscopy. Radiology 182:19–27, 1992.

Ross, B. D., Jacobson, S., Villamil, F., Korula, J., Kreis, R., Ernst, T., Shonk, T. and Moats, R. A., Subclinical hepatic encephalopathy: proton MR spectroscopic abnormalities. Radiology 193:457–463, 1994.

Taylor-Robinson, S. D., Sargentoni, J., Mallalieu, R. J., Bell, J. D., Bryant, D. J., Coutts, G. A. and Morgan, M. Y., Cerebral phosphorus-31 magnetic resonance spectroscopy in patients with chronic hepatic encephalopathy. Hepatology 20:1173–1178, 1994.

Taylor-Robinson, S. D., Sargentoni, J., Marcus, C. D., Morgan, M. Y. and Bryant, D. J., Regional variations in cerebral proton spectroscopy in patients with chronic hepatic encephalopathy. Metab. Brain Dis. 9:347–359, 1994.

Geissler, A., Lock, G., Frund, R., Held, P., Hollerbach, S., Andus, T., Scholmerich, J., Feuerbach, S. and Holstege, A., Cerebral abnormalities in patients with cirrhosis detected by proton magnetic resonance spectroscopy and magnetic resonance imaging. Hepatology 25:48–54, 1997.

Bluml, S., Zuckerman, E., Tan, J. and Ross, B. D., Proton-decoupled ^{31}P magnetic resonance spectroscopy reveals osmotic and metabolic disturbances in human hepatic encephalopathy. J. Neurochem. 71:1564–1576, 1998.

Huda, A., Guze, B. H., Thomas, M. A., Bugbee, M., Fairbanks, L., Strouse, T. and Fawzy, F. I., Clinical correlation of neuropsychological tests with 1H magnetic resonance spectroscopy in hepatic encephalopathy. Psychosom. Med. 60:550–556, 1998.

Thomas, M. A., Huda, A., Guze, B., Curran, J., Bugbee, M., Fairbanks, L., Ke, Y., Oshiro, T., Martin, P. and Fawzy, F., Cerebral ^{1}H MR spectroscopy and neuropsychologic status of patients with hepatic encephalopathy. AJR Am. J. Roentgenol. 171:1123–1130, 1998.

Behar, K. L., Rothman, D. L., Petersen, K. F., Hooten, M., Delaney, R., Petroff, O. A., Shulman, G. I., Navarro, V., Petrakis, I. L., Charney, D. S. and Krystal, J. H., Preliminary evidence of low cortical GABA levels in localized ^{1}H-MR spectra of alcohol-dependent and hepatic encephalopathy patients. Am. J. Psychiatry 156:952–954, 1999.

Wernicke and Korsakoff Syndromes

Charness, M. E. and DeLaPaz, R. L., Mamillary body atrophy in Wernicke's encephalopathy: antemortem identification using magnetic resonance imaging. Ann. Neurol. 22:595–600, 1987.

Kitaguchi, T., Kobayashi, T., Tobimatsu, S., Goto, I. and Kuroiwa, Y., Computed tomography and magnetic resonance imaging in a young patient with Wernicke's encephalopathy. J. Neurology 234:449–450, 1987.

Christie, J. E., Kean, D. M., Douglas, R. H., Engleman, H. M., St. Clair, D. and Blackburn, I. M., Magnetic resonance imaging in pre-senile dementia of the Alzheimer-type, multi-infarct dementia and Korsakoff's syndrome. Psychol. Med. 18:319–329, 1988.

Besson, J. A., Crawford, J. R., Parker, D. M. and Smith, F. W., Magnetic resonance imaging in Alzheimer's disease, multi-infarct dementia, alcoholic dementia and Korsakoff's psychosis. Acta Psychiatrica Scand. 80:451–458, 1989.

Bigler, E. D., Nelson, J. E. and Schmidt, R. D., Identification of mamillary body atrophy in Korsakoff's syndrome using magnetic resonance imaging [letter]. J. Neuropsychiatry Clin. Neurosci. 1:341–342, 1989.

Ujike, H., Matsueda, H., Kazahaya, Y., Kuroda, S. and Otsuki, S., Korsakoff's syndrome as a prominent feature of bilateral paramedian thalamic infarction: a case report. Rinsho Shinkeigaku 29:1055–1058, 1989. [Case Report] [Japanese]

Donnal, J. F., Heinz, E. R. and Buerger, P. C., MR of reversible thalamic lesions in Wernicke syndrome. AJNR Am. J. Neuroradiol. 11:893–894, 1990.

Gallucci, M., Bozzao, A., Splendiani, A., Masciocchi, C. and Passariello, R., Wernicke Encephalopathy: MR findings in five patients. AJNR Am. J. Neuroradiol. 11:887–892, 1990.

Ostertun, B., Dewes, W., Hanisch, E. and Harder, T., MR tomography and computer tomography of alcohol-induced brain tissue changes. Rofo Fortschr. Geb. Rontgenstr. Neuen Bildgeb. Verfahr 152:87–90, 1990. [German]

Squire, L. R., Amaral, D. G. and Press, G. A., Magnetic resonance imaging of the hippocampal formation and mammillary nuclei distinguish medial temporal lobe and diencephalic amnesia. J. Neurosci. 10:3106–3117, 1990.

Jernigan, T. L., Schafer, K., Butters, N. and Cermak, L. S., Magnetic resonance imaging of alcoholic Korsakoff patients. Neuropsychopharmacology 4:175–186, 1991.

Blansjaar, B. A., Vielvoye, G. J., van Dijk, J. G. and Rijnders, R. J., Similar brain lesions in alcoholics and Korsakoff patients: MRI, psychometric and clinical findings. Clin. Neurol. Neurosurg. 94:197–203, 1992.

Cole, M., Winkelman, M. D., Morris, J. C., Simon, J. E. and Boyd, T. A., Thalamic amnesia: Korsakoff syndrome due to left thalamic infarction. J. Neurol. Sci. 110:62–67, 1992.

Delis, D. C., Squire, L. R., Bihrle, A. and Massman, P., Componential analysis of problem-solving ability: performance of patients with frontal lobe damage and amnesic patients on a new sorting test. Neuropsychologia 30:683–697, 1992.

Vortmeyer, A. O., Wernicke's encephalopathy, Korsakow's amnesic state and thiamine deficient encephalopathy. Alcohol Alcohol. 28:199–200, 1993.

Emsley, R., Smith, R., Roberts, M., Kapnias, S., Pieters, H. and Maritz, S., Magnetic resonance imaging in alcoholic Korsakoff's syndrome: evidence for an association with alcoholic dementia. Alcohol Alcohol. 31:479–486, 1996.

Shear, P. K., Sullivan, E. V., Lane, B. and Pfefferbaum, A., Mammillary body and cerebellar shrinkage in chronic alcoholics with and without amnesia. Alcohol. Clin. Exp. Res. 20:1489–1495, 1996.

Welch, L. W., Nimmerrichter, A., Kessler, R., King, D., Hoehn, R., Margolin, R. and Martin, P. R., Severe global amnesia presenting as Wernicke-Korsakoff syndrome but resulting from atypical lesions. Psychol. Med. 26:421–425, 1996. [Case Report]

Kopelman, M. D., Stanhope, N. and Kingsley, D., Temporal and spatial context memory in patients with focal frontal, temporal lobe, and diencephalic lesions. Neuropsychologia 35:1533–1545, 1997.

Matsuda, K., Yamaji, S., Ishii, K., Sasaki, M., Sakamoto, S., Kitagaki, H., Imamura, T. and Mori, E., Regional cerebral blood flow and oxygen metabolism in a patient with Korsakoff syndrome. Ann. Nucl. Med. 11:33–35, 1997.

Antunez, E., Estruch, R., Cardenal, C., Nicolas, J. M., Fernandez-Sola, J. and Urbano-Marquez, A., Usefulness of CT and MR imaging in the diagnosis of acute Wernicke's encephalopathy. AJR Am. J. Roentgenol. 171:1131–1137, 1998.

Central Pontine Myelinolysis

DeWitt, L. D., Buonanno, F. S., Kistler, J. P., Zeffiro, T., DeLaPaz, R. L., Brady, T. J., Rosen, B. R. and Pykett, I. L., Central pontine myelinolysis: demonstration by nuclear magnetic resonance. Neurology 34:570–576, 1984.

Pfister, H. W., Einhaupl, K. M. and Brandt, T. Mild Central Pontine Myelinolysis: a frequently undetected syndrome. Eur. Arch. Psychiatry Neurol. Sci. 235:134–139, 1985.

Price, D. B., Kramer, J., Hotson, G. and Loh, J. P., Central Pontine Myelinolysis: report of a case with distinctive appearance on MR imaging. AJNR Am. J. Neuroradiol. 8:576–577, 1987. [Case Report]

Rippe, D. J., Edwards, M. K., D'Amour, P. G., Holden, R. W. and Roos, K. L., MR imaging of central pontine myelinolysis. J. Comput. Assist. Tomogr. 11:724–726, 1987.

Miller, G. M., Baker, H. L., Jr., Okazaki, H. and Whisnant, J. P., Central pontine myelinolysis and its imitators: MR findings. Radiology 168:795–802, 1988.

Steller, U., Koschorek, F. and Strenge, H., Cerebellar ataxia with recovery related to central pontine myelinolysis. J. Neurology 235:379–381, 1988.

Bahr, M., Sommer, N., Petersen, D., Wietholter, H. and Dichgans, J., Central pontine myelinolysis associated with low potassium levels in alcoholism. J. Neurology 237:275–276, 1990.

Brunner, J. E., Redmond, J. M., Haggar, A. M., Kruger, D. F. and Elias, S. B., Central pontine myelinolysis and pontine lesions after rapid correction of hyponatremia: a prospective magnetic resonance imaging study. Ann. Neurol. 27:61–66, 1990.

Koci, T. M., Chiang, F., Chow, P., Wang, A., Chiu, L. C., Itabashi, H. and Mehringer, C. M., Thalamic extrapontine lesions in central pontine myelinolysis. AJNR Am. J. Neuroradiol. 11:1229–1233, 1990.

Ostertun, B., Dewes, W., Hanisch, E. and Harder, T., MR tomography and computer tomography of alcohol-induced brain tissue changes. Rofo Fortschr. Geb. Rontgenstr. Neuen Bildgeb. Verfahr 152:87–90, 1990. [German]

Schmidt, J. A., Krause, A., Feddersen, C. O., Kohl, F. V., Mariss, G., Lutcke, A. and von-Wichert, P., Central pontine myelinolysis following severe hyponatremia. Klin. Wochenschr. 68:191–198, 1990. [German]

Heilemann, H., Skiba, N. and Hillemacher, A., Clinical aspects and electrophysiologic findings in an unusual course of central pontine myelinolysis. Nervenarzt 62:645–647, 1991. [German]

Adamson, D. J., Laing, R. B. and Nathwani, D., Alcoholism, hyponatraemia and central neurological damage: more than pontine myelinolysis? Scottish Med. J. 37:83–84, 1992.

Demaerel, P., Wilms, G., De Baets, P., Vanderwegen, L., Casteels, M., Carton, H. and Baert, A. L., Magnetic resonance imaging of extrapontine lesions in central pontine myelinolysis J. Belge Radiol. 75:186–187, 1992.

Dieterle, L., Buchler, G. and Pfitzer, F., Central pontine myelinolysis. Dtsch. Med. Wochenschr. 117:332–336, 1992. [German]

Tien, R., Arieff, A.I., Kucharczyk, W., Wasik, A. and Kucharczyk, J., Hyponatremic encephalopathy: is central pontine myelinolysis a component? Am. J. Med. 92:513–522, 1992.

Gille, M., Jacquemin, C., Kiame, G., Delbecq, J., Guilmot, D. and Depre, A., Central pontine myelinolysis with cerebellar ataxia and dystonia. Rev. Neurol. (Paris) 149:344–346, 1993. [French]

Laitt, R. D., Thornton, M. and Goddard, P., Pontine myelinolysis in a normonatraemic alcoholic. Clin. Radiol. 48:432–433, 1993. [Case Report]

Mascalchi, M., Cincotta, M. and Piazzini, M., Case report: MRI demonstration of pontine and thalamic myelinolysis in a normonatremic alcoholic. Clin. Radiol. 47:137–138, 1993. [Case Report]

Fuger, K., Pfadenhauer, K. and Wienbeck, M., Reversible neurologic manifestations in a 50-year-old patient with central pontine myelinolysis. Med. Klin. 89:225–228, 1994. [German]

Rouanet, F., Tison, F., Dousset, V., Corand, V. and Orgogozo, J. M., Early T_2 hypointense signal abnormality preceding clinical manifestations of central pontine myelinolysis. Neurology 44:979–980, 1994.

Laubenberger, J., Schneider, B., Ansorge, O., Gotz, F., Haussinger, D., Volk, B. and Langer, M., Central pontine myelinolysis: clinical presentation and radiologic findings. Eur. Radiol. 6:177–183, 1996.

Silver, N. C., Barker, G. J., MacManus, D. G., Miller, D. H., Thorpe, J. W. and Howard, R. S., Decreased magnetisation transfer ratio due to demyelination: a case of central pontine myelinolysis. J. Neurol. Neurosurg. Psychiatry 61:208–209, 1996.

Kelly, J., Wassif, W., Mitchard, J. and Gardner, W. N., Severe hyponatraemia secondary to beer potomania complicated by central pontine myelinolysis. Int. J. Clin. Practice 52:585–587, 1998. [Case Report]

Kosmowski, W., Rybakowski, J., Ziolkowski, M., Borkowska, A., Dubaniewicz-Wybieralska, M. and Araszkiewicz, A., The case of central pontine myelinolysis in an alcohol dependent male. Psychiatr. Pol. 32:103–111, 1998. [Polish]

Marchiafava–Bignami Disease

Kawamura, M., Shiota, J., Yagashita, T. and Hirayama, K., Marchiafava-Bignami disease: Computed tomographic scan and magnetic resonance imaging. Ann. Neurol. 18:103–104, 1985.

Bracard, S., Claude, D., Vespignani, H., Almeras, M., Carsin, M., Lambert, H. and Picard, L., Computerized tomography and MRI in Marchifava-Bignami disease. J. Neuroradiol. 13:87–94, 1986. [Case Report]

Clavier, E., Thiebot, J., Delangre, T., Hannequin, D., Samson, M. and Benozio, M., Marchiafava-Bignami disease. A case studied by CT and MR imaging. Neuroradiology 28:376, 1986. [Case Report]

Delangre, T., Hannequin, D., Clavier, E., Denis, P., Mihout, B. and Samson, M., Marchiafava-Bignami disease with favorable development. Rev. Neurol. (Paris) 142:933–936, 1986. [French]

Mayer, J. M., de Liege, P., Netter, J. M., Danze, F. and Reizine, D., Computerized tomography and nuclear magnetic resonance imaging in Marchiafava-Bignami disease. J. Neuroradiol. 14:152–158, 1987.

Meyrignac, C., Bokobza, M., Cesaro, P., and Degos, J. D., Magnetic resonance imaging in the diagnosis of Marchiafava-Bignami disease. Presse Med. 16:1863–1864, 1987. [French]

Baron, R., Heuser, K. and Marioth, G., Marchiafava-Bignami disease with recovery diagnosed by CT and MRI: demyelination affects several CNS structures J. Neurology 236:364–366, 1989.

Ikeda, A., Antoku, Y., Abe, T., Nishimura, H. and Iwashita, H., Marchiafava-Bignami disease: consecutive observation at acute stage by magnetic resonance imaging and computerized tomography Jpn. J. Med. 28:740–743, 1989.

Shiota, J., Kawamura, M., Hirayama, K., Isono, O. and Maki, T., Antemortem diagnosis of Marchiafava-Bignami disease. Rinsho Shinkeigaku 29:701–706, 1989. [Japanese]

Namba, Y., Bando, M., Takeda, K., Iwata, M. and Mannen, T., Marchiafava-Bignami disease with symptoms of the motor impersistence and unilateral hemispatial neglect. Rinsho Shinkeigaku 31:632–635, 1991. [Case Report] [Japanese]

Rosa, A., Demiati, M., Cartz, L. and Mizon, J. P., Marchiafava-Bignami disease, syndrome of interhemispheric disconnection, and right-handed agraphia in a left-hander. Arch. Neurol. 48:986–988, 1991.

Canaple, S., Rosa, A. and Mizon, J. P., Marchiafava-Bignami disease. Interhemispheric disconnection, favourable outcome, neurological aspect. Rev. Neurol. (Paris) 148:638–640, 1992. [French]

Chang, K. H., Cha, S. H., Han, M. H., Park, S. H., Nah, D. L. and Hong, J. H., Marchiafava-Bignami disease: serial changes in corpus callosum on MRI. Neuroradiology 34:480–482, 1992. [Case Report]

Humbert, T., De Guilhermier, P., Maktouf, C., Grasset, G., Lopez, F. M. and Chabrand, P., Marchiafava-Bignami disease. A case studied by structural and functional brain imaging. Eur. Arch. Psychiatry Clin. Neurosci. 242:69–71, 1992.

Izquierdo, G., Quesada, M. A., Chacon, J. and Martel, J., Neuroradiologic abnormalities in Marchiafava-Bignami disease of benign evolution. Eur. J. Radiol. 15:71–74, 1992.

Martinez-Fernandez, R., Manzano, L., Cabrera, F., Arranz, A. and Alvarez-Mon, M., Marchiafava-Bignami disease with a favorable clinical evolution (letter). Revista Clinica Espanola 190:431–432, 1992. [Spanish]

Otake, S., Mizutani, H., Ohba, S., Mitake, S. and Kureyama, Y., Marchiafava-Bignami disease: CT and MRI findings. Eur. Radiol. 2:382–384, 1992.

Kamaki, M., Kawamura, M., Moriya, H. and Hirayama, K., "Crossed homonymous hemianopia" and "crossed left hemispatial neglect" in a case of Marchiafava-Bignami disease. J. Neurol. Neurosurg. Psychiatry 56:1027–1032, 1993.

Tomasini, P., Guillot, D., Sabbah, P., Brosset, C., Salamand, P. and Briant, J. F., Marchiafava-Bignami's disease with a favourable course. Apropos of a case. Ann. Radiol. (Paris) 36:319–322, 1993. [French]

Berek, K., Wagner, M., Chemelli, A. P., Aichner, F. and Benke, T., Hemispheric disconnection in Marchiafava-Bignami disease: clinical, neuropsychological and MRI findings. J. Neurol. Sci. 123:2–5, 1994.

Caparros-Lefebvre, D., Pruvo, J. P., Josien, E., Pertuzon, B., Clarisse, J. and Petit, H., Marchiafava-Bignami disease: use of contrast media in CT and MRI. Neuroradiology 36:509–511, 1994.

Kalckreuth, W., Zimmermann, P., Preilowski, B. and Wallesch, C. W., Incomplete split-brain syndrome in a patient with chronic Marchiafava-Bignami disease. Behav. Brain Res. 64:219–228, 1994.

Marjama, J., Yoshino, M. T. and Reese, C., Marchiafava-Bignami disease. Premortem diagnosis of an acute case utilizing magnetic resonance imaging. J. Neuroimaging 4:106–109, 1994.

Nicoli, F., Vion-Dury, J., Chave, B., Houallah, T., Confort-Gouny, S., Cozzone, P. J. and Gastaut, J. L., Marchiafava-Bignami disease: interhemispheric disconnection, Balint syndrome, spontaneously favourable outcome. Rev. Neurol. (Paris) 150:157–161, 1994. [French]

Pappata, S., Chabriat, H., Levasseur, M., Legault-Demare, F. and Baron, J. C., Marchiafava-Bignami disease with dementia: severe cerebral metabolic depression revealed by PET. J. Neural. Transm. Park. Dis. Dement. Sect. 8:131–137, 1994.

Kamaki, M., Kawamura, M., Moriya, H. and Hirayama, K., Callosal bleeding in a case of Marchiafava-Bignami disease. J. Neurol. Sci. 136:86–89, 1996. [Case Report]

Logak, M., Feve, A., Samson, Y., Guillard, A. and Rancurel, G., Contribution of position emission tomography in a case of Marchiafava Bignami disease: Morel's laminar sclerosis? Rev. Neurol. (Paris) 152:47–50, 1996. [Case Report] [French]

Tobita, M., Mochizuki, H., Takahashi, S., Onodera, H., Itoyama, Y. and Iwasaki, Y., A case of Marchiafava-Bignami disease with complete recovery: sequential imaging documenting improvement of callosal lesions. Tohoku J. Exp. Med. 182:175–179, 1997.

Yamashita, K., Kobayashi, S., Yamaguchi, S., Koide, H. and Nishi, K., Reversible corpus callosum lesions in a patient with Marchiafava-Bignami disease: serial changes on MRI. Eur. Neurol. 37:192–193, 1997.

Gass, A., Birtsch, G., Olster, M., Schwartz, A. and Hennerici, M. G., Marchiafava-Bignami disease: reversibility of neuroimaging abnormality. J. Comput. Assist. Tomogr. 22:503–504, 1998.

Ferracci, F., Conte, F., Gentile, M., Candeago, R., Foscolo, L., Bendini, M. and Fassetta, G., Marchiafava-Bignami disease: computed tomographic scan, ^{99m}Tc HMPAO-SPECT, and FLAIR MRI findings in a patient with subcortical aphasia, alexia, bilateral agraphia, and left-handed deficit of constructional ability. Arch. Neurol. 56:107–110, 1999. [Case Report]

Prenatal Exposure

Gabrielli, O., Salvolini, U., Coppa, G. V., Catassi, C., Rossi, R., Manca, A., Lanza, R. and Giorgi, P. L., Magnetic resonance imaging in the malformative syndromes with mental retardation. Pediatr. Radiol. 21:16–19, 1990.

Schaefer, G. B., Shuman, R. M., Wilson, D. A., Saleeb, S., Domek, D. B., Johnson, S. F. and Bodensteiner, J. B., Partial agenesis of the anterior corpus callosum: correlation between appearance, imaging, and neuropathology. Pediatr. Neurol. 7:39–44, 1991. [Case Report]

Mattson, S. N., Riley, E. P., Jernigan, T. L., Ehlers, C. L., Delis, D. C., Jones, K. L., Stern, C., Johnson, K. A., Hesselink, J. R. and Bellugi, U., Fetal alcohol syndrome: a case report of neuropsychological, MRI and EEG assessment of two children. Alcohol. Clin. Exp. Res. 16:1001–1003, 1992. [Case Report]

Mattson, S. N., Riley, E. P., Jernigan, T. L., Garcia, A., Kaneko, W. M., Ehlers, C. L. and Jones, K. L., A decrease in the size of the basal ganglia following prenatal alcohol exposure: a preliminary report. Neurotoxicol. Teratol. 16:283–289, 1994.

Astley, S. J., Weinberger, E., Shaw, D. W., Richards, T. L. and Clarren, S. K., Magnetic resonance imaging and spectroscopy in fetal ethanol exposed Macaca nemestrina. Neurotoxicol. Teratol. 17:523–530, 1995. [Nonhuman Primate]

Riley, E. P., Mattson, S. N., Sowell, E. R., Jernigan, T. L., Sobel, D. F. and Jones, K. L., Abnormalities of the corpus callosum in children prenatally exposed to alcohol. Alcohol. Clin. Exp. Res. 19:1198–1202, 1995.

Johnson, V. P., Swayze, V. W., II., Sato, Y. and Andreasen, N. C., Fetal alcohol syndrome: craniofacial and central nervous system manifestations. Am. J. Med. Genet. 61:329–339, 1996.

Mattson, S. N., Riley, E. P., Sowell, E. R., Jernigan, T. L., Sobel, D. F. and Jones, K. L., A decrease in the size of the basal ganglia in children with fetal alcohol syndrome. Alcohol. Clin. Exp. Res. 20:1088–1093, 1996.

Sowell, E. R., Jernigan, T. L., Mattson, S. N., Riley, E. P., Sobel, D. F. and Jones, K. L., Abnormal development of the cerebellar vermis in children prenatally exposed to alcohol: size reduction in lobules I-V. Alcohol. Clin. Exp. Res. 20:31–34, 1996.

Swayze, V. W., 2nd, Johnson, V. P., Hanson, J. W., Piven, J., Sato, Y., Giedd, J. N., Mosnik, D. and Andreasen, N. C., Magnetic resonance imaging of brain anomalies in fetal alcohol syndrome. Pediatrics 99:232–240, 1997.

Benzodiazepines and Alcoholism

Lingford-Hughes, A. R., Acton, P. D., Gacinovic, S., Suckling, J., Busatto, G. F., Boddington, S. J., Bullmore, E., Woodruff, P. W., Costa, D. C., Pilowsky, L. S., Ell, P. J., Marshall, E. J. and Kerwin, R. W., Reduced levels of GABA-benzodiazepine receptor in alcohol dependency in the absence of grey matter atrophy. Br. J. Psychiatry 173:116–122, 1998.

Streeter, C. C., Ciraulo, D. A., Harris, G. J., Kaufman, M. J., Lewis, R. F., Knapp, C. M., Ciraulo, A. M., Maas, L. C., Ungeheuer, M., Szulewski, S. and Renshaw, P. F., Functional magnetic resonance imaging of alprazolam-induced changes in humans with familial alcoholism. Psychiatry Res. 82:69–82, 1998.

Methanol

Koopmans, R. A., Li, D. K. and Paty, D. W., Basal ganglia lesions in methanol poisoning: MR appearance. J. Comput. Assist. Tomogr. 12:168–169, 1988. [Case Report]

Verslegers, W., Van den Kerchove, M., Crols, R., De Potter, W., Appel, B. and Lowenthal, A., Methanol intoxication. Parkinsonism and decreased Met-enkephalin levels due to putaminal necrosis. Acta Neurol. Belg. 88:163–171, 1988. [Case Report]

Bartoli, J. M., Laurent, C., Moulin, G., Vignoli, P., Graziani, N., Jean, P. and Kasbarian, M., Methanol poisoning. Report of 2 cases studied with x-ray computed tomography and magnetic resonance imaging. Ann. Radiol. (Paris) 33:257–259, 1990. [Case Report] [French]

Indakoetxea, B., Lopez de Munain, A., Marti-Masso, J. F. and Linazasoro, G., Parkinsonism after methyl alcohol poisoning. Neurologia 5:238–241, 1990. [Case Report] [Spanish]

Chen, J. C., Schneiderman, J. F. and Wortzman, G., Methanol poisoning: bilateral putaminal and cerebellar cortical lesions on CT and MR. J. Comput. Assist. Tomogr. 15:522–524, 1991. [Case Report]

Mozaz, M. J., Wyke, M. A. and Indakoetxea, B., Parkinsonism and defects of praxis following methanol poisoning. J. Neurol. Neurosurg. Psychiatry 54:843–844, 1991.

Pelletier, J., Habib, M. H., Khalil, R., Salamon, G., Bartoli, D. and Jean, P., Putaminal necrosis after methanol intoxication. J. Neurol. Neurosurg. Psychiatry 55:234–235, 1992. [Case Report]

Glazer, M. and Dross, P., Necrosis of the putamen caused by methanol intoxication: MR findings. AJR Am. J. Roentgenol. 160:1105–1106, 1993. [Case Report]

Gaul, H. P., Wallace, C. J., Auer, R. N. and Fong, T. C., MR findings in methanol intoxication. AJNR Am. J. Neuroradiol. 16:1783–1786, 1995. [Case Report]

Rubinstein, D., Escott, E. and Kelly, J. P., Methanol intoxication with putaminal and white matter necrosis: MR and CT findings. AJNR Am. J. Neuroradiol. 16:1492–1494, 1995.

Yu, F. C., Lin, S. H., Lin, Y. F., Lu, K. C., Shyu, W. C. and Tsao, W. L., Double gaps metabolic acidosis and bilateral basal ganglion lesions in methanol intoxication. Am. J. Emerg. Med. 13:369–371, 1995. [Case Report]

Anderson, C. A., Rubinstein, D., Filley, C. M. and Stears, J. C., MR enhancing brain lesions in methanol intoxication. J. Comput. Assist Tomogr. 21:834–836, 1997. [Case Report]

Hantson, P., Duprez, T. and Mahieu, P., Neurotoxicity to the basal ganglia shown by magnetic resonance imaging (MRI) following poisoning by methanol and other substances. J. Toxicol. Clin. Toxicol. 35:151–161, 1997. [Case Report]

Hsu, H. H., Chen, C. Y., Chen, F. H., Lee, C. C., Chou, T. Y. and Zimmerman, R. A., Optic atrophy and cerebral infarcts caused by methanol intoxication: MRI. Neuroradiology 39:192–194, 1997. [Case Report]

Kuteifan, K., Oesterle, H., Tajahmady, T., Gutbub, A. M. and Laplatte, G., Necrosis and haemorrhage of the putamen in methanol poisoning shown on MRI. Neuroradiology 40:158–160, 1998. [Case Report]

Onder, F., Ilker, S., Kansu, T., Tatar, T., and Kural, G., Acute blindness and putaminal necrosis in methanol intoxication. Int. Ophthalmol. 22:81–84, 1998.

Reviews

Eckardt, M. J., Rohrbaugh, J. W., Rio, D., Rawlings, R. R. and Coppola, R., Brain imaging in alcoholic patients. Adv. Alcohol. Subst. Abuse 7:59–71, 1988.

Victor, M., MR in the diagnosis of Wernicke-Korsakoff syndrome. AJR Am. J. Roentgenol. 11:895, 1990.

von Einsiedel, H. G., Magnetic resonance tomography in white matter diseases. Rontgenpraxis 44:193–199, 1991. [German]

Blansjaar, B. A., Korsakoff syndrome. Nederlands Tijdschrift voor Geneeskunde 137:1043–1048, 1993. [Dutch]

Charness, M. E., Brain lesions in alcoholics. Alcohol. Clin. Exp. Res. 17:2–11, 1993.

Freedland, E. S. and McMicken, D. B., Alcohol-related seizures, Part I: Pathophysiology, differential diagnosis, and evaluation. J. Emerg. Med. 11:463–473, 1993.

O'Carroll, R., Neuropsychological and neuroimaging aspects of latent hepatic encephalopathy (LHE). Alcohol Alcohol. Suppl. 2:191–195, 1993.

Joyce, E. M., Aetiology of alcoholic brain damage: alcoholic neurotoxicity or thiamine malnutrition? Br. Med. Bull. 50:99–114, 1994.

Mann, K., Mundle, G., Strayle, M. and Wakat, P., Neuroimaging in alcoholism: CT and MRI results and clinical correlates. J. Neural. Transm. Gen. Sect. 99:145–155, 1995.

Seery, J. P. and Taylor-Robinson, S. D., The application of magnetic resonance spectroscopy to the study of hepatic encephalopathy. J. Hepatol. 25:988–998, 1996.

Neiman, J., Alcohol as a risk factor for brain damage: neurologic aspects. Alcohol. Clin. Exp. Res. 22(7 Suppl.):346S–351S, 1998.

Roebuck, T. M., Mattson, S. N. and Riley, E. P., A review of the neuroanatomical findings in children with fetal alcohol syndrome or prenatal exposure to alcohol. Alcohol. Clin. Exp. Res. 22:339–344, 1998.

Marijuana and Hallucinogens

Marijuana

Yurgelun-Todd, D. A., Gruber, S. A., Hanson, R. A., Baird, A. A., Renshaw, P. F. and Pope, H. G., Jr., Residual effects of marijuana use: an fMRI study., College on Problems of Drug Dependence, 60th Annual Scientific Meeting. Scottsdale, AZ, p. 167, 1998. [Abstract].

Ketamine

Burdett, N. G., Menon, D. K., Carpenter, T. A., Jones, J. G. and Hall, L. D., Visualisation of changes in regional cerebral blood flow (rCBF) produced by ketamine using long TE gradient-echo sequences: preliminary results. Magn. Reson. Imaging 13:549–553, 1995. [Rodent]

Anabolic Steroids

Akhter, J., Hyder, S. and Ahmed, M., Cerebrovascular accident associated with anabolic steroid use in a young man. Neurology 44:2405–2406, 1994. [Case Report]

MDMA

Grob, C. S., Poland, R. E., Chang, L. and Ernst, T., Psychobiologic effects of 3,4-methylenedioxymethamphetamine in humans: methodological considerations and preliminary observations. Behav. Brain Res. 73:103–107, 1996.

Bitsch, A., Thiel, A., Rieckmann, P. and Prange, H., Acute inflammatory CNS disease after MDMA ('ecstasy'). Eur. Neurol. 36:328–329, 1996. [Case Report]

Chang, L., Ernst, T., Grob, C. S. and Poland, R. E., Cerebral ^{1}H MRS alterations in recreational 3,4-methylenedioxymethamphetamine (MDMA, "Ecstasy") users. J. Magn. Reson. Imaging 10:521–526, 1999.

Schlaeppi, M., Prica, A. and de Torrente, A., Cerebral hemorrhage and "ecstasy." Schweiz Rundsch. Med. Prax. 88:568–572, 1999. [Case Report] [German]

Benzodiazepines

Deicken, R. F., Calabrese, G., Raz, J., Sappey-Marinier, D., Meyerhoff, D., Dillon, W. P., Weiner, M. W. and Fein, G., A 31phosphorous magnetic resonance spectroscopy study of diazepam does not affect brain phosphorous metabolism. Biol. Psychiatry 32:628–631, 1992.

Streeter, C. C., Ciraulo, D. A., Harris, G. J., Kaufman, M. J., Lewis, R. F., Knapp, C. M., Ciraulo, A. M., Maas, L. C., Ungeheuer, M., Szulewski, S. and Renshaw, P. F., Functional magnetic resonance imaging of alprazolam-induced changes in humans with familial alcoholism. Psychiatry Res. 82:69–82, 1998.

Heroin and Opiates

Imaging

Volkow, N. D., Valentine, A. and Kulkarni, M., Radiological and neurological changes in the drug abuse patient: a study with MRI. J. Neuroradiol. 15:288–293, 1988. [Case Report]

Hungerbuhler, H. and Waespe, W., Leukoencephalopathy following inhalation of heroin pyrolysate. Schweiz. Med. Wochenschr. 120:1801–1805, 1990. [Case Report] [German]

Sempere, A. P., Posada, I., Ramo, C. and Cabello, A., Spongiform leucoencephalopathy after inhaling heroin. Lancet 338(8762):320, 1991. [Case Report]

Amass, L., Nardin, R., Mendelson, J. H., Teoh, S. K. and Woods, B. T., Quantitative magnetic resonance imaging in heroin- and cocaine- dependent men: a preliminary study. Psychiatry Res. 45:15–23, 1992.

Bartolomei, F., Nicoli, F., Swiader, L. and Gastaut, J. L., Ischemic cerebral vascular stroke after heroin sniffing. A new case. Presse Med. 21:983–986, 1992. [Case Report] [French]

Roulet Perez, E., Maeder, P., Rivier, L. and Deonna, T., Toxic leucoencephalopathy after heroin ingestion in a 21/2-year-old child. Lancet 340(8821):729, 1992. [Case Report]

Teoh, S. K., Mendelson, J. H., Woods, B. T., Mello, N. K., Hallgring, E., Anfinsen, P., Douglas, A. and Mercer, G., Pituitary volume in men with concurrent heroin and cocaine dependence. J. Clin. Endocrinol. Metab. 76:1529–1532, 1993.

Tan, T. P., Algra, P. R., Valk, J. and Wolters, E. C., Toxic leukoencephalopathy after inhalation of poisoned heroin: MR findings. AJNR Am. J. Neuroradiol. 15:175–178, 1994.

Benassi, G., Rinaldi, R., Azzimondi, G., Stracciari, A., D'Alessandro, R. and Pazzaglia, P., Acute generalized dystonia due to a bilateral lesion of basal ganglia mainly affecting the nuclei pallidi. Ital. J. Neurol. Sci. 17:71–73, 1996. [Case Report]

Celius, E. G. and Andersson, S., Leucoencephalopathy after inhalation of heroin: a case report. J. Neurol. Neurosurg. Psychiatry 60:694–695, 1996. [Case Report]

Rose, J. S., Branchey, M., Buydens-Branchey, L., Stapleton, J. M., Chasten, K., Werrell, A. and Maayan, M. L., Cerebral perfusion in early and late opiate withdrawal: a technetium-99m-HMPAO SPECT study. Psychiatry Res. 67:39–47, 1996.

Zuckerman, G. B., Ruiz, D. C., Keller, I. A. and Brooks, J., Neurologic complications following intranasal administration of heroin in an adolescent. Ann. Pharmacother. 30:778–781, 1996. [Case Report]

Chang, Y. J., Tsai, C. H. and Chen, C. J., Leukoencephalopathy after inhalation of heroin vapor. J. Formos. Med. Assoc. 96:758–760, 1997. [Case Report]

Kriegstein, A. R., Armitage, B. A. and Kim, P. Y., Heroin inhalation and progressive spongiform leukoencephalopathy. N. Engl. J. Med. 336:589–590, 1997. [Case Report]

Niehaus, L., Roricht, S., Meyer, B. U. and Sander, B., Nuclear magnetic resonance tomography detection of heroin-associated CNS lesions. Aktuelle Radiol. 7:309–311, 1997. [Case Report] [German]

Vila, N. and Chamorro, A., Ballistic movements due to ischemic infarcts after intravenous heroin overdose: report of two cases. Clin. Neurol. Neurosurg. 99:259–262, 1997. [Case Report]

Niehaus, L. and Meyer, B. U., Bilateral borderzone brain infarctions in association with heroin abuse. J. Neurol. Sci. 160:180–182, 1998. [Case Report]

Weber, W., Henkes, H., Moller, P., Bade, K. and Kuhne, D., Toxic spongiform leucoencephalopathy after inhaling heroin vapour. Eur. Radiol. 8:749–755, 1998. [Case Report]

Spectroscopy

Christensen, J. D., Kaufman, M. J., Levin, J. M., Mendelson, J. H., Holman, B. L., Cohen, B. M. and Renshaw, P. F., Abnormal cerebral metabolism in polydrug abusers during early withdrawal: A ^{31}P MR spectroscopy study. Magn. Reson. Med. 35:658–663, 1996.

Shungu, D. C., Millar, W. S., Kriegstein, A. R., Lynch, T. and DeLaPaz, R. L., "Chasing the Dragon" with multislice ^{1}H MRSI of the human brain exposed to heroin vapors. International Society for Magnetic Resonance in Medicine, Sixth Scientific Meeting and Exhibition. Sydney, Australia, p. 1713, 1998. [Abstract]

Kaufman, M. J., Pollack, M. H., Villafuerte, R. A., Kukes, T. J., Rose, S. E., Mendelson, J. H., Cohen, B. M. and Renshaw, P. F., Cerebral phosphorus metabolite abnormalities in opiate-dependent polydrug abusers in methadone maintenance. Psychiatry Res. 90:143–152, 1999.

Functional MRI

Sell, L. A., Simmons, A., Lemmens, G. M., Williams, S. C. R., Brammer, M. and Strang, J., Functional magnetic resonance imaging of the acute effect of intravenous heroin administration on visual activation in long-term heroin addicts: results from a feasibility study. Drug Alcohol Depend. 49:55–60, 1997.

Cocaine

Acute Administration

Imaging

DeVore, R. A. and Tucker, H. M., Dysphagia and dysarthria as a result of cocaine abuse. Otolaryngol. Head Neck Surg. 98:174–175, 1988. [Case Report]

Nalls, G., Disher, A., Daryabagi, J., Zant, Z. and Eisenman, J., Subcortical cerebral hemorrhages associated with cocaine abuse: CT and MR findings. J. Comput. Assist. Tomogr. 13:1–5, 1989.

Huff, J. S., Spinal epidural hematoma associated with cocaine abuse. Am. J. Emerg. Med. 12:350–352, 1994. [Case Report]

Mena, I., Giombetti, R. J., Miller, B. L., Garrett, K., Villanueva-Meyer, J., Mody, C. and Goldberg, M. A., Cerebral blood flow changes with acute cocaine intoxication: Clinical correlations with SPECT, CT and MRI. In: Imaging Techniques in Medications Development: Preclinical and Clinical Aspects, ed. by H. Sorer, H. and Rapaka, R. S. (eds.) U.S. Dept. of Health and Human Services, Rockville, MD, pp. 161–173, 1994.

Yamazaki, K., Katayama, S., Iwai, T. and Hirata, K., A case of malignant syndrome with leukoencephalopathy due to cocaine abuse. Rinsho Shinkeigaku 34:582–586, 1994. [Case Report] [Japanese]

Gradon, J. D. and Wityk, R., Diagnosis of probably cocaine-induced cerebral vasculitis by magnetic resonance angiography. Southern Med. J. 88:1264–1266, 1995. [Case Report]

Yamauchi, T., Shibata, K., Uchiyama, S., Osawa, M. and Iwata, M., A case of cerebral infarction in a young adult following an abuse of cocaine and other drugs. Rinsho Shinkeigaku 35:1256–1258, 1995. [Case Report] [Japanese]

Samkoff, L. M., Daras, M., Kleiman, A. R. and Koppel, B. S., Spontaneous spinal epidural hematoma. Another neurologic complication of cocaine? Arch. Neurol. 53:819–821, 1996. [Case Report]

Di Lazzaro, V., Restuccia, D., Oliviero, A., Profice, P., Nardone, R., Valeriani, M., Colosimo, C., Tartaglione, T., Della Corte, F., Pennisi, M. A. and Tonali, P., Ischaemic myelopathy associated with cocaine: clinical, neurophysiological, and neuroradiological features. J. Neurol. Neurosurg. Psychiatry 63:531–533, 1997. [Case Report]

Gillams, A. R., Allen, E., Hrieb, K., Venna, N., Craven, D. and Carter, A. P., Cerebral infarction in patients with AIDS. AJNR Am. J. Neuroradiol. 18:1581–1585. 1997.

Walz, R., Bianchin, M., Chaves, M. L., Cerski, M. R., Severo, L. C. and Londero, A. T., Cerebral phaeohyphomycosis caused by Cladophialophora bantiana in a Brazilian drug abuser. J. Med. Vet. Mycol. 35:427–431, 1997. [Case Report]

Kaufman, M. J., Levin, J. M., Ross, M. H., Lange, N., Rose, S. L., Kukes, T. J., Mendelson, J. H., Lukas, S. E., Cohen, B. M. and Renshaw, P. F., Cocaine-induced cerebral vasoconstriction detected in humans with magnetic resonance angiography. JAMA 279:376–380, 1998.

Leira, E. C., Bendixen, B. H., Kardon, R. H. and Adams, H. P., Jr., Brief, transient Horner's syndrome can be the hallmark of a carotid artery dissection. Neurology 50:289–290, 1998. [Case Report]

Nuytten, D., Wyffels, E., Michiels, K., Ferrante, M., Verbraeken, H., Daelemans, R., Baeck, E. and Cras, P., Drug-induced spongiform leucoencephalopathy, a case report with review of the literature. Acta Neurol. Belg. 98:32–35, 1998. [Case Report]

Spectroscopy

Christensen, J. D., Kaufman, M. J., Rose, S. L., Mendelson, J. H., Moore, C. M., Cohen, B. M. and Renshaw, P. F., ^{1}H MRS of human basal ganglia response to acute cocaine administration. International Society for Magnetic Resonance in Medicine, Fifth Scientific Meeting and Exhibition. Vancouver, B.C., p. 994, 1997. [Abstract]

Li, S.-J., Wang, Y., Risinger, R., Rainey, C., Harsch, H., Pankiewicz, J., Sperry, L., Cho, J.-K., Bloom, A. S. and Stein, E. A., Acute cocaine administration induces NAA increase detected by ^{1}H MRS. International Society for Magnetic Resonance in Medicine, Sixth Scientific Meeting and Exhibition. Sydney, Australia, p. 1714, 1998. [Abstract]

Functional MRI

Breiter, H. C., Gollub, R. L., Weisskoff, R. M., Kennedy, D. N., Makris, N., Berke, J. D., Goodman, J. M., Kantor, H. L., Gastfriend, D. R., Riorden, J. P., Mathew, R. T., Makris, N., Rosen, B. R. and Hyman, S. E., Acute effects of cocaine on human brain activity and emotion. Neuron 19:591–611, 1997.

Gollub, R. L., Breiter, H. C., Kantor, H., Kennedy, D., Gastfriend, D., Mathew, R. T., Makris, N., Guimaraes, A., Riorden, J., Campbell, T., Foley, M., Hyman, S. E., Rosen, B. and Weisskoff, R., Cocaine decreases cortical cerebral blood flow but does not obscure regional activation in functional magnetic resonance imaging in human subjects. J. Cereb. Blood Flow Metab. 18:724–734, 1998.

Kaufman, M. J., Levin, J. M., Maas, L. C., Rose, S. L., Lukas, S. E., Mendelson, J. H., Cohen, B. M. and Renshaw, P. F., Cocaine decreases relative cerebral blood volume in humans: a dynamic susceptibility contrast magnetic resonance imaging study. Psychopharmacology (Berl.) 138:76–81, 1998.

Kaufman, M. J., Levin, J. M., Kukes, T. J., Villafuerte, R. A., Hsia, S. B., Lukas, S. E., Mendelson, J. H., Cohen, B. M. and Renshaw, P. F., Menstrual cycle phase modulates cocaine-induced cerebral blood volume reduction in women. International Society of Magnetic Resonance in Medicine, Sixth Scientific Meeting and Exhibition. Sydney, Australia, p. 1581, 1998. [Abstract]

Zhang, M., Booze, R. M., Nicholls, M. A., Andersen, A. H., Welch, M. A., Strupp, B. J., Mactutus, C. F. and Avison, M. J., Cerebral response to cocaine and cocaine methiodide in the adult rat studied by fMRI. International Society for Magnetic Resonance in Medicine, Sixth Scientific Meeting and Exhibition. Sydney, Australia, p. 1580, 1998. [Abstract] [Rodent]

Levin, J. M., Kaufman, M. J., Ross, M. H., Roc, A. C., Maas, L. C., Mendelson, J. H., Cohen, B. M. and Renshaw, P. F., Cocaine Increases BOLD fMRI Response to Photic Stimulation. International Society for Magnetic Resonance in Medicine, Seventh Scientific Meeting and Exhibition. Philadelphia, PA, p. 838, 1999. [Abstract]

Chronic Administration

Imaging

Mody, C. K., Miller, B. L., McIntyre, H. B., Cobb, S. K. and Goldberg, M. A., Neurologic complications of cocaine abuse. Neurology 38:1189–1193, 1988. [Case Report]

Volkow, N. D., Valentine, A. and Kulkarni, M., Radiological and neurological changes in the drug abuse patient: a study with MRI. J. Neuroradiol. 15:288–293, 1988. [Case Report]

Goldberg, R. A., Weisman, J. S., McFarland, J. E., Krauss, H. R., Hepler, R. S. and Shorr, N., Orbital inflammation and optic neuropathies associated with chronic sinusitis of intranasal cocaine abuse. Possible role of contiguous inflammation. Arch. Ophthalmol. 107:831–835, 1989. [Case Report]

Klonoff, D., Andrews, B. and Obana, W., Stroke associated with cocaine use. Arch. Neurol. 46:989–993, 1989.

Nalls, G., Disher, A., Daryabagi, J., Zant, Z. and Eisenman, J., Subcortical cerebral hemorrhages associated with cocaine abuse: CT and MR findings. J. Comput. Assist. Tomogr. 13:1–5, 1989.

Aggarwal, S. and Byrne, B. D., Massive ischemic cerebellar infarction due to cocaine use. Neuroradiology 33:449–450, 1991. [Case Report]

Peterson, P. L., Roszler, M., Jacobs, I. and Wilner, H. I., Neurovascular complications of cocaine abuse. J. Neuropsychiatry Clin. Neurosci. 3:143–149, 1991.

Ramadan, N. M., Levine, S. R. and Welch, K. M., Pontine hemorrhage following "crack" cocaine use. Neurology 41:946–947, 1991. [Case Report]

Amass, L., Nardin, R., Mendelson, J. H., Teoh, S. K. and Woods, B. T., Quantitative magnetic resonance imaging in heroin- and cocaine- dependent men: a preliminary study. Psychiatry Res. 45:15–23, 1992.

MacKay, S., Meyerhoff, D. J., Dillon, W. P., Weiner, M .W. and Fein, G., Alteration of brain phospholipid metabolites in cocaine-dependent polysubstance abusers. Biol. Psychiatry 34:261–264, 1993.

Teoh, S. K., Mendelson, J. H., Woods, B. T., Mello, N. K., Hallgring, E., Anfinsen, P., Douglas, A. and Mercer, G., Pituitary volume in men with concurrent heroin and cocaine dependence. J. Clin. Endocrinol. Metab. 76:1529–1532, 1993.

Diez-Tejedor, E., Frank, A., Gutierrez, M. and Barreiro, P., Encephalopathy and biopsy-proven cerebrovascular inflammatory changes in a cocaine abuser. Eur. J. Neurol. 5:103–107, 1998.

Disclafani, V., Clark, H. W., Tolou-shams, M., Bloomer, C., Salas, G. A., Norman, D. and Fein, G., Premorbid brain size is a determinant of functional reserve in abstinent crack-cocaine and crack-cocaine-alcohol-dependent adults. J. Int. Neuropsychol. Soc. 4:559–565, 1998.

Disclafani, V., Truran, D. L., Bloomer, C., Toloushams, M., Clark, H. W., Norman, D., Hannauer, D. and Fein, G., Abstinent chronic crack-cocaine and crack-cocaine/alcohol abusers evidence normal hippocampal volumes on MRI despite persistent cognitive impairments. Addiction Biol. 3:261–270, 1998.

Meltzer, C. C., Wells, S. W., Becher, M. W., Flanigan, K. M., Oyler, G. A. and Lee, R. R., AIDS-related MR hyperintensity of the basal ganglia. AJNR Am. J. Neuroradiol. 19:83–89, 1998.

Bartzokis, G., Beckson, M., Hance, D. B., Lu, P. H., Foster, J. A., Mintz, J., Ling, W., Bridge, P., Magnetic resonance imaging evidence of "silent" cerebrovascular toxicity in cocaine dependence. Biol. Psychiatry 45:1203–1211, 1999.

Spectroscopy

Christensen, J. D., Kaufman, M. J., Levin, J. M., Mendelson, J. H., Holman, B. L., Cohen, B. M. and Renshaw, P. F., Abnormal cerebral metabolism in polydrug abusers during early withdrawal: a ^{31}P MR spectroscopy study. Magn. Reson. Med. 35:658–663, 1996.

Chang, L., Mehringer, C. M., Ernst, T., Melchor, R., Myers, H., Forney, D. and Satz, P., Neurochemical alterations in asymptomatic abstinent cocaine users: a proton magnetic resonance spectroscopy study. Biol. Psychiatry 42:1105–1114, 1997.

Meyerhoff, D. J., Bloomer, C., Salas, G., Schuff, N., Norman, D., Weiner, M. W. and Fein, G., Cortical metabolite alterations in recently abstinent cocaine and cocaine/alcohol dependent subjects. International Society for Magnetic Resonance in Medicine Sixth Scientific Meeting and Exhibition. Sydney, Australia, p. 1715, 1998. [Abstract]

Chang, L., Ernst, T., Strickland, T., Mehringer, C. M., Gender effects on persistent cerebral metabolite changes in the frontal lobes of abstinent cocaine users. Am. J. Psychiatry 156:716–722 1999.

Kaufman, M. J., Pollack, M. H., Villafuerte, R. A., Kukes, T. J., Rose, S. E., Mendelson, J. H., Cohen, B. M. and Renshaw, P. F., Cerebral phosphorus metabolite abnormalities in opiate-dependent polydrug abusers in methadone maintenance. Psychiatry Res. 90:143–152, 1999.

Li, S.-J., Wang, Y., Pankiewicz, J., Stein, E. A., Neurochemical adaptation to cocaine abuse: reduction of *N*-acetyl aspartate in thalamus of human cocaine abusers. Biol. Psychiatry 45:1481–1487, 1999.

Craving

Maas, L. C., Lukas, S. E., Kaufman, M. J., Weiss, R. D., Daniels, S. L., Rogers, V. W., Kukes, T. J. and Renshaw, P. F., Functional magnetic resonance imaging of human brain activation during cue-induced cocaine craving. Am. J. Psychiatry 155:124–126, 1998.

Prenatal Exposure

Heier, L. A., Carpanzano, C. R., Mast, J., Brill, P. W., Winchester, P. and Deck, M. D. F., Maternal cocaine abuse: the spectrum of radiologic abnormalities in the neonatal CNS. AJNR Am. J. Neuroradiol. 12:951–956, 1991.

Link, E. A., Weese-Mayer, D. W. and Bryd, S. E., Magnetic resonance imaging in infants exposed to cocaine prenatally: a preliminary report. Clin. Pediatr. (Phila.) 30:506–508, 1991.

Gieron-Korthals, M. A., Helal, A. and Martinez, C. R., Expanding spectrum of cocaine induced central nervous system malformations. Brain Dev. 16:253–256, 1994. [Case Report]

Gomez-Anson, B. and Ramsey, R. G., Pachygyria in a neonate with prenatal cocaine exposure: MR features. J. Comput. Assist. Tomogr. 18:637–639, 1994. [Case Report]

Konkol, R. J., Tikofsky, R. S., Wells, R., Hellman, R. S., Nemeth, P., Walsh, D. J., Heimler, R. and Sty, J. R., Normal high-resolution cerebral ^{99m}Tc-HMPAO SPECT scans in symptomatic neonates exposed to cocaine. J. Child Neurol. 9:278–283, 1994.

Reviews

Lukas, S. E. and Renshaw, P. F., Cocaine Effects on Brain Function. In: Cocaine Abuse: Behavior, Pharmacology, and Clinical Applications, ed. by S.T. Higgins and J.L. Katz, pp. 265–287, Academic Press, San Diego, CA, 1998.

Nuytten, D., Wyffels, E., Michiels, K., Ferrante, M., Verbraeken, H., Daelemans, R., Baeck, E. and Cras, P., Drug-induced spongiform leucoencephalopathy, a case report with review of the literature. Acta Neurol. Belg. 98:32–35, 1998. [Case Report]

Strickland, T. L., Miller, B. L., Kowell, A. and Stein, R., Neurobiology of cocaine-induced organic brain impairment: contributions from functional neuroimaging. Neuropsychol. Rev. 8:1–9, 1998.

Amphetamine and Other Stimulants

Amphetamine

Detre, J. A., Williams, D. S. and Koretsky, A. P., Nuclear magnetic resonance determination of flow, lactate, and phosphate metabolites during amphetamine stimulation of the rat brain. NMR Biomed. 3:272–278, 1990. [Rodent]

Lazar, E. B., Russell, E. J., Cohen, B. A., Brody, B. and Levy, R. M., Contrast-enhanced MR of cerebral arteritis: intravascular enhancement related to flow stasis within areas of focal arterial ectasia. AJNR Am. J. Neuroradiol. 13:271–276, 1992. [Case Report]

Lambrecht, G. L., Malbrain, M. L., Chew, S. L., Baeck, E. and Verbraeken, H., Intranasal caffeine and amphetamine causing stroke. Acta Neurol. Belg. 93:146–149, 1993. [Case Report]

Tsai, E. M., Lee, J. N., Chao, M. C. and Chai, C. Y., Holoprosencephaly and trisomy 13 in a fetus with maternal early gestational amphetamine abuse: a case report. Kaohsiung J. Med. Sci. 9:703–706, 1993. [Case Report]

Silva, A. C., Zhang, W., Williams, D. S. and Koretsky, A. P., Multi-slice MRI of rat brain perfusion during amphetamine stimulation using arterial spin labeling. Magn. Reson. Med. 33:209–214, 1995. [Rodent]

Heye, N. and Hankey, G. J., Amphetamine-associated stroke. Cerebrovasc. Dis. 6:149–155, 1996. [Case Report]

Howard, R. J., Ellis, C., Bullmore, E. T., Brammer, M., Mellers, J. D., Woodruff, P. W., David, A. S., Simmons, A., Williams, S. C. R. and Parkes, J. D., Functional echoplanar imaging correlates of amphetamine administration to normal subjects and subjects with the narcoleptic syndrome. Magn. Reson. Imaging 14:1013–1016, 1996.

Chen, Y. C., Galpern, W. R., Brownell, A. L., Matthews, R. T., Bogdanov, M., Isacson, O., Keltner, J. R., Beal, M. F., Rosen, B. R. and Jenkins, B. G., Detection of dopaminergic neurotransmitter activity using pharmacologic MRI: correlation with PET, microdialysis, and behavioral data. Magn. Reson. Med. 38:389–398, 1997. [Rodent]

Nuytten, D., Wyffels, E., Michiels, K., Ferrante, M., Verbraeken, H., Daelemans, R., Baeck, E. and Cras, P., Drug-induced spongiform leucoencephalopathy, a case report with review of the literature. Acta Neurol. Belg. 98:32–35, 1998. [Case Report]

Chaudhuri, C. and Salahudeen, A. K., Massive intracerebral hemorrhage in an amphetamine addict. Am. J. Med. Sci. 317:350–352, 1999. [Case Report]

Methamphetamine

Sachdeva, K. and Woodward, K. G., Caudal thalamic infarction following intranasal methamphetamine use. Neurology 39:305–306, 1989. [Case Report]

Ellis, K. L. and Speed, J., Pharmacologic management of movement disorder after midbrain haemorrhage. Brain Inj. 12:623–628, 1998. [Case Report]

Methylphenidate

Vaidya, C. J., Austin, G., Kirkorian, G., Ridlehuber, H. W., Desmond, J. E., Glover, G. H. and Gabrieli, J. D., Selective effects of methylphenidate in attention deficit hyperactivity disorder: a functional magnetic resonance study. Proc. Natl. Acad. Sci. USA 95:14494–14499, 1998.

Ephedrine

Bruno, A., Nolte, K. B. and Chapin, J., Stroke associated with ephedrine use. Neurology 43:1313–1316, 1993. [Case Report]

Solvents and Toluene

Acute Administration

Welch, L., Kirshner, H., Heath, A., Gilliland, R. and Broyles, S., Chronic neuropsychological and neurological impairment following acute exposure to a solvent mixture of toluene and methyl ethyl ketone (MEK). J. Toxicol. Clin. Toxicol. 29:435–445, 1991. [Case Report]

Lewis, L. D., Smith, B. W. and Mamourian, A. C., Delayed sequelae after acute overdoses or poisonings: cranial neuropathy related to ethylene glycol ingestion. Clin. Pharmacol. Ther. 61:692–699, 1997. [Case Report]

Chronic Administration

Rosenberg, N. L., Kleinschmidt-DeMasters, B. K., Davis, K. A., Dreisbach, J. N., Hormes, J. T. and Filley, C. M., Toluene abuse causes diffuse central nervous system white matter changes. Ann. Neurol. 23:611–614, 1988.

Rosenberg, N. L., Spitz, M. C., Filley, C. M., Davis, K. A. and Schaumburg, H. H., Central nervous system effects of chronic toluene abuse: clinical, brainstem evoked response and magnetic resonance imaging studies. Neurotoxicol. Teratol. 10:489–495, 1988.

Filley, C. M., Heaton, R. K. and Rosenberg, N. L., White matter dementia in chronic toluene abuse. Neurology 40:532–534, 1990.

Ikeda, M. and Tsukagoshi, H., Encephalopathy due to toluene sniffing. Report of a case with magnetic resonance imaging. Eur. Neurol. 30:347–349, 1990. [Case Report]

Poungvarin, N., Multifocal brain damage due to lacquer sniffing: the first case report of Thailand. J. Med. Assoc. Thai. 74:296–300, 1991. [Case Report]

Fujita, K., Koga, Y., Takemasa, K., Koike, H. and Akai, J., A case of chronic toluene intoxication with atrophy of cerebrum, cerebellum and brainstem on CT and MRI. Rinsho Shinkeigaku 32:421–425, 1992. [Case Report] [Japanese]

Leira, H. L., Myhr, G., Nilsen, G. and Dale, L. G., Cerebral magnetic resonance imaging and cerebral computerized tomography for patients with solvent-induced encephalopathy. Scand. J. Work Environ. Health 18:68–70, 1992.

Suzuki, K., Wakayama, Y., Takada, H. and Okayasu, H., A case of chronic toluene intoxication with abnormal MRI findings: abnormal intensity areas in cerebral white matter, basal ganglia, internal capsule, brain stem and middle cerebellar peduncle. Rinsho Shinkeigaku 32:84–87, 1992. [Case Report] [Japanese]

Caldemeyer, K. S., Pascuzzi, R. M., Moran, C. C. and Smith, R. R., Toluene abuse causing reduced MR signal intensity in the brain. AJR Am. J. Roentgenol. 161:1259–1261, 1993. [Case Report]

Hirai, H. and Ikeuchi, Y., MRI of chronic toluene intoxication. Rinsho Shinkeigaku 33:552–555, 1993. [Case Report] [Japanese]

Kojima, S., Hirayama, K., Furumoto, H., Fukutake, T. and Hattori, T., Magnetic resonance imaging in chronic toluene abuse, and volitional hyperkinesia. Rinsho Shinkeigaku 33:477–482, 1993. [Case Report] [Japanese]

Sodeyama, N., Orimo, S., Okiyama, R., Arai, M. and Tamaki, M., A case of chronic thinner intoxication developing hyperkinesie volitionnelle three years after stopping thinner abuse. Rinsho Shinkeigaku 33:213–215, 1993. [Case Report] [Japanese]

Xiong, L., Matthes, J. D., Li, J. and Jinkins, J. R., MR imaging of "spray heads": toluene abuse via aerosol paint inhalation. AJNR Am. J. Neuroradiol. 14:1195–1199, 1993. [Case Report]

Unger, E., Alexander, A., Fritz, T., Rosenberg, N. and Dreisbach, J., Toluene abuse: physical basis for hypointensity of the basal ganglia on T2-weighted MR images. Radiology 193:473–476, 1994.

Ashikaga, R., Araki, Y., Miura, K. and Ishida, O., Cranial MRI in chronic thinner intoxication. Neuroradiology 37:443–444, 1995. [Case Report]

Ohnuma, A., Kimura, I. and Saso, S., MRI in chronic paint-thinner intoxication. Neuroradiology 37:445–446, 1995. [Case Report]

Yamanouchi, N., Okada, S., Kodama, K., Hirai, S., Sekine, H., Murakami, A., Komatsu, N., Sakamoto, T. and Sato, T., White matter changes caused by chronic solvent abuse. AJNR Am. J. Neuroradiol. 16:1643–1649, 1995.

Caldemeyer, K. S., Armstrong, S. W., George, K. K., Moran, C. C. and Pascuzzi, R. M., The spectrum of neuroimaging abnormalities in solvent abuse and their clinical correlation. J. Neuroimaging 6:167–173, 1996. [Case Report]

del Amo, M., Berenguer, J., Pujol, T. and Mercader, J. M., MR in trichloroethane poisoning. AJNR Am. J. Neuroradiol. 17:1180–1182, 1996. [Case Report]

Noda, S., Yamanouchi, N., Okada, S., Kodama, K., Murakami, A., Sekine, H., Sakamoto, T., Komatsu, N., Sato, T., Ikehira, H. and Morita, F., Proton MR spectroscopy in solvent abusers. Ann. NY Acad. Sci. 801:441–444, 1996.

Thuomas, K. A., Moller, C., Odkvist, L. M., Flodin, U. and Dige, N., MR imaging in solvent-induced chronic toxic encephalopathy. Acta Radiol. 37:177–179, 1996.

Arai, H., Yamada, M., Miyake, S., Yamashita, S., Iwamoto, H., Aida, N. and Hara, M., Two cases of toluene embryopathy with severe motor and intellectual disabilities syndrome. No To Hattatsu 29:361–366, 1997. [Case Report] [Japanese]

Terashi, H., Nagata, K., Satoh, Y., Hirata, Y. and Hatazawa, J., Hippocampal hypoperfusion underlying dementia due to chronic toluene intoxication. Rinsho Shinkeigaku 37:1010–1013, 1997. [Case Report] [Japanese]

Yamanouchi, N., Okada, S., Kodama, K., Sakamoto, T., Sekine, H., Hirai, S., Murakami, A., Komatsu, N. and Sato, T., Effects of MRI abnormalities on WAIS-R performance in solvent abusers. Acta Neurol. Scand. 96:34–39, 1997.

Kamran, S., and Bakshi, R., MRI in chronic toluene abuse: low signal in the cerebral cortex on T2-weighted images. Neuroradiology 40:519–521, 1998. [Case Report]

Yamanouchi, N., Okada, S.-I., Kodama, K. and Sato, T., Central nervous system impairment caused by chronic solvent abuse—a review of Japanese studies on the clinical and neuroimaging aspects. Addiction Biol. 3:15–27, 1998.

Hageman, G., van der Hoek, J., van Hout, M., van der Laan, G., Steur, E. J., de Bruin, W. and Herholz, K., Parkinsonism, pyramidal signs, polyneuropathy, and cognitive decline after long-term occupational solvent exposure. J. Neurology 246:198–206, 1999.

Kitabayashi, Y., Ueda, H., Matsuda, M., Narumoto, J., Kobayashi, T. and Fukui, K., A case report of organic solvent abuse with amotivational syndrome. Nihon Arukoru Yakubutsu Igakkai Zasshi 34:130–137, 1999. [Case Report] [Japanese]

Polydrug Abuse

Imaging

Volkow, N. D., Valentine, A. and Kulkarni, M., Radiological and neurological changes in the drug abuse patient: a study with MRI. J. Neuroradiol. 15:288–293, 1988. [Case Report]

Amass, L., Nardin, R., Mendelson, J. H., Teoh, S. K. and Woods, B. T., Quantitative magnetic resonance imaging in heroin- and cocaine- dependent men: a preliminary study. Psychiatry Res. 45:15–23, 1992.

Handelsman, L., Aronson, M., Maurer, G., Wiener, J., Jacobson, J., Bernstein, D., Ness, R., Herman, S., Losonczy, M., Song, I. S., Holloway, K., Horvath, T., Donnelly, N., Hirschowitz, J. and Rowan, A. J., Neuropsychological and neurological manifestations of HIV-1 dementia in drug users. J. Neuropsychiatry Clin. Neurosci. 4:21–28, 1992.

Aasly, J., Storsaeter, O., Nilsen, G., Smevik, O. and Rinck, P., Minor structural brain changes in young drug abusers. A magnetic resonance study. Acta Neurol. Scand. 87:210–214, 1993.

Teoh, S. K., Mendelson, J. H., Woods, B. T., Mello, N. K., Hallgring, E., Anfinsen, P., Douglas, A. and Mercer, G., Pituitary volume in men with concurrent heroin and cocaine dependence. J. Clin. Endocrinol. Metab. 76:1529–1532, 1993.

Liu, X., Phillips, R. L., Resnick, S. M., Villemagne, V. L., Wong, D. F., Stapleton, J. M. and London, E. D., Magnetic resonance imaging reveals no ventriculomegaly in polydrug abusers. Acta Neurol. Scand. 92:83–90, 1995.

Bigler, E. D., Blatter, D. D., Johnson, S. C., Anderson, C. V., Russo, A. A., Gale, S. D., Ryser, D. K., MacNamara, S. E. and Bailey, B. J., Traumatic brain injury, alcohol and quantitative neuroimaging: preliminary findings. Brain Inj. 10:197–206, 1996.

Liu, X., Matochick, J. A., Cadet, J. L. and London, E. D., Smaller volume of prefrontal lobe in polysubstance abusers: a magnetic resonance imaging study. Neuropsychopharmacology 18:243–252, 1998.

Nuytten, D., Wyffels, E., Michiels, K., Ferrante, M., Verbraeken, H., Daelemans, R., Baeck, E. and Cras, P., Drug-induced spongiform leucoencephalopathy, a case report with review of the literature. Acta Neurol. Belg. 98:32–35, 1998. [Case Report]

Scheller-Gilkey, G., Lewine, R. R., Caudle, J., and Brown, F. W., Schizophrenia, substance use, and brain morphology. Schizophr. Res. 35:113–120, 1999.

Spectroscopy

MacKay, S., Meyerhoff, D. J., Dillon, W. P., Weiner, M. W. and Fein, G., Alteration of brain phospholipid metabolites in cocaine-dependent polysubstance abusers. Biol. Psychiatry 34:261–264, 1993.

Christensen, J. D., Kaufman, M. J., Levin, J. M., Mendelson, J. H., Holman, B. L., Cohen, B. M. and Renshaw, P. F., Abnormal cerebral metabolism in polydrug abusers during early withdrawal: A ^{31}P MR spectroscopy study. Magn. Reson. Med. 35:658–663, 1996.

Kaufman, M. J., Pollack, M. H., Villafuerte, R. A., Kukes, T. J., Rose, S. E., Mendelson, J. H., Cohen, B. M. and Renshaw, P. F., Cerebral phosphorus metabolite abnormalities in opiate-dependent polydrug abusers in methadone maintenance. Psychiatry Res. 90:143–152, 1999.

Neuropsychology

Alcohol and Alcoholism

Acute Administration

Parker, E. S., Birnbaum, I. M., Weingartner, H., Hartley, J. T., Stillman, R. C. and Wyatt, R. J., Retrograde enhancement of human memory with alcohol. Psychopharmacology (Berl.) 69:219–222, 1980.

Parker, E. S., Morihisa, J. M., Wyatt, R. J., Schwartz, B. L., Weingartner, H. and Stillman, R. C., The alcohol facilitation effect on memory: a dose-response study. Psychopharmacology (Berl.) 74:88–92, 1981.

Minocha, A., Barth, J. T., Roberson, D. G., Herold, D. A. and Spyker, D. A., Impairment of cognitive and psychomotor function by ethanol in social drinkers. Vet. Hum. Toxicol. 27:533–536, 1985.

Niaura, R. S., Nathan, P. E., Frankenstein, W., Shapiro, A. P. and Brick, J., Gender differences in acute psychomotor, cognitive, and pharmacokinetic response to alcohol. Addict. Behav. 12:345–356, 1987.

Schandler, S. L., Cohen, M. J. and McArthur, D. L., Event-related brain potentials in intoxicated and detoxified alcoholics during visuospatial learning. Psychopharmacology (Berl.) 94:275–283, 1988.

Schandler, S. L., Cohen, M. J., McArthur, D. L., Naliboff, B. D. and Hassell, A., Activation peaking in intoxicated and detoxified alcoholics during visuospatial learning. J. Stud. Alcohol 49:126–130, 1988.

Haut, J. S., Beckwith, B. E., Petros, T. V. and Russell, S., Gender differences in retrieval from long-term memory following acute intoxication with ethanol. Physiol. Behav. 45:1161–1165, 1989.

Lukas, S. E., Lex, B. W., Slater, J. P., Greenwald, N. E. and Mendelson, J. H., A microanalysis of ethanol-induced disruption of body sway and psychomotor performance in women. Psychopharmacology (Berl.) 98:169–175, 1989.

Gustafson, R. and Kallmen, H., Effects of alcohol on prolonged cognitive performance measured with Stroop's Color Word Test. Psychol. Rep. 67:643–650, 1990.

Linnoila, M., Stapleton, J. M., Lister, R., Moss, H., Lane, E., Granger, A., Greenblatt, D. J. and Eckardt, M. J., Effects of adinazolam and diazepam, alone and in combination with ethanol, on psychomotor and cognitive performance and on autonomic nervous system reactivity in healthy volunteers. Eur. J. Clin. Pharmacol. 38:371–377, 1990.

Linnoila, M., Stapleton, J. M., Lister, R., Moss, H., Lane, E., Granger, A. and Eckardt, M. J., Effects of single doses of alprazolam and diazepam, alone and in combination with ethanol, on psychomotor and cognitive performance and on autonomic nervous system reactivity in healthy volunteers. Eur. J. Clin. Pharmacol. 39:21–28, 1990.

Peterson, J. B., Rothfleisch, J., Zelazo, P. D. and Pihl, R. O., Acute alcohol intoxication and cognitive functioning. J. Stud. Alcohol 51:114–122, 1990.

Hindmarch, I., Kerr, J. S. and Sherwood, N., The effects of alcohol and other drugs on psychomotor performance and cognitive function. Alcohol Alcohol. 26:71–79, 1991.

Lyvers, M. F. and Maltzman, I., Selective effects of alcohol on Wisconsin Card Sorting Test performance. Br. J. Addict. 86:399–407, 1991.

Schuckit, M. A., Greenblatt, D., Gold, E. and Irwin, M., Reactions to ethanol and diazepam in healthy young men. J. Stud. Alcohol 52:180–187, 1991.
Frewer, L. J. and Lader, M., The effects of nefazodone, imipramine and placebo, alone and combined with alcohol, in normal subjects. Int. Clin. Psychopharmacol. 8:13–20, 1993.
Higgins, S. T., Rush, C. R., Bickel, W. K., Hughes, J. R., Lynn, M. and Capeless, M. A., Acute behavioral and cardiac effects of cocaine and alcohol combinations in humans. Psychopharmacology (Berl.) 111:285–294, 1993.
Kennedy, R. S., Turnage, J. J., Wilkes, R. L. and Dunlap, W. P., Effects of graded dosages of alcohol on nine computerized repeated-measures tests. Ergonomics 36:1195–1222, 1993.
Heishman, S. J., Arasteh, K. and Stitzer, M. L., Comparative effects of alcohol and marijuana on mood, memory, and performance. Pharmacol. Biochem. Behav. 58:93–101, 1997.
Pickworth, W. B., Rohrer, M. S. and Fant, R. V., Effects of abused drugs on psychomotor performance. Exp. Clin. Psychopharmacol. 5:235–241, 1997.
Anderson, S. and Dawson, J., Neuropsychological correlates of alcoholic hangover. South African J. Sci. 95:145–147, 1999.
Bruce, K. R., Pihl, R. O., Mayerovitch, J. I. and Shestowsky, J. S., Alcohol and retrograde memory effects: role of individual differences. J. Stud. Alcohol 60:130–136, 1999.
Erblich, J. and Earleywine, M., Children of alcoholics exhibit attenuated cognitive impairment during an ethanol challenge. Alcohol. Clin. Exp. Res. 23:476–482, 1999.
Quintyn, J. C., Massy, J., Quillard, M. and Brasseur, G., Effects of low alcohol consumption on visual evoked potential, visual field and visual contrast sensitivity. Acta Ophthalmol. Scand. 77:23–26, 1999.
Schneider, U., Bevilacqua, C., Jacobs, R., Karst, M., Dietrich, D. E., Becker, H., Muller-Vahl, K. R., Seeland, I., Gielsdorf, D., Schedlowski, M. and Emrich, H. M., Effects of fentanyl and low doses of alcohol on neuropsychological performance in healthy subjects. Neuropsychobiology 39:38–43, 1999.
Wegner, A. J. and Fahle, M., Alcohol and visual performance. Prog. Neuropsychopharmacol. Biol. Psychiatry 23:465–482, 1999.

Social Drinking

Parker, E. S. and Noble, E. P., Alcohol consumption and cognitive functioning in social drinkers. J. Stud. Alcohol 38:1224–1232, 1977.
MacVane, J., Butters, N., Montgomery, K. and Farber, J., Cognitive functioning in men social drinkers; a replication study. J. Stud. Alcohol 43:81–95, 1982.
Hannon, R., Butler, C. P., Day, C. L., Khan, S. A., Quitoriano, L. A., Butler, A. M. and Meredith, L. A., Alcohol use and cognitive functioning in men and women college students. Recent Dev. Alcohol 3:241–252, 1985.
Schaeffer, K. W. and Parsons, O. A., Drinking practices and neuropsychological test performance in sober male alcoholics and social drinkers. Alcohol 3:175–179, 1986.
Page, R. D. and Cleveland, M. F., Cognitive dysfunction and aging among male alcoholics and social drinkers. Alcohol. Clin. Exp. Res. 11:376–384, 1987.
Emmerson, R. Y., Dustman, R. E., Heil, J. and Shearer, D. E., Neuropsychological performance of young nondrinkers, social drinkers, and long- and short-term sober alcoholics. Alcohol. Clin. Exp. Res. 12:625–629, 1988.
Waugh, M., Jackson, M., Fox, G. A., Hawke, S. H. and Tuck, R. R., Effect of social drinking on neuropsychological performance. Br. J. Addict. 84:659–667, 1989.
Nichols, J. M., Martin, F. and Kirkby, K. C., A comparison of the effect of lorazepam on memory in heavy and low social drinkers. Psychopharmacology (Berl.) 112:475–482, 1993.
Giancola, P. R., Zeichner, A., Yarnell, J. E. and Dickson, K. E., Relation between executive cognitive functioning and the adverse consequences of alcohol use in social drinkers. Alcohol. Clin. Exp. Res. 20:1094–1098, 1996.

Sher, K. J., Martin, E. D., Wood, P. K. and Rutledge, P. C., Alcohol use disorders and neuropsychological functioning in first-year undergraduates. Exp. Clin. Psychopharmacol. 5:304–315, 1997.

Chronic Administration

Blusewicz, M. J., Dustman, R. E., Schenkenberg, T. and Beck, E. C., Neuropsychological correlates of chronic alcoholism and aging. J. Nerv. Ment. Dis. 165:348–355, 1977.

Blusewicz, M. J., Schenkenberg, T., Dustman, R. E. and Beck, E. C., WAIS performance in young normal, young alcoholic, and elderly normal groups: an evaluation of organicity and mental aging indices. J. Clin. Psychol. 33:1149–1153, 1977.

Butters, N., Cermak, L. S., Montgomery, K. and Adinolfi, A., Some comparisons of the memory and visuoperceptive deficits of chronic alcoholics and patients with Korsakoff's disease. Alcohol. Clin. Exp. Res. 1:73–80, 1977.

Glosser, G., Butters, N. and Kaplan, E., Visuoperceptual processes in brain damaged patients on the digit symbol substitution test. Int. J. Neurosci. 7:59–66, 1977.

Kapur, N. and Butters, N., Visuoperceptive deficits in long-term alcoholics and alcoholics with Korsakoff's psychosis. J. Stud. Alcohol 38:2025–2035, 1977.

Mohs, R. C., Tinklenberg, J. R., Roth, W. T. and Kopell, B. S., Slowing of short-term memory scanning in alcoholics. J. Stud. Alcohol 39:1908–1915, 1978.

Cutting, J., Differential impairment of memory in Korsakoff's syndrome. Cortex 15:501–506, 1979.

Hill, S. Y., Reyes, R. B., Mikhael, M. and Ayre, F., A comparison of alcoholics and heroin abusers: computerized transaxial tomography and neuropsychological functioning. Curr. Alcohol 5:187–205, 1979.

O'Leary, M. R., Donovan, D. M., Chaney, E. F., Walker, R. D. and Schau, E. J., Application of discriminant analysis to level of performance of alcoholics and nonalcoholics on Wechsler-Bellevue and Halstead-Reitan subtests. J. Clin. Psychol. 35:204–208, 1979.

Wolf, S. L. and Mikhael, M. A., Computerized transaxial tomographic and neuropsychol evaluations in chronic alcoholics and heroin abusers. Am. J. Psychiatry 136:598–602, 1979.

Chmielewski, C. and Golden, C. J., Alcoholism and brain damage: an investigation using the Luria-Nebraska Neuropsychological Battery. Int. J. Neurosci. 10:99–105, 1980.

Kroll, P., Seigel, R., O'Neill, B. and Edwards, R. P., Cerebral cortical atrophy in alcoholic men. J. Clin. Psychiatry 41:417–421, 1980.

Loberg, T., Alcohol misuse and neuropsychological deficits in men. J. Stud. Alcohol 41:119–128, 1980.

Lusins, J., Zimberg, S., Smokler, H. and Gurley, K., Alcoholism and cerebral atrophy: a study of 50 patients with CT scan and psychologic testing. Alcohol. Clin. Exp. Res. 4:406–411, 1980.

Carlen, P. L., Wilkinson, D. A., Wortzman, G., Holgate, R., Cordingley, J., Lee, M. A., Huszar, L., Moddel, G., Singh, R., Kiraly, L. and Rankin, J. G., Cerebral atrophy and functional deficits in alcoholics without clinically apparent liver disease. Neurology 31:377–385, 1981.

Fabian, M. S., Jenkins, R. L. and Parsons, O. A., Gender, alcoholism, and neuropsychological functioning. J. Consult. Clin. Psychol. 49:138–140, 1981.

Jenkins, R. L. and Parsons, O. A., Neuropsychological effect of chronic alcoholism on tactual-spatial performance and memory in males. Alcohol. Clin. Exp. Res. 5:26–33, 1981.

Graff-Radford, N. R., Heaton, R. K., Earnest, M. P. and Rudikoff, J. C., Brain atrophy and neuropsychological impairment in young alcoholics. J. Stud. Alcohol 43:859–868, 1982.

Ron, M. A., The alcoholic brain: CT scan and psychological findings. Psychol. Med. Monogr. Suppl. 3:1–33, 1983.

Saletu, B., Saletu, M., Grunberger, J. and Mader, R., Spontaneous and drug-induced remission of alcoholic organic brain syndrome: clinical, psychometric, and neurophysiological studies. Psychiatry Res. 10:59–75, 1983.

Tarter, R. E., Goldstein, G., Alterman, A., Petrarulo, E. W. and Elmore, S., Alcoholic seizures: intellectual and neuropsychological sequelae. J. Nerv. Ment. Dis. 171:123–125, 1983.

Fabian, M. S., Parsons, O. A. and Sheldon, M. D., Effects of gender and alcoholism on verbal and visual-spatial learning. J. Nerv. Ment. Dis. 172:16–20, 1984.

Franceschi, M., Truci, G., Comi, G., Lozza, L., Marchettini, P., Galardi, G. and Smirne, S., Cognitive deficits and their relationship to other neurological complications in chronic alcoholic patients. J. Neurol. Neurosurg. Psychiatry 47:1134–1137, 1984.

Acker, C., Performance of female alcoholics on neurophyschological testing. Alcohol Alcohol. 20:379–386, 1985.

Ciesielski, K. T., Madden, J. S., Bligh, J. G. and Schopflocher, D., Long-term brain impairment in chronic alcoholics: N2-P3 cognitive potentials in a template-matching memory task. Alcohol Alcohol. 20:403–408, 1985.

Donovan, D. M., Kivlahan, D. R., Walker, R. D. and Umlauf, R., Derivation and validation of neuropsychological clusters among men alcoholics. J. Stud. Alcohol 46:205–211, 1985.

Leber, W. R., Parsons, O. A., and Nichols, N., Neuropsychological test results are related to ratings of men alcoholics' therapeutic progress: a replicated study. J. Stud. Alcohol. 46:116–121, 1985.

Oscar-Berman, M. and Weinstein, A., Visual processing, memory, and lateralization in alcoholism and aging. Devel. Neuropsychol. 1:99–112, 1985.

Acker, C., Neuropsychological deficits in alcoholics: the relative contributions of gender and drinking history. Br. J. Addict. 81:395–403, 1986.

Bolter, J. F. and Hannon, R., Lateralized cerebral dysfunction in early and late stage alcoholics. J. Stud. Alcohol 47:213–218, 1986.

Hightower, M. G. and Anderson, R. P., Memory evaluation of alcoholics with Russell's revised Wechsler Memory Scale. J. Clin. Psychol. 42:1000–1005, 1986.

Samson, Y., Baron, J.-C., Feline, A., Bories, J. and Crouzel, C., Local cerebral glucose utilisation in chronic alcoholics: a positron tomographic study J. Neurol. Neurosurg. Psychiatry 49:1165–1170, 1986.

Schaeffer, K. W. and Parsons, O. A., Drinking practices and neuropsychological test performance in sober male alcoholics and social drinkers. Alcohol 3:175–179, 1986.

Page, R. D. and Cleveland, M. F., Cognitive dysfunction and aging among male alcoholics and social drinkers. Alcohol. Clin. Exp. Res. 11:376–384, 1987.

Dally, S., Luft, A., Ponsin, J. C., Girre, C., Mamo, H. and Fournier, E., Abnormal pattern of cerebral blood flow distribution in young alcohol addicts. Br. J. Addict. 83:105–109, 1988.

Akshoomoff, N., Delis, D. C. and Kiefner, M. G., Block constructions of chronic alcoholic and unilateral brain-damaged patients: A test of the right hemisphere vulnerability hypothesis of alcoholism. Arch. Clin. Neuropsychol. 4:275–281, 1989.

Cermak, L. S., Verfaellie, M., Letourneau, L., Blackford, S., Weiss, S. and Numan, B., Verbal and nonverbal right hemisphere processing by chronic alcoholics. Alcohol. Clin. Exp. Res. 13:611–616, 1989.

Harker, J. O. and Riege, W. H., Memory impairments in alcoholism: effects of age and education. J. Subst. Abuse 1:417–430, 1989.

Kramer, J. H., Blusewicz, M. J. and Preston, K. A., The premature aging hypothesis: old before its time? J. Consult. Clin. Psychol. 57:257–262, 1989.

Malloy, P., Noel, N., Rogers, S., Longabaugh, R. and Beattie, M., Risk factors for neuropsychological impairment in alcoholics: antisocial personality, age, years of drinking and gender. J. Stud. Alcohol 50:422–426, 1989.

Muuronen, A., Bergman, H., Hindmarsh, T. and Telakivi, T., Influence of improved drinking habits on brain atrophy and cognitive performance in alcoholic patients: a 5-year follow-up study. Alcohol. Clin. Exp. Res. 13:137–141, 1989.

Drake, A. I., Hannay, H. J. and Gam, J., Effects of chronic alcoholism on hemispheric functioning: an examination of gender differences for cognitive and dichotic listening tasks. J. Clin. Exp. Neuropsychol. 12:781–797, 1990.
Jacobson, R. R., Acker, C. F. and Lishman, W. A., Patterns of neuropsychological deficit in alcoholic Korsakoff's syndrome. Psychol. Med. 20:321–334, 1990.
Hewett, L. J., Nixon, S. J., Glenn, W. and Parsons, O. A., Verbal fluency deficits in female alcoholics. J. Clin. Psychol. 47:716–720, 1991.
Richardson, E. D., Malloy, P. F., Longabaugh, R., Williams, J., Noel, N. and Beattie, M. C., Liver function tests and neuropsychologic impairment in substance abusers. Addict. Behav. 16:51–55, 1991.
Bowden, S. C., Benedikt, R. and Ritter, A. J., Delayed matching to sample and concurrent learning in nonamnesic humans with alcohol dependence. Neuropsychologia 30:427–435, 1992.
Glenn, S. W. and Parsons, O. A., Neuropsychological efficiency measures in male and female alcoholics. J. Stud. Alcohol 53:546–552, 1992.
Beatty, W. W., Katzung, V. M., Nixon, S. J. and Moreland, V. J., Problem-solving deficits in alcoholics: evidence from the California Card Sorting Test. J. Stud. Alcohol 54:687–692, 1993.
Mallick, J. L., Kirkby, K. C., Martin, F., Philp, M. and Hennessy, M. J., A comparison of the amnesic effects of lorazepam in alcoholics and non-alcoholics. Psychopharmacology (Berl.) 110:181–186, 1993.
Nicolas, J. M., Catafau, A. M., Estruch, R., Lomena, F. J., Salamero, M., Herranz, R., Monforte, R., Cardenal, C. and Urbano-Marquez, A., Regional cerebral blood flow-SPECT in chronic alcoholism: relation to neuropsychological testing. J. Nucl. Med. 34:1452–1459, 1993.
Wang, G. J., Volkow, N. D., Roque, C. T., Cestaro, V. L., Hitzemann, R. J., Cantos, E. L., Levy, A. V. and Dhawan, A. P., Functional importance of ventricular enlargement and cortical atrophy in healthy subjects and alcoholics as assessed with PET, MR imaging, and neuropsychologic testing. Radiology 186:59–65, 1993.
Alderdice, F. A., McGuinness, C. and Brown, K., Identification of subtypes of problem drinkers based on neuropsychological performance. Br. J. Clin. Psychol. 33:483–498, 1994.
Amir, T. and Bahri, T., Effect of substance abuse on visuographic function. Percept. Mot. Skills 78:235–241, 1994.
Jha, S. and Nag, D., Some observations on clinical, cognitive and neurophysiological changes in subjects consuming indigenous alcohol. Indian J. Physiol. Pharmacol. 38:277–280, 1994.
Molina, J. A., Bermejo, F., del Ser, T., Jimenez-Jimenez, F. J., Herranz, A., Fernandez-Calle, P., Ortuno, B., Villanueva, C. and Sainz, M. J., Alcoholic cognitive deterioration and nutritional deficiencies. Acta Neurol. Scand. 89:384–390, 1994.
Moss, H. B., Kirisci, L., Gordon, H. W. and Tarter, R. E., A neuropsychologic profile of adolescent alcoholics. Alcohol. Clin. Exp. Res. 18:159–163, 1994.
Ciesielski, K. T., Waldorf, A. V. and Jung, R. E., Jr., Anterior brain deficits in chronic alcoholism. Cause or effect? J. Nerv. Ment. Dis. 183:756–761, 1995.
Drake, A. I., Butters, N., Shear, P. K., Smith, T. L., Bondi, M., Irwin, M. and Schuckit, M. A., Cognitive recovery with abstinence and its relationship to family history for alcoholism. J. Stud. Alcohol 56:104–109, 1995.
Nixon, S. J., Tivis, R. and Parsons, O. A., Behavioral dysfunction and cognitive efficiency in male and female alcoholics. Alcohol. Clin. Exp. Res. 19:577–581, 1995.
Sullivan, E. V., Marsh, L., Mathalon, D. H., Lim, K. O. and Pfefferbaum, A., Anterior hippocampal volume deficits in nonamnesic, aging chronic alcoholics. Alcohol. Clin. Exp. Res. 19:110–122, 1995.
Tivis, R., Beatty, W. W., Nixon, S. J. and Parsons, O. A., Patterns of cognitive impairment among alcoholics: are there subtypes? Alcohol. Clin. Exp. Res. 19:496–500, 1995.
Brunfaut, E. and d'Ydewalle, G., A comparison of implicit memory tasks in Korsakoff and alcoholic patients. Neuropsychologia 34:1143–1150, 1996.

Nixon, S. J. and Bowlby, D., Evidence of alcohol-related efficiency deficits in an episodic learning task. Alcohol. Clin. Exp. Res. 20:21–24, 1996.

Nixon, S. J., Hallford, H. G. and Tivis, R. D., Neurocognitive function in alcoholic, schizophrenic, and dually diagnosed patients. Psychiatry Res. 64:35–45, 1996.

Bowden, S. C., Dodds, B., Whelan, G., Long, C., Dudgeon, P., Ritter, A. and Clifford, C., Confirmatory factor analysis of the Wechsler Memory Scale-Revised in a sample of clients with alcohol dependency. J. Clin. Exp. Neuropsychol. 19:755–762, 1997.

Carpenter, K. M. and Hittner, J. B., Cognitive impairment among the dually-diagnosed: substance use history and depressive symptom correlates. Addiction 92:747–759, 1997.

Dent, O. F., Sulway, M. R., Broe, G. A., Creasey, H., Kos, S. C., Jorm, A. F., Tennant, C. and Fairley, M. J., Alcohol consumption and cognitive performance in a random sample of Australian soldiers who served in the Second World War. Bmj 314:1655–1657, 1997.

Dufouil, C., Ducimetiere, P. and Alperovitch, A., Sex differences in the association between alcohol consumption and cognitive performance. EVA Study Group. Epidemiology of Vascular Aging. Am. J. Epidemiol. 146:405–412, 1997.

Estruch, R., Nicolas, J. M., Salamero, M., Aragon, C., Sacanella, E., Fernandez-Sola, J. and Urbano-Marquez, A., Atrophy of the corpus callosum in chronic alcoholism. J. Neurol. Sci. 146:145–151, 1997.

Johnson-Greene, D., Adams, K. M., Gilman, S., Kluin, K. J., Junck, L., Martorello, S. and Heumann, M., Impaired upper limb coordination in alcoholic cerebellar degeneration. Arch. Neurol. 54:436–439, 1997.

Keenan, E., O'Donnell, C., Sinanan, K. and O'Callaghan, E., Severity of alcohol dependence and its relationship to neurological soft signs, neuropsychological impairment and family history. Acta Psychiatr. Scand. 95:272–276, 1997.

Nicolas, J. M., Estruch, R., Salamero, M., Orteu, N., Fernandez-Sola, J., Sacanella, E. and Urbano-Marquez, A., Brain impairment in well-nourished chronic alcoholics is related to ethanol intake. Ann. Neurol. 41:590–598, 1997.

Sher, K. J., Martin, E. D., Wood, P. K. and Rutledge, P. C., Alcohol use disorders and neuropsychological functioning in first-year undergraduates. Exp. Clin. Psychopharmacol. 5:304–315, 1997.

Sullivan, E. V., Shear, P. K., Zipursky, R. B., Sagar, H. J. and Pfefferbaum, A., Patterns of content, contextual, and working memory impairments in schizophrenia and nonamnesic alcoholism. Neuropsychology 11:195–206, 1997.

Adams, K. M., Gilman, S., Johnson-Greene, D., Koeppe, R. A., Junck, L., Kluin, K. J., Martorello, S., Johnson, M. J., Heumann, M. and Hill, E., The significance of family history status in relation to neuropsychological test performance and cerebral glucose metabolism studied with positron emission tomography in older alcoholic patients. Alcohol. Clin. Exp. Res. 22:105–110, 1998.

Bondi, M. W., Drake, A. I. and Grant, I., Verbal learning and memory in alcohol abusers and polysubstance abusers with concurrent alcohol abuse. J. Intl. Neuropsychol. Soc. 4:319–328, 1998.

Dao-Castellana, M. H., Samson, Y., Legault, F., Martinot, J. L., Aubin, H. J., Crouzel, C., Feldman, L., Barrucand, D., Rancurel, G., Feline, A. and Syrota, A., Frontal dysfunction in neurologically normal chronic alcoholic subjects: metabolic and neuropsychological findings. Psychol. Med. 28:1039–1048, 1998.

Nixon, S. J., Paul, R. and Phillips, M., Cognitive efficiency in alcoholics and polysubstance abusers. Alcohol. Clin. Exp. Res. 22:1414–1420, 1998.

Selby, M. J. and Azrin, R. L., Neuropsychological functioning in drug abusers. Drug Alcohol Depend. 50:39–45, 1998.

Tiihonen, J., Vilkman, H., Rasanen, P., Ryynanen, O. P., Hakko, H., Bergman, J., Hamalainen, T., Laakso, A., Haaparanta-Solin, M., Solin, O., Kuoppamaki, M., Syvalahti, E. and Hietala,

J., Striatal presynaptic dopamine function in type 1 alcoholics measured with positron emission tomography. Mol. Psychiatry 3:156–161, 1998.

van Gorp, W. G., Altshuler, L., Theberge, D. C., Wilkins, J. and Dixon, W., Cognitive impairment in euthymic bipolar patients with and without prior alcohol dependence. A preliminary study. Arch. Gen. Psychiatry 55:41–46, 1998.

van Thriel, C., Zupanic, M., Sietmann, B., Demes, P., Willer, H. and Seeber, A., Association of biochemical and subjective indicators of drinking habits with performance on different neurobehavioral tasks. Neurotoxicology 19:713–720, 1998.

Special Syndromes Associated with Alcoholism

Hepatic Encephalopathy

Tarter, R. E., Hegedus, A. M., Van Thiel, D. H., Gavaler, J. S. and Schade, R. R., Hepatic dysfunction and neuropsychological test performance in alcoholics with cirrhosis. J. Stud. Alcohol 47:74–77, 1986.

Tarter, R. E., Van Thiel, D. H., Arria, A. M., Carra, J. and Moss, H., Impact of cirrhosis on the neuropsychological test performance of alcoholics. Alcohol. Clin. Exp. Res. 12:619–621, 1988.

Moore, J. W., Dunk, A. A., Crawford, J. R., Deans, H., Besson, J. A., De Lacey, G., Sinclair, T. S., Mowat, N. A. and Brunt, P. W., Neuropsychological deficits and morphological MRI brain scan abnormalities in apparently healthy non-encephalopathic patients with cirrhosis. A controlled study. J. Hepatology 9:319–325, 1989.

Kulisevsky, J., Pujol, J., Balanzo, J., Junque, C., Deus, J., Capdevilla, A. and Villanueva, C., Pallidal hyperintensity on magnetic resonance imaging in cirrhotic patients: clinical correlations. Hepatology 16:1382–1388, 1992.

Kulisevsky, J., Pujol, J., Junque, C., Deus, J., Balanzo, J. and Capdevila, A., MRI pallidal hyperintensity and brain atrophy in cirrhotic patients: two different MRI patterns of clinical deterioration? Neurology 43:2570–2573, 1993.

Lockwood, A. H., Murphy, B. W., Donnelly, K. Z., Mahl, T. C. and Perini, S., Positron-emission tomographic localization of abnormalities of brain metabolism in patients with minimal hepatic encephalopathy. Hepatology 18:1061–1068, 1993.

Ross, B. D., Jacobson, S., Villamil, F., Korula, J., Kreis, R., Ernst, T., Shonk, T. and Moats, R. A., Subclinical hepatic encephalopathy: proton MR spectroscopic abnormalities. Radiology 193:457–463, 1994.

Kapczinski, F., Curran, H. V., Przemioslo, R., Williams, R., Fluck, E., Fernandes, C. and File, S. E., Cognitive impairments of alcoholic cirrhotic patients: correlation with endogenous benzodiazepine receptor ligands and increased affinity of platelet receptors. J. Neurol. Neurosurg. Psychiatry 60:676–680, 1996.

Quero, J. C., Hartmann, I. J., Meulstee, J., Hop, W. C. and Schalm, S. W., The diagnosis of subclinical hepatic encephalopathy in patients with cirrhosis using neuropsychological tests and automated electroencephalogram analysis. Hepatology 24:556–560, 1996.

Walton, N. H. and Bowden, S. C., Does liver dysfunction explain neuropsychological status in recently detoxified alcohol-dependent clients? Alcohol Alcohol. 32:287–295, 1997.

Huda, A., Guze, B. H., Thomas, M. A., Bugbee, M., Fairbanks, L., Strouse, T. and Fawzy, F. I., Clinical correlation of neuropsychological tests with 1H magnetic resonance spectroscopy in hepatic encephalopathy. Psychosom. Med. 60:550–556, 1998.

Schomerus, H. and Hamster, W., Neuropsychological aspects of portal-systemic encephalopathy. Metab. Brain. Dis. 13:361–377, 1998.

Thomas, M. A., Huda, A., Guze, B., Curran, J., Bugbee, M., Fairbanks, L., Ke, Y., Oshiro, T., Martin, P. and Fawzy, F., Cerebral ^{1}H MR spectroscopy and neuropsychologic status of patients with hepatic encephalopathy. AJR Am. J. Roentgenol. 171:1123–1130, 1998.

Wernicke and Korsakoff Syndromes

Oscar-Berman, M., Hypothesis testing and focusing behavior during concept formation by amnesic Korsakoff patients. Neuropsychologia 11:191–198, 1973.

Butters, N., Cermak, L. S., Montgomery, K. and Adinolfi, A., Some comparisons of the memory and visuoperceptive deficits of chronic alcoholics and patients with Korsakoff's disease. Alcohol. Clin. Exp. Res. 1:73–80, 1977.

Glosser, G., Butters, N. and Kaplan, E., Visuoperceptual processes in brain damaged patients on the digit symbol substitution test. Int. J. Neurosci. 7:59–66, 1977.

Kapur, N. and Butters, N., Visuoperceptive deficits in long-term alcoholics and alcoholics with Korsakoff's psychosis. J. Stud. Alcohol 38:2025–2035, 1977.

Cutting, J., Differential impairment of memory in Korsakoff's syndrome. Cortex 15:501–506, 1979.

Carlen, P. L., Wilkinson, D. A., Wortzman, G., Holgate, R., Cordingley, J., Lee, M. A., Huszar, L., Moddel, G., Singh, R., Kiraly, L. and Rankin, J. G., Cerebral atrophy and functional deficits in alcoholics without clinically apparent liver disease. Neurology 31:377–385, 1981.

Markowitsch, H. J., Kessler, J. and Denzler, P., Recognition memory and psychophysiological responses to stimuli with neutral or emotional content: a study of Korsakoff patients and recently detoxified and longterm abstinent alcoholics. Int. J. Neurosci. 29:1–35, 1986.

Blackwood, D. H., St. Clair, D. M., Blackburn, I. M. and Tyrer, G. M., Cognitive brain potentials and psychological deficits in Alzheimer's dementia and Korsakoff's amnesic syndrome. Psychol. Med. 17:349–358, 1987.

Christie, J. E., Kean, D. M., Douglas, R. H., Engleman, H. M., St. Clair, D. and Blackburn, I. M., Magnetic resonance imaging in pre-senile dementia of the Alzheimer-type, multi-infarct dementia and Korsakoff's syndrome Psychol. Med. 18:319–329, 1988.

Shimamura, A. P., Jernigan, T. L. and Squire, L. R., Korsakoff's syndrome: radiological (CT) findings and neuropsychological correlates. J. Neurosci. 8:4400–4410, 1988.

Besson, J. A., Crawford, J. R., Parker, D. M. and Smith, F. W., Magnetic resonance imaging in Alzheimer's disease, multi-infarct dementia, alcoholic dementia and Korsakoff's psychosis. Acta Psychiatr. Scand. 80:451–458, 1989.

Hunter, R., McLuskie, R., Wyper, D., Patterson, J., Christie, J. E., Brooks, D. N., McCulloch, J., Fink, G. and Goodwin, G. M., The pattern of function-related regional cerebral blood flow investigated by single photon emission tomography with 99mTc-HMPAO in patients with presenile Alzheimer's disease and Korsakoff's psychosis. Psychol. Med. 19:847–855, 1989.

Jacobson, R. R., Acker, C. F. and Lishman, W. A., Patterns of neuropsychological deficit in alcoholic Korsakoff's syndrome. Psychol. Med. 20:321–334, 1990.

Jernigan, T. L., Schafer, K., Butters, N. and Cermak, L. S., Magnetic resonance imaging of alcoholic Korsakoff patients. Neuropsychopharmacology 4:175–186, 1991.

Blansjaar, B. A., Takens, H. and Zwinderman, A. H., The course of alcohol amnestic disorder: a three-year follow-up study of clinical signs and social disabilities. Acta Psychiatr. Scand. 86:240–246, 1992.

Cave, C. B. and Squire, L. R., Intact verbal and nonverbal short-term memory following damage to the human hippocampus. Hippocampus 2:151–163, 1992.

Cole, M., Winkelman, M. D., Morris, J. C., Simon, J. E. and Boyd, T. A., Thalamic amnesia: Korsakoff syndrome due to left thalamic infarction. J. Neurol. Sci. 110:62–67, 1992.

Delis, D. C., Squire, L. R., Bihrle, A. and Massman, P., Componential analysis of problem-solving ability: performance of patients with frontal lobe damage and amnesic patients on a new sorting test. Neuropsychologia 30:683–697, 1992.

Hunkin, N. M. and Parkin, A. J., Recency judgements in Wernicke-Korsakoff and post-encephalitic amnesia: influences of proactive interference and retention interval. Cortex 29:485–499, 1993.

Joyce, E. M. and Robbins, T. W., Memory deficits in Korsakoff and non-Korsakoff alcoholics following alcohol withdrawal and the relationship to length of abstinence. Alcohol Alcohol. 2:501–505, 1993.

Parkin, A., Dunn, J. C., Lee, C., O'Hara, P. F. and Nussbaum, L., Neuropsychological sequelae of Wernicke's encephalopathy in a 20-year-old woman: selective impairment of a frontal memory system. Brain Cogn. 21:1–19, 1993. [Case Report]

Moffoot, A., O'Carroll, R. E., Murray, C., Dougall, N., Ebmeier, K. and Goodwin, G. M., Clonidine infusion increases uptake of 99mTc-Exametazime in anterior cingulate cortex in Korsakoff's psychosis. Psychol. Med. 24:53–61, 1994.

Molina, J. A., Bermejo, F., del Ser, T., Jimenez-Jimenez, F. J., Herranz, A., Fernandez-Calle, P., Ortuno, B., Villanueva, C. and Sainz, M. J., Alcoholic cognitive deterioration and nutritional deficiencies. Acta Neurol. Scand. 89:384–390, 1994.

Benson, D. F., Djenderedjian, A., Miller, B. L., Pachana, N. A., Chang, L., Itti, L. and Mena, I., Neural basis of confabulation. Neurology 46:1239–1243, 1996. [Case Report]

Brunfaut, E. and d'Ydewalle, G., A comparison of implicit memory tasks in Korsakoff and alcoholic patients. Neuropsychologia 34:1143–1150, 1996.

Welch, L. W., Nimmerrichter, A., Kessler, R., King, D., Hoehn, R., Margolin, R. and Martin, P. R., Severe global amnesia presenting as Wernicke-Korsakoff syndrome but resulting from atypical lesions. Psychol. Med. 26:421–425, 1996. [Case Report]

Kopelman, M. D., Stanhope, N. and Kingsley, D., Temporal and spatial context memory in patients with focal frontal, temporal lobe, and diencephalic lesions. Neuropsychologia 35:1533–1545, 1997.

Welch, L. W., Cunningham, A. T., Eckardt, M. J. and Martin, P. R., Fine motor speed deficits in alcoholic Korsakoff's syndrome. Alcohol. Clin. Exp. Res. 21:134–139, 1997.

Welch, L. W., Nimmerrichter, A., Gilliland, R., King, D. E. and Martin, P. R., "Wineglass" confabulations among brain-damaged alcoholics on the Wechsler Memory Scale-Revised visual reproduction subtest. Cortex 33:543–551, 1997.

Withdrawal and Early Abstinence

Weingartner, H., Faillace, L. A. and Markley, H. G., Verbal information retention in alcoholics. Q. J. Stud. Alcohol 32:293–303, 1971.

Eckardt, M. J., Ryback, R. S. and Pautler, C. P., Neuropsychological deficits in alcoholic men in their mid thirties. Am. J. Psychiatry 137:932–936, 1980.

Kish, G. B., Hagen, J. M., Woody, M. M. and Harvey, H. L., Alcoholics' recovery from cerebral impairment as a function of duration of abstinence. J. Clin. Psychol. 36:584–589, 1980.

Sanchez-Craig, M., Drinking pattern as a determinant of alcoholics' performance on the trail making test. J. Stud. Alcohol 41:1082–1090, 1980.

de Obaldia, R., Leber, W. R. and Parsons, O. A., Assessment of neuropsychological functions in chronic alcoholics using a standardized version of Luria's Neuropsychological Technique. Int. J. Neurosci. 14:85–93, 1981.

Leber, W. R., Jenkins, R. L., Parsons, O. A., Recovery of visual-spatial learning and memory in chronic alcoholics. J. Clin. Psychol. 37:192–197, 1981.

Albert, M., Butters, N., Rogers, S., Pressman, J. and Geller, A., A preliminary report: nutritional levels and cognitive performance in chronic alcohol abusers. Drug Alcohol Depend. 9:131–142, 1982.

Saletu, B., Saletu, M., Grunberger, J. and Mader, R., Spontaneous and drug-induced remission of alcoholic organic brain syndrome: clinical, psychometric, and neurophysiological studies. Psychiatry Res. 10:59–75, 1983.

Tarter, R. E., Goldstein, G., Alterman, A., Petrarulo, E. W. and Elmore, S., Alcoholic seizures: intellectual and neuropsychological sequelae. J. Nerv. Ment. Dis. 171:123–125, 1983.

Franceschi, M., Truci, G., Comi, G., Lozza, L., Marchettini, P., Galardi, G. and Smirne, S., Cognitive deficits and their relationship to other neurological complications in chronic alcoholic patients. J. Neurol. Neurosurg. Psychiatry 47:1134–1137, 1984.

Hannon, R., Butler, C. P., Day, C. L., Khan, S. A., Quitoriano, L. A., Butler, A. M. and Meredith, L. A., Alcohol use and cognitive functioning in men and women college students. Recent Dev. Alcohol 3:241–252, 1985.

Kivlahan, D. R., Harris, M. D., Moore, J. E., Powel, J. and Donovan, D. M., Validation of the Luria-Nebraska Intellectual Processes Scale as a measure of intelligence in male alcoholics. J. Clin. Psychol. 41:287–290, 1985.

Spehr, W. and Stemmler, G., Postalcoholic diseases: diagnostic relevance of computerized EEG. Electroencephalogr. Clin. Neurophysiol. 60:106–114, 1985.

Hillbom, M. and Holm, L., Contribution of traumatic head injury to neuropsychological deficits in alcoholics. J. Neurol. Neurosurg. Psychiatry 49:1348–1353, 1986.

Markowitsch, H. J., Kessler, J. and Denzler, P., Recognition memory and psychophysiological responses to stimuli with neutral or emotional content: a study of Korsakoff patients and recently detoxified and longterm abstinent alcoholics. Int. J. Neurosci. 29:1–35, 1986.

Berglund, M., Hagstadius, S., Risberg, J., Johanson, T. M., Bliding, A. and Mubrin, Z., Normalization of regional cerebral blood flow in alcoholics during the first 7 weeks of abstinence. Acta Psychiatr. Scand. 75:202–208, 1987.

Eckardt, M. J., Rawlings, R. R., Graubard, B. I., Faden, V., Martin, P. R. and Gottschalk, L. A., Neuropsychological performance and treatment outcome in male alcoholics. Alcohol. Clin. Exp. Res. 12:88–93, 1988.

Emmerson, R. Y., Dustman, R. E., Heil, J. and Shearer, D. E., Neuropsychological performance of young nondrinkers, social drinkers, and long- and short-term sober alcoholics. Alcohol. Clin. Exp. Res. 12:625–629, 1988.

Glenn, S. W., Parsons, O. A., Sinha, R. and Stevens, L., The effects of repeated withdrawals from alcohol on the memory of male and female alcoholics. Alcohol Alcohol. 23:337–342, 1988.

Romani, A. and Cosi, V., Event-related potentials in chronic alcoholics during withdrawal and abstinence. Neurophysiol. Clin. 19:373–384, 1989.

Vischer, A. and Hell, D., Cognitive deficits, vitamin status and controlled thiamine substitution in alcohol dependent patients in withdrawal treatment. Nervenarzt 60:633–640, 1989. [German]

Kozaric-Kovacic, D., Skocilic, Z., Sila, A. and Buranji, I., Neuropsychological defects in alcoholics with the withdrawal syndrome. Acta Med. Iugosl. 44:325–333, 1990. [Serbo-Croatian (Roman)]

Dupont, R. M., Rourke, S. B., Grant, I., Lehr, P. P., Reed, R. J., Challakere, K., Lamoureux, G. and Halpern, S., Single photon emission computed tomography with iodoamphetamine-123 and neuropsychological studies in long-term abstinent alcoholics. Psychiatry Res. 67:99–111, 1996.

Sullivan, E. V., Marsh, L., Mathalon, D. H., Lim, K. O. and Pfefferbaum, A., Relationship between alcohol withdrawal seizures and temporal lobe white matter volume deficits. Alcohol. Clin. Exp. Res. 20:348–354, 1996.

Bates, M. E., Stability of neuropsychological assessments early in alcoholism treatment. J. Stud. Alcohol 58:617–621, 1997.

Bergman, H., Engelbrektson, K., Fransson, A., Herlitz, K., Hindmarsh, T. and Neiman, J., Alcohol-induced cognitive impairment is reversible: neuropsychological tests but not MRT show improvement after abstinence. Lakartidningen 95:4228,4231–4236, 1998. [Swedish]

Horner, M. D., Waid, L. R., Johnson, D. E., Latham, P. K., and Anton, R. F., The relationship of cognitive functioning to amount of recent and lifetime alcohol consumption in outpatient alcoholics. Addict. Behav. 24:449–453. 1999.

Mann, K., Gunther, A., Stetter, F. and Ackermann, K., Rapid recovery from cognitive deficits in abstinent alcoholics: a controlled test–retest study. Alcohol Alcohol. 34:567–574, 1999.

Prolonged Abstinence and Relapse

Jones, B. and Parsons, O. A., Impaired abstracting ability in chronic alcoholics. Arch. Gen. Psychiatry 24:71–75, 1971.

Weingartner, H., Faillace, L. A. and Markley, H. G., Verbal information retention in alcoholics. Q. J. Stud. Alcohol 32:293–303, 1971.

Tarter, R. E., An analysis of cognitive deficits in chronic alcoholics. J. Nerv. Ment. Dis. 157:138–147, 1973.

Hill, S. Y., Reyes, R. B., Mikhael, M. and Ayre, F., A comparison of alcoholics and heroin abusers: computerized transaxial tomography and neuropsychological functioning. Curr. Alcohol 5:187–205, 1979.

Berglund, M., Bliding, G., Bliding, A. and Risberg, J., Reversibility of cerebral dysfunction in alcoholism during the first seven weeks of abstinence: a regional cerebral blood flow study. Acta Psychiatr. Scand. Suppl. 286:119–127, 1980.

Eckardt, M. J., Ryback, R. S. and Pautler, C. P., Neuropsychological deficits in alcoholic men in their mid thirties. Am. J. Psychiatry 137:932–936, 1980.

Eckardt, M. J., Parker, E. S., Pautler, C. P., Noble, E. P. and Gottschalk, L. A., Neuropsychological consequences of posttreatment drinking behavior in male alcoholics. Psychiatry Res. 2:135–147, 1980.

Kish, G. B., Hagen, J. M., Woody, M. M. and Harvey, H. L., Alcoholics' recovery from cerebral impairment as a function of duration of abstinence. J. Clin. Psychol. 36:584–589, 1980.

de Obaldia, R., Leber, W. R. and Parsons, O. A., Assessment of neuropsychological functions in chronic alcoholics using a standardized version of Luria's Neuropsychological Technique. Int. J. Neurosci. 14:85–93, 1981.

Leber, W. R., Jenkins, R. L., Parsons, O. A., Recovery of visual-spatial learning and memory in chronic alcoholics. J. Clin. Psychol. 37:192–197, 1981.

Becker, J. T., Butters, N., Hermann, A. and D'Angelo, N., Learning to associate names and faces. Impaired acquisition on an ecologically relevant memory task by male alcoholics. J. Nerv. Ment. Dis. 171:617–623, 1983.

Saletu, B., Saletu, M., Grunberger, J. and Mader, R., Spontaneous and drug-induced remission of alcoholic organic brain syndrome: clinical, psychometric, and neurophysiological studies. Psychiatry Res. 10:59–75, 1983.

Acker, W., Ron, M. A., Lishman, W. A. and Shaw, G. K., A multivariate analysis of psychological, clinical and CT scanning measures in detoxified chronic alcoholics. Br. J. Addict. 79:293–301, 1984.

Adams, K. M. and Grant, I., Failure of nonlinear models of drinking history variables to predict neuropsychological performance in alcoholics. Am. J. Psychiatry 141:663–667, 1984.

Grant, I., Adams, K. M. and Reed, R., Aging, abstinence, and medical risk factors in the prediction of neuropsychologic deficit among long-term alcoholics. Arch. Gen. Psychiatry 41:710–718, 1984.

DeFranco, C., Tarbox, A. R. and McLaughlin, E. J., Cognitive deficits as a function of years of alcohol abuse. Am. J. Drug Alcohol Abuse 11:279–293, 1985.

Donovan, D. M., Kivlahan, D. R., Walker, R. D. and Umlauf, R., Derivation and validation of neuropsychological clusters among men alcoholics. J. Stud. Alcohol 46:205–211, 1985.

Kivlahan, D. R., Harris, M. D., Moore, J. E., Powel, J. and Donovan, D. M., Validation of the Luria-Nebraska Intellectual Processes Scale as a measure of intelligence in male alcoholics. J. Clin. Psychol. 41:287–290, 1985.

Pishkin, V., Lovallo, W. R. and Bourne, L. E., Jr., Chronic alcoholism in males: cognitive deficit as a function of age of onset, age, and duration. Alcohol. Clin. Exp. Res. 9:400–406, 1985.

Spehr, W. and Stemmler, G., Postalcoholic diseases: diagnostic relevance of computerized EEG. Electroencephalogr. Clin. Neurophysiol. 60:106–114, 1985.

Yohman, J. R., Parsons, O. A. and Leber, W. R., Lack of recovery in male alcoholics' neuropsychological performance one year after treatment. Alcohol. Clin. Exp. Res. 9:114–117, 1985.

Markowitsch, H. J., Kessler, J. and Denzler, P., Recognition memory and psychophysiological responses to stimuli with neutral or emotional content: a study of Korsakoff patients and recently detoxified and longterm abstinent alcoholics. Int. J. Neurosci. 29:1–35, 1986.

Svanum, S. and Schladenhauffen, J., Lifetime and recent alcohol consumption among male alcoholics. Neuropsychological implications. J. Nerv. Ment. Dis. 174:214–220, 1986.

Tarbox, A. R., Connors, G. J. and McLaughlin, E. J., Effects of drinking pattern on neuropsychological performance among alcohol misusers. J. Stud. Alcohol 47:176–179, 1986.

Berglund, M., Hagstadius, S., Risberg, J., Johanson, T. M., Bliding, A. and Mubrin, Z., Normalization of regional cerebral blood flow in alcoholics during the first 7 weeks of abstinence. Acta Psychiatr. Scand. 75:202–208, 1987.

Hannon, R., Butler, C. P., Day, C. L., Khan, S. A., Quitoriano, L. A., Butler, A. M. and Meredith, L. A., Social drinking and cognitive functioning in college students: a replication and reversibility study. J. Stud. Alcohol 48:502–506, 1987.

Nixon, S. J., Kujawski, A., Parsons, O. A. and Yohman, J. R., Semantic (verbal) and figural memory impairment in alcoholics. J. Clin. Exp. Neuropsychol. 9:311–322, 1987.

Page, R. D. and Cleveland, M. F., Cognitive dysfunction and aging among male alcoholics and social drinkers. Alcohol. Clin. Exp. Res. 11:376–384, 1987.

Emmerson, R. Y., Dustman, R. E., Heil, J. and Shearer, D. E., Neuropsychological performance of young nondrinkers, social drinkers, and long- and short-term sober alcoholics. Alcohol. Clin. Exp. Res. 12:625–629, 1988.

Miller, T. P., Taylor, J. L. and Tinklenberg, J. R., A comparison of assessment techniques measuring the effects of methylphenidate, secobarbital, diazepam and diphenhydramine in abstinent alcoholics. Neuropsychobiology 19:90–96, 1988.

Ryan, J. J. and Lewis, C. V., Comparison of normal controls and recently detoxified alcoholics on the Wechsler Memory Scale-Revised. The Clinical Neuropsychologist 2:173–180, 1988. [Abstract]

Schandler, S. L., Cohen, M. J., McArthur, D. L., Naliboff, B. D. and Hassell, A., Activation peaking in intoxicated and detoxified alcoholics during visuospatial learning. J. Stud. Alcohol 49:126–130, 1988.

Schandler, S. L., Cohen, M. J. and McArthur, D. L., Event-related brain potentials in intoxicated and detoxified alcoholics during visuospatial learning. Psychopharmacology (Berl.) 94:275–283, 1988.

Chick, J. D., Smith, M. A., Engleman, H. M., Kean, D. M., Mander, A. J., Douglas, R. H. and Best, J. J., Magnetic resonance imaging of the brain in alcoholics: cerebral atrophy, lifetime alcohol consumption, and cognitive deficits. Alcohol. Clin. Exp. Res. 13:512–518, 1989.

Harker, J. O. and Riege, W. H., Memory impairments in alcoholism: effects of age and education. J. Subst. Abuse 1:417–430, 1989.

Irwin, M., Smith, T. L., Butters, N., Brown, S., Baird, S., Grant, I. and Schuckit, M. A., Graded neuropsychological impairment and elevated gamma-glutamyl transferase in chronic alcoholic men. Alcohol. Clin. Exp. Res. 13:99–103, 1989.

Muuronen, A., Bergman, H., Hindmarsh, T. and Telakivi, T., Influence of improved drinking habits on brain atrophy and cognitive performance in alcoholic patients: a 5-year follow-up study. Alcohol. Clin. Exp. Res. 13:137–141, 1989.

Romani, A. and Cosi, V., Event-related potentials in chronic alcoholics during withdrawal and abstinence. Neurophysiol. Clin. 19:373–384, 1989.

Vischer, A. and Hell, D., Cognitive deficits, vitamin status and controlled thiamine substitution in alcohol dependent patients in withdrawal treatment. Nervenarzt 60:633–640, 1989. [German]

Hambidge, D. M., Intellectual impairment in male alcoholics. Alcohol Alcohol. 25:555–559, 1990.

Parsons, O. A., Schaeffer, K. W. and Glenn, S. W., Does neuropsychological test performance predict resumption of drinking in posttreatment alcoholics? Addict. Behav. 15:297–307, 1990.

Parsons, O. A., Sinha, R. and Williams, H. L., Relationships between neuropsychological test performance and event-related potentials in alcoholic and nonalcoholic samples. Alcohol. Clin. Exp. Res. 14:746–755, 1990.

Glenn, S. W. and Parsons, O. A., Impaired efficiency in female alcoholics' neuropsychological performance. J. Clin. Exp. Neuropsychol. 13:895–908, 1991.

Jernigan, T. L., Butters, N., DiTraglia, G., Schafer, K., Smith, T., Irwin, M., Grant, I., Schuckit, M. and Cermak, L. S., Reduced cerebral grey matter observed in alcoholics using magnetic resonance imaging. Alcohol. Clin. Exp. Res. 15:418–427, 1991.

Schafer, K., Butters, N., Smith, T., Irwin, M., Brown, S., Hanger, P., Grant, I. and Schuckit, M., Cognitive performance of alcoholics: A longitudinal evaluation of the role of drinking history, depression, liver function, nutrition and family history. Alcohol. Clin. Exp. Res. 15:653–660, 1991.

Tuck, R. R. and Jackson, M., Social, neurological and cognitive disorders in alcoholics. Med. J. Aust. 155:225–229, 1991.

Reed, R. J., Grant, I. and Rourke, S. B., Long-term abstinent alcoholics have normal memory. Alcohol. Clin. Exp. Res. 16:677–683, 1992.

Adams, K. M., Gilman, S., Koeppe, R. A., Kluin, K. J., Brunberg, J. A., Dede, D., Berent, S. and Kroll, P. D., Neuropsychological deficits are correlated with frontal hypometabolism in positron emission tomography studies of older alcoholic patients. Alcohol. Clin. Exp. Res. 17:205–210, 1993.

Caspari, D., Trabert, W., Heinz, G., Lion, N., Henkes, H. and Huber, G., The pattern of regional cerebral blood flow during alcohol withdrawal—a single photon emission tomography study with 99mTc-HMPAO. Acta Psychiatr. Scand. 87:414–417, 1993.

Joyce, E. M. and Robbins, T. W., Memory deficits in Korsakoff and non-Korsakoff alcoholics following alcohol withdrawal and the relationship to length of abstinence. Alcohol Alcohol. 2:501–505, 1993.

Rummans, T. A., Davis, L. J., Jr., Morse, R. M. and Ivnik, R. J., Learning and memory impairment in older, detoxified, benzodiazepine-dependent patients. Mayo Clin. Proc. 68:731–737, 1993.

Davila, M. D., Shear, P. K., Lane, B., Sullivan, E. V. and Pfefferbaum, A., Mammillary body and cerebellar shrinkage in chronic alcoholics: an MRI and neuropsychological study. Neuropsychology 8:433–444, 1994.

Glenn, S., Parsons, O. A. and Sinha, R., Assessment of recovery of electrophysiological and neuropsychological functions in chronic alcoholics. Biol. Psychiatry 36:443–452, 1994.

Parsons, O. A., Neuropsychological measures and event-related potentials in alcoholics: interrelationships, long-term reliabilities, and prediction of resumption of drinking. J. Clin. Psychol. 50:37–46, 1994.

Beatty, W. W., Katzung, V. M., Moreland, V. J. and Nixon, S. J., Neuropsychological performance of recently abstinent alcoholics and cocaine abusers. Drug Alcohol Depend. 37:247–253, 1995.

Di Sclafani, V., Ezekiel, F., Meyerhoff, D. J., MacKay, S., Dillon, W. P., Weiner, M. W. and Fein, G., Brain atrophy and cognitive function in older abstinent alcoholic men. Alcohol. Clin. Exp. Res. 19:1121–1126, 1995.

Drake, A. I., Butters, N., Shear, P. K., Smith, T. L., Bondi, M., Irwin, M. and Schuckit, M. A., Cognitive recovery with abstinence and its relationship to family history for alcoholism. J. Stud. Alcohol 56:104–109, 1995.

Eckardt, M. J., Stapleton, J. M., Rawlings, R. R., Davis, E. Z. and Grodin, D. M., Neuropsychological functioning in detoxified alcoholics between 18 and 35 years of age. Am. J. Psychiatry 152:53–59, 1995.

Beatty, W. W., Hames, K. A., Blanco, C. R., Nixon, S. J. and Tivis, L. J., Visuospatial perception, construction and memory in alcoholism. J. Stud. Alcohol 57:136–143, 1996.

Blusewicz, M. J., Kramer, J. H. and Delmonico, R. L., Interference effects in chronic alcoholism. J. Int. Neuropsychol. Soc. 2:141–145, 1996.

Dupont, R. M., Rourke, S. B., Grant, I., Lehr, P. P., Reed, R. J., Challakere, K., Lamoureux, G. and Halpern, S., Single photon emission computed tomography with iodoamphetamine-123 and neuropsychological studies in long-term abstinent alcoholics. Psychiatry Res. 67:99–111, 1996.

Hutner, N. and Oscar-Berman, M., Visual laterality patterns for the perception of emotional words in alcoholic and aging individuals. J. Stud. Alcohol 57:144–154, 1996.

O'Mahony, J. F. and Doherty, B., Intellectual impairment among recently abstinent alcohol abusers. Br. J. Clin. Psychol. 35:77–83, 1996.

Bates, M. E., Stability of neuropsychological assessments early in alcoholism treatment. J. Stud. Alcohol 58:617–621, 1997.

Beatty, W. W., Blanco, C. R., Hames, K. A. and Nixon, S. J., Spatial cognition in alcoholics: influence of concurrent abuse of other drugs. Drug Alcohol Depend. 44:167–174, 1997.

Easton, C. and Bauer, L. O., Neuropsychological differences between alcohol-dependent and cocaine-dependent patients with or without problematic drinking. Psychiatry Res. 71:97–103, 1997.

Ham, H. P. and Parsons, O. A., Organization of psychological functions in alcoholics and nonalcoholics: a test of the compensatory hypothesis. J. Stud. Alcohol 58:67–74, 1997.

Johnson-Greene, D., Adams, K. M., Gilman, S., Koeppe, R. A., Junck, L., Kluin, K. J., Martorello, S. and Heumann, M., Effects of abstinence and relapse upon neuropsychological function and cerebral glucose metabolism in severe chronic alcoholism. J. Clin. Exp. Neuropsychol. 19:378–385, 1997.

Bergman, H., Engelbrektson, K., Fransson, A., Herlitz, K., Hindmarsh, T. and Neiman, J., Alcohol-induced cognitive impairment is reversible: neuropsychological tests but not MRT show improvement after abstinence. Lakartidningen 95:4228, 4231–4236, 1998. [Swedish]

Disclafani, V., Truran, D. L., Bloomer, C., Toloushams, M., Clark, H. W., Norman, D., Hannauer, D. and Fein, G., Abstinent chronic crack-cocaine and crack-cocaine/alcohol abusers evidence normal hippocampal volumes on MRI despite persistent cognitive impairments. Addiction Biol. 3:261–270, 1998.

Weingartner, H. J., Rawlings, R., George, D. T. and Eckardt, M., Triazolam-induced changes in alcoholic thought processes. Psychopharmacology (Berl.) 138:311–317, 1998.

Mann, K., Gunther, A., Stetter, F. and Ackerman, K., Rapid recovery from cognitive deficits in abstinent alcoholics: a controlled test–retest study. Alcohol Alcohol. 34:567–574; 1999.

Rourke, S. B. and Grant, I., The interactive effects of age and length of abstinence on the recovery of neuropsychological functioning in chronic male alcoholics: a 2-year follow-up study. J. Int. Neuropsychol. Soc. 5:234–246, 1999.

Family History of Alcoholism

Schandler, S. L., Brannock, J. C., Cohen, M. J., Antick, J. and Caine, K., Visuospatial learning in elementary school children with and without a family history of alcoholism. J. Stud. Alcohol 49:538–545, 1988.

Parsons, O. A., Schaeffer, K. W. and Glenn, S. W., Does neuropsychological test performance predict resumption of drinking in posttreatment alcoholics? Addict. Behav. 15:297–307, 1990.

Parsons, O. A., Sinha, R. and Williams, H. L., Relationships between neuropsychological test performance and event-related potentials in alcoholic and nonalcoholic samples. Alcohol. Clin. Exp. Res. 14:746–755, 1990.

Rodriguez, M., Cognitive functioning, family history of alcoholism, and antisocial behavior in female polydrug abusers. Psychol. Rep. 73:19–26, 1993.

Rodriguez, M., Cognitive functioning in male polydrug abusers with and without family history of alcoholism. Percept. Mot. Skills 77:483–488, 1993.

Deckel, A. W., Hesselbrock, V. and Bauer, L., Relationship between alcohol-related expectancies and anterior brain functioning in young men at risk for developing alcoholism. Alcohol. Clin. Exp. Res. 19:476–481, 1995.

Drake, A. I., Butters, N., Shear, P. K., Smith, T. L., Bondi, M., Irwin, M. and Schuckit, M. A., Cognitive recovery with abstinence and its relationship to family history for alcoholism. J. Stud. Alcohol 56:104–109, 1995.

Keenan, E., O'Donnell, C., Sinanan, K. and O'Callaghan, E., Severity of alcohol dependence and its relationship to neurological soft signs, neuropsychological impairment and family history. Acta Psychiatr. Scand. 95:272–276, 1997.

Ozkaragoz, T., Satz, P. and Noble, E. P., Neuropsychological functioning in sons of active alcoholic, recovering alcoholic, and social drinking fathers. Alcohol 14:31–37, 1997.

Sher, K. J., Martin, E. D., Wood, P. K. and Rutledge, P. C., Alcohol use disorders and neuropsychological functioning in first-year undergraduates. Exp. Clin. Psychopharmacol. 5:304–315, 1997.

Adams, K. M., Gilman, S., Johnson-Greene, D., Koeppe, R. A., Junck, L., Kluin, K. J., Martorello, S., Johnson, M. J., Heumann, M. and Hill, E., The significance of family history status in relation to neuropsychological test performance and cerebral glucose metabolism studied with positron emission tomography in older alcoholic patients. Alcohol. Clin. Exp. Res. 22:105–110, 1998.

Bauer, L. O. and Hesselbrock, V. M., Subtypes of family history and conduct disorder: effects on P300 during the stroop test. Neuropsychopharmacology 21:51–62, 1999.

Erblich, J. and Earleywine, M., Children of alcoholics exhibit attenuated cognitive impairment during an ethanol challenge. Alcohol. Clin. Exp. Res. 23:476–482, 1999.

Other Risk Factors for Alcoholism

Deckel, A. W., Bauer, L. and Hesselbrock, V., Anterior brain dysfunctioning as a risk factor in alcoholic behaviors. Addiction 90:1323–1334, 1995.

Deckel, A. W., Hesselbrock, V. and Bauer, L., Relationship between alcohol-related expectancies and anterior brain functioning in young men at risk for developing alcoholism. Alcohol. Clin. Exp. Res. 19:476–481, 1995.

Giancola, P. R., Zeichner, A., Yarnell, J. E. and Dickson, K. E., Relation between executive cognitive functioning and the adverse consequences of alcohol use in social drinkers. Alcohol. Clin. Exp. Res. 20:1094–1098, 1996.

Bauer, L. O. and Hesselbrock, V. M., Subtypes of family history and conduct disorder: effects on P300 during the stroop test. Neuropsychopharmacology 21:51–62, 1999.

Deckel, A. W., Tests of executive functioning predict scores on the MacAndrew Alcoholism Scale. Prog. Neuropsychopharmacol. Biol. Psychiatry 23:209–223, 1999.

Treatment

Saletu, B., Saletu, M., Grunberger, J. and Mader, R., Spontaneous and drug-induced remission of alcoholic organic brain syndrome: clinical, psychometric, and neurophysiological studies. Psychiatry Res. 10:59–75, 1983.

Kupke, T. and O'Brien, W. Neuropsychological impairment and behavioral limitations exhibited within an alcohol treatment program. J. Clin. Exp. Neuropsychol. 7:292–304, 1985.

Vischer, A. and Hell, D., Cognitive deficits, vitamin status and controlled thiamine substitution in alcohol dependent patients in withdrawal treatment. Nervenarzt 60:633–640, 1989. [German]

Gilman, S., Adams, K. M., Johnson-Greene, D., Koeppe, R. A., Junck, L., Kluin, K. J., Martorello, S., Heumann, M. and Hill, E., Effects of disulfiram on positron emission tomography and neuropsychological studies in severe chronic alcoholism. Alcohol. Clin. Exp. Res. 20:1456–1461, 1996.

Prenatal Exposure

Streissguth, A. P., Bookstein, F. L., Sampson, P. D. and Barr, H. M., Neurobehavioral effects of prenatal alcohol: Part III. PLS analyses of neuropsychologic tests. Neurotoxicol. Teratol. 11:493–507, 1989.

Conry, J., Neuropsychological deficits in fetal alcohol syndrome and fetal alcohol effects. Alcohol. Clin. Exp. Res. 14:650–655, 1990.

Mattson, S. N., Riley, E. P., Jernigan, T. L., Ehlers, C. L., Delis, D. C., Jones, K. L., Stern, C., Johnson, K. A., Hesselink, J. R. and Bellugi, U., Fetal alcohol syndrome: a case report of neuropsychological, MRI and EEG assessment of two children. Alcohol. Clin. Exp. Res. 16:1001–1003, 1992. [Case Report]

Korkman, M., Hilakivi-Clarke, L. A., Autti-Ramo, I., Fellman, V. and Granstrom, M. L., Cognitive impairments at two years of age after prenatal alcohol exposure or perinatal asphyxia. Neuropediatrics 25:101–105, 1994.

Streissguth, A. P., Sampson, P. D., Olson, H. C., Bookstein, F. L., Barr, H. M., Scott, M., Feldman, J. and Mirsky, A. F., Maternal drinking during pregnancy: attention and short-term memory in 14-year-old offspring—a longitudinal prospective study. Alcohol. Clin. Exp. Res. 18:202–218, 1994.

Janzen, L. A., Nanson, J. L. and Block, G. W., Neuropsychological evaluation of preschoolers with fetal alcohol syndrome. Neurotoxicol. Teratol. 17:273–279, 1995.

Kopera-Frye, K., Dehaene, S. and Streissguth, A. P., Impairments of number processing induced by prenatal alcohol exposure. Neuropsychologia 34:1187–1196, 1996.

Mattson, S. N., Riley, E. P., Delis, D. C., Stern, C. and Jones, K. L., Verbal learning and memory in children with fetal alcohol syndrome. Alcohol. Clin. Exp. Res. 20:810–816, 1996.

Uecker, A. and Nadel, L., Spatial locations gone awry: object and spatial memory deficits in children with fetal alcohol syndrome. Neuropsychologia 34:209–223, 1996.

Kerns, K. A., Don, A., Mateer, C. A. and Streissguth, A. P., Cognitive deficits in nonretarded adults with fetal alcohol syndrome. J. Learn. Disabil. 30:685–693, 1997.

Aronson, M. and Hagberg, B., Neuropsychological disorders in children exposed to alcohol during pregnancy: a follow-up study of 24 children to alcoholic mothers in Goteborg, Sweden. Alcohol. Clin. Exp. Res. 22:321–324, 1998.

Mattson, S. N., Riley, E. P., Gramling, L., Delis, D. C. and Jones, K. L., Neuropsychological comparison of alcohol-exposed children with or without physical features of fetal alcohol syndrome. Neuropsychology 12:146–153, 1998.

Olson, H. C., Feldman, J. J., Streissguth, A. P., Sampson, P. D. and Bookstein, F. L., Neuropsychological deficits in adolescents with fetal alcohol syndrome: clinical findings. Alcohol. Clin. Exp. Res. 22:1998–2012, 1998.

Sex Differences

Fabian, M. S., Jenkins, R. L. and Parsons, O. A., Gender, alcoholism, and neuropsychological functioning. J. Consult. Clin. Psychol. 49:138–140, 1981.

Fabian, M. S., Parsons, O. A. and Sheldon, M. D., Effects of gender and alcoholism on verbal and visual-spatial learning. J. Nerv. Ment. Dis. 172:16–20, 1984.

Minocha, A., Barth, J. T., Roberson, D. G., Herold, D. A. and Spyker, D. A., Impairment of cognitive and psychomotor function by ethanol in social drinkers. Vet. Hum. Toxicol. 27:533–536, 1985.

Acker, C., Neuropsychological deficits in alcoholics: the relative contributions of gender and drinking history. Br. J. Addict. 81:395–403, 1986.

Niaura, R. S., Nathan, P. E., Frankenstein, W., Shapiro, A. P. and Brick, J., Gender differences in acute psychomotor, cognitive, and pharmacokinetic response to alcohol. Addict. Behav. 12:345–356, 1987.

Haut, J. S., Beckwith, B. E., Petros, T. V. and Russell, S., Gender differences in retrieval from long-term memory following acute intoxication with ethanol. Physiol. Behav. 45:1161–1165, 1989.

Malloy, P., Noel, N., Rogers, S., Longabaugh, R. and Beattie, M., Risk factors for neuropsychological impairment in alcoholics: antisocial personality, age, years of drinking and gender. J. Stud. Alcohol 50:422–426, 1989.

Drake, A. I., Hannay, H. J. and Gam, J., Effects of chronic alcoholism on hemispheric functioning: an examination of gender differences for cognitive and dichotic listening tasks. J. Clin. Exp. Neuropsychol. 12:781–797, 1990.

Gustafson, R. and Kallmen, H., Effects of alcohol on prolonged cognitive performance measured with Stroop's Color Word Test. Psychol. Rep. 67:643–650, 1990.

Jacobson, R. R., Acker, C. F. and Lishman, W. A., Patterns of neuropsychological deficit in alcoholic Korsakoff's syndrome. Psychol. Med. 20:321–334, 1990.

Nixon, S. J., Tivis, R. and Parsons, O. A., Behavioral dysfunction and cognitive efficiency in male and female alcoholics. Alcohol. Clin. Exp. Res. 19:577–581, 1995.

Nixon, S. J. and Bowlby, D., Evidence of alcohol-related efficiency deficits in an episodic learning task. Alcohol. Clin. Exp. Res. 20:21–24, 1996.

Dufouil, C., Ducimetiere, P. and Alperovitch, A., Sex differences in the association between alcohol consumption and cognitive performance. EVA Study Group. Epidemiology of Vascular Aging. Am. J. Epidemiol. 146:405–412, 1997.

Benzodiazepines and Alcohol

Miller, T. P., Taylor, J. L. and Tinklenberg, J. R., A comparison of assessment techniques measuring the effects of methylphenidate, secobarbital, diazepam and diphenhydramine in abstinent alcoholics. Neuropsychobiology 19:90–96, 1988.

Linnoila, M., Stapleton, J. M., Lister, R., Moss, H., Lane, E., Granger, A., Greenblatt, D. J. and Eckardt, M. J., Effects of adinazolam and diazepam, alone and in combination with ethanol, on psychomotor and cognitive performance and on autonomic nervous system reactivity in healthy volunteers. Eur. J. Clin. Pharmacol. 38:371–377, 1990.

Linnoila, M., Stapleton, J. M., Lister, R., Moss, H., Lane, E., Granger, A. and Eckardt, M. J., Effects of single doses of alprazolam and diazepam, alone and in combination with ethanol, on psychomotor and cognitive performance and on autonomic nervous system reactivity in healthy volunteers. Eur. J. Clin. Pharmacol. 39:21–28, 1990.

Schuckit, M. A., Greenblatt, D., Gold, E. and Irwin, M., Reactions to ethanol and diazepam in healthy young men. J. Stud. Alcohol 52:180–187, 1991.

Mallick, J. L., Kirkby, K. C., Martin, F., Philp, M. and Hennessy, M. J., A comparison of the amnesic effects of lorazepam in alcoholics and non-alcoholics. Psychopharmacology (Berl.) 110:181–186, 1993.

Nichols, J. M., Martin, F. and Kirkby, K. C., A comparison of the effect of lorazepam on memory in heavy and low social drinkers. Psychopharmacology (Berl.) 112:475–482, 1993.

Kapczinski, F., Curran, H. V., Przemioslo, R., Williams, R., Fluck, E., Fernandes, C. and File, S. E., Cognitive impairments of alcoholic cirrhotic patients: correlation with endogenous benzodiazepine receptor ligands and increased affinity of platelet receptors. J. Neurol. Neurosurg. Psychiatry 60:676–680, 1996.

Weingartner, H. J., Rawlings, R., George, D. T. and Eckardt, M., Triazolam-induced changes in alcoholic thought processes. Psychopharmacology (Berl.) 138:311–317, 1998.

Methanol

Cook, M. R., Bergman, F. J., Cohen, H. D., Gerkovich, M. M., Graham, C., Harris, R. K. and Siemann, L. G., Effects of methanol vapor on human neurobehavioral measures. Res. Rep. Health Eff. Inst. 42:1–45, 1991.

Mozaz, M. J., Wyke, M. A. and Indakoetxea, B., Parkinsonism and defects of praxis following methanol poisoning. J. Neurol. Neurosurg. Psychiatry 54:843–844, 1991.

Chuwers, P., Osterloh, J., Kelly, T., D'Alessandro, A., Quinlan, P. and Becker, C., Neurobehavioral effects of low-level methanol vapor exposure in healthy human volunteers. Environ. Res. 71:141–150, 1995.

Reviews

Tarter, R. E., Brain damage associated with chronic alcoholism. Dis. Nerv. Syst. 36:185–187, 1975.

Carlin, A. S., Stauss, F. F., Adams, K. M. and Grant, I., The prediction of neuropsychological impairment in polydrug abusers. Addict. Behav. 3:5–12, 1978.

Carlen, P. L. and Wilkinson, D. A., Assessment of neurological dysfunction and recovery in alcoholics: CT scanning and other techniques. Subst. Alcohol Actions Misuse 4:191–197, 1983.

Goldman, M. S., Cognitive impairment in chronic alcoholics: some cause for optimism. Am. Psychol. 38:1045–1054, 1983.

Johnson, J. L., Adinoff, B., Bisserbe, J. C., Martin, P. R., Rio, D., Rohrbaugh, J. W., Zubovic, E. and Eckardt, M. J., Assessment of alcoholism-related organic brain syndromes with positron emission tomography. Alcohol. Clin. Exp. Res. 10:237–240, 1986.

Parsons, O. A., Cognitive functioning in sober social drinkers: a review and critique. J. Stud. Alcohol 47:101–114, 1986.

Carlen, P. L. and Wilkinson, D. A., Alcohol-induced brain damage: confounding variables. Alcohol Alcohol. Suppl.:37–41, 1987.

Grant, I., Alcohol and the brain: neuropsychological correlates. J. Consult. Clin. Psychol. 55:310–324, 1987.

Eckardt, M. J., Rohrbaugh, J. W., Rio, D. E. and Martin, P. R., Positron emission tomography as a technique for studying the chronic effects of alcohol on the human brain. Ann. Med. 22:341–345, 1990.

Hesselbrock, V., Bauer, L. O., Hesselbrock, M. N. and Gillen, R., Neuropsychological factors in individuals at high risk for alcoholism. Recent Dev. Alcohol. 9:21–40, 1991.

Solomon, D. A. and Malloy, P. F., Alcohol, head injury, and neuropsychological function. Neuropsychology Rev. 3:249–280, 1992.

Coles, C. D. and Platzman, K. A., Behavioral development in children prenatally exposed to drugs and alcohol. Int. J. Addict. 28:1393–1433, 1993.

Coles, C. D., Impact of prenatal alcohol exposure on the newborn and the child. Clin. Obstet. Gynecol. 36:255–266, 1993.

O'Carroll, R., Neuropsychological and neuroimaging aspects of latent hepatic encephalopathy (LHE). Alcohol Alcohol. Supppl 2:191–195, 1993.

Oscar-Berman, M., A comparative neuropsychological approach to alcoholism and the brain. Alcohol Alcohol. Suppl. 2:281–289, 1994.

Weingartner, H. J., Eckardt, M. J., Hommer, D. and Johnson, D. N., Impairments in reflective cognitive functions in alcoholics: a neuropharmacological model. Alcohol Alcohol. Suppl. 2:291–298, 1994.

Nixon, S. J. and Glenn, S. W., Cognitive psychosocial performance and recovery in female alcoholics. Recent. Dev. Alcohol. 12:287–307, 1995.

Krupitsky, E. M. and Grinenko, A. Y., Ketamine psychedelic therapy (KPT): a review of the results of ten years of research. J. Psychoactive Drugs 29:165–183, 1997.

Jacobson, S. W., Specificity of neurobehavioral outcomes associated with prenatal alcohol exposure. Alcohol. Clin. Exp. Res. 22:313–320, 1998.

Mattson, S. N. and Riley EP., A review of the neurobehavioral deficits in children with fetal alcohol syndrome or prenatal exposure to alcohol. Alcohol. Clin. Exp. Res. 22:279–294, 1998.

Neiman, J., Alcohol as a risk factor for brain damage: neurologic aspects. Alcohol. Clin. Exp. Res. 22(7 Suppl.):346S–351S, 1998.

Parsons, O. A., Neurocognitive deficits in alcoholics and social drinkers—a continuum. Alcohol. Clin. Exp. Res. 22:954–961, 1998.

Parsons, O. A. and Nixon, S. J., Cognitive functioning in sober social drinkers: a review of the research since 1986. J. Stud. Alcohol 59:180–190, 1998.

Marijuana

Acute Administration

Darley, C. F., Tinklenberg, J. R., Roth, W. T., Hollister, L. E. and Atkinson, R. C., Influence of marijuana on storage and retrieval processes in memory. Memory Cognition 1:196–200, 1973.

Borg, J., Gershon, S. and Alpert, M., Dose effects of smoked marihuana on human cognitive and motor functions. Psychopharmacologia 42:211–218, 1975.

Miller, L. L., McFarland, D. J., Cornett, T. L., Brightwell, D. R. and Wikler, A., Marijuana: effects on free recall and subjective organization of pictures and words. Psychopharmacology (Berl.) 55:257–262, 1977.

Miller, L. L., McFarland, D., Cornett, T. L. and Brightwell, D., Marijuana and memory impairment: effect on free recall and recognition memory. Pharmacol. Biochem. Behav. 7:99–103, 1977.

Parker, E. S., Birnbaum, I. M., Weingartner, H., Hartley, J. T., Stillman, R. C. and Wyatt, R. J., Retrograde enhancement of human memory with alcohol. Psychopharmacology (Berl.) 69:219–222, 1980.

Braff, D. L., Silverton, L., Saccuzzo, D. P. and Janowsky, D. S., Impaired speed of visual information processing in marijuana intoxication. Am. J. Psychiatry 138:613–617, 1981.

Hooker, W. D. and Jones, R. T., Increased susceptibility to memory intrusions and the Stroop interference effect during acute marijuana intoxication. Psychopharmacology (Berl.) 91:20–24, 1987.

Heishman, S. J., Stitzer, M. L. and Yingling, J. E., Effects of tetrahydrocannabinol content on marijuana smoking behavior, subjective reports, and performance. Pharmacol. Biochem. Behav. 34:173–179, 1989.

Heishman, S. J., Huestis, M. A., Henningfield, J. E. and Cone, E. J., Acute and residual effects of marijuana: profiles of plasma THC levels, physiological, subjective, and performance measures. Pharmacol. Biochem. Behav. 37:561–565, 1990.

Wilson, W. H., Ellinwood, E. H., Mathew, R. J. and Johnson, K., Effects of marijuana on performance of a computerized cognitive-neuromotor test battery. Psychiatry Res. 51:115–125, 1994.

Solowij, N., Grenyer, B. F., Chesher, G. and Lewis, J., Biopsychosocial changes associated with cessation of cannabis use: a single case study of acute and chronic cognitive effects, withdrawal and treatment. Life Sci. 56:2127–2134, 1995. [Case Report]

Heishman, S. J., Arasteh, K. and Stitzer, M. L., Comparative effects of alcohol and marijuana on mood, memory, and performance. Pharmacol. Biochem. Behav. 58:93–101, 1997.

Pickworth, W. B., Rohrer, M. S. and Fant, R. V., Effects of abused drugs on psychomotor performance. Exp. Clin. Psychopharmacol. 5:235–241, 1997.

Kurzthaler, I., Hummer, M., Miller, C., Sperner-Unterweger, B., Gunther, V., Wechdorn, H., Battista, H. J. and Fleischhacker, W. W., Effect of cannabis use on cognitive functions and driving ability. J. Clin. Psychiatry 60:395–399, 1999.

Chronic Administration

Culver, C. M. and King, F. W., Neuropsychological assessment of undergraduate marihuana and LSD users. Arch. Gen. Psychiatry 31:707–711, 1974.
Soueif, M. I., Chronic cannabis users: Further analysis of objective test results. Bull. Narc. 27:1–26, 1975.
Satz, P., Fletcher, J. M. and Sutker, L. S., Neuropsychologic, intellectual, and personality correlates of chronic marijuana use in native Costa Ricans. Ann. NY Acad. Sci. 282:266–306, 1976.
Soueif, M. I., Some determinants of psychological deficits associated with chronic cannabis consumption. Bull. Narc. 28:25–42, 1976.
Wig, N. N. and Varma, V. K., Patterns of long-term heavy cannabis use in north India and its effects on cognitive functions: a preliminary report. Drug Alcohol Depend. 2:211–219, 1977.
Carlin, A. S., Stauss, F. F., Adams, K. M. and Grant, I., The prediction of neuropsychological impairment in polydrug abusers. Addict. Behav. 3:5–12, 1978.
Mendhiratta, S. S., Wig, N. N. and Verma, S. K., Some psychological correlates of long-term heavy cannabis users. Br. J. Psychiatry 132:482–486, 1978.
Mendhiratta, S. S., Varma, V. K., Dang, R., Malhotra, A. K., Das, K. and Nehra, R., Cannabis and cognitive functions: a re-evaluation study. Br. J. Addict. 83:749–753, 1988.
Varma, V. K., Malhotra, A. K., Dang, R., Das, K. and Nehra, R., Cannabis and cognitive functions: a prospective study. Drug Alcohol Depend. 21:147–152, 1988.
Schwartz, R. H., Gruenewald, P. J., Klitzner, M. and Fedio, P., Short-term memory impairment in cannabis-dependent adolescents. Am. J. Dis. Child. 143:1214–1219, 1989.
Block, R. I. and Ghoneim, M. M., Effects of chronic marijuana use on human cognition. Psychopharmacology (Berl.) 110:219–228, 1993.
Bernal, B., Ardila, A. and Bateman, J. R., Cognitive impairments in adolescent drug-abusers. Int. J. Neurosci. 75:203–212, 1994.
Solowij, N., Grenyer, B. F., Chesher, G. and Lewis, J., Biopsychosocial changes associated with cessation of cannabis use: a single case study of acute and chronic cognitive effects, withdrawal and treatment. Life Sci. 56:2127–2134, 1995. [Case Report]
Easton, C. and Bauer, L. O., Neuropsychological correlates of urine toxicology results. Prog. Neuro-Psychopharmacol. Biol. Psychiatry 20:969–982, 1996.
Fletcher, J. M., Page, J. B., Francis, D. J., Copeland, K., Naus, M. J., Davis, C. M., Morris, R., Krauskopf, D. and Satz, P., Cognitive correlates of long-term cannabis use in Costa Rican men. Arch. Gen. Psychiatry 53:1051–1057, 1996.
Pope, H. G., Jr. and Yurgelun-Todd, D., The residual cognitive effects of heavy marijuana use in college students. JAMA 275:521–527, 1996.
Beatty, W. W., Blanco, C. R., Hames, K. A. and Nixon, S. J., Spatial cognition in alcoholics: influence of concurrent abuse of other drugs. Drug Alcohol Depend. 44:167–174, 1997.
Elwan, O., Hassan, A. A., Abdel Naseer, M., Elwan, F., Deif, R., El Serafy, O., El Banhawy, E. and El Fatatry, M., Brain aging in a sample of normal Egyptians cognition, education, addiction and smoking. J. Neurol. Sci. 148:79–86, 1997.

Abstinence

Solowij, N., Do cognitive impairments recover following cessation of cannabis use? Life Sci. 56:2119–2126, 1995.
Solowij, N., Grenyer, B. F., Chesher, G. and Lewis, J., Biopsychosocial changes associated with cessation of cannabis use: a single case study of acute and chronic cognitive effects, withdrawal and treatment. Life Sci. 56:2127–2134, 1995. [Case Report]

Sex Differences

Pope, H. G., Jr., Jacobs, A., Mialet, J. P., Yurgelun-Todd, D. and Gruber, S., Evidence for a sex-specific residual effect of cannabis on visuospatial memory. Psychother. Psychosom. 66:179–184, 1997.

Prenatal Exposure

Day, N. L., Richardson, G. A., Goldschmidt, L., Robles, N., Taylor, P. M., Stoffer, D. S., Cornelius, M. D. and Geva, D., Effect of prenatal marijuana exposure on the cognitive development of offspring at age three. Neurotoxicol. Teratol. 16:169–175, 1994.

Fried, P. A., Watkinson, B. and Gray, R., Differential effects on cognitive functioning in 9- to 12-year olds prenatally exposed to cigarettes and marihuana. Neurotoxicol. Teratol. 20:293–306, 1998.

Hallucinogens

PCP

Cosgrove, J. and Newell, T. G., Recovery of neuropsychological functions during reduction in use of phencyclidine. J. Clin. Psychol. 47:159–169, 1991.

Ketamine

Ghoneim, M. M., Hinrichs, J. V., Mewaldt, S. P. and Petersen, R. C., Ketamine: behavioral effects of subanesthetic doses. J. Clin. Psychopharmacol. 5:70–77, 1985.

Krystal, J. H., Karper, L. P., Seibyl, J. P., Freeman, G. K., Delaney, R., Bremner, J. D., Heninger, G. R., Bowers, M. B. J. and Charney, D. S., Subanesthetic effects of the noncompetitive NMDA antagonist, ketamine, in humans. Psychotomimetic, perceptual, cognitive, and neuroendocrine responses. Arch. Gen. Psychiatry 51:199–214, 1994.

Malhotra, A. K., Pinals, D. A., Weingartner, H., Sirocco, K., Missar, C. D., Pickar, D. and Breier, A., NMDA receptor function and human cognition: the effects of ketamine in healthy volunteers. Neuropsychopharmacology 14:301–307, 1996.

Krupitsky, E. M. and Grinenko, A. Y., Ketamine psychedelic therapy (KPT): a review of the results of ten years of research. J. Psychoactive Drugs 29:165–183, 1997.

Adler, C. M., Goldberg, T. E., Malhotra, A. K., Pickar, D. and Breier, A., Effects of ketamine on thought disorder, working memory, and semantic memory in healthy volunteers. Biol. Psychiatry 43:811–816, 1998.

Krystal, J. H., Karper, L. P., Bennett, A., D'Souza, D. C., Abi-Dargham, A., Morrissey, K., Abi-Saab, D., Bremner, J. D., Bowers, M. B., Jr., Suckow, R. F., Stetson, P., Heninger, G. R. and Charney, D. S., Interactive effects of subanesthetic ketamine and subhypnotic lorazepam in humans. Psychopharmacology (Berl.) 135:213–229, 1998.

Radant, A. D., Bowdle, T. A., Cowley, D. S., Kharasch, E. D. and Roy-Byrne, P. P., Does ketamine-mediated *N*-methyl-D-aspartate receptor antagonism cause schizophrenia-like oculomotor abnormalities? Neuropsychopharmacology 19:434–444, 1998.

Newcomer, J. W., Farber, N. B., Jevtovic-Todorovic, V., Selke, G., Melson, A. K., Hershey, T., Craft, S. and Olney, J. W., Ketamine-induced NMDA receptor hypofunction as a model of memory impairment and psychosis. Neuropsychopharmacology 20:106–118, 1999.

MDMA

McCann, U. D. and Ricaurte, G. A., Lasting neuropsychiatric sequelae of (+–) methylenedioxymethamphetamine ('ecstasy') in recreational users. J. Clin. Psychopharmacol. 11:302–305, 1991. [Case Report]

Krystal, J. H., Price, L. H., Opsahl, C., Ricaurte, G. A. and Heninger, G. R., Chronic 3,4-methylenedioxymethamphetamine (MDMA) use: effects on mood and neuropsychological function? Am. J. Drug Alcohol Abuse 18:331–341, 1992.

Curran, H. V. and Travill, R. A., Mood and cognitive effects of +/–3,4-methylenedioxymethamphetamine (MDMA, "ecstasy"): week-end 'high' followed by mid-week low. Addiction 92:821–831, 1997.

Bolla, K. I., McCann, U. D. and Ricaurte, G. A., Memory impairment in abstinent MDMA ("Ecstasy") users. Neurology 51:1532–1537, 1998.

Morgan, M. J., Recreational use of "ecstasy" (MDMA) is associated with elevated impulsivity. Neuropsychopharmacology 19:252–264, 1998.

Parrott, A. C., Lees, A., Garnham, N. J., Jones, M. and Wesnes, K., Cognitive performance in recreational users of MDMA of 'ecstasy': evidence for memory deficits. J. Psychopharmacol. 12:79–83, 1998.

Vollenweider, F. X., Gamma, A., Liechti, M. and Huber, T., Psychological and cardiovascular effects and short-term sequelae of MDMA ("Ecstasy") in MDMA-naive healthy volunteers. Neuropsychopharmacology 19:241–251, 1998.

Dafters, R. I., Duffy, F., O'Donnell, P. J. and Bouquet, C., Level of use of 3,4-methylenedioxymethamphetamine (MDMA or Ecstasy) in humans correlates with EEG power and coherence. Psychopharmacology (Berl.) 145:82–90, 1999.

McCann, U. D., Mertyl, M., Eligulashvili, V. and Ricaurte, G. A., Cognitive performance in (+/-) 3,4-methylenedioxymethamphetamine (MDMA, "ecstasy") users: a controlled study. Psychopharmacology (Berl.) 143:417–425, 1999.

Morgan, M. J., Memory deficits associated with recreational use of "ecstasy" (MDMA). Psychopharmacology (Berl.) 141:30–36, 1999.

Semple, D. M., Ebmeier, K. P., Glabus, M. F., O'Carroll, R. E. and Johnstone, E. C., Reduced in vivo binding to the serotonin transporter in the cerebral cortex of MDMA ('ecstasy') users. Br. J. Psychiatry 175:63–69, 1999.

LSD

Goldberger, L., Cognitive test performance under LSD-25, placebo and isolation. J. Nerv. Ment. Dis. 142:4–9, 1966.

Cohen, S. and Edwards, A. E., LSD and organic brain impairment. Drug Dependence 2:1–4, 1969.

Wright, M. and Hogan, T. P., Repeated LSD ingestion and performance on neuropsychological tests. J. Nerv. Ment. Dis. 154:432–438, 1972.

Culver, C. M. and King, F. W., Neuropsychological assessment of undergraduate marihuana and LSD users. Arch. Gen. Psychiatry 31:707–711, 1974.

Mescaline

Culver, C. M. and King, F. W., Neuropsychological assessment of undergraduate marihuana and LSD users. Arch. Gen. Psychiatry 31:707–711, 1974.

Oepen, G., Fuenfgeld, M., Harrington, A., Hermle, L. and Botsch, H., Right hemisphere involvement in mescaline-induced psychosis. Psychiatry Res. 29:335–336, 1989.

Hermle, L., Funfgeld, M., Oepen, G., Botsch, H., Borchardt, D., Gouzoulis, E., Fehrenbach, R. A. and Spitzer, M., Mescaline-induced psychopathological, neuropsychological, and neurometabolic effects in normal subjects: experimental psychosis as a tool for psychiatric research. Biol. Psychiatry 32:976–991, 1992.

Hoasca

Grob, C. S., McKenna, D. J., Callaway, J. C., Brito, G. S., Neves, E. S., Oberlaender, G., Saide, O. L., Labigalini, E., Tacla, C., Miranda, C. T., Strassman, R. J. and Boone, K. B., Human psychopharmacology of hoasca, a plant hallucinogen used in ritual context in Brazil. J. Nerv. Ment. Dis. 184:86–94, 1996.

Unspecified

Acord, L. D. and Barker, D. D., Hallucinogenic drugs and cerebral deficit. J. Nerv. Ment. Dis. 156:281–283, 1973.

Review

Halpern, J. H. and Pope, H. G., Jr., Do hallucinogens cause residual neuropsychological toxicity? Drug Alcohol Depend. 53:247–256, 1999.

Benzodiazepines

Acute Administration

Alprazolam

Blom, M. W., Bartel, P. R., de Sommers, K., Van der Meyden, C. H. and Becker, P. J., The effects of alprazolam, quazepam and diazepam on saccadic eye movements, parameters of psychomotor function and the EEG. Fundam. Clin. Pharmacol. 4:653–661, 1990.

Linnoila, M., Stapleton, J. M., Lister, R., Moss, H., Lane, E., Granger, A. and Eckardt, M. J., Effects of single doses of alprazolam and diazepam, alone and in combination with ethanol, on psychomotor and cognitive performance and on autonomic nervous system reactivity in healthy volunteers. Eur. J. Clin. Pharmacol. 39:21–28, 1990.

Barbee, J. G., Black, F. W., Kehoe, C. E. and Todorov, A. A., A comparison of the single-dose effects of alprazolam, buspirone, and placebo upon memory function. J. Clin. Psychopharmacol. 11:351–356, 1991.

Bourin, M., Colombel, M. C. and Guitton, B., Alprazolam 0.125 mg twice a day improves aspects of psychometric performance in healthy volunteers. J. Clin. Psychopharmacol. 18:364–372, 1998.

Diazepam

Golombok, S., and Lader, M., The psychopharmacological effects of premazepam, diazepam and placebo in healthy human subjects. Br. J. Clin. Pharmacol. 18:127–133, 1984.

Funderburk, F. R., Griffiths, R. R., McLeod, D. R., Bigelow, G. E., Mackenzie, A., Liebson, I. A. and Nemeth-Coslett, R., Relative abuse liability of lorazepam and diazepam: an evaluation in 'recreational' drug users. Drug Alcohol Depend. 22:215–222, 1988.

Miller, T. P., Taylor, J. L. and Tinklenberg, J. R., A comparison of assessment techniques measuring the effects of methylphenidate, secobarbital, diazepam and diphenhydramine in abstinent alcoholics. Neuropsychobiology 19:90–96, 1988.

Blom, M. W., Bartel, P. R., de Sommers, K., Van der Meyden, C. H. and Becker, P. J., The effects of alprazolam, quazepam and diazepam on saccadic eye movements, parameters of psychomotor function and the EEG. Fundam. Clin. Pharmacol. 4:653–661, 1990.

Linnoila, M., Stapleton, J. M., Lister, R., Moss, H., Lane, E., Granger, A., Greenblatt, D. J. and Eckardt, M. J., Effects of adinazolam and diazepam, alone and in combination with ethanol, on psychomotor and cognitive performance and on autonomic nervous system reactivity in healthy volunteers. Eur. J. Clin. Pharmacol. 38:371–377, 1990.

Linnoila, M., Stapleton, J. M., Lister, R., Moss, H., Lane, E., Granger, A. and Eckardt, M. J., Effects of single doses of alprazolam and diazepam, alone and in combination with ethanol, on psychomotor and cognitive performance and on autonomic nervous system reactivity in healthy volunteers. Eur. J. Clin. Pharmacol. 39:21–28, 1990.

Anthenelli, R. M., Monteiro, M. G., Blunt, B. and Schuckit, M. A., Amnestic effects of intravenous diazepam in healthy young men. Am. J. Drug Alcohol Abuse 17:129–136, 1991.

Hennessy, M. J., Kirkby, K. C. and Montgomery, I. M., Comparison of the amnesic effects of midazolam and diazepam. Psychopharmacology (Berl.) 103:545–550, 1991.

Schuckit, M. A., Greenblatt, D., Gold, E. and Irwin, M., Reactions to ethanol and diazepam in healthy young men. J. Stud. Alcohol 52:180–187, 1991.
King, D. J. and Henry, G., The effect of neuroleptics on cognitive and psychomotor function. A preliminary study in healthy volunteers. Br. J. Psychiatry 160:647–653, 1992.
Unrug-Neervoort, A., van Luijtelaar, G. and Coenen, A., Cognition and vigilance: differential effects of diazepam and buspirone on memory and psychomotor performance. Neuropsychobiology 26:146–150, 1992.
Gorenstein, C., Bernik, M. A. and Pompeia, S., Differential acute psychomotor and cognitive effects of diazepam on long-term benzodiazepine users. Int. Clin. Psychopharmacol. 9:145–153, 1994.
Coull, J. T., Middleton, H. C., Robbins, T. W. and Sahakian, B. J., Contrasting effects of clonidine and diazepam on tests of working memory and planning. Psychopharmacology (Berl.) 120:311–321, 1995.
Coull, J. T., Middleton, H. C., Robbins, T. W. and Sahakian, B. J., Clonidine and diazepam have differential effects on tests of attention and learning. Psychopharmacology (Berl.) 120:322–332, 1995.
Cloyd, J. C., Lalonde, R. L., Beniak, T. E. and Novack, G. D., A single-blind, crossover comparison of the pharmacokinetics and cognitive effects of a new diazepam rectal gel with intravenous diazepam. Epilepsia 39:520–526, 1998.
Swift, R., Davidson, D., Rosen, S., Fitz, E. and Camara, P., Naltrexone effects on diazepam intoxication and pharmacokinetics in humans. Psychopharmacology (Berl.) 135:256–262, 1998.

Lorazepam

Funderburk, F. R., Griffiths, R. R., McLeod, D. R., Bigelow, G. E., Mackenzie, A., Liebson, I. A. and Nemeth-Coslett, R., Relative abuse liability of lorazepam and diazepam: an evaluation in 'recreational' drug users. Drug Alcohol Depend. 22:215–222, 1988.
Sunderland, T., Weingartner, H., Cohen, R. M., Tariot, P. N., Newhouse, P. A., Thompson, K. E., Lawlor, B. A. and Mueller, E. A., Low-dose oral lorazepam administration in Alzheimer subjects and age-matched controls. Psychopharmacology (Berl.) 99:129–133, 1989.
Tulen, J. H., Moleman, P., Boomsma, F., van Steenis, H. G. and van den Heuij, V. J., Dose-dependent effects of intravenous lorazepam on cardiovascular activity, plasma catecholamines and psychological function during rest and mental stress. Psychopharmacology (Berl.) 105:77–83, 1991.
Mallick, J. L., Kirkby, K. C., Martin, F., Philp, M. and Hennessy, M. J., A comparison of the amnesic effects of lorazepam in alcoholics and non-alcoholics. Psychopharmacology (Berl.) 110:181–186, 1993.
Nichols, J. M., Martin, F. and Kirkby, K. C., A comparison of the effect of lorazepam on memory in heavy and low social drinkers. Psychopharmacology (Berl.) 112:475–482, 1993.
Rush, C. R., Higgins, S. T., Bickel, W. K. and Hughes, J. R., Acute effects of triazolam and lorazepam on human learning, performance and subject ratings. J. Pharmacol. Exp. Ther. 264:1218–1226, 1993.
Bourin, M., Couetoux du Tertre, A., Colombel, M. C. and Auget, J. L., Effects of low doses of lorazepam on psychometric tests in healthy volunteers. Int. Clin. Psychopharmacol. 9:83–88, 1994.
Hanks, G. W., O'Neill, W. M., Simpson, P. and Wesnes, K., The cognitive and psychomotor effects of opioid analgesics. II. A randomized controlled trial of single doses of morphine, lorazepam and placebo in healthy subjects. Eur. J. Clin. Pharmacol. 48:455–460, 1995.
O'Neill, W. M., Hanks, G. W., White, L., Simpson, P. and Wesnes, K., The cognitive and psychomotor effects of opioid analgesics. I. A randomized controlled trial of single doses of dextropropoxyphene, lorazepam and placebo in healthy subjects. Eur. J. Clin. Pharmacol. 48:447–453, 1995.

Stewart, S. H., Rioux, G. F., Connolly, J. F., Dunphy, S. C. and Teehan, M. D., Effects of oxazepam and lorazepam on implicit and explicit memory: evidence for possible influences of time course. Psychopharmacology (Berl.) 128:139–149, 1996.

Fluck, E., File, S. E., Springett, J., Kopelman, M. D., Rees, J. and Orgill, J., Does the sedation resulting from sleep deprivation and lorazepam cause similar cognitive deficits? Pharmacol. Biochem. Behav. 59:909–915, 1998.

Krystal, J. H., Karper, L. P., Bennett, A., D'Souza, D. C., Abi-Dargham, A., Morrissey, K., Abi-Saab, D., Bremner, J. D., Bowers, M. B., Jr., Suckow, R. F., Stetson, P., Heninger, G. R. and Charney, D. S., Interactive effects of subanesthetic ketamine and subhypnotic lorazepam in humans. Psychopharmacology (Berl.) 135:213–229, 1998.

Other Benzodiazepines

Rosenfeld, W. E., Beniak, T. E., Lippmann, S. M. and Loewenson, R. B., Adverse behavioral response to clonazepam as a function of Verbal IQ-Performance IQ discrepancy. Epilepsy Res. 1:347–356, 1987.

Hennessy, M. J., Kirkby, K. C. and Montgomery, I. M., Comparison of the amnesic effects of midazolam and diazepam. Psychopharmacology (Berl.) 103:545–550, 1991.

Weingartner, H. J., Hommer, D., Lister, R. G., Thompson, K. and Wolkowitz, O., Selective effects of triazolam on memory. Psychopharmacology (Berl.) 106:341–345, 1992.

Rush, C. R., Higgins, S. T., Bickel, W. K. and Hughes, J. R., Acute effects of triazolam and lorazepam on human learning, performance and subject ratings. J. Pharmacol. Exp. Ther. 264:1218–1226, 1993.

Greenblatt, D. J., Harmatz, J. S., Gouthro, T. A., Locke, J. and Shader, R. I., Distinguishing a benzodiazepine agonist (triazolam) from a nonagonist anxiolytic (buspirone) by electroencephalography: kinetic-dynamic studies. Clin. Pharmacol. Ther. 56:100–111, 1994.

Roehrs, T., Merlotti, L., Zorick, F. and Roth, T., Sedative, memory, and performance effects of hypnotics. Psychopharmacology (Berl.) 116:130–134, 1994.

Rush, C. R. and Griffiths, R. R., Zolpidem, triazolam, and temazepam: behavioral and subject-rated effects in normal volunteers. J. Clin. Psychopharmacol. 16:146–157, 1996.

Davis, C. M., Ambros-Ingerson, J., Granger, R., Wu, J., Zabaneh, R., Abdelnaby, M. and Lynch, G., Triazolam impairs delayed recall but not acquisition of various everyday memory tasks in humans. Exp. Neurol. 148:124–134, 1997.

Veselis, R. A., Reinsel, R. A., Feshchenko, V. A., and Wronski, M., The comparative amnestic effects of midazolam, propofol, thiopental, and fentanyl at equisedative concentrations. Anesthesiology 87:749–764, 1997.

Weingartner, H. J., Rawlings, R., George, D. T. and Eckardt, M., Triazolam-induced changes in alcoholic thought processes. Psychopharmacology (Berl.) 138:311–317, 1998.

Chronic Administration

Bergman, H., Borg, S. and Holm, L., Neuropsychological impairment and exclusive abuse of sedatives or hypnotics. Am. J. Psychiatry 137:215–217, 1980.

Brooker, A. E., Wiens, A. N. and Wiens, D. A., Impaired brain functions due to diazepam and meprobamate abuse in a 53-year-old-male. J. Nerv. Ment. Dis. 172:498–501, 1984. [Case Report]

Lucki, I., Rickels, K. and Geller, A. M., Chronic use of benzodiazepines and psychomotor and cognitive test performance. Psychopharmacology (Berl.) 88:426–433, 1986.

Golombok, S., Moodley, P. and Lader, M., Cognitive impairment in long-term benzodiazepine users. Psychol. Med. 18:365–374, 1988.

Sakol, M. S. and Power, K. G., The effects of long-term benzodiazepine treatment and graded withdrawal on psychometric performance. Psychopharmacology (Berl.) 95:135–138, 1988.

Bergman, H., Borg, S., Engelbrektson, K. and Vikander, B., Dependence on sedative-hypnotics: neuropsychological impairment, field dependence and clinical course in a 5-year follow-up study. Br. J. Addict. 84:547–553, 1989.

Bourin, M., Couetoux du Tertre, A., Colombel, M. C. and Auget, J. L., Effects of low doses of lorazepam on psychometric tests in healthy volunteers. Int. Clin. Psychopharmacol. 9:83–88, 1994.

Gorenstein, C., Bernik, M. A. and Pompeia, S., Differential acute psychomotor and cognitive effects of diazepam on long-term benzodiazepine users. Int. Clin. Psychopharmacol. 9:145–153, 1994.

Saxena, S., Psychological deficits with long-term benzodiazepine use. Natl. Med. J. India 8:68–69, 1995.

Tonne, U., Hiltunen, A. J., Vikander, B., Engelbrektsson, K., Bergman, H., Bergman, I., Leifman, H. and Borg, S., Neuropsychological changes during steady-state drug use, withdrawal and abstinence in primary benzodiazepine-dependent patients. Acta Psychiatr. Scand. 91:299–304, 1995.

Gilman, S., Adams, K. M., Johnson-Greene, D., Koeppe, R. A., Junck, L., Kluin, K. J., Martorello, S., Heumann, M. and Hill, E., Effects of disulfiram on positron emission tomography and neuropsychological studies in severe chronic alcoholism. Alcohol. Clin. Exp. Res. 20:1456–1461, 1996.

Bourin, M., Colombel, M. C. and Guitton, B., Alprazolam 0.125 mg twice a day improves aspects of psychometric performance in healthy volunteers. J. Clin. Psychopharmacol. 18:364–372, 1998.

Withdrawal

Lader, M., Benzodiazepine dependence. Prog. Neuropsychopharmacol. Biol. Psychiatry 8:85–95, 1984.

Sakol, M. S. and Power, K. G., The effects of long-term benzodiazepine treatment and graded withdrawal on psychometric performance. Psychopharmacology (Berl.) 95:135–138, 1988.

Tonne, U., Hiltunen, A. J., Vikander, B., Engelbrektsson, K., Bergman, H., Bergman, I., Leifman, H. and Borg, S., Neuropsychological changes during steady-state drug use, withdrawal and abstinence in primary benzodiazepine-dependent patients. Acta Psychiatr. Scand. 91:299–304, 1995.

Abstinence

Rummans, T. A., Davis, L. J., Jr., Morse, R. M. and Ivnik, R. J., Learning and memory impairment in older, detoxified, benzodiazepine-dependent patients. Mayo Clin. Proc. 68:731–737, 1993.

Tata, P. R., Rollings, J., Collins, M., Pickering, A. and Jacobson, R. R., Lack of cognitive recovery following withdrawal from long-term benzodiazepine use. Psychol. Med. 24:203–213, 1994.

Tonne, U., Hiltunen, A. J., Vikander, B., Engelbrektsson, K., Bergman, H., Bergman, I., Leifman, H. and Borg, S., Neuropsychological changes during steady-state drug use, withdrawal and abstinence in primary benzodiazepine-dependent patients. Acta Psychiatr. Scand. 91:299–304, 1995.

Treatment

Hendler, N., Cimini, C., Ma, T. and Long, D., A comparison of cognitive impairment due to benzodiazepines and to narcotics. Am. J. Psychiatry 137:828–830, 1980.

Review

Barbee, J. G., Memory, benzodiazepines, and anxiety: integration of theoretical and clinical perspectives. J. Clin. Psychiatry 54 Suppl:86–97, 1993.

Barbiturates

Carlin, A. S., Stauss, F. F., Adams, K. M. and Grant, I., The prediction of neuropsychological impairment in polydrug abusers. Addict. Behav. 3:5–12, 1978.

Mohs, R. C., Tinklenberg, J. R., Roth, W. T. and Kopell, B. S., Sensitivity of some human cognitive functions to effects of methamphetamine and secobarbital. Drug Alcohol Depend. 5:145–150, 1980.

Miller, T. P., Taylor, J. L. and Tinklenberg, J. R., A comparison of assessment techniques measuring the effects of methylphenidate, secobarbital, diazepam and diphenhydramine in abstinent alcoholics. Neuropsychobiology 19:90–96, 1988.

Pickworth, W. B., Rohrer, M. S. and Fant, R. V., Effects of abused drugs on psychomotor performance. Exp. Clin. Psychopharmacol. 5:235–241, 1997.

Veselis, R. A., Reinsel, R. A., Feshchenko, V. A., and Wronski, M., The comparative amnestic effects of midazolam, propofol, thiopental, and fentanyl at equisedative concentrations. Anesthesiology 87:749–764, 1997.

Heroin and Opiates

Acute Administration

Morphine

Jarvik, L. F., Simpson, J. H., Guthrie, D. and Liston, E. H., Morphine, experimental pain, and psychological reactions. Psychopharmacology (Berl.) 75:124–131, 1981.

Kerr, B., Hill, H., Coda, B., Calogero, M., Chapman, C. R., Hunt, E., Buffington, V. and Mackie, A., Concentration-related effects of morphine on cognition and motor control in human subjects. Neuropsychopharmacology 5:157–166, 1991.

Hanks, G. W., O'Neill, W. M., Simpson, P. and Wesnes, K., The cognitive and psychomotor effects of opioid analgesics. II. A randomized controlled trial of single doses of morphine, lorazepam and placebo in healthy subjects. Eur. J. Clin. Pharmacol. 48:455–460, 1995.

Zacny, J. P., Hill, J. L., Black, M. L. and Sadeghi, P., Comparing the subjective, psychomotor and physiological effects of intravenous pentazocine and morphine in normal volunteers. J. Pharmacol. Exp. Ther. 286:1197–1207, 1998.

Propoxyphene

O'Neill, W. M., Hanks, G. W., White, L., Simpson, P. and Wesnes, K., The cognitive and psychomotor effects of opioid analgesics. I. A randomized controlled trial of single doses of dextropropoxyphene, lorazepam and placebo in healthy subjects. Eur. J. Clin. Pharmacol. 48:447–453, 1995.

Hydromorphone

Pickworth, W. B., Rohrer, M. S. and Fant, R. V., Effects of abused drugs on psychomotor performance. Exp. Clin. Psychopharmacol. 5:235–241, 1997.

Heroin

Zuckerman, G. B., Ruiz, D. C., Keller, I. A. and Brooks, J., Neurologic complications following intranasal administration of heroin in an adolescent. Ann. Pharmacother. 30:778–781, 1996. [Case Report]

Fentanyl

Veselis, R. A., Reinsel, R. A., Feshchenko, V. A. and Wronski, M., The comparative amnestic effects of midazolam, propofol, thiopental, and fentanyl at equisedative concentrations. Anesthesiology 87:749–764, 1997.

Schneider, U., Bevilacqua, C., Jacobs, R., Karst, M., Dietrich, D. E., Becker, H., Muller-Vahl, K. R., Seeland, I., Gielsdorf, D., Schedlowski, M. and Emrich, H. M., Effects of fentanyl and low doses of alcohol on neuropsychological performance in healthy subjects. Neuropsychobiology 39:38–43, 1999.

Pentazocine

Zacny, J. P., Hill, J. L., Black, M. L. and Sadeghi, P., Comparing the subjective, psychomotor and physiological effects of intravenous pentazocine and morphine in normal volunteers. J. Pharmacol. Exp. Ther. 286:1197–1207, 1998.

Chronic Administration

Fields, F. R. J. and Fullerton, J. R., Influence of heroin addiction on neuropsychological functioning. J. Consult. Clin. Psychol. 43:114, 1975.

Carlin, A. S., Stauss, F. F., Adams, K. M. and Grant, I., The prediction of neuropsychological impairment in polydrug abusers. Addict. Behav. 3:5–12, 1978.

Grant, I., Adams, K. M., Carlin, A. S., Rennick, P. M., Judd, L. L., Schooff, K. and Reed, R., Organic impairment in polydrug users: risk factors. Am. J. Psychiatry 135:178–184, 1978.

Hill, S. Y., Reyes, R. B., Mikhael, M. and Ayre, F., A comparison of alcoholics and heroin abusers: computerized transaxial tomography and neuropsychological functioning. Curr. Alcohol 5:187–205, 1979.

Wolf, S. L. and Mikhael, M. A., Computerized transaxial tomographic and neuropsychol evaluations in chronic alcoholics and heroin abusers. Am. J. Psychiatry 136:598–602, 1979.

Rounsaville, B. J., Jones, C., Novelly, R. A. and Kleber, H., Neuropsychological functioning in opiate addicts. J. Nerv. Ment. Dis. 170:209–216, 1982.

Guerra, D., Sole, A., Cami, J. and Tobena, A., Neuropsychological performance in opiate addicts after rapid detoxification. Drug Alcohol Depend. 20:261–270, 1987.

Strang, J. and Gurling, H., Computerized tomography and neuropsychological assessment in long-term high-dose heroin addicts. Br. J. Addict. 84:1011–1019, 1989.

Holman, B. L., Carvalho, P. A., Mendelson, J., Teoh, S. K., Nardin, R., Hallgring, E., Hebben, N. and Johnson, K. A., Brain perfusion is abnormal in cocaine-dependent polydrug users: a study using technetium-99m-HMPAO and ASPECT. J. Nucl. Med. 32:1206–1210, 1991.

Woods, S. W., O'Malley, S. S., Martini, B. L., McDougle, C. J., Price, L. H., Krystal, J. H., Hoffer, P. B. and Kosten, T. R., SPECT regional cerebral blood flow and neuropsychological testing in non-demented HIV-positive drug abusers. Prog. Neuropsychopharmacol. Biol. Psychiatry 15:649–662, 1991.

Rodriguez, M., Cognitive functioning, family history of alcoholism, and antisocial behavior in female polydrug abusers. Psychol. Rep. 73:19–26, 1993.

Amir, T. and Bahri, T., Effect of substance abuse on visuographic function. Percept. Mot. Skills 78:235–241, 1994.

Celius, E. G. and Andersson, S., Leucoencephalopathy after inhalation of heroin: a case report. J. Neurol. Neurosurg. Psychiatry 60:694–695, 1996. [Case Report]

Concha, M., Selnes, O. A., Vlahov, D., Nance-Sproson, T., Updike, M., Royal, W., Palenicek, J. and McArthur, J. C., Comparison of neuropsychological performance between AIDS-free injecting drug users and homosexual men. Neuroepidemiology 16:78–85, 1997.

Gerra, G., Calbiani, B., Zaimovic, A., Sartori, R., Ugolotti, G., Ippolito, L., Delsignore, R., Rustichelli, P. and Fontanesi, B., Regional cerebral blood flow and comorbid diagnosis in abstinent opioid addicts. Psychiatry Res. 83:117–126, 1998.

Abstinence

Hill, S. Y., Reyes, R. B., Mikhael, M. and Ayre, F., A comparison of alcoholics and heroin abusers: computerized transaxial tomography and neuropsychological functioning. Curr. Alcohol 5:187–205, 1979.

Treatment

Gritz, E. R., Shiffman, S. M., Jarvik, M. E., Haber, J., Dymond, A. M., Coger, R., Charuvastra, V. and Schlesinger, J., Physiological and psychological effects of methadone in man. Arch. Gen. Psychiatry 32:237–242, 1975.

Guerra, D., Sole, A., Cami, J. and Tobena, A., Neuropsychological performance in opiate addicts after rapid detoxification. Drug Alcohol Depend. 20:261–270, 1987.

HIV

Silberstein, C. H., McKegney, F. P., O'Dowd, M. A., Selwyn, P. A., Schoenbaum, E., Drucker, E., Feiner, C., Cox, C. P. and Friedland, G., A prospective longitudinal study of neuropsychological and psychosocial factors in asymptomatic individuals at risk for HTLV-III/LAV infection in a methadone program: preliminary findings. Int. J. Neurosci. 32:669–676, 1987.

Woods, S. W., O'Malley, S. S., Martini, B. L., McDougle, C. J., Price, L. H., Krystal, J. H., Hoffer, P. B. and Kosten, T. R., SPECT regional cerebral blood flow and neuropsychological testing in non-demented HIV-positive drug abusers. Prog. Neuropsychopharmacol. Biol. Psychiatry 15:649–662, 1991.

Concha, M., Selnes, O. A., Vlahov, D., Nance-Sproson, T., Updike, M., Royal, W., Palenicek, J. and McArthur, J. C., Comparison of neuropsychological performance between AIDS-free injecting drug users and homosexual men. Neuroepidemiology 16:78–85, 1997.

Prenatal Exposure

van Baar, A. and de Graaff, B. M., Cognitive development at preschool-age of infants of drug-dependent mothers. Dev. Med. Child Neurol. 36:1063–1075, 1994.

Cocaine

Acute Administration

Higgins, S. T., Bickel, W. K., Hughes, J. R., Lynn, M., Capeless, M. A. and Fenwick, J. W., Effects of intranasal cocaine on human learning, performance and physiology. Psychopharmacology (Berl.) 102:451–458, 1990.

Higgins, S. T., Rush, C. R., Bickel, W. K., Hughes, J. R., Lynn, M. and Capeless, M. A., Acute behavioral and cardiac effects of cocaine and alcohol combinations in humans. Psychopharmacology (Berl.) 111:285–294, 1993.

Johnson, B., Overton, D., Wells, L., Kenny, P., Abramson, D., Dhother, S., Chen, Y. R. and Bordnick, P., Effects of acute intravenous cocaine on cardiovascular function, human learning, and performance in cocaine addicts. Psychiatry Res. 77:35–42, 1998.

Chronic Administration

Manschreck, T. C., Schneyer, M. L., Weisstein, C. C., Laughery, J., Rosenthal, J., Celada, T. and Berner, J., Freebase cocaine and memory. Compr. Psychiatry 31:369–375, 1990.

Ardila, A., Rosselli, M. and Strumwasser, S., Neuropsychological deficits in chronic cocaine abusers. Int. J. Neurosci. 57:73–79, 1991.

Holman, B. L., Carvalho, P. A., Mendelson, J., Teoh, S. K., Nardin, R., Hallgring, E., Hebben, N. and Johnson, K. A., Brain perfusion is abnormal in cocaine-dependent polydrug users: a study using technetium-99m-HMPAO and ASPECT. J. Nucl. Med. 32:1206–1210, 1991.

O'Malley, S., Adamse, M., Heaton, R. K. and Gawin, F. H., Neuropsychological impairment in chronic cocaine abusers. Am. J. Drug Alcohol Abuse 18:131–144, 1992.

Bernal, B., Ardila, A. and Bateman, J. R., Cognitive impairments in adolescent drug-abusers. Int. J. Neurosci. 75:203–212, 1994.

Easton, C. and Bauer, L. O., Neuropsychological correlates of urine toxicology results. Prog. Neuro-Psychopharmacol. Biol. Psychiatry 20:969–982, 1996.

Hoff, A. L., Riordan, H., Morris, L., Cestaro, V., Wieneke, M., Alpert, R., Wang, G.-J. and Volkow, N., Effects of crack cocaine on neurocognitive function. Psychiatry Res. 60:167–176, 1996.

Rosselli, M. and Ardila, A., Cognitive effects of cocaine and polydrug abuse. J. Clin. Exp. Neuropsychol. 18:122–135, 1996.

Carpenter, K. M. and Hittner, J. B., Cognitive impairment among the dually-diagnosed: substance use history and depressive symptom correlates. Addiction 92:747–759, 1997.

Concha, M., Selnes, O. A., Vlahov, D., Nance-Sproson, T., Updike, M., Royal, W., Palenicek, J. and McArthur, J. C., Comparison of neuropsychological performance between AIDS-free injecting drug users and homosexual men. Neuroepidemiology 16:78–85, 1997.

Selby, M. J. and Azrin, R. L., Neuropsychological functioning in drug abusers. Drug Alcohol Depend. 50:39–45, 1998.

Robinson, J. E., Heaton, R. K. and O'Malley, S. S., Neuropsychological functioning in cocaine abusers with and without alcohol dependence. J. Int. Neuropsychol. Soc. 5:10–19, 1999.

van Gorp, W. G., Wilkins, J. N., Hinkin, C. H., Moore, L. H., Hull, J., Horner, M. D. and Plotkin, D., Declarative and procedural memory functioning in abstinent cocaine abusers. Arch. Gen. Psychiatry 56:85–89, 1999.

Abstinence

Berry, J., van Gorp, W. G., Herzberg, D. S., Hinkin, C., Boone, K., Steinman, L. and Wilkins, J. N., Neuropsychological deficits in abstinent cocaine abusers: preliminary findings after two weeks of abstinence. Drug Alcohol Depend. 32:231–237, 1993.

Strickland, T. L., Mena, I., J., Villanueva-Meyer, J., Miller, B. L., Cummings, J., Mehringer, C. M., Satz, P. and Myers, H., Cerebral perfusion and neuropsychological consequences of chronic cocaine use. J. Neuropsychiatry Clin. Neurosci. 5:419–427, 1993.

Beatty, W. W., Katzung, V. M., Moreland, V. J. and Nixon, S. J., Neuropsychological performance of recently abstinent alcoholics and cocaine abusers. Drug Alcohol Depend. 37:247–253, 1995.

Easton, C. J. and Bauer, L. O., Beneficial effects of thiamine on recognition memory and P300 in abstinent cocaine-dependent patients. Psychiatry Res. 70:165–174, 1997.

Easton, C. J. and Bauer, L. O., Neuropsychological differences between alcohol-dependent and cocaine- dependent patients with or without problematic drinking. Psychiatry Res. 71:97–103, 1997.

Disclafani, V., Truran, D. L., Bloomer, C., Tolou-shams, M., Clark, H. W., Norman, D., Hannauer, D. and Fein, G., Abstinent chronic crack-cocaine and crack-cocaine/alcohol abusers evidence normal hippocampal volumes on MRI despite persistent cognitive impairments. Addiction Biol. 3:261–270, 1998.

Gillen, R. W., Kranzler, H. R., Bauer, L. O., Burleson, J. A., Samarel, D. and Morrison, D. J., Neuropsychologic findings in cocaine-dependent outpatients. Prog. Neuro-Psychopharmacol. Biol. Psychiatry 22:1061–1076, 1998.

van Gorp, W. G., Wilkins, J. N., Hinkin, C. H., Moore, L. H., Hull, J., Horner, M. D. and Plotkin, D., Declarative and procedural memory functioning in abstinent cocaine abusers. Arch. Gen. Psychiatry 56:85–89, 1999.

Treatment

Ollo, C., Alim, T. N., Rosse, R. B., Lindquist, T., Green, T., Gillis, T., Ricci, J., Khan, M. and Deutsch, S. I., Lack of neurotoxic effect of diethylpropion in crack-cocaine abusers. Clin. Neuropharmacol. 19:52–58, 1996.

Easton, C. J. and Bauer, L. O., Beneficial effects of thiamine on recognition memory and P300 in abstinent cocaine-dependent patients. Psychiatry Res. 70:165–174, 1997.

Prenatal Exposure

Struthers, J. M. and Hansen, R. L., Visual recognition memory in drug-exposed infants. J. Dev. Behav. Pediatr. 13:108–111, 1992.

Nulman, I., Rovet, J., Altmann, D., Bradley, C., Einarson, T. and Koren, G., Neurodevelopment of adopted children exposed in utero to cocaine. CMAJ 151:1591–1597, 1994.

van Baar, A. and de Graaff, B. M., Cognitive development at preschool-age of infants of drug-dependent mothers. Dev. Med. Child Neurol. 36:1063–1075, 1994.

Jacobson, S. W., Jacobson, J. L., Sokol, R. J., Martier, S. S. and Chiodo, L. M., New evidence for neurobehavioral effects of in utero cocaine exposure. J. Pediatr. 129:581–590, 1996.

Richardson, G. A., Conroy, M. L. and Day, N. L., Prenatal cocaine exposure: effects on the development of school-age children. Neurotoxicol. Teratol. 18:627–634, 1996.

Tronick, E. Z., Frank, D. A., Cabral, H., Mirochnick, M. and Zuckerman, B., Late dose-response effects of prenatal cocaine exposure on newborn neurobehavioral performance. Pediatrics 98:76–83, 1996.

Alessandri, S. M., Bendersky, M. and Lewis, M., Cognitive functioning in 8- to 18-month-old drug-exposed infants. Dev. Psychol. 34:565–573, 1998.

Bland-Stewart, L. M., Seymour, H. N., Beeghly, M. and Frank, D. A., Semantic development of African-American children prenatally exposed to cocaine. Semin. Speech Lang. 19:167–186, 1998.

Reviews

O'Malley, S. S. and Gawin, F. H., Abstinence symptomatology and neuropsychological impairment in chronic cocaine abusers. NIDA Res. Monogr. 101:179–190, 1990.

Strickland, T. L. and Stein, R., Cocaine-induced cerebrovascular impairment: challenges to neuropsychological assessment. Neuropsychol. Rev. 5:69–79, 1995.

Strickland, T. L., Miller, B. L., Kowell, A. and Stein, R., Neurobiology of cocaine-induced organic brain impairment: contributions from functional neuroimaging. Neuropsychol. Rev. 8:1–9, 1998.

Horner, M. D., Attentional functioning in abstinent cocaine abusers. Drug Alcohol Depend. 54:19–33, 1999.

Amphetamine and Other Stimulants

Acute Administration

Halliday, R., Callaway, E., Naylor, H., Gratzinger, P. and Prael, R., The effects of stimulant drugs on information processing in elderly adults. J. Gerontol. 41:748–757, 1986.

Schmedtje, J. F., Jr., Oman, C. M., Letz, R. and Baker, E. L., Effects of scopolamine and dextroamphetamine on human performance. Aviat. Space Environ. Med. 59:407–410, 1988.

Newhouse, P. A., Belenky, G., Thomas, M., Thorne, D., Sing, H. C. and Fertig, J., The effects of d-amphetamine on arousal, cognition, and mood after prolonged total sleep deprivation. Neuropsychopharmacology 2:153–164, 1989.

Halliday, R., Gregory, K., Naylor, H., Callaway, E. and Yano, L., Beyond drug effects and dependent variables: the use of the Poisson-Erlang model to assess the effects of D-amphetamine on information processing. Acta Psychol. (Amst.) 73:35–54, 1990.

Fleming, K., Bigelow, L. B., Weinberger, D. R. and Goldberg, T. E., Neuropsychological effects of amphetamine may correlate with personality characteristics. Psychopharmacol. Bull. 31:357–362, 1995.

Mattay, V. S., Berman, K. F., Ostrem, J. L., Esposito, G., Van Horn, J. D., Bigelow, L. B. and Weinberger, D. R., Dextroamphetamine enhances "neural network-specific" physiological signals: a positron-emission tomography rCBF study. J. Neurosci. 16:4816–4822, 1996.

Pickworth, W. B., Rohrer, M. S. and Fant, R. V., Effects of abused drugs on psychomotor performance. Exp. Clin. Psychopharmacol. 5:235–241, 1997.

Servan-Schreiber, D., Carter, C. S., Bruno, R. M. and Cohen, J. D., Dopamine and the mechanisms of cognition: Part II. D-Amphetamine effects in human subjects performing a selective attention task. Biol. Psychiatry 43:723–729, 1998.

Chronic Administration

Carlin, A. S., Stauss, F. F., Adams, K. M. and Grant, I., The prediction of neuropsychological impairment in polydrug abusers. Addict. Behav. 3:5–12, 1978.

Khattab, N. Y. and Amer, G., Undetected neuropsychophysiological sequelae of khat chewing in standard aviation medical examination. Aviat. Space Environ. Med. 66:739–744, 1995.

McKetin, R. and Mattick, R. P., Attention and memory in illicit amphetamine users. Drug Alcohol Depend. 48:235–242, 1997.

McKetin, R. and Mattick, R. P., Attention and memory in illicit amphetamine users: comparison with non-drug-using controls. Drug Alcohol Depend, 50:181–184, 1998.

McKetin, R. and Solowij, N., Event-related potential indices of auditory selective attention in dependent amphetamine users. Biol. Psychiatry 45:1488–1497, 1999.

Prenatal Exposure

Struthers, J. M. and Hansen, R. L., Visual recognition memory in drug-exposed infants. J. Dev. Behav. Pediatr. 13:108–111, 1992.

Methamphetamine

Siomopoulos, V., Thought disorder in amphetamine psychosis: a case report. Psychosomatics 17:42–44, 1976. [Case Report]

Mohs, R. C., Tinklenberg, J. R., Roth, W. T. and Kopell, B. S., Methamphetamine and diphenhydramine effects on the rate of cognitive processing. Psychopharmacology (Berl.) 59:13–19, 1978.

Mohs, R. C., Tinklenberg, J. R., Roth, W. T. and Kopell, B. S., Sensitivity of some human cognitive functions to effects of methamphetamine and secobarbital. Drug Alcohol Depend. 5:145–150, 1980.

Methylphenidate

Halliday, R., Callaway, E., Naylor, H., Gratzinger, P. and Prael, R., The effects of stimulant drugs on information processing in elderly adults. J. Gerontol. 41:748–757, 1986.

Miller, T. P., Taylor, J. L. and Tinklenberg, J. R., A comparison of assessment techniques measuring the effects of methylphenidate, secobarbital, diazepam and diphenhydramine in abstinent alcoholics. Neuropsychobiology 19:90–96, 1988.

Camp-Bruno, J. A. and Herting, R. L., Cognitive effects of milacemide and methylphenidate in healthy young adults. Psychopharmacology (Berl.) 115:46–52, 1994.

Elliott, R., Sahakian, B. J., Matthews, K., Bannerjea, A., Rimmer, J. and Robbins, T. W., Effects of methylphenidate on spatial working memory and planning in healthy young adults. Psychopharmacology (Berl.) 131:196–206, 1997.

Solvents and Toluene

Acute Administration

Eskelinen, L., Luisto, M., Tenkanen, L. and Mattei, O., Neuropsychological methods in the differentiation of organic solvent intoxication from certain neurological conditions. J. Clin. Exp. Neuropsychol. 8:239–256, 1986.

Dudek, B., Gralewicz, K., Jakubowski, M., Kostrzewski, P. and Sokal, J., Neurobehavioral effects of experimental exposure to toluene, xylene and their mixture. Pol. J. Occup. Med. 3:109–116, 1990.

Rahill, A. A., Weiss, B., Morrow, P. E., Frampton, M. W., Cox, C., Gibb, R., Gelein, R., Speers, D. and Utell, M. J., Human performance during exposure to toluene. Aviat. Space Environ. Med. 67:640–647, 1996.

Little, C. H., Georgiou, G. M., Shelton, M. J., Simpson, F. and Cone, R. E., Clinical and immunological responses in subjects sensitive to solvents. Arch. Environ. Health 54:6–14, 1999.

Chronic Administration

Tsushima, W. T. and Towne, W. S., Effects of paint sniffing on neuropsychological test performance. J. Abnorm. Psychol. 86:402–407, 1977.

Korman, M., Matthews, R. W. and Lovitt, R., Neuropsychological effects of abuse of inhalants. Percept. Mot. Skills 53:547–553, 1981.

Fornazzari, L., Wilkinson, D. A., Kapur, B. M. and Carlen, P. L., Cerebellar, cortical and functional impairment in toluene abusers. Acta Neurol. Scand. 67:319–329, 1983.

Filley, C. M., Heaton, R. K. and Rosenberg, N. L., White matter dementia in chronic toluene abuse. Neurology 40:532–534, 1990.

Zur, J. and Yule, W., Chronic solvent abuse. 1. Cognitive sequelae. Child Care Health Dev. 16:1–20, 1990.

Byrne, A., Kirby, B., Zibin, T. and Ensminger, S., Psychiatric and neurological effects of chronic solvent abuse. Can. J. Psychiatry 36:735–738, 1991.

Katzelnick, D. J., Davar, G. and Scanlon, J. P., Reversibility of psychiatric symptoms in a chronic solvent abuser: a case report. J. Neuropsychiatry Clin. Neurosci. 3:319–321, 1991. [Case Report]

Bernal, B., Ardila, A. and Bateman, J. R., Cognitive impairments in adolescent drug-abusers. Int. J. Neurosci. 75:203–212, 1994.

Fukui, K., Kobayashi, T., Hayakawa, S., Koga, E., Ono, I., Kawakami, F., Fukui, Y., Tani, N., Kato, A. and Nakajima, T., Amotivational syndrome of chronic organic solvent abusers—neuropsychological study. Arukoru Kenkyuto Yakubutsu Ison 30:367–374, 1995. [Japanese]

Lemmen, C. A., Holden, C. E. and Benedek, E. P., Criminal responsibility and solvent exposure. New Dir. Ment. Health Serv. 69:59–66, 1996. [Case Report]

Terashi, H., Nagata, K., Satoh, Y., Hirata, Y. and Hatazawa, J., Hippocampal hypoperfusion underlying dementia due to chronic toluene intoxication. Rinsho Shinkeigaku 37:1010–1013, 1997. [Case Report] [Japanese]

Yamanouchi, N., Okada, S., Kodama, K., Sakamoto, T., Sekine, H., Hirai, S., Murakami, A., Komatsu, N. and Sato, T., Effects of MRI abnormalities on WAIS-R performance in solvent abusers. Acta Neurol. Scand. 96:34–39, 1997.

Kitabayashi, Y., Ueda, H., Matsuda, M., Narumoto, J., Kobayashi, T. and Fukui, K., A case report of organic solvent abuse with amotivational syndrome. Nihon Arukoru Yakubutsu Igakkai Zasshi 34:130–137, 1999. [Japanese] [Case Report]

Abstinence

Mahmood, Z., Cognitive functioning of solvent abusers. Scott. Med. J. 28:276–280, 1983.

Katzelnick, D. J., Davar, G. and Scanlon, J. P., Reversibility of psychiatric symptoms in a chronic solvent abuser: a case report. J. Neuropsychiatry Clin. Neurosci. 3:319–321, 1991. [Case Report]

Occupational Exposure

Iregren, A., Effects on psychological test performance of workers exposed to a single solvent (toluene): a comparison with effects of exposure to a mixture of organic solvents. Neurobehav. Toxicol. Teratol. 4:695–701, 1982.

Cherry, N., Hutchins, H., Pace, T. and Waldron, H. A., Neurobehavioural effects of repeated occupational exposure to toluene and paint solvents. Br. J. Ind. Med. 42:291–300, 1985.

Linz, D. H., de Garmo, P. L., Morton, W. E., Wiens, A. N., Coull, B. M. and Maricle, R. A., Organic solvent-induced encephalopathy in industrial painters. J. Occup. Med. 28:119–125, 1986.

Stollery, B. T. and Flindt, M. L., Memory sequelae of solvent intoxication. Scand. J. Work Environ. Health 14:45–48, 1988.

Foo, S. C., Jeyaratnam, J. and Koh, D., Chronic neurobehavioural effects of toluene. Br. J. Ind. Med. 47:480–484, 1990.

Gupta, B. N., Kumar, P. and Srivastava, A. K., An investigation of the neurobehavioural effects on workers exposed to organic solvents. J. Soc. Occup. Med. 40:94–96, 1990.

Morrow, L. A., Ryan, C. M., Hodgson, M. J. and Robin, N., Alterations in cognitive and psychological functioning after organic solvent exposure. J. Occup. Med. 32:444–450, 1990.

Bleecker, M. L., Bolla, K. I., Agnew, J., Schwartz, B. S. and Ford, D. P., Dose-related subclinical neurobehavioral effects of chronic exposure to low levels of organic solvents. Am. J. Ind. Med. 19:715–728, 1991.

Bowler, R. M., Mergler, D., Huel, G., Harrison, R. and Cone, J., Neuropsychological impairment among former microelectronics workers. Neurotoxicology 12:87–103, 1991.

Schwartz, B. S., Ford, D. P., Bolla, K. I., Agnew, J. and Bleecker, M. L., Solvent-associated olfactory dysfunction: not a predictor of deficits in learning and memory. Am. J. Psychiatry 148:751–756, 1991.

Welch, L., Kirshner, H., Heath, A., Gilliland, R. and Broyles, S., Chronic neuropsychological and neurological impairment following acute exposure to a solvent mixture of toluene and methyl ethyl ketone (MEK). J. Toxicol. Clin. Toxicol. 29:435–445, 1991. [Case Report]

Waszkowska, M. and Bazylewicz-Walczak, B., Psychological evaluation of the effects of chronic occupational exposure of paint shop workers to the mixture of organic solvents. Med. Pr. 43:35–39, 1992. [Polish]

Callender, T. J., Morrow, L., Subramanian, K., Duhon, D. and Ristovu, M., Three-dimensional brain metabolic imaging in patients with toxic encephalopathy. Environ. Res. 60:295–319, 1993.

Chia, S. E., Ong, C. N., Phoon, W. H., Tan, K. T. and Jeyaratnam, J., Neurobehavioural effects on workers in a video tape manufacturing factory in Singapore. Neurotoxicology 14:51–56, 1993.

Kishi, R., Harabuchi, I., Katakura, Y., Ikeda, T. and Miyake, H., Neurobehavioral effects of chronic occupational exposure to organic solvents among Japanese industrial painters. Environ. Res. 62:303–313, 1993.

Damasceno, B. P. and de Capitani, E. M., Cerebellar atrophy related to chronic exposure to toluene. Case report. Arq. Neuropsiquiatr. 52:90–92, 1994. [Case Report]

White, R. F., Robins, T. G., Proctor, S., Echeverria, D. and Rocskay, A. S., Neuropsychological effects of exposure to naphtha among automotive workers. Occup. Environ. Med. 51:102–112, 1994.

Bolla, K. I., Schwartz, B. S., Stewart, W., Rignani, J., Agnew, J. and Ford, D. P., Comparison of neurobehavioral function in workers exposed to a mixture of organic and inorganic lead and in workers exposed to solvents. Am. J. Ind. Med. 27:231–246, 1995.

White, R. F., Proctor, S. P., Echeverria, D., Schweikert, J. and Feldman, R. G., Neurobehavioral effects of acute and chronic mixed-solvent exposure in the screen printing industry. Am. J. Ind. Med. 28:221–231, 1995.

Muijser, H., Geuskens, R. B., Hooisma, J., Emmen, H. H. and Kulig, B. M., Behavioral effects of exposure to organic solvents in carpet layers. Neurotoxicol. Teratol. 18:455–462, 1996.

Pauling, T. L. and Ogden, J. A., Screening and Neuropsychological Assessment of Spray Painters at Risk for Organic Solvent Neurotoxicity. Int. J. Occup. Environ. Health 2:286–293, 1996.

Boey, K. W., Foo, S. C. and Jeyaratnam, J., Effects of occupational exposure to toluene: a neuropsychological study on workers in Singapore. Ann. Acad. Med. Singapore 26:184–187, 1997.

Ellingsen, D. G., Lorentzen, P. and Langard, S., A Neuropsychological Study of Patients Exposed to Organic Solvents. Int. J. Occup. Environ. Health 3:177–183, 1997.

Morrow, L. A., Steinhauer, S. R., Condray, R. and Hodgson, M., Neuropsychological performance of journeymen painters under acute solvent exposure and exposure-free conditions. J. Int. Neuropsychol. Soc. 3:269–275, 1997.

Tsai, S. Y., Chen, J. D., Chao, W. Y. and Wang, J. D., Neurobehavioral effects of occupational exposure to low-level organic solvents among Taiwanese workers in paint factories. Environ. Res. 73:146–155, 1997.

Pelegrin, C., Ceballos, C., Baringo, T., Poza, A. and Carrero, P., Secondary encephalopathy due to exposure to organic solvents: psychopathological, neuropsychological and neuroimaging findings. An. Med. Interna 15:91–94, 1998. [Spanish] [Case Report]

Jang, J. Y., Lee, S. Y., Kim, J. I., Park, J. B., Lee, K. J. and Chung, H. K., Application of biological monitoring to the quantitative exposure assessment for neuropsychological effect by chronic exposure to organic solvents. Int. Arch. Occup. Environ. Health 72:107–114, 1999.

Reviews

Winneke, G., Acute behavioral effects of exposure to some organic solvents—psychophysiological aspects. Acta Neurol. Scand. Suppl. 92:117–129, 1982.

Ron, M. A., Volatile substance abuse: a review of possible long-term neurological, intellectual and psychiatric sequelae. Br. J. Psychiatry 148:235–246, 1986.

Chadwick, O. F. and Anderson, H. R., Neuropsychological consequences of volatile substance abuse: a review. Hum. Toxicol. 8:307–312, 1989.

Hawkins, K. A., Occupational neurotoxicology: some neuropsychological issues and challenges. J. Clin. Exp. Neuropsychol. 12:664–680, 1990.

Triebig, G. and Lang, C., Brain imaging techniques applied to chronically solvent-exposed workers: current results and clinical evaluation. Environ. Res. 61:239–250, 1993.

Yamanouchi, N., Okada, S.-I., Kodama, K. and Sato, T., Central nervous system impairment caused by chronic solvent abuse—a review of Japanese studies on the clinical and neuroimaging aspects. Addiction Biol. 3:15–27, 1998.

Polydrug Abuse

Bruhn, P. and Maage, N., Intellectual and neuropsychological functions in young men with heavy and long-term patterns of drug abuse. Am. J. Psychiatry 132:397–401, 1975.

Grant, I. and Judd, L. L., Neuropsychological and EEG disturbances in polydrug users. Am. J. Psychiatry 133:1039–1042, 1976.

Grant, I., Mohns, L., Miller, M. and Reitan, R. M., A neuropsychological study of polydrug users. Arch. Gen. Psychiatry 33:973–978, 1976.

Grant, I., Adams, K. M., Carlin, A. S. and Rennick, P. M., Neuropsychological deficit in polydrug users. A preliminary report of the findings of the collaborative neuropsychological study of polydrug users. Drug Alcohol Depend. 2:91–108, 1977.

Carlin, A. S., Stauss, F. F., Adams, K. M. and Grant, I., The prediction of neuropsychological impairment in polydrug abusers. Addict. Behav. 3:5–12, 1978.

Grant, I., Adams, K. M., Carlin, A. S., Rennick, P. M., Judd, L. L., Schooff, K. and Reed, R., Organic impairment in polydrug users: risk factors. Am. J. Psychiatry 135:178–184, 1978.

Silberstein, C. H., McKegney, F. P., O'Dowd, M. A., Selwyn, P. A., Schoenbaum, E., Drucker, E., Feiner, C., Cox, C. P. and Friedland, G., A prospective longitudinal study of neuropsychological and psychosocial factors in asymptomatic individuals at risk for HTLV-III/LAV infection in a methadone program: preliminary findings. Int. J. Neurosci. 32:669–676, 1987.

Meek, P. S., Clark, H. W. and Solana, V. L., Neurocognitive impairment: the unrecognized component of dual diagnosis in substance abuse treatment. J. Psychoactive Drugs 21:153–160, 1989.

Holman, B. L., Carvalho, P. A., Mendelson, J., Teoh, S. K., Nardin, R., Hallgring, E., Hebben, N. and Johnson, K. A., Brain perfusion is abnormal in cocaine-dependent polydrug users: a study using technetium-99m-HMPAO and ASPECT. J. Nucl. Med. 32:1206–1210, 1991.

Woods, S. W., O'Malley, S. S., Martini, B. L., McDougle, C. J., Price, L. H., Krystal, J. H., Hoffer, P. B. and Kosten, T. R., SPECT regional cerebral blood flow and neuropsychological testing in non-demented HIV-positive drug abusers. Prog. Neuropsychopharmacol. Biol. Psychiatry 15:649–662, 1991.

Pakesch, G., Loimer, N., Grunberger, J., Pfersmann, D., Linzmayer, L. and Mayerhofer, S., Neuropsychological findings and psychiatric symptoms in HIV-1 infected and noninfected drug users. Psychiatry Res. 41:163–177, 1992.

Rodriguez, M., Cognitive functioning, family history of alcoholism, and antisocial behavior in female polydrug abusers. Psychol. Rep. 73:19–26, 1993.

Rodriguez, M., Cognitive functioning in male polydrug abusers with and without family history of alcoholism. Percept. Mot. Skills 77:483–488, 1993.

Amir, T. and Bahri, T., Effect of substance abuse on visuographic function. Percept. Mot. Skills 78:235–241, 1994.

Bernal, B., Ardila, A. and Bateman, J. R., Cognitive impairments in adolescent drug-abusers. Int. J. Neurosci. 75:203–212, 1994.

Concha, M., Selnes, O. A., McArthur, J. C., Nance-Sproson, T., Updike, M. L., Royal, W., 3rd., Solomon, L. and Vlahov, D., Normative data for a brief neuropsychologic test battery in a cohort of injecting drug users. Int. J. Addict. 30:823–841, 1995.

Scheier, L. M. and Botvin, G. J., Effects of early adolescent drug use on cognitive efficacy in early-late adolescence: a developmental structural model. J. Subst. Abuse 7:379–404, 1995.

Tarter, R. E., Mezzich, A. C., Hsieh, Y. C. and Parks, S. M., Cognitive capacity in female adolescent substance abusers. Drug Alcohol Depend. 39:15–21, 1995.

Easton, C. and Bauer, L. O., Neuropsychological correlates of urine toxicology results. Prog. Neuro-Psychopharmacol. Biol. Psychiatry 20:969–982, 1996.

Rosselli, M. and Ardila, A., Cognitive effects of cocaine and polydrug abuse. J. Clin. Exp. Neuropsychol. 18:122–135, 1996.

Beatty, W. W., Blanco, C. R., Hames, K. A. and Nixon, S. J., Spatial cognition in alcoholics: influence of concurrent abuse of other drugs. Drug Alcohol Depend. 44:167–174, 1997.

Carpenter, K. M. and Hittner, J. B., Cognitive impairment among the dually-diagnosed: substance use history and depressive symptom correlates. Addiction 92:747–759, 1997.

Concha, M., Selnes, O. A., Vlahov, D., Nance-Sproson, T., Updike, M., Royal, W., Palenicek, J. and McArthur, J. C., Comparison of neuropsychological performance between AIDS-free injecting drug users and homosexual men. Neuroepidemiology 16:78–85, 1997.

Easton, C. J. and Bauer, L. O., Neuropsychological differences between alcohol-dependent and cocaine- dependent patients with or without problematic drinking. Psychiatry Res. 71:97–103, 1997.

Bondi, M. W., Drake, A. I. and Grant, I., Verbal learning and memory in alcohol abusers and polysubstance abusers with concurrent alcohol abuse. J. Intl. Neuropsychol. Soc. 4:319–328, 1998.

Disclafani, V., Truran, D. L., Bloomer, C., Toloushams, M., Clark, H. W., Norman, D., Hannauer, D. and Fein, G., Abstinent chronic crack-cocaine and crack-cocaine/alcohol abusers evidence normal hippocampal volumes on MRI despite persistent cognitive impairments. Addiction Biol. 3:261–270, 1998.

Morgan, M. J., Recreational use of "ecstasy" (MDMA) is associated with elevated impulsivity. Neuropsychopharmacology 19:252–264, 1998.

Nixon, S. J., Paul, R. and Phillips, M., Cognitive efficiency in alcoholics and polysubstance abusers. Alcohol. Clin. Exp. Res. 22:1414–1420, 1998.

Selby, M. J. and Azrin, R. L., Neuropsychological functioning in drug abusers. Drug Alcohol Depend. 50:39–45, 1998.

Bauer, L. O. and Hesselbrock, V. M., Subtypes of family history and conduct disorder: effects on P300 during the stroop test. Neuropsychopharmacology 21:51–62, 1999.

Robinson, J. E., Heaton, R. K. and O'Malley, S. S., Neuropsychological functioning in cocaine abusers with and without alcohol dependence. J. Int. Neuropsychol. Soc. 5:10–19, 1999.

Tapert, S. F., Brown, S. A., Myers, M. G. and Granholm, E., The role of neurocognitive abilities in coping with adolescent relapse to alcohol and drug use. J. Stud. Alcohol 60:500–508, 1999.

HIV

Silberstein, C. H., McKegney, F. P., O'Dowd, M. A., Selwyn, P. A., Schoenbaum, E., Drucker, E., Feiner, C., Cox, C. P. and Friedland, G., A prospective longitudinal study of neuropsychological and psychosocial factors in asymptomatic individuals at risk for HTLV-III/LAV infection in a methadone program: preliminary findings. Int. J. Neurosci. 32:669–676, 1987.

Woods, S. W., O'Malley, S. S., Martini, B. L., McDougle, C. J., Price, L. H., Krystal, J. H., Hoffer, P. B. and Kosten, T. R., SPECT regional cerebral blood flow and neuropsychological testing in non-demented HIV-positive drug abusers. Prog. Neuropsychopharmacol. Biol. Psychiatry 15:649–662, 1991.

Concha, M., Graham, N. M., Munoz, A., Vlahov, D., Royal, W., 3rd, Updike, M., Nance-Sproson, T., Selnes, O. A. and McArthur, J. C., Effect of chronic substance abuse on the neuropsychological performance of intravenous drug users with a high prevalence of HIV-1 seropositivity. Am. J. Epidemiol. 136:1338–1348, 1992.

Handelsman, L., Aronson, M., Maurer, G., Wiener, J., Jacobson, J., Bernstein, D., Ness, R., Herman, S., Losonczy, M., Song, I. S., Holloway, K., Horvath, T., Donnelly, N., Hirschowitz, J. and Rowan, A. J., Neuropsychological and neurological manifestations of HIV-1 dementia in drug users. J. Neuropsychiatry Clin. Neurosci. 4:21–28, 1992.

Kovner, R., Lazar, J. W., Lesser, M., Perecman, E., Kaplan, M. H., Hainline, B. and Napolitano, B., Use of the Dementia Rating Scale as a test for neuropsychological dysfunction in HIV-positive i.v. drug abusers. J. Subst. Abuse Treat. 9:133–137, 1992.

Pakesch, G., Loimer, N., Grunberger, J., Pfersmann, D., Linzmayer, L. and Mayerhofer, S., Neuropsychological findings and psychiatric symptoms in HIV-1 infected and noninfected drug users. Psychiatry Res. 41:163–177, 1992.

Wellman, M. C., Neuropsychological impairment among intravenous drug users in pre-AIDS stages of HIV infection. Int. J. Neurosci. 64:183–194, 1992.

Grassi, M. P., Perin, C., Clerici, F., Zocchetti, C., Cargnel, A. and Mangoni, A., Neuropsychological performance in HIV-1-infected drug abusers. Acta Neurol. Scand. 88:119–122, 1993.

Concha, M., Selnes, O. A., Vlahov, D., Nance-Sproson, T., Updike, M., Royal, W., Palenicek, J. and McArthur, J. C., Comparison of neuropsychological performance between AIDS-free injecting drug users and homosexual men. Neuroepidemiology 16:78–85, 1997.

Prenatal Exposure

van Baar, A. and de Graaff, B. M., Cognitive development at preschool-age of infants of drug-dependent mothers. Dev. Med. Child Neurol. 36:1063–1075, 1994.

Index

Introduction to the Index

The Index is constructed to provide access to topics of interest to readers of different backgrounds. Major headings include search terms that are familiar to both novices and specialists in the field. The book content may be searched by abused drug, imaging technique, drug use state (e.g., abstinence, acute, chronic, craving, relapse, withdrawal), or neuroanatomy. The Index is also designed to broaden the reader's focus. For each abused substance, citations of research findings from all imaging modalities are grouped together. This assists readers seeking to acquire a more comprehensive, cross-modal appreciation of the extant research on major drugs of abuse. Major headings for the caveats, confounds, and technical limitations confronting imaging researchers are also included, to inform readers about the complexities associated with conducting and interpreting brain imaging research studies of substance abuse. The following abbreviations are used:

BOLD, Blood Oxygen Level Dependent fMRI
CBF, Cerebral Blood Flow
CBV, Cerebral Blood Volume
CMR, Cerebral Metabolic Rate
DSC MRI, Dynamic Susceptibility Contrast MRI
EEG, Electroencephalography
ERP/EP, Event Related Potentials/Evoked Potentials
fMRI, Functional Magnetic Resonance Imaging
MRI, Magnetic Resonance Imaging
MRS, Magnetic Resonance Spectroscopy
PET, Positron Emission Tomography
SPECT, Single Photon Emission Computed Tomography

B

D

G

H

N

R

S